D1499619

Immunobiology of

TRANSPLANTATION, CANCER *and* PREGNANCY

Pergamon Titles of Related Interest

Gross ONCOGENIC VIRUSES, THIRD EDITION
ADVANCES IN MEDICAL ONCOLOGY, RESEARCH AND EDUCATION,
VOLUMES 1-12
Glauser/Klastersky THERAPY AND PREVENTION OF INFECTIONS
IN CANCER PATIENTS
Klastersky INFECTIONS IN CANCER CHEMOTHERAPY
Twycross et al. CONTINUING CARE OF TERMINAL CANCER PATIENTS
oncoLOGIC: MULTIDISCIPLINARY DECISIONS IN ONCOLOGY

Related Journals*

MEDICAL ONCOLOGY AND TUMOR PHARMACOTHERAPY
EUROPEAN JOURNAL OF CANCER AND CLINICAL ONCOLOGY
INTERNATIONAL JOURNAL OF RADIATION ONCOLOGY,
BIOLOGY, PHYSICS
CLINICAL AND INVESTIGATIVE MEDICINE
JOURNAL OF CHRONIC DISEASES
DEVELOPMENTAL AND COMPARATIVE IMMUNOLOGY
MOLECULAR IMMUNOLOGY
INTERNATIONAL JOURNAL OF APPLIED RADIATION AND ISOTOPES
COMPARATIVE IMMUNOLOGY, MICROBIOLOGY
AND INFECTIOUS DISEASES

*Free specimen copies available upon request

Immunobiology of

TRANSPLANTATION, CANCER *and* PREGNANCY

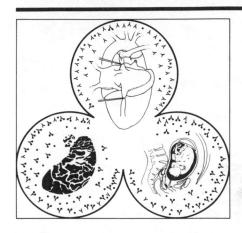

Edited by
Prasanta K. Ray
The Medical College of
Pennsylvania and Hospital

Pergamon Press New York Oxford Toronto Sydney Paris Frankfurt

Pergamon Press Offices:

U.S.A.	Pergamon Press Inc., Maxwell House, Fairview Park, Elmsford, New York 10523, U.S.A.
U.K.	Pergamon Press Ltd., Headington Hill Hall, Oxford OX3 0BW, England
CANADA	Pergamon Press Canada Ltd., Suite 104, 150 Consumers Road, Willowdale, Ontario M2J 1P9, Canada
AUSTRALIA	Pergamon Press (Aust.) Pty. Ltd., P.O. Box 544, Potts Point, NSW 2011, Australia
FRANCE	Pergamon Press SARL, 24 rue des Ecoles, 75240 Paris, Cedex 05, France
FEDERAL REPUBLIC OF GERMANY	Pergamon Press GmbH, Hammerweg 6, D-6242 Kronberg-Taunus, Federal Republic of Germany

Copyright © 1983 Pergamon Press, Inc.

Library of Congress Cataloging in Publication Data
Main entry under title:

Immunobiology of transplantation, cancer, and pregnancy.

     1. Immunological tolerance – Addresses, essays, lec-
tures.   2. Transplantation immunology – Addresses, es-
says, lectures.   3. Cancer – Immunological aspects –
Addresses, essays, lectures.   4. Pregnancy – Immuno-
logical aspects – Addresses, essays, lectures.   I. Ray,
Prasanta K.   [DNLM: 1. Transplantation immunology.
2. Pregnancy.   3. Neoplasms – Immunology.   4. Immunity.
QZ 200 I337]
QR188.4.I4 1983   616.07'9   83-2335
ISBN 0-08-025994-4

Printed in the United States of America

Dedicated to the
memory of

Labanya P. Ray
(1894–1972)

My beloved mother
My source of inspiration and encouragement

Contents

viii   Contents

Preface

During my active involvement in immunobiological research over many years, I have noted, like many others, that there is a need for a detailed and comparative discussion on the immunobiological mechanisms involved in transplantation, cancer, and pregnancy. These three areas have tremendous similarities as far as immunologic reactions are concerned, and confusion existing in one, if solved, can perhaps help in unraveling the mystery in another.

During the last two decades tremendous advancements have been made in the areas of transplantation and cancer immunology. Substantial advancement, however, is lacking in the area of immunobiology of pregnancy, although very recently this area has been given much attention. In this volume, I have attempted to bring together topics which are pertinent to compare and contrast the immunobiological mechanisms relating to these three areas. Also, I have tried to focus attention on those topics which are relatively new. Articles were solicited from experts who have long contributed in their respective fields. Therefore, I think the information provided will be up-to-date in all the areas discussed. I would feel gratified if this volume becomes helpful to both clinical and nonclinical scientists who are interested in the investigational aspects of the immunobiology of transplantation, cancer, and pregnancy. Since immunobiological concepts, hypotheses, and mechanisms have been given detailed treatment, immunologists, in particular, may find this volume useful. If this is achieved, I will consider my attempt a success.

In transplantation the chronic immunological rejection remains as the chief hindrance for the survival of the allograft. Chemotherapeutic drugs which maintain the host in a suboptimally immunosuppressed state remain the treatment of choice. Refined techniques for tissue-typing using monospecific sera allow close matching of donor and recipient tissue. Discovery of newer histocompatibility antigens and their presence on red blood cells throw more light on the complexities of typing donor and recipient tissues. The knowledge gained in this area has given the means to increase survival times of allografts, but general success in long-term maintenance of allografts has not been achieved. New attempts based on new understanding are needed to elucidate the immunological mechanisms more clearly and in depth so that allografts can be maintained in a functional state for an extended period.

In the area of tumor immunobiology the recognition of tumor-associated antigens and their ability to induce both cellular and humoral immunity indicate that tumors can be regarded as allografts. However, a transplanted tissue is rejected, while a tumor is not. Tremendous advancement has been made in recent years in describing the host response against tumors. Manipulating host immunological response occasionally results in a successful therapeutic benefit against minimal residual tumors. Fresh attempts are being made to eliminate blocking factors from tumor-bearing hosts, which should augment the immune reactivity of the host against the tumor. The role of suppressor cells in tumor-bearing animals provides a new direction of research in the area of cell-mediated immunosuppression. Controlling this mechanism might induce cell-mediated immune attack against the tumor.

In the area of pregnancy, we are just recognizing the importance of immunological reactions: histocompatibility antigens on spermatozoa; specific maternal antibody against fetal tissues; demonstration of blocking factors in the plasma of pregnant women; and evidence of immune rejection in spontaneous abortion. While data indicate that spontaneous abortion may be related to immunological rejection of the allograft, it is not certain yet whether or not delivery of the child is somehow related to the same phenomenon, in addition to the hormonal, biochemical, and physiological mechanisms which are also known to be involved in the process.

These topics, while still controversial in some aspects, are nevertheless fascinating and may arouse new research interests and approaches in these fields. Work remains to be done on the similarities of the immune response induced by fetus and tumor. Both have foreign antigens, but are not rejected. Rejection of fetus is seen in spontaneous abortion and also perhaps in delivery, and tumors, on occasion, undergo spontaneous regression. However, most of the time tumors are accepted in spite of being allografts. If the fundamental mechanism is elucidated describing how recognition of the fetus as a foreign tissue takes place on some occasions and leads to rejection of the fetus, the same might be utilized to induce rejection of tumors. In organ transplantation, new work is being reported indicating that induction of plasma-blocking factor and suppressor cell activity may be helpful in prolonging allograft survival. In view of the fascinating concepts and ideas being developed, I have attempted to bring them together through solicited articles written by recognized experts in their respective fields. This volume has been divided into five parts. Part I discusses the basic aspects of immune phenomena. Part II deals with immunobiology of organ transplantation. Part III describes immune phenomena related to tumor growth and therapy. Part IV discusses the immunologic phenomena related to the maintenance of fetal growth and to its abortion. At the end, in part V, immunologic phenomena related to transplantation, cancer, and pregnancy are discussed in order to focus their similarities and dissimilarities. I would hope this book will be helpful for all researchers interested in the immunobiology of transplantation, cancer, and pregnancy, and would be happy if the reader finds it useful, stimulating, and of unique value.

Established experts from all parts of the world have contributed in this Volume. They have made every honest effort to review the respective areas and illustrate the present status of the respective fields. The authors, themselves, are responsible for the contents, views and comments they have expressed in their chapters. Every reasonable effort has been made to provide reliable data and information. The editor and the publisher, however, cannot assume responsibility for the validity of all material or for the consequences of their use.

I thank all the authors for their stimulating and informative contributions. Thanks are due to Donald R. Cooper, M.D. and James G. Bassett, M.D. for their continuous encouragement in this effort. I thank all my colleagues who have helped me in a variety of ways to make this effort a success. I should also like to thank the staff of Pergamon Press for their unfailing efficiency and courtesy. Thanks are also due to Claire Schultz and Alan Rubin for their help in the preparation of various manuscripts. Secretarial help from Aretia Davis Duncan, Julia Holub, and Ruth Adams is highly appreciated. Grateful recognition goes to my wife, Khana, who waited patiently and worked with me in bringing this volume to fruition.

P. K. Ray
Philadelphia
June 1983

PART I
IMMUNE SYSTEM—
A UNIQUE DEVICE
TO PROTECT THE SELF

1

Immune System—A Unique Device to Protect the Self

Prasanta K. Ray

The immune system is a unique device by which the body defends itself against a hostile environment that is swarming with harmful elements such as bacteria, fungi, viruses, and various other undesirable substances.

The immune system serves a variety of purposes in the body of a living being. First, when any antigen recognized as foreign material enters the body, macrophages, previously sensitized lymphocytes, memory cells, natural killer cells, and/or preformed antibody provide an offensive attack against the invading elements. Second, biochemical reactions are induced to develop an effective armed force by the development of effector components, specific for antigens, like those mentioned above. Third, the immune system maintains a reserved force for quick response against any future attack. In this case, memory cells from both types of lymphocytes, T lymphocytes (thymus derived lymphocytes) and B lymphocytes (bone-marrow derived lymphocytes), are formed. Fourth, when the system gets overstimulated, the body initiates a feedback mechanism, so that any hyperactivity of T and B lymphocytes is controlled. This is done by way of generation of suppressor cells, which become operative against the hyperactive cell type. Antiglobulins also play a role in these autoregulatory phenomena. Thus, the immune system provides various regulatory functions in the body. The principal objective is to protect the self against intruders, that is, against non-self.

From time immemorial, through the entire process of evolution, the animal body developed a well-regulated, unique, protective device—*the immune system*. Such a system has also been detected in plants, and in nonvertebrates, though not in equal complexity, and perhaps developing in a gradual process during evolution. However, that all living things have some mechanisms to protect themselves against the environment has become more and more evident in recent years.

The immune system is regulated by a complex network of biochemical reactions and cellular interactions whose various factors cooperate with one another to effect certain specific reactions (1,2). There exists a great degree of cooperativity through which the different components of the immune

3

system react with one another, with the final development of immunity—a status in which the host is competent to mount an effective attack against the invading elements. One of the most important steps in the immunological processing of an antigen is the *recognition phenomenon*, by which an antigen is recognized as *foreign*. Ultimately, a variety of signals are transmitted; an equally large number of immunologic reactions take place for the appropriate processing of the antigen: transmission of messages from one part of the body to another; recruitment of immune components to reach the target to marshal an immune attack; destruction of the foreign body; and elimination of the products of the destruction from the body. A continuous vigilance is maintained by the immune forces of the body to protect the self.

It may be of interest to go through very quickly, without the intricate details, the various basic aspects of the immune system, before discussing the specifics of any particular mechanism. The basic information is presented in a manner that may help stir the memory of individuals who have not been in touch with the subject for a long time.

ANTIGEN

Antigens are substances that have the ability to induce the formation of antibodies or immune lymphocytes, and are able to react specifically with the antibody or the sensitized cell. Substances that can only react with the antibody or cells, but cannot cause their generation, are known as haptens. An antigen may have hundreds of different determinant groups, each of which antibodies can be formed against. Alteration of the biochemical nature of an antigen may induce the production of different forms of antibodies. The immunogenicity of an antigen is dependent upon (a) the extent of the foreignness of the molecule to the host system; (b) its molecular size; and (c) its chemical complexity. Proteins are the best antigens, while small molecular weight compounds (less than 10,000 daltons) are usually non-antigenic, as are pure lipids and long-chain hydrocarbons. However, lipopolysaccharides are good antigens. Mammalian and bacterial cells are composed of complex biomolecules and, therefore, are good antigens. The immunogenicity of an antigen may be altered by deletion or addition of antigenic or haptenic molecules.

Against each of the antigenic determinants, the body is able to produce antibody and sensitized cells which can react specifically against the antigenic markers. Thus, antigen-antibody reactions are specific. The specific antibody usually does not react against another antigenic marker. However, there are occasions when cross-reactivity between an antigen and antibody does occur. This is primarily due to close similarity between the two antigenic determinants. The similarity may be sterical and/or configurational. If the basic structure of the two molecules is the same, with the difference being in their functional groups or side chains, then antibodies produced against them may sometimes cross-react.

Although foreignness is one of the most important requirements for antigenicity, antibodies are sometimes formed against self antigens, which normally are not available for sensitization of the antibody-forming cells. These self antigens are regarded as foreign, because they are situated in occult positions normally inaccessible to the immune system. If due to damage or defect in the cell surface structure these antigens become accessible to the antibody-forming cells, then autoimmune reactions may be induced. These may become life-threatening at times.

ANTIBODY

In response to foreign antigenic material, the body produces antibody, belonging to a specific class of serum immunoglobulins, which has the specificity to react with the specific antigen. There are five different forms of antibodies, which are also known as immunoglobulins. These immunoglobulins differ in terms of their structure, sedimentation coefficient ('S' value), electrophoretic mobility, concentration in normal serum, participation in immune reactions, availability in biological fluids, and ability to cross the placenta, among others. There are five classes of immunoglobulins (Ig) termed IgG, IgM, IgA, IgD, and IgE. All the classes of immunoglobulins consist of heavy chains (γ, μ, α, δ, ξ, respectively), and light chains (κ or λ). Different subclasses have also been identified. These are IgG1, IgG2, IgG3, IgG4, IgA1, and IgA2. It is not known yet if there exists other forms of Ig. Considering the complexities of immunological reactions, and the wide variety of functions that the immune system has to perform, there exists a strong possibility that several other types of Igs may also exist in the mammalian system. With the development of more quantitative assay systems, precise identification of newer immune phenomena, and the ability to differentiate one from another, it is possible that new Igs will be identified in the future.

There may still be a number of different types of immunological reactions mediated by Igs which are unidentified, both mechanistically and developmentally. It is not known what the differences are among the Igs, which may have a common structural identity. It is also not known what signals at the gene level are responsible for the structural changes that determine new Ig specificity, and how this mechanism can be controlled. A good understanding of these mechanisms will provide deeper understanding of: (a) how a transplanted allograft can be maintained by inducing enhancing antibody; (b) how a tumor can be made to regress by inducing the formation of cytotoxic antibody and inhibiting the formation of enhancing antibody; (c) how enhancing antibodies are induced by a fetus; and (d) whether or not abortion or delivery has any relationship with cytotoxic antibody which may cause abortion by acting directly against the fetus, or against tissues surrounding the fetus.

Types of Antibody

Immunoglobulin G (IgG). Immunoglobulin G molecule has a molecular weight of approximately 150,000 daltons. It is a 7S molecule and comprises the major portion (76%) of antibody activity in the human body. It has a half life of 21 days and a valency of 2 (2 antigen-binding sites). In normal serum its concentration ranges from 700 mg% to 1500 mg%. It can cross the placenta and provide protective antibodies to the fetus and during the very early phase of independent life, until the newborn develops its own immune system.

The pioneering work of Porter provided much knowledge about the intricate structure of the IgG molecule. According to present knowledge, an IgG molecule is composed of four polypeptide chains; (a) two identical light (L) chains (about 210 to 230 amino acids) and (b) two identical heavy (H) chains (about 420 to 440 amino acids). These are connected by disulfide (S-S) bonds in a Y-shaped structure (Fig. 1.1). Using different proteolytic enzymes, structural analyses have been performed. Papain digestion splits the IgG molecule into three fragments: (1) Antigen-binding fragment (Fab: molecular weight 52,000 daltons), through which an IgG molecule binds an antigen (Fig. 1.2). The Fab fragment has two identical sites, making the molecule bivalent. With the help of these two arms, the IgG molecule can bind with two antigenic molecules (Fig. 1.2), and can form a lattice-like structure of antigen-antibody complex.

The fragment containing only heavy chain after papain digestion is termed the Fc or crystallizable fragment (molecular weight 48,000). This Fc contains some carbohydrate. Serum complement binds with this fragment through antigen-antibody complex. The unique property by which IgG can cross the placenta is located in the Fc portion of the molecule. Another fragment of IgG, Fd, is the heavy chain component of Fab. This heavy chain structure is recognized as having an N-terminal and a C-terminal end, like any other protein.

Pepsin digestion cleaves the upper portion of the IgG structure into two fragments, each called $F(ab)_2$. This portion can bind antigen, since the antigen-binding site of the original molecule remains intact.

Since the two chains of the IgG structure are polypeptide in nature, they form intrachain loops separated by domains, -S-S- bridges. There are four

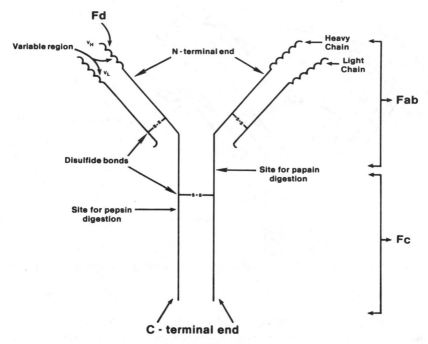

Fig.1.1. Immunoglobulin G structure.

such domains in the H chain of IgG i.e., VH, CH_1, CH_2, and CH_3 (Fig. 1.3). There are two domains i.e., V_L and C_L in the L chain of IgG. Both H and L chains have one variable domain, V_H and V_L, respectively; the rest are constant domains. IgM and IgD have one additional constant domain in their heavy chain.

The structural composition of the H and L chains varies from antibody to antibody. This is specific for the specific type of antibody formed against a specific antigen. There are two types of light chains among the different classes of Ig's—one is known as Kappa and the other as Lambda. In any one type of Ig structure the light chains do not vary.

Immunoglobulin M (IgM). IgM is the immunoglobulin with the highest molecular weight. It's molecular weight is about 900,000 daltons; sedimentation coefficient, 19S. In normal serum its concentration is usually low, about 60 to 180 mg%. It is a pentamer, made up of five units of IgG structure, giving it a valency of 10. These units are held together by a glycoprotein called the *J*-chain or joining chain. It is the first antibody formed after antigen stimulation. IgM can fix serum complement and enhance phagocytosis, but cannot cross the placental barrier, probably because of its large size. It can be detected in cord serum and may be synthesized by

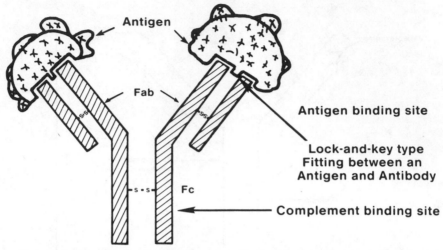

Fig.1.2. Antigen-binding through Fab region of IgG molecule. Complement binds through Fc structure.

the fetus. An increased level of IgM in cord serum may be an indicator of intrauterine infection, leading to the immunological stimulation and formation of IgM antibodies.

Immunoglobulin A (IgA). IgA can exist in a variety of forms; i.e., monomeric, dimeric, and polymeric forms of IgA can be detected in plasma.

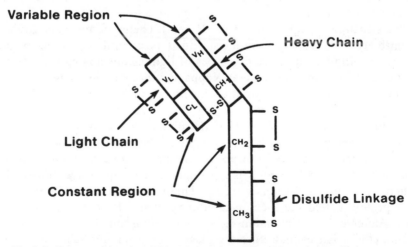

Fig.1.3. Constant (c) and variable (v) domains of H and L chain of IgG structure.

Its molecular weight ranges from 150,000 to 600,000 daltons; sedimentation coefficient, 7S to 17S; valency, 2 to 8; normal serum concentration, 150 to 250 mg%. The monomeric forms are joined together by the J-chain. Another type of IgA, known as secretory IgA, is a dimer held together by the J-chain and a secretory component which helps in the migration of these molecules from the secretory epithelial cells. IgA type antibody provides local immunity, and is present in various body fluids and/or secretions, such as saliva, tears, bronchial mucus, urinary tract secretions, and colostrum.

Immunoglobulin D (IgD). The molecular weight of IgD type antibody is about 200,000 daltons; sedimentation coefficient, 7S; valency, 2; normal serum level, 3 mg%. It is a non-complement-fixing antibody. It is found in different autoimmune disorders, and also is formed against penicillin and insulin.

Immunoglobulin E (IgE). The molecular weight of IgE is 190,000 daltons; sedimentation coefficient, 8S; valency, 2; normal serum level, insignificant. It is heat-sensitive and is labile at 56°C when heated for 4 hours. IgE can fix complement, involving the C_3-alternate pathway. Allergic and hypersensitivity disorders are related to IgE antibody activity. Atopy, hay fever, and anaphylaxis are also due to an IgE-mediated immune response.

Antibody Formation

All forms of vertebrates have immunologic capabilities, because they have organized and well-developed lymphoid organs. One of the functions of these lymphoid tissues is the production of antibodies and effector lymphocytes and/or soluble immune modulators. If, however, the balance of production and control of antibody synthesis is lost, the immune system can cause more harm than good to the host. Allergic and hypersensitivity reactions, autoimmune disease, and immunologic injury to the embryo are all examples of a defective or altered antibody response. However, the beneficial aspects of antibody undoubtedly surpass its occasional malfunction.

The route and dosage of antigen inoculation may determine the nature of antibody response. Some antigens elicit one major class of antibody molecules while others can elicit several types. Only a small amount of an antigen is necessary for the sensitization of the host for antibody production. A large dose may induce immunological tolerance, by completely inhibiting the production of antibody. The status of immune tolerance may persist for a long time and is possibly dependent upon the maintenance of a high level of antigen in the system. It is possible that the fetus induces an immunologic tolerance phenomena in the mother by shedding large amounts of fetal antigens. Tumors may also induce similar mechanisms by releasing an excess of tumor-associated antigens in the host system. There are several other mechanisms of immunologic tolerance induction which will be discussed in the last chapter of this volume. Any serious attempts to induce immunological tolerance against the donor tissue by large dose antigen immunization of donor tissue-specific antigen, including histocompatibility antigens, remain for the future in terms of prolongation of graft survival.

Certain substances, not always necessarily antigenic by themselves, can augment antibody production. These are known as adjuvants. One of the most widely used adjuvants in nonhuman experiments is Freund's adjuvant, which is a mixture of mineral oil, waxes, and killed tubercle bacilli. Freund's adjuvant is routinely used in laboratory research for the purpose of production of high titer antibody.

The capacity to form antibodies is a unique and inherent property of the mature individual. Formation of appreciable quantities of IgM antibodies begins at birth, followed by IgA antibodies after 2 weeks and IgG antibodies after 4 to 6 weeks. Usually, the capacity to produce antibodies declines in old age, and during some disease processes. Individuals suffering from immunodeficiency disease such as agammaglobulinemia produce either none or else very small amounts of Igs. These patients obviously suffer from serious infectious episodes. On the contrary, in myeloma patients, large amounts of some specific Ig is synthesized. This is a malignant disorder and is normally associated with the production of only one type of Ig, such as IgG in IgG-Myeloma, IgM in macroglobulinemia, and IgA in IgA-Myeloma, etc. During these conditions, production of other Ig is very low.

The inability to form antibodies during fetal development is unique and may be a part of the phenomenon of discrimination between self and non-self antigens. This ability to discriminate starts early in life, and involves lymphoid tissues recognizing the proper antigens as foreign. It is not known if alteration due to infection, etc., of this self-recognition phase early in fetal life can make an individual more prone to develop autoimmune disease. If this recognition of any of the self antigens does not occur, then autoimmune disease is highly likely. On the other hand, if during adult life some autologous antigens, which the host lympoid tissue does not have any knowledge of, are either unmasked or become exposed, then an autoimmune reaction may be induced. It is thus possible that autoimmune disorders may evolve secondary to a degenerative disease process.

IMMUNOLOGICAL RECOGNITION

The initial step in the immunological processing of an antigen is the recognition of non-self. This ability of the body, the discrimination between

self and non-self, has perhaps been attained step by step through the evolutionary process because of the necessity of the living being to protect the
self. It may be that development of an immune system was part of the
process which allowed the *fittest* to survive.

The general ability to recognize non-self allogeneic cells through histocompatibility differences has been described in invertebrates (3). Allograft
rejection (4), memory system (4, 5), and involvement of lymphocyte-like
cells in tissue rejection (6) have also been reported in invertebrate systems.

The role of histocompatibility antigens has been implicated in various
immune phenomena, including immune recognition (7, 8). Further, histocompatibility antigens may play a role in cell-to-cell interaction, in other
cellular communication, and differentiation in vertebrates (9). The existence
of precursors of histocompatibility antigens is also suspected in invertebrates
(10), indicating that the complex markers of immune recognition were probably developed during the evolutionary process.

All types of cells have some capacity to recognize and respond to external
stimuli. The initial step in molecular immune recognition is binding of cell
surface receptors by ligands present on non-self material. This binding may
trigger a series of molecular events: (a) activation of lymphocyte binding
of the non-self ligand; (b) interaction among immunologically competent
cells; and (c) production of specific effector T and B cells.

It is widely held that binding of a ligand onto the cell surface results in
the activation process. However, some contradictory findings have been
reported (11). Binding of anti-immunoglobulin (Ig) antibodies to murine B
cells, and concanavalin A to B cells did not result in activation of cells
(12). In the case of lymphocytes, primary binding of the ligand to the
lymphocytes has been considered to be equivalent to specific recognition
(13). Other workers (14) considered specific immune differentiation as the
definition of recognition. It has been suggested that major histocompatibility
complex (MHC)-associated surface antigenic markers may be related to the
recognition process (15), since anti-H-2 sera can block specific T-cell differentiation.

Cell surface molecules have been implicated as receptors for ligands in
the immune recognition process. These receptors may be adsorbed by the
cell from serum or the cell may produce them endogenously. Specific cell
surface molecules like F_c receptors on lymphocytes (16), macrophages (17),
and mast cells (18) are known to occur; and these receptors are known to
bind exogenously produced molecules. In the other category are cells binding
Ig subclasses (monocytes and lymphocytes) and IgE (mast cells). Cells
(mammalian phagocytes) binding C-reactive protein serving as an opsonin
have also been reported (19). This subject has been exhaustively reviewed
in a recent article by Marchalonis (20). Involvement of glycosphingolipids
(21), phospholipids (21), and cyclic AMP (21) has been reported to have
a role in the early membrane events following the primary binding of a

ligand to a cell surface receptor, but the details of the biochemical mechanisms which induce the differentiation of the cell remain to be explored.

ANTIGEN PROCESSING

The immune system in the body of an adult has the ability to process a large number of antigenic determinants (probably greater than one million). These antigenic determinants (short peptides or oligosaccharides) are present on complex biomolecules like proteins, conjugated proteins, cell membranes, and microorganisms. An antigenic determinant is recognized by a lymphocyte or an antibody molecule produced by the lymphocyte. This specificity is determined by the amino acid sequence of three to four or fewer hypervariable regions of an Ig heavy chain and three to four hypervariable regions of a light chain. Each hypervariable region consists of three to five amino acid residues. The chains are folded so that one or more of the amino acid residues from several hypervariable regions form a configuration or recognition patch which is complementary to the antigenic determinant, and binds to it by a lock-and-key type arrangement.

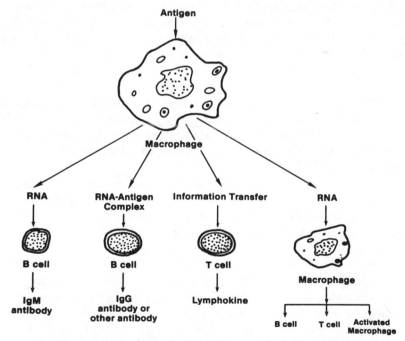

Fig.1.4. Antigen-Processing by macrophage and formation of antibody.

Antibodies are formed in lymphoid organs such as the spleen, lymph nodes, and bone marrow, but not in areas where lymphoid elements are lacking, such as the central nervous system. When the host becomes exposed to an antigen for the first time, antibodies are formed within a few days, attain a peak level slowly, and then decline. During the secondary response to the same antigen, antibodies are produced very quickly and then increase sharply.

After the antigen enters into the system, macrophages process it and present information to T cells, B cells, or other macrophages. When the information (RNA or RNA-antigen complexes) is presented to the B cell, antibodies are formed; T cells are stimulated to form lymphokines; and macrophages are activated, causing increased phagocytic reactions (Fig.1.4).

Humoral Immunity

When a B cell is stimulated by antigen or an informational molecule is transferred to it by either macrophages or T cells, the B cell undergoes blastogenic transformation, differentiates into a plasma cell, and synthesizes a particular type of antibody, which is released into the circulation (Fig.1.5).

Cell-Mediated Immunity

When an antigen is presented to a T cell, several types of reactions may occur (Fig.1.6). The T cell can assist the B cell in its antibody-forming ability by way of its helper cell (T_H) activity, which involves a thymic hormone, called thymosin. Activated effector lymphocytes (T_E) can produce (a) some lymphokine molecules to act as suppressor of antibody formation by a B cell; (b) a mitogenic agent which causes blastogenic transformation of other T cells; (c) a chemotactic factor for attracting macrophages to the site of antigens; (d) some lymphokines which call forth activated macrophages to the antigen site; (e) macrophage migration inhibition factor(s) to inhibit macrophages from leaving the areas of antigen-processing; (f) lymphokines like interferon, which confer on the host ability to resist viral or parasitic infection; and (g) a lymphokine called lymphotoxin, which can exert cytolytic action on cells like tumor cells. Another class of T cells, T suppressor cells (TS) can suppress immune reactions by interaction with T_H, with B cells, or possibly with antigen in association with these other cell types.

Upon immunization, T lymphocytes proliferate, progeny cells are formed and then circulated in the system. Later they mediate helper or suppressor effect on B or T cells by direct cell-cell interaction, or act cytotoxically against foreign cells or organisms through cell-target contact (22–25). Various

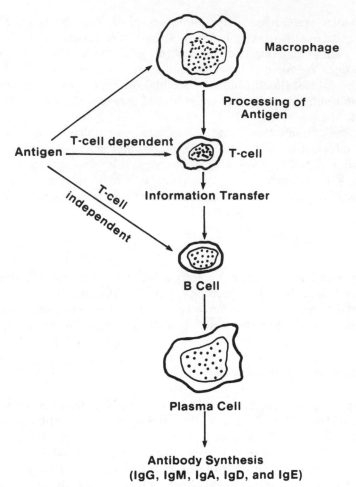

Fig.1.5. Antibody Synthesis by B Cell.

factors isolated from cells *in vitro* or from culture media can substitute for
or replace activity provided by intact lymphocytes, but it is not known
whether such factors are released *in vivo* and act at a distance from the cells
producing them (26–28). Binding of an antigenic determinant to a lymphocyte
receptor is required for the specificity of these interactions, but the binding
itself is not sufficient to trigger the entire sequence of events leading to
either activation or suppression of an immune response. The different factors
responsible for triggering the various kinds of responses are not exactly
known. However, different factors which may influence the responses have
been recognized. They are the form, amount, route of exposure to the

antigen, previous exposure to the antigen, and the size of the responding clones of cells.

Interaction Between Antigen and Cell

After immunization antigens are localized in macrophages in the spleen or lymph nodes. After phagocytosis the antigens are rapidly degraded, although some demonstrable immunogenic material is retained (29–31). Lymphocytes specifically sensitized against an antigen are recruited from the blood and lymph so that 24 hours after immunization there is a selective depletion of

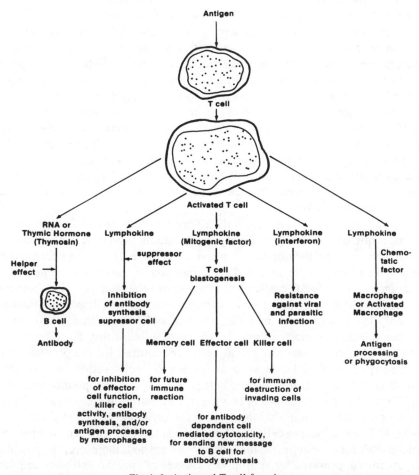

Fig.1.6. Activated T cell function.

these sensitized lymphocytes from the lymph and blood, and an enrichment of such in the spleen and lymph nodes. Antibody to an antigen, when administered passively, can markedly suppress formation of the specific antibody, perhaps by combining with the circulatory pool of antigen and making it unavailable for sensitization of the immune system. However, with passive immnunization, lymphocytes specific for the antigen remain in the lymph and blood and are normally responsive when transferred to another animal (32,33). Thus, a small amount of antigenic material localized in some critical sites is responsible for the selective recruitment of specific lymphocytes, and for the induction of certain cooperative immunological reactions between other lymphocytes.

Cells that phagocytize antigen can be separated from lymphocytes because they have the ability to adhere to plastic or other surfaces. Almost all of these cells (greater than 95%) can phagocytize a wide variety of foreign particles, such as carbon particles and foreign cells. Adherent cells obtained from mice recently injected with antigen stimulate a high antibody response when normal B and T lymphocytes are added to them. Adherent cells exposed to antigen *in vitro* or *in vivo* and then treated with antibody to the antigen and washed do not stimulate a response from normal B and T lymphocytes. Similarly, adherent cells fed antigen first and then treated chemically to inactivate the antigen did not stimulate normal lymphocytes, although the adherent cells that were refed the antigen were effective. Both the phagocytic and immunologic function of adherent cells are quite resistant to X-irradiation, and the number and function of these cells do not change measurably after immunization, indicating that the adherent cells do not proliferate in an immune response (34–36).

Several studies indicate that only a very few adherent cells may suffice for the required immunological responses, and that too many adherent cells can actually prevent the immune response (37, 38) i.e., can exert a suppressive effect. Such findings are expected if the function of cells that have interacted with antigen is to focus cell-cell interaction of relatively few lymphocytes. Adherent cells may be nonspecific in both ingestion and display of antigen, but only the combination of adherent cells and antigen that results in recruitment of B lymphocytes may be effective in recruiting T_H cells specific for carrier determinants. Adherent cells are required for the production of antigen-specific T cells, as well as for B-cell proliferation *in vitro* (39–43). It is not known, however, whether the different subpopulations of B and T lymphocytes responding to antigenic stimulation are triggered by the same or a different population of adherent cells that have interacted with antigen. Thus, adherent cells that have interacted with antigen are probably crucial sites for connection in the immune system and, therefore, are potential targets for suppression by appropriate classes of specific antibody and subpopulations of T_S lymphocytes.

ANTIGEN-ANTIBODY REACTIONS

An antibody molecule binds with an antigen in order to allow it to be cleared from the system. Five types of reactions may occur, depending upon the nature of the antigenic material.

1. *Agglutination*. With particulate antigen (intact cells, white blood cells, red blood cells, bacteria, etc.) specific antibody binds to form aggregates or clumps. When bacteria enter the system, antibodies (performed) agglutinate these bacteria, a process known as opsonization, to facilitate their destruction by phagocytes. Large aggregates or clumps of particulate antigens are formed because of the bivalent nature of the antibody molecule, which can bind with numerous antigenic determinant sites on the antigen to form a lattice-like structure. Eventually, these can form large aggregates which are detectable to the naked eye.

2. *Precipitation*. When a soluble antigen reacts with soluble antibody, precipitation occurs. With optimal concentration of both antigen and antibody, large amounts of precipitate are formed. However, in the presence of excess antigen or antibody, the amount of precipitate formed is less than maximal.

3. *Lysis*. An antibody can bind with antigen on cell membrane and, with the help of serum complement, cause lysis of the cell. Bacteria, virus, or any cell of non-self origin is lysed by the immune components (antibody and complement) of the body by this procedure. Cancer cells can also be destroyed by the lytic process. It is believed by many that occasionally a few cancer cells may be formed within the animal body, but usually the host can destroy them by specific antibody and complement action or by effector lymphocytes and natural killer cells.

4. *Toxin neutralization*. An antibody against a toxin (elaborated by a bacterium) can neutralize the toxic action. Against diphtheria or tetanus toxin, for example, inoculation of antitoxin helps neutralize their action.

5. *Flocculation reaction*. If an antigen is neither soluble nor cellular, but is in an insoluble particulate form, flocculation reaction occurs with antibody. This type of test is performed for the diagnosis of syphilis. A heterophile antigen shared between the spirochete of syphilis and beef heart is used for this test. The antigen used in this test is cardiolipin, a water insoluble material, which can bind with reaginic antibody present in the serum of patients suffering from syphilis, to form visible aggregates of flocculated material.

COMPLEMENT REACTION

Complement (C) cascade comprises a group of nine serum proteins, which can bind to antigen-antibody complex to give rise to cytolytic activity.

Complement components C_1 through C_9, bind to the antigen-antibody complex in a specific manner: C_1, C_4, C_2, and C_3 bind one after another in this order, followed by C_5 through C_9. Lysis cannot take place until C_9 is fixed on the large complex. Detailed information on this mechanism may be found in any textbook on immunology. There are several other subfractions of C having important biological activity. These are C_{3a}, C_{3b}, C_{5a}, and C_{5b}. C_{3a} and C_{5a} act on mast cells and basophils to release some soluble factors, causing an increase in capillary permeability and the contraction of smooth muscle. They also have chemotactic properties for basophils. Cells having C_{3b} attached on their surfaces are very easily phagocytized, a process known as opsonization of cells. These cells also can aggregate together, a process known as immune adherence. C_{5b} can complex with C_6 and C_7, chemotactically attracting neutrophils. Several regulatory components are available to control the action of complement. These are C_1 esterase inhibitor, C_{3b} inactivator, and anaphylatoxin inactivator.

Unlike the classical complement pathway, where C_1 through C_9 components of complement are required to effect lysis, lysis may also occur through the alternate pathway of complement. In the latter case, only C_3 through C_9' are required for complement action . IgA, IgE, IgG, cobra venom factor, and bacterial endotoxin can trigger complement action by the alternate pathway.

Complement molecules take part in the lysis of bacteria and viruses, and perhaps in the immune clearance of defective or damaged cells in the body, thus serving a vital function in the overall immune system. Complement deficiency has been observed in patients suffering from various disorders, including malignancy.

HYPERSENSITIVITY REACTIONS

Sensitization of a host against an antigen is not always beneficial. Sometimes synthesis of antibodies against some antigens and their later reaction with the specific antigen can be harmful to the host. During the second exposure to the antigen, several unusual reactions can sometimes occur. Such reactions are termed *allergic* or *hypersensitive* reactions. Hypersensitivity means heightened reactivity to an antigen, the nature of such reaction being immunologic. At the initial stage, exposure to an antigen or to an autocomplexing haptenic molecule is necessary. After a certain lag period, the individual is in a position to produce humoral and cellular factors against the sensitizing antigen, thus becoming sensitive to that antigen. When a second dose of antigen is administered, the animal responds either immediately (immediate hypersensitivity), or later (delayed type of hypersensitivity). In general, the immediate reaction is mediated by humoral factors.

Immediate Hypersensitivity

Immediate hypersensitivity type reactions may occur very quickly following the binding of an antibody to a specific antigen. Two types of reactions may occur—(a) anaphylaxis and (b) atopy. Anaphylaxis type reaction may be either systemic or local. It is manifested by smooth muscle contraction, increased capillary permeability, edema, and obstruction of the respiratory tract. This may lead to death, sometimes within a very short period of time.

Atopic reactions tend to occur in individuals having a hereditary predisposition. Allergic asthma, dermatitis, urticaria, and rhinitis are different types of atopic reactions. The most common symptoms in these situations are itching, sneezing, watery nasal discharge, nasal obstruction, shortness of breath, tightness in the chest, bronchospasm, erythema, and angioedema.

Reaginic type antibodies (IgE) have been implicated in immediate hypersensitivity reactions. When an individual having reaginic antibodies fixed on his mast cells is exposed to the sensitizing antigen (allergen), an antigen-antibody reaction (between the allergen and IgE antibody) occurs, triggering a series of events that leads to the release of a number of pharmacologically active components, which cause the different types of reactions discussed above. The released components include histamine, bradykinin, platelet-activating factor, eosinophil chemotactic factor, and slow-reacting substance.

Delayed Hypersensitivity

Delayed hypersensitivity is the manifestation of cell-mediated immunity against an antigen. It is involved in drug allergy, contact dermatitis, allergic response to insect venoms, rejection of tissues or grafts (allografts), and tumor rejection; although humoral mechanisms are also involved in some of these reactions. Delayed hypersensitivity reactions are mediated by T cells and occur 24 to 48 hours or later following the exposure to the antigen. The tuberculin skin test is an example of a delayed hypersensitivity reaction. It is believed that the antigen binds with antigen-specific T lymphocytes, followed by the release of a variety of soluble mediators, called lymphokines. A number of such lymphokines have been described. They include transfer factor, macrophage migration inhibitory factor, macrophage activating factor, macrophage chemotactic factor, mitogenic factor, and lymphotoxin. Corticosteroids, antilymphocyte serum, and other immunosuppressive drugs can inhibit delayed type hypersensitivity reactions. Immunomodulators, such as BCG, *C. parvum*, protein A of *S. aureus* and Levamisole can augment delayed hypersensitivity reaction.

REGULATION OF IMMUNE RESPONSE

Evidence that cooperativity in the immune functions exists comes in part from the demonstration that specific amplification or suppression of the immune response is possible using isolated antibody or cells. Thus, an antibody to an antigenic determinant can be extremely immunosuppressive when inoculated before or up to 24 hours after initial immunization. It is possible that this suppression is due to interference with the interaction between the antigenic determinants and the responding cells, and not simply to masking of the antigen. Much less antibody is required to suppress than to mask all antigenic determinants present on an antigen; indeed, washed antigen-antibody complexes formed in antibody excess can suppress responses to free antigen. The F_c portion of the antibody molecule is important because some classes of immunoglobulin (IgA) suppress poorly or not at all, while other classes having the same idiotype (IgG) are effective. F(ab)$_2$ fragments that retain full combining activity are ineffective immunosuppressants (44–47). In most of these studies, antisera to complex antigens used to suppress immunization probably contained antibodies to antigenic determinants to which T_H lymphocytes were directed, so that the suppression observed may have resulted from the summation of inhibition of the interaction of both T_H and B lymphocytes with antigenic determinants. However, in recent studies, homogeneous antibody was shown to be effective in suppressing immunization *in vitro* and *in vivo* (48). Presumably, the antibody that has suppressor activity links antigenic determinants and F_c receptors on adherent cells and/or B lymphocytes, so that it is possible that immune complexes (specific or nonspecific) may interfere with this process.

During an infection or on re-exposure to the agent, antibodies should not turn off the immune response to the antigen, and in fact, antibody is a much less effective immunosuppressant when given more than 24 hours after a first immunization or before a second immunization, even if the second immunization is weeks or months after the first one. Along with other factors, the changing mixture of antibodies produced, the formation of antibody-antigen complexes, and the generation of T_H and T_S cells, probably account for this change. At present, however, it is impossible to assess the combined interactions of the reactants in the functioning of the network during the course of an immune response.

The potential for regulation through complementary antibody is great. Antigen stimulates the production of antibody, and an antibody stimulates production of complementary clones that regulate, directly or indirectly through their products, the interaction with cells having the idiotype of the original responding cells. Several findings are consistent with these possibilities (49–51).

The mechanisms of regulation by complementary idiotypes, however, must be more complex than simple binding of an antibody to receptors. $F(ab)_2$ fragments of antibody to one specific antigen do not suppress immunization to another specific antigen *in vitro*. Under these experimental conditions, fragments are not eliminated and retain full binding activity. These findings strongly suggest that cross-linking of antigen with Fc receptors may be required for suppression (52). Also, when mice are intentionally immunized simultaneously with the two antigens, reciprocal regulation does not occur; each response is undiminished, and circulating complexes of the complementary antibodies are formed. This absence of regulation cannot be accounted for by a shift in idiotypes of either of the complementary responses. At first, the stimulated clones of cells should proliferate and synthesize antibody in the absence of appreciable complementary idiotype. With progression of responses, released antibody, which can be considered a shed antigen, may shield cells from being targets for complementary antibody. Alternatively, complexes of complementary antibody may bind to F_c receptors that are required for regulation by complementary antibody, and prevent regulation in this way (53). Thus, the role of autogenous complementary antibody in regulation is not simple or obvious. Future efforts should be directed to elucidate the exact role of this type of molecule in immune regulation. The question would remain, however, whether anti-idiotype antibody generation is a phenomenon of autoregulation, or is a type of feedback to control an excessive immune response that the host cannot handle. Further study in two areas, tumor growth and fetal development, may throw new light and more understanding on the subject. At least theoretically, humoral regulation of maintenance of continued growth of tumor and fetus, in the otherwise hostile immune environment of the host, appears a more likely possibility.

The regulatory role of T_H and T_S lymphocytes has also been shown to be important in a large number of studies. T_H and T_S lymphocytes are stimulated by appropriate host immunization with a complex antigen. The subsequent response to a new antigenic determinant coupled with that antigen is strongly modified by the previous sensitization of the animal, which correlates directly with the presence of T_H and T_S lymphocytes. A regulatory effect of T_H or B lymphocytes may be involved in triggering B-lymphocyte proliferation. T_H lymphocytes may also be involved in the generation of T_S or T_E lymphocytes. Different populations of T_S lymphocytes that are generated during the course of continuous immunization, or during hyperimmunization (54–56), may be directed against sites that include determinants of antigen in association with adherent cells or in association with B lymphocytes. It has been demonstrated that a population of T lymphocytes can shut off secretion of antibody by B lymphocytes (57). A strong possibility is that this class of T lymphocytes is of the T_S type. The target for T_S lymphocytes may be the V domains of receptors of B or T lymphocytes. This view is supported by the results of Cooke et al. (58), where a self-limitation phenomenon against an experimentally-induced autoimmune hemolytic anemia has been described. Various other self-limiting phenomena have also been found to be related to the presence of T_S lymphocytes.

SUMMARY

The immune system comprises a very complex network of biochemical reactions and cellular interactions where soluble serum factors and cells function with one another. These reactions and interactions are specifically connected by the complementarity of receptors for antigens and receptors for receptors. The complex network includes multiple positive and negative feedback mechanisms which determine the type, magnitude, and duration of responses. The great challenge is to devise ways and means to manipulate the immune system, specifically to induce effective autoimmunity to cancer, to prevent allograft rejection, and to turn off undersirable reactions, such as allergies and autoimmune disorders. Recognition of the complexity of the immune system explains why these objectives are so difficult to reach and why manipulation of the multiple components of the immune system to achieve a desired regulation is so difficult. Manipulation is usually focused on one or several aspects of the immune response, without giving attention to the many different mechanisms involved in the immune response. This perhaps is the cause of frustration in many of the attempts at immunologic modulation as a form of therapy. Extensive studies involving careful intervention in the complex network of immune mechanisms as related to many known and as yet unknown forms of immunologic diseases may provide some fruitful therapeutic regimen for immunologic therapy of various disorders.

REFERENCES

1. Jerne, N. A., *Ann. Immunol. Inst. Pasteur* **125C**:373, 1974.
2. Jerne, N. K., *Harvey Lect.* **70**:93, 1976.
3. De Pasquier, L., *Arch. Biol.* **85**:91, 1974.
4. Coffaro, K. A., and Hinegardner, R. T., *Science*, **197**:1389, 1977.
5. Hildemann, W. H., *Immunogenetics* **5**:193, 1977.
6. Karp, R. D., and Hildemann, W. H., *Transplantation* **22**:434, 1976.
7. Bodmer, W. F., *Nature* **237**:139, 1972.
8. Burnet, F. M., *Nature* **245**:259, 1973.

9. Katz, D. H., T lymphocyte receptors and cell interactions in the immune system. In B. R. Brinkley and K. R. Portu (Eds.), *International Cell Biology*, pp. 112–118. New York: Rockefeller University Press, 1975.
10. Peterson, P. A., Rask, L., Sege, K., Klareskog, L., Amundi, H., and Ostberg, L., *Proc. Natl. Acad. Sci. USA* **72**:1612, 1975.
11. Clarke, A., and Knox, R. B., *Q. Rev. Biol.* **53**:3, 1978.
12. Greaves, M. F., Janossy, G., Feldman, M., and Doenhoff, M., Polyclonal mitogens and the nature of B lymphocyte activation mechanism. In E. E. Sercarz, A. R. Williamson, and C. F. Fox (Eds.), *The Immune System: Genes, Receptors and Signals*, pp. 271–297. New York: Academic Press, 1974.
13. Marchalonis, J. J., and Warr, G. W., Antigen receptors on thymus-derived lymphocytes. In J. J. Marchalonis, M. G. Hanna, Jr., and I. J. Fidler (Eds.), *Cancer Biology Reviews*, Vol. 1, pp. 1–47. New York: Marcel Dekker, 1981.
14. Paul, W. E., and Benacerraf, B., *Science* **195**:1293, 1977.
15. Bluestein, H., *J. Exp. Med.* **140**:481, 1974.
16. Dickler, H.B., *Adv. Immunol.* **24**:167, 1976.
17. Warner, N. L., *Adv. Immunol.* **19**:67, 1974.
18. Metzger, H., Early molecular events in immunoglobulin E mediated mast cell exocytosis. In E. E. Sercarz, A. R. Williamson, and C. F. Fox (Eds.), *The Immune System: Genes, Receptors and Signals*, pp. 679–690. New York: Academic Press, 1974.
19. Kindmark, C. O., *Clin. Exp. Immunol.* **8**:941, 1971.
20. Marchalonis, J. J., Molecular interactions and recognition specificity of surface receptors. In J. J. Marchalonis, and N. Cohen (Eds.), *Contemporary Topics in Immunobiology*, pp. 255–288. New York: Plenum Press, 1980.
21. Curtain, C. C., *Immunology* **36**:805, 1979.
22. Golub, E. S., *The Cellular Basis of the Immune Response: An Approach to Immunobiology*. Sunderland, MA: Sinauer Associates, 1977.
23. Marchalonis, J. J., Decker, J. M., Deluka, D., Moseley, J. M., Smith, P., and Warr, G. W., *Cold Spring Harbor Symp. Quant. Biol.* **61**:261, 1976.
24. Evans, R. L., Breard, J. M., Lazarus, H., Schlossman, S. F., and Chess, L., *J. Exp. Med.* **145**:221, 1977.
25. Owen, F. L., Ju, S. T., and Nisonoff, A., *J. Exp. Med.* **145**:1559, 1977.
26. Munro, A. F., and Taussig, M. J., *Nature* **256**:103, 1975.
27. Kindred, B., and Corley, R. B., *Nature* **268**:531, 1977.
28. Diamanstein, H., and Naher, H., *Nature* **271**:275, 1978.
29. Franzl, R. E., *Inf. Immun.* **6**:469, 1972.
30. Unanue, E. R., and Askonsas, B. A., *J. Exp. Med.* **127**:915, 1968.
31. Pike, B. L., and Nossal, J.V., *J. Exp. Med.* **44**:568, 1976.
32. Rowley, D. C., Gowans, J. L., Atkins, R. C., Ford, W. L., and Smith, W. E., *J. Exp. Med.* **136**:499, 1972.
33. Ford, W. L., *Prog. Allergy* **19**:1, 1975.
34. Rowley, D. A., Cosenza, H., Leserman, L.D., and Fitch, F. W., The third cell type in the macrophage population required for the antibody response. In R. VanFurth (Ed.), *Mononuclear Phagocytes in Immunology, Infection and Pathology*, pp. 755–763. Oxford: Blackwell Scientific, 1975.
35. Lee, K. C., Shiozara, C., Shaw, A., and Diener, E., *Eur. J. Immunol.* **6**:63, 1976.
36. Landahl, C. A., *Eur. J. Immunol.* **6**:130, 1976.
37. Mosier, D. E., and Coppleson, L. W., *Proc. Natl. Acad. Sci. USA* **61**:542, 1968.
38. Weiss, A., and Fitch, F. W., *J. Immunol* **120**:357, 1978.
39. Moller, G.: The role of macrophages in the immune response. In G. Moller (Ed.), *Immunological Reviews.*, Vol. 40. Copenhagen: Munksgaard, 1978.

40. Rosenthal, A. S., Barcinski, M. A., and Rosenwasser, L. J., *Fed. Proc. Fed. Am. Soc. Exp. Biol.* **37**:79, 1978.
41. Beller, D. I., Farr, A. G., and Unanue, E. R., *Fed. Proc. Fed. Am. Soc. Exp. Biol.* **37**:91, 1978
42. Pierce, C. W., and Kapp, J. A., *Fed. Proc. Fed. Am. Soc. Exp. Biol.* **37**:86, 1978.
43. Erb, P., Gasser, M., Strasser, S., Kontiainen, S., and Feldman, M., *Fed. Proc. Fed. Am. Soc. Exp. Biol.* **37**:2032, 1978.
44. Rowley, D. A., Fitch, F. W., Stuart, F. P., Kohler, H., and Cosenza, H., *Science* **181**:1133, 1973.
45. Moretta, L., Mingari, M. C., and Romanzi, C. A., *Nature* **272**:618, 1978.
46. Fitch, F. W., *Prog. Allergy.* **19**:195, 1975.
47. Sidman, C. L., and Unanue, E. R., *J. Exp. Med.* **144**:882, 1976.
48. McKearn, T. J., Weiss, A., Stuart, F. P., and Fitch, F. W., *Transpl. Proc.* **11**:932, 1979.
49. Rowley, D. A., Kohler, H., Schreiber, H., Kaye, S. T., and Lorbach, I., *J. Exp. Med.* **144**:946, 1976.
50. Cosenza, H., *Eur. J. Immunol.* **6**:114, 1976.
51. Bona, C., Lieberman, R., Chien, C. C., Mond, J., House, S., Green, I., and Paul, W. E., *J. Immunol.* **120**:1436, 1978.
52. Kohler, H., Richardson, B. C., Rowley, D. A., and Smyk, S., *J. Immunol.* **119**:1979, 1978.
53. Rowley, D. A., Miller, G. W., and Lorbach, I., *J. Exp. Med.* **148**:148, 1978.
54. Ray, P. K., and Raychaudhuri, S., *Fed. Am. Soc. Exp. Biol.* **39**(3):696, 1980.
55. Saha, S., and Ray, P. K., *Fed. Am. Soc. Exp. Biol.* **41**(3):411, 1982.
56. Raychaudhuri, S., Ray, P. K., Bassett, J. G., and Cooper, D. R., *Fed. Am. Soc. Exp. Biol.* **39**(3):2263, 1980.
57. Warren, R. W., and Davie, J. M., *J. Immunol.* **119**:1806, 1977.
58. Cooke, A., Hutchings, P. R., and Playfair, J. H. L., *Nature* **273**:154, 1978.

PART II
IMMUNOBIOLOGY OF TRANSPLANTATION— A PHENOMENON OF REJECTION OF NON-SELF

2
Mammalian Cell-Surface Antigens

C. John Abeyounis and Felix Milgrom

SPECIES-SPECIFIC ANTIGENS

A species-specific antigen may be defined as an antigen that is present in all members of a given species and which differs from an analogous antigen of other species. The studies on species specificity were initiated at the turn of this century by demonstration of differences in antigenic structure of milk originating from various mammalian species (1, 2). Pioneering experiments were conducted by Nuttall (3), who studied several hundred serum specimens by means of 30 antisera that were obtained in rabbits by immunization with sera of various species origin. Each antiserum gave the strongest reaction with the serum of the same species as the serum used for immunization. Cross-reactions, many of which were noted, were strong for closely related species and weak for biologically distant species. Practically no cross-reactions were seen between sera originating from different vertebrate classes.

In the studies by Nuttall, the serum was treated as if it were an antigenic entity. Several decades later, when it became obvious that serum is composed of 30-odd proteins, it was also observed that all these proteins are impregnated with species specificity and that they show similar behavior as that observed by Nuttall for whole serum, i.e., strong cross-reactions between analogous proteins of closely related species and weak or no cross-reactions between such proteins of distant species. Furthermore, even fragments of a protein molecule, e.g., Fc piece of IgG, show definite species specificity. It also became obvious that not only serum proteins but also cytoplasmic proteins, e.g., thyroglobulin, show definite species specificity. As shown by Rose and Witebsky (4), thyroglobulins of human, porcine, and bovine origin show distinct specificities even though they also demonstrate cross-reactions.

Species-specific characteristics are limited, by and large, to protein antigens. Carbohydrate antigens, however, may appear in completely unpredictable fashion. They may be shared by remote species without being shared by closely related species. Carbohydrates are responsible for heterophile reactions, which may be defined as unpredictable cross-reactions. The best known heterophile specificity was described by Forssman in 1911 (5).

In parallel with studies on species specificity, studies on tissue specificity were conducted. (The terms tissue and organ specificity have been used as synonyms. This may be somewhat annoying for a morphologist, but is not resented by immunologists who have used this nomenclature for over half a century.) They were initiated in 1903 by the experiments of Uhlenhuth on the lens of the eye (6). Tissue-specific antigen may be defined as an antigen restricted to one organ or tissue and absent from other organs and tissues. Thyroglobulin is a tissue-specific antigen characteristic for thyroid gland and it is virtually absent in any other place of the body (7). In a similar way, basic protein is characteristic for brain (8). Tissue-specific antigens have been described for practically every organ of the body. They usually have well-pronounced species specificity (e.g., thyroglobulin), however, some tissue-specific antigens have hardly any species specificity.

The above quoted studies were performed, by and large, on antigenic substances present in body fluids or readily extracted from tissues. Analysis of cell-membrane antigens, most of which are nonextractable in saline, has been largely neglected except for investigations on erythrocytes which can be easily studied by means of agglutination tests. The species-specific antigens of the erythrocyte surface were readily detected by means of heteroimmune sera. On the other hand, very little information has been available concerning cell-surface antigens of nucleated cells. A very important step forward towards studying these antigens was made by the procedure of mixed agglutination (9). The procedure developed by Fagraeus and Espmark (10) involving mixed agglutination with cell cultures proved to be especially convenient. In this procedure, monolayer cell cultures are incubated with a serum that presumably contains antibodies to the cell-surface antigens. Following removal of unbound proteins by washing, the adherence of antibody immunoglobulins to the monolayer surface is detected by means of indicator erythrocytes. These are usually sheep erythrocytes sensitized by antisheep erythrocyte antibodies of the same species origin as the serum tested against the cell culture. The sensitized erythrocytes are agglutinated by an excess of the proper anti-gamma-globulin serum. If antibodies of the test serum are bound to the cell cultures, indicator erythrocytes adhere to the cell monolayer through the anti-gamma-globulin cross linkings, otherwise, they remain free. The result of the test is assessed by inspection of the cell monolayer with a microscope at low magnification (11).

The results of these studies showed that the predominant antigens of living mammalian cells are apparently devoid of tissue specificity (11). It

Table 2.1. Mixed Agglutination with Cell Cultures of Bovine Adrenal Medulla

Antiserum Dilution 1:	Antiserum against Bovine				
	Adrenal Suspension	Brain Suspension	Liver Suspension	Liver Extract	Serum
10	+ + + +	+ + + +	+ + + +	±	+ +
100	+ + + +	+ + + +	+ + + +	±	+
1,000	+ + + +	+ + + +	+ + +	−	−
10,000	+ + + +	+ + +	+ + +	−	−
100,000	+ +	+ +	+	−	−
1,000,000	−	±	−	−	−

may be seen in Table 2.1 that cultures of bovine adrenal medulla gave equally strong reactions with antisera to bovine adrenal, brain, and liver suspensions. It may be noted also that the antigens participating in these reactions were saline nonextractable since immunization with saline extracts of liver resulted in an antiserum which virtually failed to combine with the cell cultures. Antiserum to bovine serum gave a very weak reaction which, with all likelihood, was not produced by antibodies to any soluble antigens, but by antibodies to small fragments of lymphocytes or platelets that had not been removed from the serum used for immunization. Antisera to erythrocytes also reacted with cultures of nucleated cells, but these reactions were considerably weaker than those produced by antisera to tissue suspensions containing nucleated cells, e.g., liver suspension. Furthermore, antisera to tissue suspensions could be extensively absorbed with bovine erythrocytes without losing any significant activity against nucleated cell cultures. Very similar results were obtained with cell cultures of other species origin including man, dog, guinea pig, hamster, rat, and mouse. Antisera produced in a foreign species (most frequently in rabbits) by immunization with crude organ suspension or suspension of any nucleated cells including blood leukocytes or various cell cultures were successfully employed for these studies. The reactions observed showed very pronounced species specificity, as shown in Table 2.2. It may be noted that antisera to bovine, hamster, and human cells gave the strongest reactions with bovine, hamster, and human cell cultures respectively. Interspecies cross-reactions were observed but they were 100 to 1000 times weaker than the reaction

Table 2.2. Mixed Agglutination with Ox, Hamster, and Human Cell Cultures

		Titer of mixed agglutination with antisera against suspension of tissues originating from:		
		Ox	Hamster	Man
Cell cultures originating from:	Ox	100,000	100	1,000
	Hamster	100	100,000	1,000
	Man	100	1,000	1,000,000

with cell cultures originating from the species that donated the tissues used for immunization. Furthermore, these interspecies cross-reactions could be readily removed by proper absorptions without influencing the intraspecific reactions. It was concluded from these studies that the predominant antigens of mammalian cell cultures are species-specific antigens.

Rewarding experiments were obtained in studies on interspecific hybrid cells such as man-mouse hybrids. It could be clearly shown that the hybrid contains species-specific antigens of both parents (12).

From the beginning of these studies, it appeared rather obvious that the species-specific reactions under study were not due to one antigen but were caused by a multiplicity of cell-surface antigens, all impregnated with species specificity. The majority of these antigens was apparently of protein nature since tissues used for absorption of the antibodies under investigation would lose their absorbing capacity after exposure to the temperature of 80°C for one-half hour. Further characterization of the antigens under study was not attempted.

No chemical approaches were used to isolate individual species-specific antigens from the cell surface, but evidence for the multiplicity of these antigens was obtained from genetic studies (13) which were a continuation of the above-mentioned research on man-mouse hybrids. Clones of cells were obtained in which the appearance of the human species-specific antigens was encoded only by chromosome 21. On these clones, expression of species antigens was much weaker than on human cells or other hybrid cells where many chromosomes were responsible for encoding these antigens. Still, evidence was obtained from absorption studies that the single human chromosome 21 was responsible for the appearance of more than one antigen on the cell surface.

It is tempting to compare the present status of the studies on species antigens of the cell surface to the studies of Nuttall (3) in which serum was treated as if it were a single antigen. There is little doubt that in the near future individual cell-surface antigen will be isolated and characterized.

Heterophile Antigens

As mentioned, the above discussed features of species specificity pertain to protein antigens. In contrast, carbohydrate antigens are characterized by haphazard appearance in various species of the animal and plant kingdoms irrespective of the biological relationship among the species. Accordingly, carbohydrates are frequently responsible for unexpected cross-reactions, which were named heterophile or heterologous cross-reactions to distinguish them from interspecies cross-reactions among proteins, which parallel the evolutionary pathway. Heterophile antibodies are defined as antibodies which, in an unpredictable fashion, act upon an antigen related to the antigen which elicited their formation. Heterophile antigens are antigens that stimulate formation of or enter into reaction with heterophile antibodies.

We will limit our discussion just to four heterophile systems which are of major interest to students of biology and medicine.

Forssman Antigen

One of the first heterophile systems was described by Forssman (5), who noticed that sera of rabbits injected with a suspension of guinea pig organs combined with sheep erythrocytes. The precise structure of the Forssman antigen as ceramid pentasaccharide was only recently elucidated (14). All the animal kingdom may be divided into Forssman-positive species, of which the most important are guinea pig, horse, sheep, goat, dog, cat, and chicken, and into Forssman-negative species, as exemplified by rabbit, rat, ox, pig, and pigeon. Man is a Forssman-negative species even though the structure of human blood group A antigen is related to the Forssman antigen. Also, many investigators claimed that some human tumors acquire the structure of Forssman antigens. The most recent studies along these lines were made by Hakomori et al. (15). Further data on this fascinating topic are expected. Forssman antigen is distributed in most cells and tissues of Forssman-positive animals. In addition to its intracellular localization, Forssman antigen is present on cell membranes (11, 16). Because of its localization on the cell surface, the reaction of antibodies with the Forssman antigen results in most dramatic pathologic events. These were mostly studied in the guinea pig. Intravenous injection of even very small amounts of Forssman antisera into a guinea pig results in an immediate shock that resembles anaphylactic shock and terminates within a few minutes with the animal's death. Doerr and Pick (17) called this shock inverse anaphylaxis to indicate that, in this instance, antigen was in the animal and antibody was injected intravenously, in contrast to the usual anaphylactic shock.

Paul-Bunnell Antigens

In 1932, Paul and Bunnell (18) described antibodies characteristic for infectious mononucleosis. These antibodies are almost exclusively of the IgM variety; they react with an antigen present on erythrocytes and other tissues of sheep, ox, horse, and several other animal species. Under normal conditions, human tissues are devoid of Paul-Bunnell antigen. (This statement may be an oversimplification in view of our recent observations on the possible *allo* nature of the Paul-Bunnell antigen [unpublished].) The Paul-

Bunnell antigen is a glycoprotein (19, 20). This antigen differs from the Forssman antigen in that it is present on tissues of some Forssman-negative species, e.g., ox, but it is absent from tissues of many Forssman-positive animals, e.g., guinea pig (21).

The mode of formation of Paul-Bunnell antibodies has been a mystery. The possible cross-reactions between Paul-Bunnell antigen and a virus responsible for infectious mononucleosis seem unlikely since evidence was presented that the Epstein-Barr virus is responsible for infectious mononucleosis (22) and since numerous studies showed that this virus gives no cross-reactions with Paul-Bunnell antigen. Several years ago a hypothesis was forwarded proposing that formation of Paul-Bunnell antibodies is stimulated by a novel antigen that appears on human cells as the result of the pathological process (23). Evidence for this hypothesis was only recently presented by demonstrating the Paul-Bunnell antigen in tissues of a patient who died of a heart attack in the very early stage of infectious mononucleosis (24). Furthermore, it was also recently demonstrated that Paul-Bunnell antigen can be extracted from the buffy coat of patients suffering from infectious mononucleosis (unpublished data). Studies from our laboratory also showed that Paul-Bunnell antigen appears in tissues and serum of patients suffering from various diseases, primarily lymphomas and leukemias, but also other malignancies, as well as other diseases accompanied by extensive tissue destruction (25–27).

Paul-Bunnell antigen is present on the surface of erythrocytes and lymphocytes of animals bearing this antigen, as readily shown by reactions of agglutination and lysis with infectious mononucleosis sera.

It appears quite likely that formation of Paul-Bunnell antibodies plays an important role in the course of infectious mononucleosis. These antibodies may contribute to the recovery from infectious mononucleosis by eliminating aberrant cells. Significantly, in other diseases in which Paul-Bunnell antigen was demonstrated, formation of its corresponding antibodies has never been encountered. Apparently, this antigen is released in an immunogenic form only in infectious mononucleosis, and not in other diseases (e.g., lymphoma or leukemia).

Hanganutziu-Deicher Antigens

In the 1920s, antibodies, which were referred to as *serum sickness antibodies* and which combine with sheep and bovine erythrocytes, were repoted by Hanganutziu (28) and Deicher (29). The first descriptions of these antibodies were made in studying sera of patients injected with a foreign species serum for serum therapy of diphtheria and serum prophylaxis of tetanus. Since some of these patients also had symtoms of serum sickness, the name of serum-sickness antibodies was used, which obviously was a misnomer since formation of these antibodies was independent from the symptoms of serum sickness. The corresponding antigen differs from the Forssman and the Paul-Bunnell antigen and is present on both bovine erythrocytes and guinea pig tissues.

Recent studies from this laboratory (30) "unearthed" this antigen by demonstrating antibodies directed against it in sera of patients suffering from various diseases, even though in low frequency. Immunochemical studies (31) showed that the major specificity of the Hanganutziu-Deicher antigen resides on a ganglioside and that the determinant is n-glycolylneuraminic acid. Further investigations showed that in additon to the ganglioside, Hanganutziu-Deicher specificity resides also in a high molecular weight glycoprotein fraction of an extract from bovine erythrocyte stromata (32).

Interestingly, the Hanganutziu-Deicher antigen could be demonstrated frequently in pathologic human sera, e.g., in malignancies 30 to 35% of sera were shown to contain this antigen (33).

Heterophile Transplantation Antigens

Our own studies as well as studies by other investigators (33–39) have shown that many sera of human allograft recipients, both volunteers who received skin grafts and patients after kidney transplantation, contained antibodies that combined with erythrocytes of several animal species. In our research, the strongest reactions were obtained with bovine erythrocytes (39). According to the evidence obtained from our studies, human nucleated cells contain alloantigens shared with bovine erythrocytes. Interestingly, the bovine erythrocytes apparently cover all the antigenic repertoire of this system and, therefore, alloantibodies of various individual specificities all react with bovine erythrocytes. Some evidence for the role of these antigens in allograft rejection has been presented by McDonald (37, 38).

ALLOANTIGENS

Alloantigens are those antigens that appear in some, but not in all individuals of a given species. Alloantigens are present on soluble molecules such as immunoglobulins, as well as on membrane-bound constituents of the cell surface. Only antigens of the latter type are pertinent to this discussion.

Each vertebrate species has many genetic loci bearing alleles that determine cell-membrane alloantigens. These consist of genes governing erythrocyte or blood group alloantigens, such as ABO and Rh in man and Ea in the mouse; genes that control lymphocyte markers, such as the Ly, Thy-1, and TL systems in mice; genes that control antigens detectable by activating or stimulating lymphocytes, and finally, genes that govern the appearance of transplantation antigens such as HLA in man and H-2 in mice.

Membrane alloantigens may be limited to a single cell type, e.g., erythrocytes, or they may have wider distribution and be shared by a variety of cell types. Some of these specificities may be found in other animal species and even in microorganisms.

Relationship of Alloantigens to Species-Specific Antigens

This interesting and important relationship was recognized in studying allotypes, i.e., alloantigens of serum protein. Here, a clearly defined serum

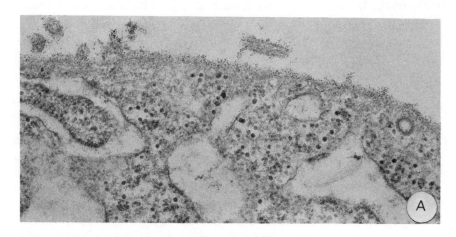

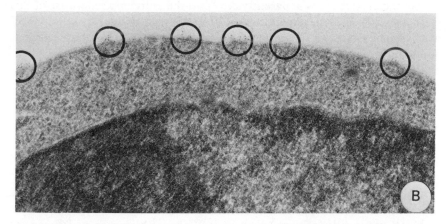

Fig. 2.1. (A) Uniform localization of ferritin-conjugated antibodies to rabbit IgG on HEp-2 cells sensitized with rabbit antiserum to human species antigens. (B) Patchy distribution of ferritin-conjugated antibodies to human IgG on human lymphocyte sensitized with human anti-HLA-A2 antibodies.

protein such as gamma globulin carries definite species specificity, and in addition, allotypic specificities, some of which are now defined in terms of amino acid sequences. There is good reason to believe that alloantigens of nucleated cells are also *riding* on molecules which carry definite species specificity. It has been shown (40) that alloantibodies to HLA antigens can be displaced from the cell surface by an excess of heteroimmune serum containing antibodies to human species-specific antigens. In contrast, displacement of species-specific antibodies by HLA antibodies could not be achieved. Very similar results were obtained from studies on alloantibodies to H-2 antigens and heteroantisera to murine species-specific antigens. These findings are completely consistent with the previously discussed thesis of multiplicity of species-specific antigens. Apparently, antigens of the HLA system are associated only with some species-specific molecules such as β_2-microglobulin. A similar situation prevails for H-2 alloantigens and murine species antigens. This trend of thought is further supported by electron microscopic studies that showed dense distribution of species-specific antigens and patchy distribution of alloantigens, such as HLA antigens (Fig. 2.1). Very strong evidence for association of cell-surface alloantigens with species antigens stemmed from studies on man-mouse hybrid cells. It was clearly shown (40) that in such hybrid cells, HLA antigens remained associated with human species-specific antigens and H-2 antigens remained associated with murine species-specific antigens and there was no *shuffling* of antigens.

Blood Group Antigens

The first alloantigens to be described on mammalian cells were the human blood group antigens present on erythrocytes. Studies of these antigens have been conducted for over 80 years, beginning with the discovery of the ABO blood group system by Landsteiner in 1900 (41). Since that time, more than 15 different blood group systems with over 160 specificities have been described in man (42).

It would be beyond the scope of the present review to go into any lengthy discussion of the enormous impact that studies of blood group antigens have had on medicine and biology. It appears, however, that stressing a few points is not out of place:

1. Blood transfusion became feasible only after the discovery of ABO blood groups and became safer when other human blood group systems, primarily the Rh system, became known (43,44).
2. Discovery of inheritance of ABO blood groups (45) initiated the most fruitful field of immunogenetics and provided the practical application of blood group examinations in cases of dubious parenthood.

3. The discovery of the different frequency of A and B antigens among various races, followed by similar studies for other alloantigens enriched anthropological research most remarkably (46).
4. Discovery of the role of Rh incompatibility in hemolytic disease of the newborn (47,48) gave impetus to investigations on immunological relations between the mother and her fetus.

Prophylactic measures against hemolytic disease of the newborn in the form of injection of anti-Rh antibodies constitute one of the most spectacular applications of immunology for human welfare (for references, see 49).

The most thoroughly characterized of the human blood groups is the ABO system. This system is composed of four phenotypes, O, A, B, and AB and six genotypes, *OO, AO, AA, BO, BB*, and *AB*. The two antigens of this system, A and B, are detectable by proper antisera. Blood group A and B antigens appear in two molecular forms, as alcohol-soluble glycolipids which are present on cell membranes and as water-soluble glycoproteins which are found in body fluids, such as saliva. Individuals in whom the water-soluble form is present are referred to as secretors. Secretion of the antigens is an inherited trait found in approximately 80% of human beings (50).

Biochemical studies have revealed that blood group A antigen is formed by addition of N-acetyl galactosamine to the erythrocyte surface by the enzyme α-N-acetyl-D-galactosaminyltransferase. Blood group B antigen is formed by the addition of galactose by the enzyme, α-D-galactosyltransferase. Presence of these enzymes, which actually determines the blood group, is coded for by the *A* and *B* alleles respectively. The *O* allele is silent (51, 52).

An important and peculiar feature of the ABO system is the regular occurrence of natural antibodies, anti-A and anti-B, whenever the corresponding antigen is absent.

Antigens of the ABO system have wider tissue distribution, being present not only on erythrocytes, but also on a variety of nucleated cells. The ubiquity of the antigens of the ABO system and the occurrence of natural antibodies explain the importance of the ABO system in the transplantion of organs and tissues in man.

As may be expected of polysaccharide moieties, the antigenic determinants of the ABO system are also found in other animals and even in microorganisms.

The Rh antigens, unlike those of the ABO system, are tissue restricted, being found only on erythrocytes. Several specificities are recognized in this system, the strongest and most important of which is the Rh_0 or D specificity. The presence of this specificity identifies the Rh-positive individual. This specificity is by far the most important for the feto-maternal conflict in which an Rh− mother responds with antibody formation to the erythrocytes of an Rh+ fetus. This can result in fetal abnormalities, stillbirth, and hemolytic disease of the newborn. Chemical studies of the Rh antigens have shown them to be of lipoprotein nature (53).

The Lewis blood group system is unique in that it is the only blood group system in man in which the antigens are found principally in body fluids and only secondarily on erythrocytes. The antigens, which are water-soluble glycoproteins with high carbohydrate content, are acquired by erythrocytes from the blood plasma (54, 55). A similar situation prevails in the blood groups of several other animals, most notable of which is the J blood group of cattle (56).

Antigens of the Major Histocompatibility System

Starting with the pioneering studies of Gorer on murine H-2 antigens (57), it became obvious that rejection of allografts is caused by an immune response to cell-surface alloantigens. These antigens became known as transplantation or histocompatibility antigens.

Many cell-surface alloantigens have been identified serologically and are frequently referred to as transplantation or histocompatibility antigens with insufficient evidence that the serologically detected alloantigens are identical to the targets of graft rejection.

In mice and other animals including man, evidence has been obtained for the existence of many histocompatibility genes. Those histocompatibility genes that encode antigens leading to the most rapid and violent graft rejection form the major histocompatibility complex (MHC).

In the 1960s and 1970s, a clear picture emerged for the existence of an MHC in each animal species thus far studied. The present discussion will be limited to man and mouse, the two species in which the most extensive knowledge of this complex has been gained. The subject of murine transplantation antigens including those encoded by genes of the MHC has been reviewed in numerous excellent monographs (for more recent reviews, see 58–63).

MHC of the Mouse. Studies in the mouse have identified over 45 different genetic loci that control cell-membrane alloantigens. The most important genes are those of the *H-2* complex (the murine MHC) which together with several other genes are located on the seventeenth chromosome. The H-2 complex consists of 4 regions (K, I, S, D). Other regions of interest on this chromosome for this discussion are Qa and T1a (Fig. 2.2).

All these regions, except S, control the expression of cell-surface glycoproteins. The S region contains genes that determine production of certain complement components. This region will not be considered further in this discussion.

Genes of the K and D regions of H-2 determine cell-surface structures that are potent alloantigens. These H-2 antigens are glycoproteins with a molecular weight of approximately 44,000. On the cell membrane they are believed to be linked noncovalently in a 1 to 1 ratio with β_2-microglobulin, a small protein weighing 11,600 daltons and bearing species specificity, but apparently no allospecificity. The 44,000 dalton moiety is about 90% protein and 10% carbohydrate. The allospecific determinants are on the protein portion of the molecule and the carbohydrate portion seems to be identical for all H-2 molecules. Three to 10 determinants or specificities may be found on the typical H-2 molecule. There are specificities that are unique for H-2K molecules and specificities that are unique for H-2D molecules. These specificities are termed private specificities. Each molecule also carries one or more specificities that are found on other H-2K and/or H-2D molecules. These are called public specificities (58). All these features account for the highly polymorphic nature of the H-2 system.

H-2 antigens are distributed widely and are present in virtually all cells. Highest concentrations are found in lymphoid tissue such as spleen and lymph node. In contrast, erythrocytes, skeletal muscle, and brain contain low concentrations. However, the amount of H-2 antigens on erythrocytes is sufficient to perform H-2 typing by hemagglutination tests.

Aside from functioning as serological markers, H-2 molecules are intimately involved in interactions among cells underlying a variety of immune phenomena. It is known that H-2 incompatibility between cells, even one limited to H-2K or H-2D molecules, gives rise to a mixed lymphocyte reaction (MLR). This reaction is believed to be an *in vitro* response of T lymphocytes to lymphocyte-activating determinants of allogeneic lymphocytes. Some investigators believe that H-2 molecules themselves act as stimulating molecules. Others believe that the lymphocyte-activating determinants may be encoded by genes termed *Lad* genes, closely linked to but distinct from H-2K or H-2D genes.

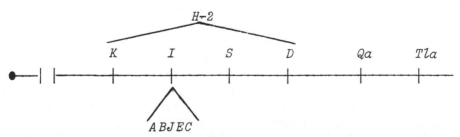

Fig. 2.2. Schematic representation of the H-2 complex on a portion of murine chromosome 17 (not drawn to scale).

Most investigators agree that H-2 molecules serve as targets of cytotoxic T lymphocytes both *in vivo* and *in vitro*. However, evidence suggests that the serological determinants on the H-2 molecule are not identical to the target structures for cytotoxic T cells.

In recent years, it has become apparent that H-2K and H-2D molecules play a significant role in the effector function of cytotoxic lymphocytes and that this function for various antigens is restricted by H-2 molecules (62). It was shown that lymphocytes of H-2^a mice sensitized to vaccinia virus would kill vaccinia virus-infected cells from an H-2^a mouse, but not vaccinia virus-infected cells from an H-2^b mouse. Apparently, the cytotoxic lymphocytes recognize the *primary* antigen, vaccinia virus, only in the proper H-2 context, i.e., the H-2 molecule restricts the activity of cytotoxic lymphocytes to the H-2 milieu in which the initial stimulation took place. These observations have been extended and it appears that mature cytotoxic lymphocytes recognize not only viral antigens, but also autoantigens, and tumor antigens only in the H-2 context in which the stimulating antigens are presented.

The I region of the H-2 complex is divided into five subregions, A, B, J, E, and C. Some of these subregions bear genes that control immune responses (Ir genes) to a variety of antigens. In addition, these subregions bear genes that determine cell-surface alloantigens, termed Ia antigens.

Unlike H-2 molecules, Ia antigens have restricted tissue distribution. B cells are the principal bearers of these antigens, in that about 90% of B cells carry Ia. These antigens are also present on up to 50% of macrophages. Originally, T cells were thought to be lacking in Ia. However, it has been recently demonstrated that a small population of T cells expresses low concentrations of these antigens. Ia antigens also have been detected on epidermal cells, sperm, and even certain tumors.

Ia molecules are glycoproteins consisting of two subunits, an α chain of 35,000 to 38,000 daltons and a β chain of 25,000 to 28,000 daltons. Unlike H-2 molecules, Ia antigens are not associated with β_2-microglobulin.

I region differences between donor and recipient can result in graft rejection, with subsequent appearance of strong anti-Ia antibodies. I region differences also give rise to strong MLR. The evidence suggests that Ia molecules, themselves, act as lymphocyte activating determinants, since MLR can be blocked by antibodies to Ia antigens of the stimulating cells. However, the possibility of steric hindrance has not been ruled out.

It appears that Ia antigens play a role in antigen-specific T cell-macrophage interactions, as well as T cell and B cell interactions. Ia molecules restrict the specific action of helper T cells in the same way as H-2 molecules restrict the specific action of cytotoxic lymphocytes.

Recent studies in inbred mice have suggested that Ia molecules of F1 hybrids may possess antigenic determinants, termed hybrid determinants, that are not demonstrable in either parent. It has been proposed that multiple hybrid determinants can arise by random assembly in the hybrid animal of the parental α and β chains. These hybrid determinants may be in part responsible for the multiplicity of structures that are involved in recognition and presentation of foreign antigens to the immune system (64).

MHC in Man. Knowledge of the human MHC, HLA, stemmed from the work of Dausset (65) and others on cell-surface alloantigens on human leukocytes. Review of the HLA system has been discussed recently in several monographs (63,66–69). Genes of the HLA system are on chromosome 6 and are found at four loci, A, B, C, and D (Fig. 2.3). Products of genes at the A, B, and C loci are usually detected serologically, but can also give rise to MLR. Determinants encoded by genes at the D locus are demonstrated by MLR. Similar to the H-2 system of mice, the HLA system is characterized by extensive polymorphism. There are 20 alleles known at the A locus, 31 at the B locus, 6 at the C locus, and 11 at the D locus. Recently, serologically detectable determinants, termed DR (D-related), have been ascribed to alleles in or very near the D locus. Thus far, 7 DR antigens have been described. It is not yet clear whether DR antigens are identical to the lymphocyte-activating determinants that evoke MLR and are encoded by D genes. The HLA-A and HLA-B loci are considered counterparts of the murine H-2K and H-2D loci. Their genes determine strong transplantation antigens which elicit production of cytotoxic antibodies. Antigens determined by genes of the C locus are apparently much less important than those determined by genes at the A and B loci and they will not be discussed further.

Antigens encoded by the A and B genes are found in practically all cells of the body. Lymphoid organs are particularly rich in HLA antigens. Lower concentrations are found in lung, liver, and kidney, and minute amounts are found in brain and muscle. HLA antigens are detectable also in soluble form or as very small particles in plasma and milk. Unlike H-2 antigens in mice, HLA antigens are not detectable on erythrocytes.

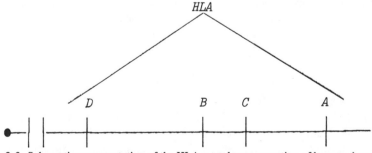

Fig. 2.3. Schematic representation of the HLA complex on a portion of human chromosome 6 (not drawn to scale).

Studies have shown that the biochemical nature of HLA antigens is similar to that of H-2 antigens. They consist of glycoprotein of approximately 44,000 daltons to which β_2-microglobulin of 11,600 daltons is attached noncovalently. The antigenic determinants reside in the polypeptide moiety of the glycoprotein. No biologic activity has been ascribed to the carbohydrate.

The alleles at the A and B loci that encode HLA antigens are inherited codominantly. The HLA genotype of an individual consists of two haplotypes. (A haplotype is a set of genes that occupy a given chromosome or its segment.) Each haplotype contains the loci that constitute the MHC. One haplotype is inherited from the father and the other from the mother. Somatic cells from an individual heterozygous at both A and B loci possess four HLA antigens, two controlled by A alleles and two controlled by B alleles. Individuals heterozygous at one locus and homozygous at the other locus have three HLA antigens and individuals homozygous at both loci possess two HLA antigens. Most of the specificities ascribed to the A and B antigens are analogous to the private specificities of the H-2 system. However, some cross-reacting specificities (or public specificities) which are shared by individuals having different private specificities have been described.

The importance of the HLA system in rejection of human allografts was first demonstrated by tracing the outcome of experimental skin grafts (66, 70). These studies showed that skin grafts from HLA-identical siblings survived significantly longer than grafts from HLA-non-identical siblings. This observation was further confirmed on extensive clinical material in which the outcome of renal graft has been most favorable when the donor was an HLA-identical sibling, less favorable when the graft originated from a parental or sibling donor with one identical HLA haplotype, and least favorable when it originated from a sibling differing from the recipient in two HLA haplotypes.

Serological tests for HLA identity, e.g., of family members, are performed by the lymphocytotoxicity procedure using a panel of sera that detect all known HLA specificities and are operationally monospecific, i.e., each serum detects only one HLA specificity. An example of such a determination is given in Table 2.3.

By inspection, one can determine that children I, II and IV possess paternal antigens A2 and B5 which were inherited together, and children III and V possess paternal antigens A10 and B14. So the paternal haplotypes are A2, B5 and A10, B14. Similarly, the maternal haplotypes are A1-B12 and A3-B7. The children can have only four genotypes. The genotypes of the children may be ac, ad, bc, and bd, if one designates the paternal haplotypes as a and b and the maternal haplotypes as c and d. Thus, the likelihood is 25% that two siblings will have identical genotypes for A and B, i.e., they will be HLA identical. In the example shown in the table, the best donor-recipient combination based on the serological tests would be children I and II.

In addition to serological tests for HLA-A and HLA-B antigens, identity of HLA-D determinants established by means of MLR is important for donor-recipient matching. Individuals whose lymphocytes give a negative MLR are HLA-D identical. In contrast, a positive MLR is given by lymphocytes of individuals with different HLA-D genes. The vast majority of siblings who are HLA-A and HLA-B identical are also HLA-D identical, but approximately 1% are not. Consequently, the best donor-recipient combination is one that is identical at all three loci, HLA-A, HLA-B, and HLA-D. Significantly, lymphocytes from individuals that are HLA-A and HLA-B identical but differ for HLA-D gives stronger MLR than lymphocytes from individuals who are HLA-D identical, but differ for HLA-A and HLA-B.

Recent studies have shown that HLA molecules, similar to H-2 molecules, can function as restricting factors. Products of the HLA-A, B, and C genes restrict activity of cytotoxic T cells and products of the HLA-D (DR) genes restrict activity of helper and amplifier T cells.

The Role of Cellular and Humoral Immunity in Transplantation

In the late 1950s and early 1960s, most investigators agreed that rejection of a solid tissue graft is accomplished by cell-mediated rather than humoral immunity. This was supported by the results of passive transfer experiments in which the hypersensitivity to the graft from a sensitized animal to a normal animal was successfully accomplished by transfer of lymphoid cells but not by antibody-containing serum (71–73). Allograft rejection is a violent necrotic reaction that is characterized by infiltration of the graft by mononuclear cells (lymphocytes and macrophages). Incompatibility at the MHC results in rejection in 6 to 9 days in an unprimed recipient (first set rejection). If the recipient is confronted with a second graft from the same or a related donor, the rejection is more rapid, occurring in 4 to 6 days (second-set rejection). If the donor and recipient differ in minor histocompatibility antigens, the first-set rejection may take several weeks or even several months. In spite of numerous experiments, the precise mechanism of rejection of a solid graft such as a skin graft never has been unraveled. It appears likely that cytotoxic lymphocytes generated upon confrontation of the recipient with the foreign tissues of the donor play the important role in graft rejection (74). The paramount role of antigens encoded by the MHC appears, however, proven beyond any doubt.

The subject of allograft rejection by humoral antibodies was revised in connection with studies on hyperacute rejection of renal grafts. This name was given by surgeons to a catastrophic rejection of a renal graft, which occurs within a few minutes or a few hours after establishing vascular

Table 2.3. Determination of HLA Haplotypes

	A locus				B locus			
	A1	A2	A3	A10	B5	B7	B12	B14
Father	−	+	−	+	+	−	−	+
Mother	+	−	+	−	−	+	+	−
Children:								
I	+	+	−	−	+	−	+	−
II	+	+	−	−	+	−	+	−
III	+	−	−	+	−	−	+	+
IV	−	+	+	−	+	+	−	−
V	−	−	+	+	−	+	−	+

anastomoses. Histologic hallmarks of this rejection are accumulation of polymorphonuclear neutrophils in glomerular and peritubular capillaries and, if the graft is left long enough *in situ*, renal cortical necrosis (75, 76). The hyperacute rejection of renal grafts could be related to the appearance of preformed humoral antibodies (76). This role of humoral antibodies was further substantiated by animal experiments (77).

The late deterioration of human renal grafts that occurs after several months or several years of satisfactory graft function constitutes now the major problem of clinical transplantation. In some instances, such late rejection is elicited by the recurrence of the original renal disease. In many other cases, however, there is a *de novo* process which accounts for the rejection. A possible role of humoral transplantation antibodies in the late deterioration of renal grafts has been considered (78).

Cell markers

As an outgrowth of serological analysis of antisera produced in a foreign species, e.g., antisera to thymocytes of lymphocytes used for studies on suppression of the immune response, several species-specific antigens showing restricted tissue distribution have been described, primarily on murine cells (59). These include the mouse-specific lymphocyte antigen (MSLA) (79) and the mouse bone-marrow-derived lymphocyte antigen (MBLA) (80). Mention should also be made of the H-Y antigen, which is present on spermatocytes, lymphoid, and skin cells of all male mice. H-Y is detectable by serological tests and plays a role in graft rejection (81).

In addition to tissue-restricted species-specific antigens, murine lymphoid cells bear a number of cell-surface antigenic markers that show allospecificity. The most thoroughly studied are the antigens of the Thy-1, TL, Ly, (Ly, Lyt, and Lyb), and Qa systems. These alloantigens are also known as differentiation antigens. They serve as markers for lymphocytes or subpopulations of lymphocytes and, in many cases, are associated with a particular developmental stage of the lymphocyte and thus with its function.

One of the first of these antigens to be described was the thymus-leukemia antigen (TL) shared by normal thymocytes and leukemia cells (82, 83). Subsequent studies showed that TL antigens are thymus-restricted alloantigens, being present on normal thymocytes of several, but not all strains of mice. Five specificities (59), TL.1 to TL.5, encoded by alleles at the T1a complex, have been described. TL antigens also appear on murine leukemia cells as tumor antigens and this characteristic will be discussed below.

Recent work has shown an interesting relationship between TL antigens and the H-2 antigens, H-2K and H-2D. All three molecules are linked noncovalently to β_2-microglobulin (84). There also appears to be a close structural relationship between TL and H-2D antigens. TL− thymocytes have a much higher concentration of H-2D antigens than do TL+ cells (85). During antigenic modulation (see below), the concentration of TL antigen on the surface decreases, the concentration of H-2D increases, and the amount of H-2K remains constant (86). Also, when T cells leave the thymus, TL antigen is lost and the amount of H-2D increases on the cell surface (87).

Thy-1 antigens, discovered in 1964 and originally termed θ (88), were the first markers described for peripheral lymphocytes in mice. Subsequently, these markers were crucial in studies that served to identify T cells and B cells as the two major populations of lymphocytes (89). The Thy-1 system in mice consists of two specificities, Thy-1.1 and Thy-1.2 encoded by alleles at the Thy-1 locus, which is on chromosome 9. Thy-1 antigens are present on thymocytes and peripheral T cells. Distribution of Thy-1 is not completely restricted to T cells, since they are also found in brain tissue as well as epithelial cells (90) and fibroblasts (91). Nevertheless, Thy-1 antigens have served as most useful T cell markers. Anti-Thy-1 sera are frequently used to remove T cells from a mixed population of cells. Interestingly, in the differentiation of T cells from immature thymocytes to mature thymocytes, the concentration of Thy-1 antigens decreases.

Thy-1 antigens have also been described in the rat (92, 93). Rat Thy-1 antigen bears two determinants, one specific for rat and a second that cross-reacts with murine Thy-1 (59). Rat Thy-1 is not considered a T cell marker since it is also present on some B cells.

Recently, a Thy-1-like antigen has been described in man. The antigen was present in lymphoid organs such as thymus, spleen, and lymph nodes. Curiously, it was not detectable on dispersed cells of lymphoid organs including the thymus. The evidence suggests that human Thy-1 is a marker for early or immature T cells (94).

Discovery of the TL and Thy-1 antigens stimulated the search for other lymphocyte markers, a search which led to the identification of the Ly group of alloantigens (95). Originally termed LyA and LyB, these were the first known antigenic markers that were truly lymphocyte specific. Several Ly antigens have now been described. They are termed Ly if they appear on both T and B cells, Lyt if they appear predominantly or exclusively on T cells, and Lyb if they appear primarily on B cells. The Ly antigens have been useful not only in identifying T and B cells, but also in identifying subpopulations of T cells. For example, Lyt-1 is found on 30 to 35% of peripheral T cells. These T cells, known as helper cells, augment the activity of other lymphoid cells such as B cells, killer T cells, and macrophages. Lyt-2,3 is present in 10% of peripheral T cells, a population that includes suppressor T cells and killer T cells that are directed against allogeneic determinants. Lyt-1,2,3 T cells are believed to be the precursors of Lyt-1 and Lyt-2,3 T cells (59).

In addition to TL, Thy-1, and Ly, a number of other antigenic cell markers have been described on murine cells. These include the Qa antigens of T cells; A1C, which is found on activated T and B cells; and Mph, which is present on macrophages. Qa antigens, notably Qa-1, can distinguish subsets within the Lyt-1 population and Lyt-1,2,3 population of T cells (59). There are also several antigens, termed Ea, that appear predominantly on erythrocytes (58).

In man, Ly-like specificities, i.e., lymphocyte differentiation antigens, have been recently identified. Similar to the mouse, some of these specificities are shared by T and B cells (96) and others are restricted to T cells (97) or B cells (98). Subpopulations of T cells can also be identified (99).

Mention should be made of several other cell-surface components that are not part of this discussion, but that serve, nevertheless, as cell markers. These include Fc receptors, complement receptors, receptors for sheep erythrocytes, membrane-bound immunoglobulins, and enzymes such as terminal deoxynucleotidyl transferase (100).

TUMOR ANTIGENS

The search for antigens that would aid in the diagnosis and therapy of malignancy has been long and arduous. Today's promise too often has transpired into tomorrow's disappointment. Yet, effort has not been totally fruitless. Most information concerning tumor antigens has been gained from studies of experimental animals, particularly the mouse, a species in which inbred animals are readily available. This discussion will focus on the tumor antigens of this species and of man.

Malignancy oftentimes is accompanied by antigenic alteration. The alteration may be quantitative, whereby a given normal antigen may decrease in concentration or become deleted altogether, e.g., blood group specificities in certain tumors (101, 102). Conversely, normal antigens may increase in tumors, e.g., carcinoembryonic antigen (CEA) (103). Antigens of the latter type are known as tumor-associated antigens (TAA). Antigenic alteration also may be qualitative, as seen by the appearance of new antigens that are foreign to the host. These should be termed tumor-specific antigens (TSA). TSA may arise as intracellular structures in the cytoplasm or nucleus. Alternatively, TSA may be present as new cell-surface structures, and because of this location they may make the cells vulnerable to the effects of the immune system.

Convincing evidence for the existence of TSA began accumulating almost 40 years ago when Gross reported that mice immunized with a syngeneic tumor that had been induced with the chemical carcinogen, methylcholanthrene, were resistant to subsequent inoculation of the same tumor (104). Later studies showed that (a) mice treated in such a manner were not resistant to another syngeneic tumor (105), (b) mice immunized and subsequently resistant to a syngeneic methylcholanthrene-induced tumor would readily accept a syngeneic skin graft (106), and (c) tumor resistance could be induced with an autochthonous tumor (107).

The tumor antigens involved in the above described results were detected by transplantation experiments and have been termed tumor-specific transplantation antigens (TSTA). Subsequently, TSTA were demonstrated on carcinomas and hepatomas induced in several experimental animals, including mice, rats, and guinea pigs, by a variety of chemical and physical agents such as polycyclic hydrocarbons, plastic films, and ultraviolet irradiation (108).

A striking feature concerning TSTA induced by chemical or physical agents is the individual specificity exhibited by them. For example, two distinct tumors, A and B, induced by the same chemical carcinogen and even induced in the same animal, possess TSTA that are unique for each tumor. Syngeneic animals immunized with A are resistant to A, but not to B, and those immunized with B are resistant to B, but not to A (108, 109).

In 1961, resistance to virus-induced tumors was shown by Sjøgren and his co-workers (110) and by Habel (111). They reported that animals immunized with a tumor induced by polyoma virus (a DNA virus) were resistant to this tumor. Subsequently, resistance was demonstrated to tumors induced with other DNA viruses such as SV_{40} and Shope papilloma, and by oncogenic RNA virus including the mammary tumor virus (MTV) and the murine leukemia viruses (MuLV).

Resistance to virus-induced tumors is virus specific. Immunization with a tumor induced by one virus, e.g., polyoma virus, elicits resistance to polyoma virus-induced tumors, even if the tumor arises in a different species, but it does not elicit resistance to tumors induced by other viruses. Immunological studies on tumors induced in experimental animals by various chemical agents and viruses have been reviewed extensively in several monographs (108, 112–115).

In addition to the TSTA discussed above, which are detected by rejection of tumors, TSA have been demonstrated on the cell surface by serological procedures. For example, the individual specificity of chemically-induced tumors has been shown by serological tests (116). However, it is not clear whether these antigens are the same as the TSTA. The relationship of TSTA to TSA that are detectable serologically is frequently obscure, consequently, we propose to call the latter antigens tumor-specific cell-surface antigens (TSCSA) without prejudicing their role in tumor graft rejection.

In addition to determinants that are unique for individual tumors, chemically-induced tumors also possess determinants that are shared by a variety of tumors, including those induced by different carcinogens. Many of these cross-reacting antigens are also detectable on fetal tissues (see below).

Serological analysis of tumor antigens has been most rewarding in studies on virus-induced tumors. The cell surface of tumors induced by DNA viruses contains TSCSA which does not act as TSTA (114). Still, these TSCSA are virus specific, i.e., they are absent from normal cells and from tumors induced by unrelated viruses. Evidence suggests that TSCSA of DNA-virus-induced tumors may be distinct from TSTA. Tumors bearing TSCSA but lacking TSTA have been described (117). TSCSA can also be exposed by treatment of normal cells with trypsin, making it conceivable that some TSCSA are normal cell structures that are revealed by viral transformation (118).

Serological studies of RNA-virus-induced tumors have shown that the tumor cell surface bears TSCSA, which are related to but are not part of the virion, as well as viral envelope antigens (VEA).

Infection by virtually all MuLV gives rise to the virus-specific TSCSA. In addition, there are TSCSA that are shared by MuLV-induced leukemia cells. For example, there are TSCSA that are characteristic for leukemia cells induced by the Friend virus, TSCSA characteristic for leukemia cells induced by the Maloney virus, and TSCSA that are shared by leukemia cells induced by these viruses. Similar to TSCSA, some VEA of MuLV-induced tumor cells may be virus specific, whereas others may be shared by several viruses. Immunoelectron microscopy studies have shown that TSCSA are distinct from VEA on the leukemia cell surface (119, 113). Tumor resistance demonstrable in transplantation tests is believed to be due to VEA.

Both chemically-induced and virus-induced tumors possess TSCSA that are present in fetal tissue. Such antigens that are shared by tumor and fetal tissues are known as oncofetal antigens. These antigens are absent from or are in extremely low concentration in normal adult tissue. The appearance of oncofetal antigens in tumor tissue is believed to result from derepression of proper genes. Oncofetal antigens expressed in chemically-induced tumors as well as in DNA-and RNA-virus-induced tumors are frequently widely distributed in tumors within these three groups. Whether these oncofetal TSCSA can induce tumor resistance is not clear; much evidence suggests that they elicit weak protection, if any (120).

Of particular interest is a group of TSA that may also occur as normal alloantigens. The classic example of this group is the TL antigens discussed previously. TL antigens were demonstrated by immunization of C57BL/6 mice with a spontaneous leukemia of strain A mice. The antiserum was cytotoxic for the strain A leukemia cells and several leukemias of C57BL/6 origin, but it did not react with normal C57BL/6 tissue. Subsequent studies showed that TL antigens are present on normal thymocytes of some murine strains (TL+) and absent from those of other strains (TL−). TL antigens may also appear on leukemia cells of TL+ mice, and significantly, on leukemia cells of TL− mice. Thus, in TL− strains, the TL antigen is a TSA (83).

Expression of TL antigens on TL+ leukemia cells can be suppressed, i.e., TL+ cells become TL−, when the leukemia cells are grown in the presence of anti-TL antibodies. TL antigen expression is restored by growth of the tumor cells in the absence of anti-TL antibodies. This phenomenon is know as antigenic modulation (121). Significantly, antigenic modulation has been observed with other antigens and is not unique for TL (122, 123).

Since these observations, other examples of normal alloantigens appearing . as TSA have been noted. These include the G_{ix} antigen (124, 83) and the X.1 antigen (125, 83). The G_{ix} antigen is a tissue-restricted antigen present only on thymocytes and spermatocytes of some ($G_{ix}+$) but not of other strains of mice ($G_{ix}-$). Similar to TL antigens, the G_{ix} antigen may be present on leukemia cells of both $G_{ix}+$ and $G_{ix}-$ mice. Interestingly, in mice infected with MuLV-Gross, G_{ix} is present in all lymphoid tissues. Significantly, the G_{ix} antigen is very similar to or identical with the glycoprotein gp 70 that is a major structural compenent of MuLV.

Of particular interest is the recent observation by a number of workers that tumor cells may bear H-2-like specificities that are absent from normal cells of the tumor-bearing animal (126, 127). For example, it has been shown that immunization of mice with normal tissues from an H-2 incompatible strain rendered the mice resistant to a syngeneic tumor. These observations have led to the suggestion that somatic cells of mice bear structural genes for all H-2 specificities, and that expression of a particular specificity is encoded by regulatory genes (128). A similar concept has been suggested for TL antigens (83).

TSA in human malignancies have been sought since the early days of immunology. Progress has been slow, in large measure because of the genetic heterogeneity of man. In recent years several TAA have been described and some of them have proven to be useful in the diagnosis and management of malignant diseases. These include hormones such as human chorionic gonadotropin, which can be an ectopic secretion of certain tumors and is useful in the diagnosis of those malignancies, as well as enzymes such as alkaline phosphatase.

Considerable interest has been focused recently on a group of TAA that are classed as oncofetal antigens (for reviews see 120, 129, 130). These include α-fetoprotein (131), associated with primary hepatoma, pancreatic oncofetal antigen (132), which appears to be associated with pancreatic malignancy, and CEA. This discussion will be limited to the last-mentioned antigen.

CEA was originally described as an antigen present in adenocarcinomas of the intestinal tract and in embryonic tissue of man, but absent from normal adult tissue (for reviews see 130, 133–135). Later studies showed that CEA is also found in nonintestinal malignancies (136), nonmalignant pathologic tissue, and even at very low concentrations in normal adult tissues (137,138). Thus it should be considered a TAA.

CEA is a glycoprotein of the cell-surface glycocalyx and is aproximately 50% carbohydrate. The molecule has the electrophoretic mobility of a β globulin and weighs approximately 200,000 daltons. CEA is extractable from tissue by perchloric acid or even physiologic saline solution. The antigen was originally detected by precipitation tests in agar gel using absorbed rabbit antisera, but is presently most often studied by radioimmunoassay and by enzyme immunoassay. It is detectable in patient's serum in nanogram quantities.

Patients with a variety of malignancies and patients with noncancerous conditions such as chronic lung disease, pancreatitis, and cirrhosis of the liver often have elevated serum levels of CEA. Above normal levels are also seen in a significant percentage of healthy individuals, the majority of whom are heavy smokers.

Most investigators agree that tests for CEA should not be used for screening purposes, or to confirm the diagnosis of malignancy. However, CEA tests are useful in the prognosis of cancer and in monitoring the effectiveness of cancer therapy (130).

Many claims of TSCSA and TAA on human tumors have been reported over the years, but convincing evidence has been provided for very few. Promising results have been obtained in studies on some malignant diseases (139) including malignant melanoma (140), osteogenic sarcoma (140), bladder carcinoma (141), and Burkitt's lymphoma (142).

In Burkitt's lymphoma, which is associated with Epstein-Barr virus infection, the lymphoma cells bear surface antigens related to the virus and a cytoplasmic antigen that is a virus-related nonvirion antigen known as early antigen (EA). Antibodies in patients' sera to the surface antigens (143) and to EA (144) are useful in the diagnosis and prognosis of the disease (142).

Finally, TAA have been identified for leukemic cells from patients with acute lymphocytic leukemia (ALL). These antigens are useful in distinguishing T-cell ALL from non-T-cell ALL; a distinction that is important for therapy. Recently developed monoclonal antibodies to these antigens have provided better diagnostic reagents and may be promising for use in serotherapy (145, 146).

SUMMARY

Mammalian cells bear numerous cell-surface determinants that are detectable by immunological techniques. The presence of many of these, such as the species antigens and the blood group antigens, have been known for several decades, yet their precise biological role is still not clear. Most investigators agree that the species-specific determinants are important in maintaining the integrity of the species; that the tissue-specific determinants are a consequence of cell differentiation and are related to specialized cell function; and that alloantigens reflect the uniqueness of the individual and play a significant role in the preservation of self.

Recent identification of cell markers on lymphoid cells has permitted better understanding of the immunological functions of various subpopulations of these cells. This, in turn, has allowed the demonstration that certain histocompatibility antigens of the MHC are important in cell-cell interactions in the immune system.

One can anticipate that the biological function of other cell-surface determinants, including those on cells of solid organs will be clarified in the next few years.

REFERENCES

1. Fisch, C., *St. Louis Courier of Medicine* **22**:90, 1900.
2. Wasserman, A., and Schütze, A., *Berl. klin. Wschr.* **38**:187, 1901.
3. Nuttall, G. H. F., *Blood immunity and blood relationship*. Cambridge: University Press, England, 1904.
4. Rose, N. R., and Witebsky, E., *J. Immunol.* **75**:282, 1955.
5. Forssman, J., *Handbuch der pathogenen Mikroorganismen* 3/1:469, 1930.
6. Uhlenhuth, P., Zur Lehre von der Unterscheidung verschiedener Eiweissarten mit Hilfe spezifischer Sera. In *Festschrift zum Sechzigsten Geburtstage von Robert Koch*, p. 49. Jena: Fischer, 1930.
7. Hektoen, L., and Schulhof, K., *Proc. Natl. Acad. Sci. USA* **11**:481, 1925.

8. Kies, M. W., and Alvord, E. C., Jr., Encephalitogenic activity in guinea pigs of water-soluble protein fractions of nervous tissues. In M. W. Kies, and E. C. Alvord, Jr. (Eds.), *Allergic encephalomyelitis*, p. 293. Springfield: Charles C. Thomas, 1959.
9. Coombs, R. R. A., and Franks, D., *Prog. Allergy* 13:174, 1969.
10. Fagraeus, A., and Espmark, A., *Nature* 190:370, 1961.
11. Milgrom, F., Kano, K., Barron, A. L., et al., *J. Immunol.* 92:8, 1964.
12. Kano, K., Knowles, B. B., Koprowski, H., et al., *Eur. J. Immunol.* 2:198, 1972.
13. Chan, M. M., Kano, K., Dorman, B., et al., *Immunogenetics* 8:265, 1979.
14. Siddiqui, B., and Hakomori, S., *J. Biol. Chem.* 246:5766, 1971.
15. Hakomori, S., Wang, S. -M., and Young, W. W., Jr., *Proc. Natl. Acad. Sci. USA* 74:3023, 1977.
16. Hawes, M. D., and Coombs, R. R. A., *J. Immunol.* 84:586, 1960.
17. Doerr, R., and Pick, R., *Ztschr. f. Immunitätsforsch. u. exper. Therap.* 19:251, 1913.
18. Paul, J. R., and Bunnell, W. W., *Am. J. Med. Sci.* 183:90, 1932.
19. Fletcher, M. A., and Woolfolk, B. J., *J. Immunol.* 107:842, 1971.
20. Merrick, J. M., Schifferle, R., Zadarlik, K., et al., *J. Supramol. Struct.* 6:275, 1977.
21. Davidsohn, I., *Am. J. Clin. Path.* 8:56, 1938.
22. Henle, G., Henle, W., and Diehl, V., *Proc. Natl. Acad. Sci. USA* 59:94, 1968.
23. Milgrom, F., *Transfusion* 4:407, 1964.
24. Andres, G. A., Kano, K., Elwood, C., et al., *Int. Arch. Allergy Appl. Immunol.* 52:136, 1976.
25. Milgrom, F., Kano, K., and Fjelde, A., *Int. Arch. Allergy Appl. Immunol.* 45:631, 1973.
26. Nishimaki, T., Kano, K., and Milgrom, F. *Int. Arch. Allergy Appl. Immunol.* 60:115, 1979.
27. Masaki, M., Kano, K., Merrick, J. M., et al., *Int. Arch. Allergy Appl. Immunol.* 65:313, 1981.
28. Hanganutziu, M., *C.R. Soc. Biol.* (Paris) 91:1457, 1924.
29. Deicher, H., *Z. Hyg. Infekt-Kr.* 106:561, 1926.
30. Kasukawa, R., Kano, K., Bloom, M. L., et al., *Clin. Exp. Immunol.* 25:122, 1976.
31. Merrick, J. M., Zadarlik, K., and Milgrom, F., *Int. Arch. Allergy Appl. Immunol.* 57:477, 1978.
32. Nowak, J. A., Jain, N. K., and Merrick, J. M., Abstr. Annual Meeting Soc. Complex Carbohydrates. 1982.
33. Nishimaki, T., Kano, K., and Milgrom, F., *J. Immunol.* 122:2314, 1979.
34. Rapaport, F. T., Kano, K., and Milgrom, F., *Lancet* 2:1131, 1966.
35. Iwasaki, Y., Talmage, D., and Starzl, T. E., *Transplantation* 5:191, 1967.
36. Rapaport, F. T., Heterologous antigens and antibodies in transplantation. In F. T. Rapaport and J. Dausset (Eds.), *Human transplantation*, p. 635. New York: Grune and Stratton, 1968.
37. McDonald, J. C., *Transplantation* 15:116, 1973.
38. McDonald, J. C., *Transplantation* 15:123, 1973.
39. Kano, K., Loza, U., Gerbasi, J. R., et al., *Transplantation* 19:20, 1975.
40. Kano, K., Andres, G. A., Hsu, K. C., et al., *Int. Arch. Allergy Appl. Immunol.* 43:608, 1972.
41. Landsteiner, K., *Zbl. Bakt.* 27:357, 1900.
42. Race, R. R., and Sanger, R., *Blood groups in man.* 6th ed. Oxford: Blackwell Scientific, 1975.
43. Levine, P., and Stetson, R. E., *J. Am. Med. Assoc.* 113:126, 1939.
44. Landsteiner, K., and Wiener, A. S., *Proc. Soc. Exp. Biol. Med.* 43:223, 1940.
45. von Dungern, E., and Hirszfeld, L., *Z. für Immunitätsforsch. und exper. Therapie* 4:531, 1910.

46. Hirszfeld, L., and Hirschfeld, H., *Lancet* **2**:675, 1919.
47. Levine, P., Katzin, E. M., and Burnham, L., *J. Am. Med. Assoc.* **116**:825, 1941.
48. Levine, P., Vogel., P., Katzin, E. M., et al., *Science* **94**:371, 1941.
49. Pollack, W., Gorman, J. G., and Freda, V. J., Prevention of Rh hemolytic disease. In E. Brown and C. V. Moore (Eds.), *Progress in Hematology*, Vol. 6, p. 121. London: Heinemann Medical Books, 1969.
50. Schiff, F., and Sasaki, H., *Klin. Woch.* **11**:1426, 1932.
51. Morgan, W. T. J., *Proc. Roy. Soc., B.* **151**:308, 1960.
52. Watkins, W. M., *Science* **152**:172, 1966.
53. Lorusso, D. J., and Green, F. A., *Science* **188**:66, 1975.
54. Grubb, R., *Acta Path. Microbiol. Scand.* **28**:61, 1951.
55. Ceppellini, R., *Proc. 5th Congr. Int. Soc. Blood Transf.*, p. 207. Paris, 1955.
56. Stormont, C., *Proc. Natl. Acad. Sci. USA* **35**:232, 1949.
57. Gorer, P. A., *J. Path Bact.* **44**:691, 1937.
58. Klein, J., *Biology of the mouse histocompatibility-2 complex.* New York: Springer-Verlag, 1975.
59. McKenzie, I. F. C., and Potter, T., *Adv. Immunol.* **27**:179, 1979.
60. Vitetta, E. A., and Capra, J. D., *Adv. Immunol.* **26**:147, 1978.
61. Forman, J., Antigens and the major histocompatibility complex. In S. Sell (Ed.), *Cancer Markers*, p. 133. Clifton, NJ: Humana Press, 1980.
62. Zinkernagel, R. M., and Doherty, P. C., *Adv. Immunol.* **27**:51, 1979.
63. Zaleski, M., Abeyounis, C. J., and Kano, K. (Eds.), *Immunobiology of the major histocompatibility complex. 7th International Convocation on Immunology*, Basel: S. Karger, 1981.
64. David, C. S., and Lafuse, W. P., Hybrid Ia antigens: identification, characterization and role in immune response. In M. Zaleski, C. J. Abeyounis, and K. Kano (Eds.), *Immunobiology of the major histocompatibility complex. 7th International Convocation on Immunology*, p. 28. Basel: S. Karger, 1981.
65. Dausset, J., *Acta Haematol.* **120**:156, 1958.
66. Amos, D. B., Hattler, G., MacQueen, J. M., et al., An interpretation and application of cytotoxicity typing. In J. Dausset, J. Hamburger, and G. Mathe (Eds.), *Advances in transplantation*, p. 203. Copenhagen: Munksgaard, 1967.
67. Cepellini, R., and van Rood, J. J., *Semin. Haematol.* **11**:233, 1974.
68. Snell, G. D., Dausset, J., and Nathenson, S., *Histocompatibility.* New York: Academic Press, 1976.
69. Bodmer, W. F., *Br. Med. Bull.* **34**:213, 1978.
70. Ceppellini, R., The genetic basis of transplantation. In F. T. Rapaport and J. Dausset (Eds.), *Human transplantation*, p. 21. New York: Grune and Stratton, 1968.
71. Medawar, P. B., *Harvey Lect.* **52**:144, 1958.
72. Hasek, M., Lengerova, A., and Hraba, T., *Adv. Immunol.* **1**:1, 1961.
73. Stetson, C. A., *Adv. Immunol.* **3**:97, 1963.
74. Berke, G., *Prog. Allergy* **27**:69, 1980.
75. Williams, G. M., Hume, D. M., Kano, K., et al., *JAMA* **204**:119, 1968.
76. Williams, G. M., Hume, D. M., Hudson, R. P., Jr., et al., *New Engl. J. Med.* **279**:611, 1968.
77. Klassen, J., and Milgrom, F., *Transplantation* **8**:566, 1969.
78. Milgrom, F., *Transpl. Proc.* **12**:557, 1980.
79. Shigeno, N., Arpels, C., Hämmerling, U., et al., *Lancet* **2**:320, 1968.
80. Raff, M. C., Nase, S., and Mitchison, N. A., *Nature* **230**:50, 1971.
81. Wachtel, S. S., *Immunol. Rev.* **33**:33, 1977.
82. Old, L. J., Boyse, E. A., and Stockert, E., *J. Natl. Cancer Inst.* **31**:977, 1963.

83. Old, L. J., and Stockert, E., *Ann. Rev. Genet.* **17**:127, 1977.
84. Ostberg, L., Rask, L., Wigzell, H., et al., *Nature* **253**, 735, 1975.
85. Boyse, E. A., Stockert, E., and Old, L. J., *J. Exp. Med.* **128**:85, 1968.
86. Old, L. J., Stockert, E., Boyse, E. A., et al., *J. Exp. Med.* **127**:523, 1968.
87. Mathieson, B. J., Sharrow, S. O., Campbell, P. S., et al., *Nature* **277**:478, 1979.
88. Reif, A. E., and Allen, J. M. V., *J. Exp. Med.* **120**:413, 1964.
89. Raff, M. C., *Transpl. Rev.* **6**:52, 1971.
90. Scheid, M., Boyse, E. A., Carswell, E. A., et al., *J. Exp. Med.* **135**:938, 1972.
91. Stern, P. L., *Nature (London) New Biol.* **246**:76, 1973.
92. Douglas, T. C., *J. Exp. Med.* **136**:1054, 1972.
93. Michael, B., Pasternak, G., and Steuden, J., *Nature (London) New Biol.* **241**:222, 1973.
94. McKenzie, J. L., and Fabre, J. W., *J. Immunol.* **126**:843, 1981.
95. Boyse, E. A., Meijazawa, M., Aoki, T., et al., *Proc. Roy. Soc. Biol.* (Ser. B) **170**:175, 1968.
96. Pizzolo, G., Sloane, J., Beverley, P., et al., *Cancer* **46**:2640, 1980.
97. Martin, P. J., Hansen, J. A., Nowinski, R. C., et al., *Immunogenetics* **11**:429, 1980.
98. Stashenko, P., Nadler, L. M., Hardy, R., et al., *J. Immunol.* **125**:1678, 1980.
99. Reinherz, E. L., Kung, P. C., Goldstein, G., et al., *Proc. Natl. Acad. Sci. USA* **76**:4061, 1979.
100. Leventhal, B. G., Civin, C. I., and Reaman, G., Markers in human lymphoid tumors. In S. Sell (Ed.), *Cancer markers*, p. 89. Clifton, NJ: Humana Press, 1980.
101. Davidsohn, I., Kovarik, S., and Ni, L. Y., *Arch. Pathol.* **84**:306, 1969.
102. Yogeeswaran, G., Surface glycolipid and glycoprotein antigens. In S. Sell (Ed.), *Cancer markers*, p. 371. Clifton, NJ: Humana Press, 1980.
103. Gold, P., and Freedman, S. O., *J. Exp. Med.* **121**:439, 1965.
104. Gross, L., *Cancer Res.* **3**:326, 1943.
105. Foley, E. J., *Cancer Res.* **13**:835, 1953.
106. Prehn, R. T., and Main, J. M., *J. Natl. Cancer Inst.* **18**:769, 1957.
107. Klein, G., Sjögren, H. O., Klein, E., et al., *Cancer Res.* **20**:1561, 1960.
108. Klein, G., *Ann. Rev. Microbiol.* **20**:223, 1966.
109. Globerson, A., and Feldman, M., *J. Natl. Cancer Inst.* **32**:1229, 1964.
110. Sjögren, H. O., Hellström, I., and Klein, G., *Cancer Res.* **21**:329, 1961.
111. Habel, K., *Proc. Soc. Exp. Biol. Med.* **106**:722, 1961.
112. Baldwin, R. W., *Adv. Cancer Res.* **18**:1, 1973.
113. Old, L. J., and Boyse, E. A., *Harvey Lect.* **67**:273, 1973.
114. Tevethia, S., and Tevethia, M. J.: DNA virus (SV40) induced antigens. In F. F. Becker (Ed.), *Comprehensive treatise.* Vol. 4. *Biology of tumors: surfaces, immunology and comparative pathology*, p. 185. New York: Plenum Press, 1979.
115. Aoki, T., and Sibal, L. R., RNA oncogenic virus-associated antigens and host immune response to them. In F. F. Becker (Ed.), *Cancer. Comprehensive treatise.* Vol. 4. *Biology of tumors: surfaces, immunology and comparative pathology*, p. 159. New York: Plenum Press, 1979.
116. Baldwin, R. W., and Moore, M., Tumour-specific antigens and tumour-host interactions. In N. W. Nisbet and M. W. Elves (Eds.), *Immunological tolerance to tissue antigens*, p. 299. Oswestry, England: Orthopaedic Hospital, 1971.
117. Tevethia, S. S., Diamandopoulos, G. T., Rapp, F., et al., *J. Immunol.* **101**:1192, 1968.
118. Hayry, P., and Defendi, V., *Virology* **41**:22, 1970.
119. Aoki, T., Boyse, E. A., Old, L. J., et al., *Proc. Natl. Acad. Sci. USA* **65**:569, 1970.
120. Chism, S. E., Oncofetal transplantation antigens. In. S. Sell (Ed.), *Cancer markers*, p. 115. Clifton, NJ: Humana Press, 1980.

121. Boyse, E. A., Old, L. J., and Luell, S., *J. Natl. Cancer Inst.* **31**:987, 1963.
122. Joseph, B. S., and Oldstone, M. B. A., *J. Exp. Med.* **142**:864, 1975.
123. Ritz, J., Pesando, J. M., Notis-McConarty, J., et al., *J. Immunol.* **125**:1506, 1980.
124. Stockert, E., Old, L. J., and Boyse, E. A., *J. Exp. Med.* **133**:1334, 1971.
125. Sato, H., Boyse, E. A., Aoki, T., et al., *J. Exp. Med.* **138**:593, 1973.
126. Parmiani, G., and Invernizzi, G., *Int. J. Cancer* **16**:756, 1975.
127. Garrido, F., Schirrmacher, V., and Festenstein, H., *J. Immunogenet.* **4**:15, 1977.
128. Festenstein, H., The role of histocompatibility antigens in the development and growth of tumors. In M. Zaleski, C. J. Abeyounis, and K. Kano (Eds.), *Immunobiology of the major histocompatibililty complex. 7th International Convocation on Immunology*, p. 338. Basel: S. Karger, 1981.
129. Baldwin, R. W., Embleton, M. J., Price, M. R., et al., *Transpl. Rev.* **20**:77, 1974.
130. Terry, W. D., Henkart, P. A., Coligan, J. E., et al., *Transpl. Rev.* **20**:100, 1974.
131. Sell, S., Alphafetoprotein. In S. Sell (Ed.), *Cancer markers*, p. 249. Clifton, NJ: Humana Press, 1980.
132. Banwo, O., Versey, T., and Hobbs, J. R., *Lancet* **1**:643, 1974.
133. Fuks, A., Banjo, C., Shuster, J., et al., *Biochem. Biophys. Acta* **417**:123, 1974.
134. Shively, J. E., and Todd, C. W., Carcinoembryonic antigen A: chemistry and biology. In S. Sell (Ed.), *Cancer markers*, p. 295. Clifton, NJ: Humana Press, 1980.
135. Fuks, A., Shuster, J., and Gold, P., Theoretical and practical consideration of the utility of the radioimmunoassay for carcinoembryonic antigen (CEA) in clinical medicine. In S. Sell (Ed.), *Cancer markers*, p. 315. Clifton, NJ: Humana Press, 1980.
136. Lo Gerfo, P., Krupey, J., and Hansen, H. J., *New Engl. J. Med.* **285**:138, 1971.
137. Martin, F., and Martin, M. S., *Int. J. Cancer* **6**:352, 1970.
138. Abeyounis, C. J., and Milgrom, F., *Int. Arch. Allergy Appl. Immunol.* **43**:30, 1972.
139. Gold, D. U., and Goldenberg, D. M., Antigens associated with human solid tumors. In S. Sell (Ed.), *Cancer markers*, p. 329. Clifton, NJ: Humana Press, 1980.
140. Morton, D. L., Eilber, F. R., and Malmgren, R. A., *Prog. Exp. Tumor Res.* **14**:25, 1971.
141. Bubenik, J., Perlmann, P., Helmstein, K., et al., *Int. J. Cancer* **5**:310, 1970.
142. Klein, G., *Adv. Immunol.* **14**:187, 1971.
143. Kleink, G., Clifford, P., Klein, E., et al., *Proc. Natl. Acad. Sci. USA* **55**:1628, 1966.
144. Henle, W., Henle, G., Zajac, B. A., et al., *Science* **169**:188, 1970.
145. Ritz, J., Pesando, J. M., Notis-McConarty, J., et al., *Nature* **283**, 583, 1980.
146. Ritz, J., Pesando, J. M., Notis-McConarty, J., et al., *Cancer Res.* **41**:4771, 1981.

3

Tissue Typing: Recent Advances*

Charles B. Carpenter and Edmond J. Yunis

The immunologic apparatus in animals is a complex network of amplifying and suppressing systems that function in a well-integrated fashion to produce an immune response. This immune network is regulated by molecules that are encoded by genes within the major histocompatibility complex (MHC). These genes (1) are mapped in the mouse on chromosome 17 within H-2 region and, in man, on chromosome 6, the analogous region is called HLA. The term major histocompatibility complex (MHC) more precisely refers to the closely-linked genes of H-2 or HLA responsible for the induction and expression of the immune response. In particular, the MHC controls the recognition of antigens by T lymphocytes. As defined by Klein (1) "The MHC is a group of loci, the products of which restrict the specificity of antigen-recognition by T lymphocytes." Mitchison (2) prefers the term *guide* instead of *restrict* to refer to the crucial role of MHC gene products in the control of antigen recognition, antibody production, lymphocyte proliferation, cytotoxicity, and suppression (1–4).

At present, the nature of the T-cell receptor for antigen and the precise manner in which positive and negative regulatory signals are generated and perceived is unknown. MHC nomenclature has evolved to ascribe functional and serological properties to regions and loci which are separable by laboratory observations of chromosomal crossing-over (recombination) of marker characteristics. Unfortunately, there is little similarity in nomenclature for the MHC of mouse and man, even when analogous gene products are being described. It is useful, therefore, to employ a more general classification into which MHC gene products of mouse, man, rat, guinea pig, or any other creature can be placed (1). *Class I molecules*, broadly distributed glycoproteins on the surfaces of most tissues, consist of a 44,000 dalton glycoprotein noncovalently bound to a 12,000 dalton polypeptide and are most important in the effector phases of immunity. *Class II molecules*, glycoproteins restricted in expression to certain tissues, consist of noncovalently bound 34,000 and 29,000 dalton chains and are most important in the rec-

*This work was supported by grants from the NIH # CA 20531, AG 02329 and CA 06516.

ognition or initiation phases of the immune response. As further details of the MHC are presented in the following text, the terms class I and class II will be added to the official mouse or human MHC nomenclature (Table 3.1).

Immunoregulation can be mediated by the major cell types of the immune system, i.e., T cells, B cells, and macrophages (4, 5). These regulatory cells and their products are influenced intrinsically by a complex regulatory system of positive and negative factors that are under genetic control especially by genes of the MHC. Therefore, it is not surprising that the MHC per se or the alleles encoded by their loci are found associated or linked to several diseases (7,8). These regulatory components of the immune system can be manipulated extrinsically by therapeutic and environmental factors. The net effect of intrinsic and extrinsic immunoregulation is reflected by the state of health and ultimate life span of an individual.

INTRINSIC IMMUNOREGULATORY FACTORS

The immune system provides the host with resistance against a broad spectrum of infections. The operation and maintenance of the immune system requires the differentiation, interaction, and regulation of multiple cell types. The activities of many genes and their products are required for the development and maintenance of a functional immune system. Biozzi and his associates (9) have shown that at least 10 independent polymorphic loci can influence

Table 3.1. Homology Between Human and Mouse MHC

Description and Biologic Activity	Genetic Region and Phenotypes	
	Human	Mouse
Broad distribution of bimolecular glycoproteins (12,000 and 44,000 daltons) Class I	HLA-A, B, C	H-2D, K and L
Restricted distribution		
Bimolecular glycoproteins (29,000 and 34,000 daltons) Class II	HLA-DR	H-2I-A, -E/C
Bimolecular glycoproteins (12,000 and approx. 38,000 daltons)	HT?	TL-Qa
Immunoregulatory genes	HLA-D?	I-A, E/C, Qa
Mixed lymphocyte stimulatory determinants (MLR-S)	HLA-D	I-A, I-E/C
Antigen presentation by macrophages to T lymphocytes	HLA-DR	I-A, I-E/C
Helper factor	HLA-DR	I-A,?-E/C
Suppressor factor	?	I-J
Cellular interactions of T and B lymphocytes	HLA-D	I-A, I-E/C
Complement associated proteins	BF, C2, C4	C4, BF

the immune response. However, one genetic system, the major histocompatibility complex, has a predominant influence on the immune response. Thus, the major histocompatibility complex (MHC) can control the ability to respond to selected antigens in an all-or-none fashion (10).

The Major Histocompatibility Complex

Humoral and cellular immune responses depend upon carefully integrated cooperative cellular interactions involving macrophages, T lymphocytes, and B lymphocytes (11, 12). Studies in animals using molecules with single (or at most a few) antigenic determinants have revealed that these immune responses are under control of genes within at least two separate linkage groups, those controlling idiotypic specificities (closely linked to immunoglobulin heavy chain genetic loci) and those of the major histocompatibility complex (MHC) (13, 14). Idiotypic specificities are related to the unique structural specificities of antibody combining sites on immunoglobulin molecules (7), whereas, the genes of the MHC that control the presence, absence, and magnitude of the antibody response are called Ir genes (13). In the animal with the best characterized MHC, the mouse, Ir genes have been localized within the MHC on the seventeenth chromosome between H-2K (class I), and the S (Ss-Slp) region, the latter, controlling the synthesis of the fourth component of murine complement, C4 or Ss, and a closely similar molecule without C4 function, Slp (14, 15). The I region (class II) contains the Ir genetic loci and has been subdivided (proceeding from H-2K toward the S region and H-2D) into I-A,I-B,I-J, and I-E/C (16). By immunizing inbred strains of mice with lymphocytes from other inbred strains differing genetically only in their I regions, antibodies have been obtained that react with surface determinants, Ia antigens, produced by I-region genes (17, 18). It is now known that genes within I-A, I-B, and I-E/C code for structures on helper T lymphocytes, whereas those in I-J control molecules on suppressor T cells (19). I-A and I-E/C gene products are class II, while the structure of the I-J gene product is unknown. Even more remarkably, both antigen-specific helper and suppressor factors secreted by the respective subsets of T lymphocytes, carry Ia antigenic determinants and idiotypic determinants without constant regions of heavy or light immunoglobulin chains (20). These factors, of about 45 to 50,000 daltons, are critical in the regulation of production of specific antibody by B cells and their progeny, plasma cells. The recognition of viral antigens for cytotoxicity requires their presentation to the immune system in conjunction with MHC-produced class I self-antigens, H-2D or K (21, 22).

Much of what we now know of the genetic control of the immune response comes from the study in experimental animals, particularly the mouse, guinea pig, and rat, of the antibody response to three kinds of restricted antigenic determinants (13): (a) synthetic polypeptides of limited structural heterogeneity such as (T, G) -A -L and GAT; (b) slight differences in structure of autologous antigens as in allotypic determinants or slightly chemically-modified autologous proteins; and (c) complex heterologous antigens given at such low doses that only one or a few antigenic determinants are recognized. The evidence obtained from such studies shows that the MHC-linked genes controlling the response to different antigens are distinct from each other and map separately (23).

The MHC's of different mammalian species show striking similarities except that there has been an apparent inversion in murine species (mouse and rat). In the mouse seventeenth chromosome the I-region (class II) is between the two major serologically defined class I histocompatibility loci (H-2K and H-2D) rather than outside. In the rhesus monkey, a probable model for man, Ir genes map outside RhLA (24). Figure 3.1 shows that the

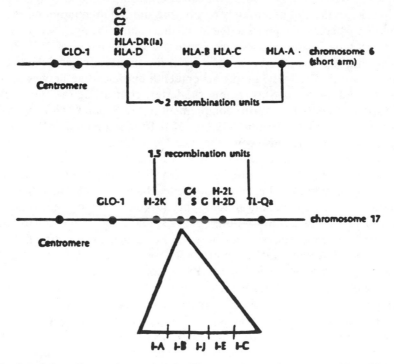

Fig. 3.1. Schematic genetic maps of the HLA complex on chromosome 6 in man and the H-2 complex on chromosome 17 in the mouse. In man, the loci are: PGM$_3$, phosphoglucomutase-3; GLO-1, glyoxylase-1; C2 and C4, component factors; Bf factor B of properdin system; HLA-D; HLA-DR; HLA-B; HLA-C; and HLA-A. In the mouse the loci are: GLO-1, glyoxylase-1; H-2K of the K region; I-A, I-B, I-J, I-E and I-C of the I region; C4 complement component of the S region; H-2D of the D region; H-2L of the L region; and TL-Qa of the T region.

precise positions of the MHC-linked genes for the complement proteins C4, B (BF), and C2 in man are not settled, but they are either between HLA-B and HLA-D/DR or outside of HLA-D/DR. It is agreed that the complement loci C4A (Rodgers), C4B (Chido), BF, and C2 are very closely linked to each other and no crossover has yet been observed (25). Although Ir genes are presumed to be present in man, their clear cut identification has been difficult.

There are a number of common diseases of unknown etiology, with possible precipitation by viral infection and, strongly suspected of occurring only in genetically susceptible individuals, of unclear mode of inheritance. As a group, they are characterized by *autoimmunity* either against single cell types, such as pancreatic β cells in insulin-dependent juvenile-onset diabetes mellitus (IDDM) and the hepatocyte in chronic active hepatitis; or certain neurons in multiple sclerosis (MS); or a number of organs, as in rheumatoid arthritis or systematic lupus erythematosus (SLE). Logically, they have been regarded as possibly being at least partly determined by postulated specific immune response genes in susceptible individuals.

These considerations led to the search for HLA-disease associations, particularly among patients with this group of disorders. Such associations have been found (26, 27). For the diseases mentioned above, these associations are in general weak for HLA-A and HLA-B (class I) types and stronger for HLA-D and HLA-DR (class II) types (7). In contrast, other HLA-associated diseases without suspected immunopathogenesis are more markedly associated with HLA-A (hemochromatosis) (28) or HLA-B (21 hydroxylase deficiency) (29). In addition, a particularly strong association has been found between HLA-B27 and ankylosing spondylitis (32,33).

There is evidence for the association of certain immunoglobulin (km and/ or Gm) genetic markers with a high or low antibody response to flagellin (34) to the polyribose phosphate antigen of *H. influenzae* or to pneumococcal C-polysaccharide (35) and to the acetyl choline receptor in patients with myasthenia gravis (36).

The Classical Loci of the Major Histocompatibility Complex

*Genetic organization.*The alloantigens of mouse H-2 were first described by Peter Gorer in the late 1930s (37, 38). The MHC of man and other mammals consists of a series of genetic loci which produce membrane-associated proteins (38). There are a number of alleles at each locus and specific alleles of each locus are inherited with alleles of other loci in the region, a phenomenon termed *linkage disequilibrium*. Together these genes appear to function as a *supergene*. These antigens are found on all nucleated cells except the trophoblast and some are also found on platelets. Antibodies reactive to HLA alloantigens are found in the sera of recipients of organ transplants or blood transfusions, and, also, commonly in healthy multiparous women who make an immune response in the normal course of pregnancy to the paternal HLA antigens of the fetus. At least five of these loci are closely linked on the short arm of chromosome 6. The MHC of man has been localized to the short arm of chromosome 6 by cell hybridization and family studies and by chromosome banding techniques (6p21–6p22) which have defined specific bands associated with metaphase. Designated HLA-A, HLA-C, HLA-B, HLA-D, and HLA-DR, they have been found to be homologous to systems of cell surface antigens found in mouse (H-2), guinea pig (GPLA), rhesus (RhLA), chimpanzee (ChLA), rat (RTI), chicken (B), dog (DLA), pig (SL-A), rabbit (RL-A), and all other mammals thus far studied (Fig.3.1). The MHC of mouse, H-2, is the most studied system and has several regions coding for traits homologous to those found in man, though there appears to have been a reorganization of their chromosomal order. In mouse, the class I H-2K and D regions appear homologous to human HLA-A and HLA-B loci while the H-2I region appears homologous to human HLA-D and HLA-DR class II loci. As will be mentioned later, the human complement components BF, C2, C4A, and C4B appear to be coded close to HLA-D and DR , while the mouse H-2S region, which codes for C4, has been localized between H-2 and D (Fig.3.1).

Functions. The genes of HLA region code for glycoproteins which are important in diverse aspects of regulation of the immune response such as:

1. the production of antibodies,
2. the production of various classes of T lymphocytes (cytotoxic, suppressor, or helper),
3. the strength of the immune response,
4. the biosynthesis of several components of the complement system,
5. the control of embryogenesis,

as well as the regulation of the synthesis of certain steroid hormones. Perhaps more important, these antigens may serve as substrates for elimination of pathogens in immune surveillance or as markers for genes important in the pathogenesis of certain diseases, especially those with *autoimmune etiology*.

Genetic and Structural Studies. Initially, these antigens were a tangle of specificities each identified in a single laboratory. They have been defined by a series of international workshops beginning in 1964, the most recent one in 1980. No attempt is made to provide complete references which are to be found in reviews of the MHC (39) or in the Workshop Proceedings (40–46). In general, the most important discoveries that led to the description of a number of important aspects of the human MHC are:

1. Recombination between four different regions (HLA-A, B, C, and D) and probably a fifth (HLA-DR), hence demonstrating the MHC to be a genetic complex (48), and the production in mouse of congenic strains of mice with description of separate regions of the H-2 called D, S, I, and K.
2. Cytogenetic techniques for banding chromosomes that permit morphological identification of chromosomes and fine structural analysis of segments of chromosome, as in translocations.
3. The development of cell hybrids between human and other animal cells which permits identification of enzymes and antigens marking one or another of human or animal chromosomes and the demonstration of the maintenance of synteny of this linkage group among all mammals thus far studied (49).
4. The discovery of linkage between enzyme, red cell, and complement genes of chromosome 6 of man with markers of the HLA system and the similar finding in mouse that the Ss protein is C4.
5. The identification of various classes of lymphocytes; the development of methods for producing continuous culture lines of pure lymphocyte subsets, and development of methods for fractionation of different subsets of lymphocytes.
6. The finding of specific alloantigenic systems restricted to lymphocyte subsets such as those of the class II region of the mouse and the HLA-DR region in man.
7. The chemical characterization of two different classes of molecules isolated from the membranes of cells.

> Class I—Associated with HLA-A, B, and probably C, and H-2K and D consisting of a 44,000 dalton glycoprotein and a molecule of β2m (a 12,000 dalton glycoprotein coded on chromosome 15 in man).

> Class II—Associated with HLA-D, DR, and H-2I molecules consisting of 29,000 and 34,000 dalton subunits (29, 34 molecules) and the discovery of the association of Ia (antigen of the I region) and Ia-like molecules in man with B lymphocytes; and in mouse, studies of the genetic control of immune responsiveness (Ir), immune suppression (Is), and other aspects of the immune regulation by the MHC involving interaction of T lymphocytes, macrophages, and B lymphocytes. Because of the preservation of synteny such functions are presumed to occur in man.

8. Description of methods for production of hybridomas with myeloma cells allowing production of monoclonal antibodies of high titer.

HLA Terminology. This has been determined by a committee of the World Health Organization and the International Union of Immunological Societies

(46). There are more than 20 HLA-A antigens, 33 HLA-B, 8 HLA-C, 12 HLA-D, and 10 HLA-DR antigens which are officially numbered in the WHO-IUIS report. Many of these are well agreed upon and designated by numbers, while others are given provisional numbers prefixed by *w*. In addition, a number of antigenic variants have been *split* producing two or more new specificities.

The HLA-A,B, C antigens are determined by a microlymphocytotoxicity assay. Antisera obtained from multiple-immunized individuals (multiparous women, patients receiving multiple transfusions, or deliberately immunized) are incubated with lymphocytes and rabbit serum (as a source of complement). Lymphocytes are obtained by sedimentation on Ficoll-Hypaque gradients; killing of lymphocytes in the presence of complement is determined by eosin or trypan blue exclusion.

Because the genes are closely linked, HLA-A, -B, -C, -D, -DR antigens are inherited as haplotypes except in the rare case of crossovers during meiosis. Hence, each child receives a haplotype from each parent. On some occasions, a crossover can be demonstrated as illustrated in Fig.3.2. These crossover events are valuable in assigning the relative positions of these loci as described later.

In assigning specificities to HLA-A, -B, and -C antisera, numerous problems have been associated with the existence of supertypic specificities which react with and include a number of other subtypic specificities and with the general phenomenon of cross reaction between certain HLA specificities.

There are 3 HLA-A supertypic specificities: Aw19 encompasses A29, Aw30, Aw31, Aw32, Aw33, and Aw34; A9 encompasses Aw23 and Aw24; A10 encompasses A25 and A26. There are 10 supertypic specificities of HLA-B and 34 subtypic ones: Bw16 encompasses Bw38 and Bw39; B12 encompasses Bw44 and Bw45; Bw21 includes Bw49 and Bw50; B5 includes Bw57 and Bw58; B40 includes Bw60 and Bw61; B15 includes Bw62 and Bw63. In addition, two specificities, Bw4 and Bw6, include all the antigens of the B locus and are of help in defining the specificity of new antisera. There are 8 HLA-C specificities.

Figure 3.3 demonstrates some of the known cross reactions of HLA antisera (known as CREG's). These may be of use in the study of the evolution of these antigens, in the selection of grafts and in the transfusion of platelets.

HLA-D codes for the antigenic determinants responsible for the stimulation *in vitro* of mixed cultures of lymphocytes from different individuals. In the mixed culture (MLC), one cell population is inactivated by X-irradiation so that the other proliferative response can be assessed. The HLA-D determinants are operationally defined by lymphocytes obtained from individuals homozygous for one allele. Responding cells having the same antigen as the homozygous stimulating cells are not stimulated to divide and proliferate

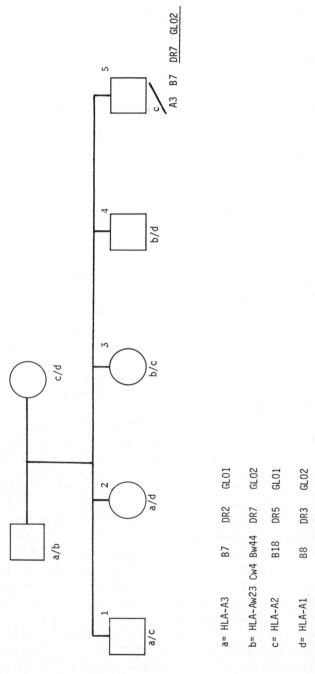

a = HLA-A3   B7   DR2   GL01

b = HLA-Aw23 Cw4 Bw44 DR7   GL02

c = HLA-A2   B18   DR5   GL01

d = HLA-A1   B8   DR3   GL02

Fig. 3.2. The figure depicts the inheritance of the paternal and maternal chromosomes in the first four siblings and the inheritance of a paternal recombinant chromosome in the fifth sibling. This recombination occurred between HLA-B and D, GLO.

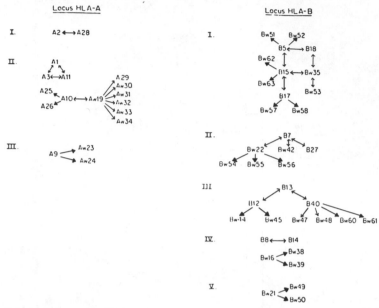

Fig. 3.3. Antisera used in HLA typing are not strictly monospecific. There are cross reactions between HLA antigens and these antisera. Arrows show both cross reactivity and one way reactivity between antibodies.

(an event evaluated by radioactive tritium incorporation). For instance, a cell of type Dw1 and Dw3 will give a good response to homozygous cells of the type Dw2 or Dw4, but not to cells of the type Dw1 or Dw3. There are 12 defined HLA-D specificities.

The specificities of HLA-DR are characterized serologically by antibodies reacting with antigens found on B lymphocytes or monocytes. These antigens are also expressed on macrophages, Langerhans cells of the skin, melanocytes, Kupffer cells, normoblasts (50, 51), and myeloid precursors (52) and to a variable degree on T lymphocytes and cytotoxic T cells (53). The DR antigens in man are structurally homologous to class II, Ia antigens in mouse. Several specificities originally believed to belong to the DR locus are probably coded for by separate closely-linked loci (54–56). No recombination has been detected, but biochemical evidence suggests that these molecules differ from Ia or DR antigens (57–60). These are termed MB, MT, and DC. There are several alleles of MB and MT and at best two of DC. Antibodies to MB1, MT1 and DC1 react with cells of phenotype DR1, DR2, DRw6 and DRw8, while those to MB2 and MB3 react with cells of phenotypes DR3 and DR7, and phenotypes DR4, DR5, DRw6 and DRw9, respectively and those to MT2 and MT3 with phenotypes DR3, 5, 6 or 8, and phenotypes 4, 7 and 9, respectively. HLA-DR antigens can be resolved into at least five molecular species by the technique of two dimensional isoelectric focusing (61).

Several other genetic systems are associated with HLA. As discussed below, several enzymes and complement components are associated with this system. In mouse, genes distal to H2-D (TL and Qa) expressed on thymocytes and immature lymphocytes are also known. It is probable that there is a human analog distal to HLA-A known as HT. It appears that HT molecules are Klein's class I. The amino acid sequences of β2m and IgG suggest homology as do the sequences of HLA and IgG (62). Molecules of Klein's class II include HLA-D and H-2Ia molecules (Table 3.1).

In man, it has been difficult to demonstrate genetically separable serological determinants on B lymphocytes or macrophages but immunoprecipitation has enabled identification of several class II molecules encoded in the HLA-D region (54–60, 63). Monoclonal antibodies have been produced by immunizing Balb/c mice with purified β2m, with Burkitt's lymphoma tumor cells, or with tumor cells obtained from a patient with diffuse poorly differentiated lymphocytic lymphoma. Three of several monoclonal antibodies that react with Ia molecules have been studied extensively and are known to identify different complexes on human cell lines produced from HLA homozygous cells. By immune precipitation and cross-absorption experiments with metabolically labeled cells, complete extraction of the Ia complexes identified by one antibody left unprecipitated was recognized by the two remaining antisera. These experiments suggested the existence of three nonallelic genes coding for these complexes. One of these (I-LR1 antibody) showed alloreactivity with a panel of homozygous typing cells which do not fit any of the three known serological systems (DR, MB, or MT) encoded by the HLA-D region (55). This antibody has been shown to block reactivity of SB antigens (63a). SB is an additional class II locus mapping between HLA-DR and ALO-1, and has six alleles detected by primed lymphocyte testing (63b, 63c). Monoclonal antibodies or polyclonal xenoantibodies against Ia, HLA heavy chain, or β2m have been used to block the corresponding framework molecules with respect to their reaction with alloantibodies. The lymphocytes activated by lectins or by alloreactive cells can be shown to synthesize Ia molecules. Since in the mouse the MHC encodes for other (non-H2) class I glycoproteins such as those of the TL-Qa systems (18), and since human anti-HLA sera produced by planned immunization contain alloantibodies against subset of T lymphocytes (64), it was not surprising to discover similar membrane glycoproteins in man. The use of a combination of antibodies against membrane components such as the antibodies against framework molecules (HLA heavy chain, β2m, and 29, 34 bipeptides) to block these determinants permits localization of the reactions with other antibodies. Two such antisera react with alloantigens which were named HT and are inherited with HLA-A (65).

Functional Studies. MHC molecules appear to function in cellular communication and regulation of the immune response. For instance, cytotoxic T cells preferentially kill a virus when it is presented on a target cell sharing a class I, HLA-A or -B or H-2K or D specificity with the T cell which originally presented the antigen (21, 22, 66, 67). On the other hand, antigen recognition by T cells and T-cell helper and suppressor factors are determined by the interaction of class II gene products of the I region in mouse (and probably HLA-DR products in man) (68). These products control the presentation of antigen by macrophages to T cells, whether these T cells respond, and which subset of T cells proliferate in response. As mentioned, in the mouse, specific separable Ir genes are known which determine the response to synthetic polypeptides. These have been identified as those that produce class II, Ia molecules homologous to human HLA-D/DR products. The strongest evidence that Ir gene products are the Ia molecules on the surface of macrophages or other antigen presenting cells is related to the analysis of Ir genes in systems in which two distinct MHC-linked genes were required for immune responsiveness (69, 70). This gene complementation has been explained at the molecular level. Two loci of the I region, I-A and I-E/C, code for serologically and structurally distinct polypeptide chains which constitute Ia molecules. The heavier of the chains produced by the genes in I-A, bind noncovalently to either an I-A encoded, or an I-E/C encoded light chain to form the two chain Ia molecule. Hence, complementation is intramolecular and can occur when I-A and I-E/C genes are cis (same haplotype) or trans (different haplotypes, one from each parent).

It appears that these molecules can be synthesized and secreted by activated T cells (53) and that these molecules can amplify or modulate the immune response as part of helper or suppressor factors (68, 71). In this regard, a general requirement for T-cell activation involves the interaction between the lymphocyte and the macrophage in which the T cell recognizes an antigen through specific receptors on its surface, together with the recognition of the Ia antigen represented on the surface of the macrophages (72). Therefore, it is quite possible that the genetic control of the immune response (activation or suppression) is elicited through these molecules (73).

In the mouse, recognition of Ia antigens (represented on the surface of the macrophage) together with the interaction of a T lymphocyte with a specific receptor on the macrophage, results in T-cell activation. This appears to be an absolute requirement; depletion of macrophages or blocking macrophage Ia determinants with anti-Ia antisera results in the failure of antigen to trigger T cells (74–75).

Likewise, anti-HLA-DR antisera inhibit macrophage-dependent antigen-induced T-cell proliferation in man, primarily by masking HLA-DR determinants on the surface of macrophages (72).

In the mouse, there are T-independent antigens which directly trigger

B cells, while in man they are unknown. Indeed, patients with pure thymic aplasia (Nezelof's Syndrome) have normal B-cell populations and IgG serum levels, but no antibody activity. T-cell factors derived from the supernatants of antigen-activated T cells replace the T-cell effect required for B-cell antibody production. At least two types of helper factors are known. Non-specific T-cell factors trigger autologous and allogeneic B cells to proliferate and secrete antibodies to a number of antigens. The antigen-specific helper factors induce specific antibodies (76) and can be absorbed in immunoabsorbent columns containing antisera to class II, Ia determinants or HLA-DR antigens expressed on cells of the donor which produced the factor (73, 77). Similarly, T-cell suppressor activity can be mediated by soluble factors which contain both antigen-binding capacity and gene products of the I-J subregion of the I region (78). Suppressor cells have also been demonstrated in man (79), in an experiment with supraoptimal antigen stimulation of T cells. Suppressor-cells are specific to the HLA-DR antigens presented by stimulator lymphocytes and these probably release suppressor factor when confronted with the specific HLA-DR antigen (80). In man suppression by a soluble T-cell factor of the MLR is highly specific for HLA-D products of the responder cell and requires HLA-D identity of suppressor and responder cells (81) (Table 3.1).

As mentioned previously in this section specificity of cytotoxic T lymphocytes is governed by gene products of class I, K and D region antigens in the mouse and HLA-A, -B, and -C regions in man. From studies of families with recombinations in the HLA region it appears that HLA-B determinants are more important than HLA-A determinants in the recognition of targets by cytotoxic T cells (82).

As will be discussed later, specific alleles of the loci of the MHC appear to be important in the generation and regulation of the immune response and may be responsible for the associations of specific responses and diseases with HLA. In the mouse, certain H-2 haplotypes of congenic strains are associated with long or short life span (83). For instance, $H-2^b$ confers longer life than $H-2^m$. This factor affecting aging appears to be coded in the I-C region. Finally, it appears that the MHC antigens participate in the initial selection of T cells (in the thymus as they differentiate) which are specific for autologous MHC antigens (84, 85). Subsequent loss of regulation of these clones may lead to autoaggression (86).

Immune Surveillance. In a more fundamental sense, one of the probable functions of MHC products in the immune response is the recognition of altered self, specifically neoplastic cells (87). While the role of the immune system in immune surveillance has been challenged because of the lack of increase in frequency of solid neoplasms in immunosuppressed or immunodeficient hosts and other observations, this may be because there are other mechanisms for suppression of neoplastic growth (21, 88–89). MHC products appear to be recognized as altered self in the presence of virus or hapten. In such cases, T cells recognize modified syngeneic MHC antigens. In the cases of postinfectious (reactive) arthritis following infection with Yersinia, Salmonella, Chlamydia, or Shigella, along with ankylosing spondylitis, Reiter's Syndrome, and anterior uveitis, a great proportion of patients have the antigen HLA-B27. In each case, the immune response may be against the membrane component altered by a virus or bacterial product. A factor has been identified in Klebsiella culture filtrates which modified an HLA-B27 associated cell-surface component (90, 91). In a family study in man, *in vitro* cytotoxic T-cell responses to influenza-virus-infected autologous cells showed T-cell recognition of influenza virus (by cytotoxicity) to be dependent upon HLA type (92).

The TL-Qa Genetic Region. The TL-Qa genetic region in the mouse is located on chromosome 17 next to the H2-D region of the MHC. Present data indicate that nine loci map in this region and are designated Qa-1, Qa-2, Qa-3, Qa-4, Qa-5, H-2T, H-31, H-32, and TL (18). These gene products are of interest since they are expressed on particular subpopulations of lymphocytes and thymocytes. While the TL-Qa genetic region is not considered a part of the H-2 region, TL-Qa loci determine serologically detectable differentiation antigens, skin and tumor graft rejection, and cell-mediated lympholysis not restricted by the H-2 haplotype. Thus, gene products of both the TL-Qa and H-2 regions are associated with similar functions. Further, TL-Qa and H-2 gene products possess similar molecular properties i.e., a two polypeptide chain complex with a common β2 microglobulin determinant of 12,000 daltons and a variable heavy chain of 43,000 to 45,000 daltons. The TL-Qa region may be quite important for understanding how the lymphocyte functions within the complex immune system.

The possible existence of a human analog to the TL-Qa system is under active investigation (65). Our efforts in this regard have resulted in the identification of human alloantiserums that react with cell-surface determinants expressed on mitogen-activated lymphocytes, but not expressed on resting T cells. The alloantigens identified, referred to as HT, are different from the classical HLA-A, -B, -C, and -DR antigens, but are associated with β2 microglobulin. These determinants may be encoded by genes which appear to segregate with the HLA-A region, the counterpart of the murine H-2D region, and may represent the TL-Qa-like region in man (65).

EXTRINSIC IMMUNOREGULATORY FACTORS

There are several means by which one can modulate the immune response to specific antigens. Many of the procedures appear to preferentially eliminate or reduce helper-suppressor cell activity. One approach involves the induction of antigen-mediated immune suppression. Intravenous administration of syngeneic spleen cells, coupled with the palmitoyl-derivative of protein antigens, results in a state of carrier-specific tolerance in mice (93). Such antigen-induced immunosuppression is thought to be due to mechanisms involving the induction of both T-cell tolerance and T-cell suppression. The generation of T-suppressor cells apparently has the effect of decreasing T-cell help needed by the specific B cells.

Elimination of suppressor activity can also be demonstrated experimentally. Suppressor T cells (94) and factors (95, 96) produced by such cells contain antigenic products encoded by the I-J subregions of the H-2 complex in mice. Identification of these I-J products led to another approach by which immunoregulation was manipulated *in vivo*. Benacerraf and associates (97) reasoned that administration of antiserum directed against I-J determinants on suppressor T cells should eliminate the activity of this T-cell subset. They examined this hypothesis in tumor-bearing mice and found that tumor growth did not progress in mice treated daily with small quantities of anti-I-J serum (98). Apparently, the immunologic balance in these mice shifted in favor of immunity following elimination of specific suppressor T cells by anti-I-J serum. Identification of I-J like molecules on human suppressor T cells and the development of related antibody would allow for the possible elimination of suppressor cell activity associated with immunologic hyporesponsiveness in tumor-bearing patients.

Nonsensitized lymphoid cells referred to as natural killer cells are capable of lysing malignant cells (99). Such natural killer-cell activity works independently of antibody, complement, and phagocytosis. NK cells, with characteristics of T cells, B cells and macrophages, are present in both normal and athymic mice. Athymic mice lack a T-cell system, but do not demonstrate a high incidence of spontaneous tumors (100). NK cells are capable of spontaneous cytotoxic activity directed against both normal cells and tumor targets *in vitro*. Thus, it is hypothesized that such cells play an important role in immunologic surveillance against neoplastic growth in athymic mice, as well as with a normal T-cell system. However, their control of spontaneous tumor development is open to question. Nevertheless, NK activity, like helper and suppressor T-cell activity, is subject to manipulation. Antiserum that is specific for Ly5 antigens on NK cells allows for positive selection of such cells from nonimmune mice. These NK cells, upon adoptive transfer, can protect syngeneic mice against local growth of two different types of tumor cells (101). NK-cell activity can also be influenced by agents with opposing effects, such as interferon and glucan. Interferon, which can affect many different aspects of the immune response (102), augments NK activity (103). Tilorone is a drug which augments NK activity through stimulation of interferon production (104). Glucan, a β1,3-glucosidic polyglucose, is a potent reticuloendothelial stimulant; however, this immunomodulating agent apparently causes significant depression of NK-cell activities in mice (105).

The thymus and lymphoid cells derived from this organ have an important influence on immunoregulation, as evidenced by the effect of adult thymectomy on the generation of suppressor T cells. When thymectomy is performed in adult life, humoral and cell-mediated immune responses are increased (106), while T-suppressor activity directed against malignant tissue *in vivo* is abrogated (107). Furthermore, spleen cells from mice that are thymectomized as adults exhibit an enhanced capacity to lyse syngeneic tumor cells *in vitro* (108). These findings demonstrate that thymectomy serves as an important approach for analysis of function controlled by thymus-derived T-cell subpopulations.

The nutritional state of an individual plays an important role in the function of the immune system. The influence of nutritional factors on malignancy, longevity, and immunity in experimental animals and man has been investigated extensively for years (109). Most dietary manipulations shown to have an effect on immunity as it relates to disease and aging involved either a caloric restriction (110, 111), a deficiency in essential amino acids (112, 113), or a reduction of protein intake (114). Polysaturated fatty acids (PUFA) also have been noted to have an apparent immunoregulatory effect (115). In contrast to caloric and protein restriction, the immunoregulation observed with PUFA dietary manipulation appeared to have a dual nature, immunoinhibition was observed with a deficiency of PUFA and immunopotentiation resulted with an excess of PUFA. Indeed, numerous studies have attempted to understand the immunoregulatory influence of nutrition on immune function and disease (116).

Conclusion. The immune system is composed of a complex network of amplifying and suppressing systems that function in a controlled manner to produce an immune response. Immune responsiveness requires the interactions of lymphoid cells and macrophages with antigen. The immune network, which is regulated by cells and mediators within the system, is primarily under genetic control by the major histocompatibility complex. Gene products of the MHC control antigen recognition, antibody production, lymphocyte proliferation, cytotoxicity, and suppression. Many of the intrinsic and extrinsic factors which influence immune responsiveness change with age. Such changes are reflected by the immunologic vigor and the state of health of the individual.

Practical Aspects of Tissue-Typing of MHC

From the discussion presented thus far, it should be clear that the MHC is a genetic region in the midportion of chromosome 6 comprising approximately seven recombinant units or cM (centimorgans) encoding several loci: HLA-A, B, C, D-DR, complement (C2, C4, Bf) and GLO-1. All these loci are polymorphic and are inherited as a gametic unit named a haplotype composed of alleles which are codominant. It follows that any of the loci could be used as markers (phenotypes, alleles). These alleles are transmitted genetically to the children. If the inheritance of the gametes is at random, the combinations of four haplotypes of the parents will be represented in an equal number of the siblings giving four possible genotypes: ac, ad, bc, and bd. It is possible to determine the HLA genotype of an individual using serological reactions against alleles of HLA-A, B, or C and by using cellular typing by homozygous typing cells. In addition, by electrophoretic techniques, we can identify the HLA genotypes using the alleles of C2, C4, Bf. These reactions are represented in Table 3.2: the paternal chromosomes (a and b) and the maternal chromosomes (c and d). Since each of the markers are polymorphic (several alleles), many individuals are heterozygotes for each position and therefore the children inherit the factors of each of the chromosomes. In the example depicted in Table 3.2, siblings 1 and 4 have inherited the chromosomal region haplotype a of the father and c of the mother. Each child possesses 25% of the probabilities to have an HLA identical sibling.

Family analysis with recombination within HLA have shown four loci: A, C, B, and D which are illustrated in Figure 3.2.

Table 3.2. Inheritance of MHC Markers

	Father	Mother	Siblings 1	2	3	4	5	Chromosomal Markers
Microlymphocytotoxicity or Electrophoresis	+	−	+	−	+	+	−	a
	+	−	−	+	−	−	+	b
	−	+	+	+	−	+	−	c
	−	+	−	−	+	−	+	d
Genotype	ab	cd	ac	bc	ad	ac	bd	

The genetic markers of polymorphic genes (HLA-A, B, C, D/DR or C4, C2, BF, GLO) are represented by letters a or b of the father, and c or d of the mother. There is a 25% probability of two children being identical as are siblings 1 and 4.

The chromosomal region of HLA is approximately two centimorgans long, or two units of recombination. This means that there are two recombinants in 100 meioses. During meiosis the homologous chromosomes pair and crossing-over occurs between them before reduction of the number of chromosomes from 46 (diploid) to 23 (haploid). This mechanism is called recombination. The frequency of recombinations between HLA-A and HLA-D is less than 2 percent. The progeny in a family usually inherit all the alleles of the HLA complex from each parent. One group of the alleles of each chromosome is called a haplotype and the two haplotypes constitute one genotype (Fig. 3.3).

Bone Marrow. The HLA genotypically identical sibling is clearly the preferred appropriate donor for bone marrow or organ transplantation. Because of the fact that only approximately 35% of the patients needing bone marrow will have an identical sibling donor and significantly less in kidney transplants, a large group of transplant patients require unrelated donors. It is of interest that although the expected Mendelian ratios of haplotype inheritance would predict a 25% chance for an HLA-identical sibling, the actual number is close to 35% for leukemic bone-marrow recipients. These findings suggest that an HLA-linked factor(s) which promote genetic survival may also affect susceptibility to leukemia, at least in some families. The incentive to pursue the issue of bone-marrow donor selection from individuals other than HLA genotypically identical siblings came from the study of allogeneic bone-marrow transplantation in severe combined immunodeficiency (SCID). The selection of allogeneic bone-marrow donors for SCID patients lacking an HLA-identical sibling has been based on the assumption that compatibility between donor and recipient for the determinants responsible for stimulation in the mixed lymphocyte culture (MLC) plays a major role in prevention of severe graft-versus-host disease (GVHD). The subsequent selection of marrow donors for patients with aplastic anemia and leukemia who lack an HLA-identical sibling has been based on the additional assumption that compatibility for MLC-stimulating determinants plays a major role in the prevention of graft rejection as well as GVHD. A number of successful bone-marrow transplants have now been performed in patients with SCID, aplastic anemia, and leukemia, using non-HLA genotypically identical related donors. Most of these related transplants are between HLA phenotypically identical pairs (117,118).

Compatibility in the MLC and at HLA-D provides, at present, the best indicator test for successful outcome of allogeneic bone-marrow transplantation when donor and recipient are not HLA genotypically identical. Typing for HLA-D could, therefore, serve as a method for identification of donor-recipient pairs (119, 120).

Typing for the closely related DR antigens does, however, provide a more rapid method of identification of potential unrelated donors for allogeneic bone-marrow transplantation. This indicates a promising direction for future attempts to select HLA phenotypically identical donors for patients lacking in HLA-identical sibling. Alternatively, the possibility now exists for bone marrow transplantation with HLA haploidentical related, or HLA identical unrelated, donors, by removal of immunocompetent T cells from donor marrow using lectins (119) or monoclonal antibodies (120).

Kidney Transplantation. Matching for antigens of the HLA major histocompatibility gene complex has long been accepted as an ideal criterion for selection of donors for renal allografts. Other antigens called *minor*, may nevertheless play crucial roles, especially the ABH blood groups and a newly defined endothelial monocyte antigen (121,122). The main evidence for designation of HLA as the genetic region encoding strong transplantation antigens comes from the success rate in living related donor renal and bone-marrow transplantation, with superior results in HLA-identical sibling pairs. Nevertheless, 10 to 15% of HLA-identical renal allografts are rejected, and often within the first weeks after transplantation (123). It is likely, though not proven, that these failures represent states of prior sensitization to non-HLA antigens. Normally, non-HLA antigens, other than ABH, are considered to be relatively weak and, therefore, suppressible by conventional immunosuppressive therapy. Once priming has occurred, however, secondary responses are much more refractory to treatment. This is the true situation with ABH incompatibilities, since it is the preformed natural anti-A and anti-B antibodies which constitute the barrier to graft success.

Living-Related Donors. Among first degree relatives, the general level of expected graft success was long thought to be in direct proportion to matching for 2, 1, or no HLA haplotypes, as defined by HLA serologic typing and the presence or absence of a proliferative response in the mixed lymphocyte culture (124). HLA incompatible siblings do little better than the overall average with cadaveric donors (50 to 60% at 1-year), while HLA semi-identicals (haploidentical) are in the 70 to 75% range. Since a number of poorly matched grafts do quite well, it is apparent that mere typing does not necessarily provide a measure of the strength of an incompatibility in a given case. Furthermore, incompatible haplotypes may on occasion share antigens or cross-react. Several studies show that intrafamilial MLCs amongst haploidenticals can have a range of response from high to low, and that low responders have a 1-year graft survival of 90%, while high responders have a 1-year graft survival of 55% (125-129). The MLC is a relatively imprecise technique, with center-to-center variation in the optimal method for performance and interpretation of results. Also, one can expect to find intermediate responders of indeterminant prognosis. However, it seems established that the MLC, when carefully controlled, can be used to select those living related HLA haploidentical donors who will be tolerated as well as HLA identicals, while discerning those donors which are little better than cadaveric donors. Careful study of the reasons for low and high MLC response in relation to matching for the various components of the HLA-D region (e.g., D, DR, MB, MT) (130), as well as for the generation of suppressor cells which could down-modulate an early vigorous response, should permit both some understanding of this phenomenon and more precise means of measuring it. We feel it is premature to rule out a living donor simply because of a high MLC until the risk relative to a cadaveric graft for long-term success can be more clearly predicted.

Cadaveric Donors. It has been extremely difficult to assess the role of HLA-A, B, C matching in cadaveric donor grafting because of considerable variation in overall results from center to center (124), including, until recently, high mortality rates. It should be clear that the so called *full-house* match of 2 HLA-A and 2 HLA-B antigens between unrelated individuals has only a small statistical chance of matching for other loci adjacent to HLA-A and B in contrast to first degree relatives where simple HLA-A and B typing is an excellent marker system for the other linked loci. The degree to which 2A and 2B antigen matching improves cadaveric renal graft survival, perhaps as much as 10%, is most likely attributable to the fact that some of these matches will also include compatibility for HLA-D, because of the non-randomness of the association of linked alleles (linkage disequilibrium) in the population. Of course, the more racially homogeneous the population, the greater the chances that any given marker will be in linkage disequilibrium with another. The cadaver matching results reported in recent surveys range from good in France and England to moderate in Scandinavia to fair in the United States. These discrepancies may be partly accounted for by the incomplete definition of the HLA region, population heterogeneity, and the possible role of additional unknown histocompatibility loci. Other factors include variability among transplant centers in the protocols and sensitivities of the crossmatch procedures used to detect preexisting immunity in the recipients and, finally, differences in the immunosuppressive regimens used. The probability of finding an HLA phenotypical and seroidentical cadaveric kidney for a patient awaiting kidney transplantation depends on the sizes of the donor and recipient pools.

The availability of reagents to type for HLA-DR antigens, as expressed on peripheral blood and tissue B lymphocytes and monocytes, now makes direct approximation of HLA-D compatibility feasible. The results thus far seem to confirm the importance of matching for both DR alleles, with 15% or more improvement over one or no matches (131). Although some additional benefit may be gained by HLA-A, B matching, the major effect so far seems to be with consideration of DR alone. HLA-D and DR are not strictly identical, and in some cases are clearly dissociated, as in a rare number of individuals with disparate D and DR antigens, and in the fact that DR4 includes Dw4, Dw10, and at least two other new D antigens (132). Taken together with the MLC data which show that cadaveric transplants also survive much better when the donor-specific MLC reactivity is low, it is apparent that rapid assessment (e.g., 24 hours) of MLC response could be a very successful technical advance. So far, reports of protein synthesis as a marker of early activation have not been reproducible, while the expression of insulin receptors on responding T cells 24 hours into the MLC has indeed been shown to correlate with the standard ^{3}HTDR uptake at 6 to 7 days (133).

Presensitization. A positive crossmatch of recipient serum with donor T lymphocytes is usually predictive of an acute vasculitic tragedy called *hyperacute* rejection. A few years ago it was thought that patients making such antibodies against a surrogate panel of normal lymphocytes were at high risk for accelerated, if not hyperacute, rejection, even when the donor-specific crossmatch was negative. That this is no longer so can be attributed to the greater efforts being made in monitoring patients while on dialysis, defining not only the presence or absence of antibodies, but the HLA antigens to which they are directed. Patients sustained by hemodialysis often show fluctuating antibody levels and specificity patterns, sometimes, but not always, related to receipt of blood transfusions. At the time of assignment of a cadaveric kidney, crossmatches are performed with more than one highly reactive serum, and the previously analyzed antibody specificities are also taken into account. Another advance has been the finding that presensitization to antigens expressed on B lymphocytes, but not T lymphocytes, is not a contraindication to transplantation (134). Many of these antibodies are not actually anti-DR, but are non-HLA IgM antibodies active in the cold and at room temperature, which may also be auto-reactive. Recognition of all of the above has permitted successful transplantation of a number of chronic dialysis patients previously stigmatized because of their *high responder* status.

Increased sensitivity of the crossmatch procedure by augmentation of complement-dependent cytotoxicity with anti-T-cell antibodies, or by antiimmunoglobulin reagents, is frequently of value in detecting low levels of antibodies. Other techniques, such as the antibody-dependent cell-mediated cytotoxicity (ADCC) assay for IgG antibodies is also very sensitive (135). However, the precise cutoff point for sensitivity in the antibody crossmatch has not been determined. Too sensitive a technique may exclude potentially successful grafts, particularly if irrelevant non-HLA antibodies are detected. Tests for preformed killer cells to donor cells may also be performed; however, in our experience such a positive lymphocyte-mediated cytotoxicity

(LMC) assay is not a good predictor of graft failure (136), possibly because immunosuppressive drugs are effective upon cells, whereas they cannot block the effect of IgG molecules already formed.

Endothelial-Monocyte System. Both cadaveric and living related, including HLA-identical, grafts may be rejected in an accelerated fashion. In some of these cases antibodies with reactivity to renal endothelium and blood monocytes have been found, both in the circulation and in eluates from rejected grafts (121). Although not yet proven, it is possible that the rare incidence of accelerated rejection in the face of a positive B-lymphocyte crossmatch may well be due to the additional presence of an endothelial-monocyte antibody. Our on-going study of this system in the inbred rat model shows it to be genetically distinct from major histocompatibility complex antigens, that it is poorly immunogenic presented as a single incompatibility, but that once an antibody response is made it produces a dramatic, accelerated vasculitis. Practical techniques of typing and crossmatching for this system need development as 10 to 20% of all early (4 to 6 weeks) failures may be attributable to presensitization to this non-HLA antigen system. Second transplants, following rapid loss of the first graft, may be particularly at risk.

Blood transfusions and cadaveric grafts. At a time when it appeared that transfusion-induced sensitization against a random lymphocyte panel was predictive of a high graft failure rate, a number of units undertook a policy of withholding blood from as many dialysis patients as possible. The clinical need for blood had been found to be less than originally thought, especially in non-nephrectomized patients. The overall experience with the nontransfused patients has been a dramatic one, confirmed many times over; such patients are at the highest risk for graft failure (131, 137). Still at issue is the number of transfused units needed for optimal graft survival, with the bulk of the evidence showing that more than 10 units is optimal, although some claim an effect with 1 or 2 units given in advance or at the time of transplantation. Our own transplant group currently follows a policy of giving at least 5 units during the pretransplant period for patients awaiting first grafts, although more may well be optimal. Further study is needed, including data on the unresolved question of fresh-vs-frozen-vs-washed cells, as well as the precise methods of storage employed. As in many areas of clinical transplantation, one lacks sufficient numbers of cases and/or carefully randomized trials. Nevertheless, the large numbers of cases included in two prospective studies compiled by Opelz and Terasaki provide impressive evidence that the larger the numbers of transfusions, the better the graft survival (131, 137).

The mechanisms of the transfusion effect are possibly two-fold. First, exposure of a potential recipient to a large menu of potentially strong HLA antigens allows him to select those of greatest interest, and these preferences are detected by monthly screens for antibodies. Future organ donors are thereby selected in a negative fashion. About 30% of randomly transfused end stage renal disease patients develop cytotoxic antibodies. Second, priming with HLA antigens may induce antigen-specific unresponsiveness in some recipients, presumably by induction of suppressor cell systems. Ample precedent for this effect exists in animal models of graft enhancement, while nonspecific immunosuppressive effects of blood transfusion are also known to occur in man. Although the screening out phenomenon (negative selection) is easily documented in the tissue-typing laboratory, no direct evidence exists that an organ allograft covered by immunosuppressive therapy would suffer the same fate as a blood transfusion bearing the same HLA antigens. On the other hand, there is little direct evidence for the transfusion-induced suppressor cell activity. The transfusion effect is a clinical finding which requires explanation in modern immunological terms.

Since both transfusions and HLA-DR matching have beneficial effects upon cadaveric graft survival, and particularly since presensitization to HLA-DR antigens seems not to prejudice graft success, it is of considerable importance to assess the combined effects of transfusions and DR matching. Patients receiving two DR matched kidneys, or 10 to 20 units of blood prior to transplantation do well, but the effects are not additive (131). From a practical standpoint, one may opt to do either; however, patients receiving less than 10 blood units do receive benefit from two DR matching. Further data are needed to confirm these studies from the recent eighth International Histocompatibility Workshop. Theoretically, these data point again to a key role for the HLA-D region in the immunogeneticity of allografts. The argument would state that if one can match for these antigens, prior priming to induce low responsiveness is unnecessary, while mismatches can be overcome only by priming with suppressor cell induction, coupled with some element of negative selection. Future studies must not only explain the immunological phenomena, but also take into account the triage effect of both transfusion and DR matching policies.

Blood transfusions and living related donors. Because the logistics of planning these transplants are so different from cadaveric grafting, one tends to think of them as entirely different immunologically. Except for the HLA-identicals, living donor haploidentical grafts actually do provide strong histocompatibility barriers and also appear to benefit from blood transfusions. In particular, the use of donor-specific blood on three occasions prior to transplantation results in superior graft survival in those 70% of recipients who do not become sensitized (138). Again, the effect is one of negative selection of the nonresponders, while an additional degree of specific unresponsiveness may also be induced. In these studies (138), the MLC high responders have been selected for the protocol, improving survival from an expected 60% to the 90% range. Fortunately, those making antidonor antibody responses are not generally sensitized to a random panel, and are excellent candidates for a kidney from another crossmatch negative donor. In a sense, this protocol provides a relatively harmless test of a recipient's responsiveness to a given set of HLA antigens. It should be noted that although the selectivity of the anti-HLA response may well be under genetic control there is no evidence to date that one can define high and low responders to a given HLA antigen by the individual's HLA phenotype.

Overview of Renal Transplantation Immunogenetics. In addition to the ABH blood groups, the important histocompatibility antigens presently known are HLA-A, B, C, the class I, β2-microglobulin-containing structures present on virtually all body cells; HLA-DR, the class II, Ia-like antigens restricted to B lymphocytes, monocytes, sperm, and some activated T lymphocytes; and the endothelial-monocyte system (Table 3.3). The best current data suggest that major immunogenicity lies in the DR antigens, while A, B, C and endothelial-monocyte antigens provide the major targets for effector antibodies, and in the case of A,B,C, at least, for killer lymphocytes. Hence, the current emphasis is on A,B,C crossmatching and DR matching. Addition of practical methods for ruling out presensitization to the endothelialmonocyte system are needed, as well as ways of determining which donor-recipient combinations are most likely to work because of induction of suppressor cells.

The Rejection Process. In considering the nature of alloimmune response, the interface between host and alloantigen-bearing tissue is of some importance. A skin allograft is nourished by the ingrowth of host capillaries, while the kidney presents a large surface area of donor endothelium to the

**Table 3.3. Relative Importance of Histocompatibility Antigens
in Renal Transplantation**

	Primary Role		Phenotype Matching	Serum-Target Cell Cross-Matching
	Induction (Immunogenicity)	Targets for Effectors		
HLA-A, -B, -C	+ +	+ + + +	+	+ + + +
HLA-DR	+ + + +	+	+ + + +	−
Endothelial/ Monocyte	±	+ + + +	? −	+ + + +

circulating blood of the host. In contrast, the fetus is apparently protected by the trophoblastic barrier. Sensitization of the host occurs in all three cases, and it has been shown that lymphocytic drainage via lymphatic channels plays an important role in each. For example, if prior to the establishment of host capillary ingrowth 48 hours after skin transplantation the graft is removed, the host remains unsensitized. In murine pregnancy the uterine regional lymph nodes are activated and become immune to paternal antigens. Normal human pregnancy often results in the development of a clear-cut anti-HLA antibody response directed to paternal antigens. About 10% of multipara are antibody positive and some of these are sufficiently monospecific to be used as HLA-typing reagents. No clear evidence exists for a harmful effect of such antibodies upon fertility or fetal survival. When more sensitive techniques are employed, all normal pregnancies can be shown to involve maternal sensitization to paternal cells, hence, the modern medical artifacts of transplantation and transfusion are not unique examples of alloimmunization. Furthermore, the fact of making an alloimmune response does not in itself indicate that target tissue will be destroyed immunologically.

Rejection of a vascularized organ allograft is associated with a variety of pathological and clinical patterns. This heterogeneity reflects the variable effects of the responsiveness of a given host to a given set of histocompatibility antigens, states, of prior sensitization, and responsiveness to therapeutic manipulation.

Sensitization can occur by either the lymphatic or venous route, and the host has a number of options in developing an effector response. The resulting spectrum from cell-mediated to immunoglobulin-mediated lesions attests to the repertoire available for rejection of a renal allograft. Presumably, the fetus could be similarly assaulted if it were not for the trophoblastic barrier and other modifying influences upon the alloimmune response. The conservation through evolution of the MHC attests to its central role in immune reactivity to non-self invaders. The efficiency of the T-cell response when it is guided (restricted) by MHC gene products on the surfaces of lymphoid cells and macrophages must be of primary evolutionary importance. In this view, the fetus requires special protection from the case of mistaken identity when the host's T cells perceive fetal MHC antigens as altered self.

All alloimmune responses are not harmful per se to an allograft as evidenced by the apparent beneficial effects of deliberate preimmunization with blood transfusion, at least in most cases. Experimentally, such priming has been termed *enhancement*. Rat renal allografts, for example, can enjoy long-term successful function, even in the presence of infiltrating cytotoxic T cells in the graft, provided that the IgG antibodies to the vascular endothelium are suppressed by protocols involving passive transfer of small amounts of IgG directed to donor antigens. Some understanding of the corrrelates of graft rejection with certain qualitative and quantitative aspects of the immune response to the donor has been gained recently. Although a variety of cell types are present in rejection lesions, recovery of these cells and elution of antibodies bound to graft cells have shown that both cytotoxic T cells and IgG antibodies are specifically accumulated in grafts. Information on the other subsets of T cells is lacking in detail thus far. Recruitment of very large numbers of B lymphocytes, null cells, and macrophages, as well as cells capable of mediating antibody-dependent cell-mediated cytotoxicity (ADCC) into rejecting grafts, has been clearly documented and shows that the final effector pathways may be multiple. Most studies of human cases have been performed on failed grafts. The promise of performing analyses on small biopsy specimens has not yet been fully realized.

Immunological Monitoring of Renal Transplant Recipients. A number of assays of immunological function can be performed on peripheral blood samples, and include both quantitative and qualitative aspects of cellular and antibody responses. There are two potential limitations on such studies: (a) not all immune responses are necessarily harmful to a graft, and (b) the peripheral blood may not be an accurate reflection of events within the graft. Only by careful correlative study with the clinical course of a transplant will it be possible to answer these concerns. A number of important observations have already been made, and they do indicate that considerable progress in the understanding of the alloimmune response will be possible by study of venous blood samples.

Two basic types of assays exist, those which reflect specific host antidonor immune activity, and those which reflect nonspecific host responses.

After renal transplantation in hosts treated with azathioprine and steroids, cytotoxic T cells are detectable in blood between the fourth and fifth days after grafting. They reach an initial peak by day seven and then decline by the end of the second week only to reappear in the circulation in varying degrees with rejection activity (139). There is not a complete correlation between rejection activity and circulating donor-specific cytotoxic cells, however, reflecting differing mechanisms of rejection in some individuals. Furthermore, in experimental models it is clear that cytotoxic T cells are first concentrated in the grafts, and only secondarily are detectable in the circulation. Therefore, direct measurement of such lymphocyte-mediated cytotoxicity (LMC) is more useful in definition of the immune mechanisms being activated than in providing a reliable early warning system for a rejection episode.

As described earlier, ADCC is a very sensitive assay for IgG antibodies directed against cell surface antigens. ADCC is able to detect both HLA as well as non-HLA antibodies. A positive ADCC against donor cells is closely associated with acute rejection, i.e., in 29 of 34 rejection episodes (140). Pathologic study of biopsy material revealed humoral rejection in all 29 cases with varying degrees of arteritis ranging from necrotizing arteritis and acute proliferative arteritis to subacute fibro-obliterative arteritis (141). A positive ADCC was detected in only 27 of 74 sera during periods of clinical *quiescence*.

Antidonor antibodies may induce lysis of donor target cells by complement activation (complement-dependent cytotoxicity, CDC). Many groups have employed ^{51}Cr-labeled target cells to detect complement-dependent cytotoxic antibodies, which are often detectable after transplantation and are associated with rejection and a comprised prognosis. In our studies both the ADCC and CDC assays were positive during 24 of 34 rejection episodes, but more importantly, they were both negative in only 1 of 34 rejection episodes. Negative results in both assays may exclude the diagnosis of rejection (142).

Further evidence of the important role of antibody relates to the correlation of *in vitro* assays for antidonor antibody with response to rejection therapy (143). Among 14 patients whose ADCC remained positive after a steroid pulse, 13 lost graft function within 3 months, only 2 of 12 who became ADCC negative after a pulse lost graft function within a similar period. These results suggested that the adequacy of treatment for rejection may be approached through the use of objective measurements of immune function.

Donor specific anti-B-cell antibodies have been shown to develop post-transplant in association with rejection. In our own experience (144), donor specific cytotoxic B-cell antibodies were found in 13 of 35 sera collected during acute or sustained rejection periods and in only 1 of 35 sera from quiescent periods. Since these antibodies have been eluted from rejected grafts (145) and their persistence in the circulation after steriod therapy for rejection has also been associated with a high incidence of graft failure (146), it is possible that these antibodies are important in the actual events of rejection.

Utilizing indirect immunofluorescent staining techniques on umbilical cord derived cells, sections of renal and/or intercostal arteries, and renal biopsy sections, the appearance of antiendothelial antibodies after transplantation has been established. The vast majority of antiendothelial antibodies, however, are detected after graft nephrectomy; possibly negating the value of detecting these antibodies in the diagnosis of rejection.

Donor specific immunologic assays have clearly shown that specific immunologic activity can be dissected during rejection episodes.Due to the need for donor tissue, the number of assays that can be performed is limited. Nevertheless, the data indicate that the continued presence of antidonor antibody in the circulation after treatment for rejection (ADCC, or anti-B-cell antibody) is a poor prognostic sign. These assays may be of greater use to indicate treatment failure.

Measurements of the spontaneous rate of DNA synthesis in recipients' peripheral blood mononuclear cells can be utilized to assess the *in vivo* response to allogeneic stimulation. Since transformed, thymidine-incorporating host blast cells appear in the draining lymph and peripheral blood as well as the parenchyma of transplanted kidneys, measurements of blood as well as the parenchyma of transplanted kidneys, measurements of activated peripheral blood lymphocytes have been undertaken by a number of laboratories. These investigators have found a significant increase in DNA or RNA synthesis either prior to or concomitant with clinical signs of early and late rejection (147, 148). Numerous false positive responses have been noted to occur and are well documented, e.g., surgical trauma and stress, infection and recovery from azathioprine myelosuppression. A recent report (149) described three different levels of reactivity that correlate with the patient's clinical status. Minimal spontaneous blastogenesis (680 cpm) was observed in pretransplant patients. A moderate elevation (2300 to 5300 cpm) was noted in posttransplant during clinically quiescent intervals and following the onset of easily reversible rejection. Marked elevations (310,000 cpm) were frequently observed within 6 days prior to and during vigorous rejection episodes.

Several groups (150, 151) have found that administration of ATG in the early posttransplant period causes a profound reduction in total T cells as measured by the sheep RBC rosette technique. If total T rosette forming cells are reduced to <300 cells/mm^3 or 10% of pretransplant values, early cellular rejections are unusual. In patients not receiving ATG a generalized lymphopenia is seen with little correlation between total T-cell levels and rejection activity. However, the active T rosette forming cell may be useful in this situation (152). Decreased percentage of active T rosette forming cells (A-T RFC) when associated with an increase in spontaneous blastogenesis was noted to occur with each of 90 acute rejection episodes experienced by 72 non-ATG treated patients.

Identification of T-cell subset patterns may be useful. Preliminary results (153) suggest that when the normal ratio of T helper cells to T cytotoxic/suppressor cells of 2 to 1 is present despite immunosuppressive therapy, rejection is highly likely. A diminished T helper to cytotoxic/suppressor ratio, correlates well with clinical quiescence.

Thus, several assays that do not measure antidonor immunity, per se, may be used in the assessment and diagnosis of rejection episodes while the donor specific assays may be most helpful in determining when the immune response has been adequately controlled by immunosuppressive treatment.

Chronic rejection is the usual cause of progressive late failure of long surviving renal allografts. Serum creatinine levels slowly, inexorably rise in the absence of obvious physical symptoms or signs. Protracted humoral injury manifested by intimal fibro-obliterative arterial lesions are common, and may reflect a dominant cause of allograft failure. These intimal abnormalities are thought to represent repetitive cycles of chronic immune injury to vascular endothelium, with focal thrombosis and incorporation of thrombus into the arterial wall (154). Similarly, cellular rejection may occur after many years. Although late acute cellular rejection usually follows discontinuation of immunosuppressive therapy, acute cellular rejection may occasionally develop in the absence of any known precipitating factor.

REFERENCES

1. Klein, J., *Immunology Today* 2:166, 1981.
2. Mitchison, N. A., *Immunology Today* 2:167, 1981.
3. Klein, J., Biology of the Mouse Histocompatibility-2 Complex. New York: Springer-Verlag, 1975.
4. Fifth International Workshop on Human Gene Mapping (Edinburgh Conference, 1979) *Human gene*. Daniel Bergsma (Ed.), The National Foundation–March of Dimes, 1981.
5. Benacerraf, B.,*Transplant Proc.* 9:825, 1977.
6. Yunis, E. J., and Dupont, B., The HLA System. In D. Nathan and F. A. Aski (Eds.), *Hematology of Infancy and Childhood*. Philadelphia: W. B. Saunders, 1438, 1981.
7. Dausset, J., and Svejgarrd, A., (Eds.), *HLA and Disease*, Copenhagen, 1977.
8. Bodmer, W., (Ed.), *Histocompatibility testing 1977*, Copenhagen: Munskgaard.
9. Biozzi, G., Moutou, D., Heumann, A. M., et al., *Immunology* 36:427, 1979.
10. Benacerraf, B., and McDevitt, H. O., *Science* 175:273, 1972.
11. Katz, D. H., and Benacerraf, B., *The Role of Products of the Histocompatibility Gene Complex in the Human Response*. New York: Academic Press, 1976.
12. Rosenthal, A. S., *Immunological Rev.* 40:136, 1978.
13. Benacerraf, B., and McDevitt, H. O., *Science* 175:273, 1972.
14. Roos, M. H., Atkinson, J. P., and Shreffler, D. C., *J. Immunol.* 121:1106, 1978.
15. Parker, K. L., Atkinson, J. P., Roos, M. H., et al., *Immunogenetics* 11:55, 1980.
16. Klein, J., Flaherty, L., Van de Berg, J. L., et al., *Immunogenetics* 6:489, 1978.
17. David, C. S., Shreffler, D. C., and Frelinger, J. A., *Proc. Natl. Acad. Sci. USA* 70:2509, 1973.
18. Hammerling, G. J., Hammerling, U., and Flaherty, L., *J. Exp. Med.* 150:108, 1979.
19. Murphy, D. B., Herzenberg, L. A., Okumura, K., et al., *J. Exp. Med.* 144:699, 1976.
20. Mozes, E. and Haimovich, J., *Nature* 278:56, 1979.
21. Doherty, P. C., Blanden, R. V., and Zinkernagel, R. M., *Transplant. Rev.* 29:89, 1976.
22. Doherty, P. C., Biddison, W. E., Bennick, J. R., et al., *J. Exp. Med.* 148:534, 1978.
23. Lieberman, R., Paul, W. E., and Humphrey, W., *J. Exp. Med.* 136:1231, 1972.
24. Dorf, M. E., Balner, H., and Benacerraf, B. J., *Exp. Med.* 142:673, 1975.
25. Raum, D., Awdeh, Z. L., and Glass, D., et al., *Immunogenetics* 12:59, 1981.
26. Vladatiu, A. O., and Rose, N. R., *Science* 174:1137, 1971.
27. Dixon, F. J., Andrews, B.S., and Eisenberg, R. A., et al., *Arthritis and Rheum.* (Suppl. 5), 21:864, 1978.
28. Simon, M., Bourel, M., Genetet, B., et al. *N. Engl. J. Med.* 297:1017, 1977.
29. Dupont,B., Oberfield, S. E., Smithwick, E. M., et al., *Lancet* 2:1309, 1977.
30. Weitkamp, L.R., Bryson, M. R., and Bacon, G. E., *Lancet* 1:931, 1978.
31. Grosse-Wilde, H., Weil, J., Albert, E., et al., *Immunogenetics* 8:41–49, 1979.
32. Brewerton, D. A., Hart, F. D., Nicholls, A., et al., *Lancet* 1:904–907, 1973.
33. Schlosstein, L., Terasaki, P. I., Bluestone, R., et al., *N. Engl. J. Med,* 288:704, 1973.
34. Wells, J. V., Fudenberg, H. H., and Mackay, I. R., *J. Immunol.* 107:1505, 1971.
35. Pandey, J. P., Fudenberg, H. H., Virella, G., et al., *Lancet* 1:190, 1979.

36. Nakao, Y., Miyaski, T., Ota, K., et al., *Lancet* **1**:677, 1980.
37. Gorer, P. A., *J. Pathol. Bacteriol.* **47**:231, 1938.
38. Gorer, P. A., Lyman, S., and Snell, G. D., *Proc. R. Soc. Lond. B. Biol. Sci.* **135**:499, 1948.
39. Raum, D., Awdeh, Z., Yunis, E. J., and Alper, C. A., Major Histocompatibility Markers in Disease. In A. S. Fauci (Ed.), *Clinics in Immunology and Allergy*, Philadelphia: W. B.Saunders, June 1981, p. 305.
40. Russell, P. S., and Winn, H. J., (Eds.), *Histocompatibility Testing*. Washington, D.C. Natl. Acad. Sci. USA, Publ., 1965, p. 1229.
41. Balner, H., Cleton, F. J., and Eernisse, J. G., (Eds.), *Histocompatibility Testing 1965*. Baltimore: Williams and Wilkins, 1966, p. 288.
42. Curtoni, E.S., Mattiuz, P. L., and Tosi, R. M., (Eds.), *Histocompatibility Testing 1967*. Copenhagen: Munksgaard, 1967, p. 458.
43. Terasaki, P. I., (Ed.), *Histocompatibility Testing 1972*. Copenhagen: Munksgaard, 1973, p. 778.
44. Dausset, J., and Colombani, J. (Eds.), *Histocompatibility Testing 1972*. Copenhagen: Munksgaard, 1973, p. 778.
45. Kissmeyer-Nielsen, F., (Ed.), *Histocompatibility Testing 1975*. Copenhagen: Munksgaard, 1975, p. 1035.
46. Bodmer, W. F., Batchelor, J. R., Bodmer, J. G., et al. (Eds.), *Histocompatibility Testing 1977*. Copenhagen: Munksgaard, 1978.
47. Terasaki, P. I., (Ed.), *Histocompatibility Testing 1980*. Copenhagen: Munksgaard, 1980, p. 1227.
48. Yunis, E. J. and Amos, D. B., *Proc. Natl. Acad. Sci. USA* **68**:3031, 1971.
49. Lalley, P. A., Francke, U., and Minna, J. D., *Proc. Natl. Acad. Sci. USA* **75**:2283, 1978.
50. Thorsby, E., Albrechtsen, D. L., Hirschberg, H., et al., *Transplant. Proc.* **9**:393, 1977.
51. Robinson, J., Sieff, C., Delia, D., et al., *Nature* **289**:68, 1981.
52. Fitchen, J. H., Ferrone, S., Quaranta, U., et al., *J. Immunol.* **125**:2004, 1980.
53. Evans, R. L., Faldetta, T. J., Humphreys, D. M., et al., *J. Exp. Med.* **148**:1440, 1978.
54. Tosi, R., Tanigaki, N., Center, D., et al., *J. Exp. Med.* **148**:1592, 1978.
55. Nadler, L., Stashenko, P., Hardy, R., et al., *Monoclonal antibodies defining serologically distinct HLA-D/DR related Ia-like antigens in man. Human Immunology* **1**, 77, 1981.
56. Pesando, J. M., Nadler, L. M., Lazarus, H., et al., *Human Immunology*. **3**:67, 1981.
57. Crumpton, M. J., Snary, D., Walsh, F. S., et al., *Proc. R.Soc. Lond. B. Biol. Sci.* **202**:159, 1978.
58. Giphart, M. J., Kaufman, J. F., Fuks, A., et al., *Natl. Acad. Sci. USA* **74**:3533, 1977.
59. Charron, D. J., and McDevitt, H. O., *Proc. Natl. Acad.Sci. USA* **76**:6567, 1979.
60. Shackelford, D. A., and Strominger, J. L., *J. Exp. Med.* **151**:144, 1980.
61. van Rood, J. J., van Leeuwen, A., Keuning, J. J., et al., *Scand. J. Immunol.* **6**, 373–384, 1977.
62. Orr, H. T., Lancet, D., Robb, R. J., et al., *Nature* **282**:266, 1979.
63. Lampson, L. A., and Levy,R., *J. Immunol.* **125**:293, 1980.
63a. Nodler, L. M., Stashenko, P., Hardy, R. *Nature* **290**:591, 1981.
63b. Shaw, S., Johnson, A. H., and Shearer, G. M., *J. Exp. Med.* **152**:565, 1980.
63c. Shaw, S., Kavathas, P., Pollack, M. S. et al., *Nature* **293**:745, 1981.
64. Ferrara, G. B., Strelkauskas, A. J., Longo, A., et al., *J. Immunol.* **123**:1272, 1979.
65. Gazit, E., Terhorst, C., and Yunis, E. J., *Nature* **284**:275, 1980.
66. Bevan, M. J., *J. Exp. Med.* **142**:1349, 1975.
67. Shaw, S., Shearer, G. M., and Biddison, W. E., *J.Exp. Med.* **151**:235, 1980.

68. Dorf, M.E., and Benacerraf, B., *Behringwerke Institute Mitteilungen* **63**:56, 1979.
69. Dorf, M. E., and Benacerraf, B., *Proc. Natl. Acad. Sci. USA* **72**:3671, 1975.
70. Benacerraf, B., and Dorf, M. E., *Cold Spring Harbor Symp. Quant.Biol.* **41**:465, 1976.
71. Tada, T., In Immune System Genetics and Regulations. *ICN-UCLA Symposia on Molecular and Cellular Biology.* **6**:345, 1979.
72. Geha, R. S., Milgrom, H. F., Broff, M., et al., *Proc. Natl. Acad. Sci. USA* **76**:4038, 1979.
73. Mudawar, F., Yunis, E. J., and Geha, R. S., *J. Exp. Med.* **148**:1032, 1978.
74. Ruhl, H., and Shevach, E. M., *J. Immunol.* **115**:1493, 1975.
75. Schwartz, R. H., David, C. S., Sachs, D. H., et al., *J. Immunol.* **117**:531, 1976.
76. Geha, R. S., Schneeberger, E., Rosen, F. S., et al., *J. Exp.Med.* **138**:1230, 1973.
77. Munro, A., Taussig, M., Campbell, B., et al., *J.Exp. Med.* **140**:1579, 1974.
78. Tada, T. M., Taniguchi, M., and David, C. S., *Cold Spring Harbor Sym. Quant. Biol.* **41**:119, 1976.
79. UytdeHaag,F., B cell activation *in vitro*: Regulation by antigen specific human suppressor T-cells. In A. S. Fauci and R. S.Ballieux (Eds.), *Antibody Production in Man. In Vitro Synthesis and Clinical Complications*, pp. 141–158. New York: Academic press, 1979.
80. Sasportes, M., Wollman, E., Cohen, D., et al., *J. Exp. Med.* **152**:270 (Suppl) 1980.
81. Engleman, E.G., and McDevitt, H. O., *J. Clin. Invest.* **61**:828, 1978.
82. Geha, R. S., Malakian, A., Geha, O., et al., *J. Immunol.* **118**:1286, 1977.
83. Smith, G. S., and Walford, R. L., *Nature* **270**:727, 1977.
84. Benacerraf, B., *J. Immunol.* **120**:1809, 1978.
85. Katz, D. H., *Adv. Immunol.* **29**:137, 1980.
86. Lemonnier, F., Burakoff, S. J., Germain, R. N., et al., *Proc. Natl. Acad. Sci. USA* **74**:1229, 1977.
87. Burnett, F. M., *Immunological Surveillance.* New York: Pergamon Press, 1970.
88. Lilly, F., *J. Exp. Med.* **127**:465, 1968.
89. Zinkernagel, R. M., and Doherty, P. C., *Nature* **251**:574, 1974.
90. Geczy, A. F., Alexander, K., Bashir, II. V., *Nature* **283**:782, 1980.
91. Geczy, A. F., Alexander, K., Bashir, H. V., et al., *J. Exp. Med.* (Suppl. 331s) **152,** 1980.
92. Biddison, W. E., Payne, S. M., Shearer, G. M., et al., *J. Exp. Med.* (Suppl. 204s) **152,** 1980.
93. Sherr, D. H., Heghinian, K. M., Benacerraf, B., et al., *J. Immunol.* **123**:2682, 1979.
94. Murphy, D. B., Herzenberg, L. A., Okumura, K., et al., *J. Exp. Med.* **144**:699, 1976.
95. Tada, T., Taniguchi, M., David, C. S., *J. Exp. Med.* **144**:713, 1976.
96. Theze, J., Waltenbaugh, C., Dorf, M. E., et al., *J. Exp. Med.* **146**:287, 1977.
97. Pierres, M., Germain, R. N., Dorf, M. E., et al., *J.Exp. Med.* **147**:656, 1978.
98. Greene, M. I., Dorf, M. E., Pierres, M., et al., *Acad. Sci. USA* **74**:5118, 1977.
99. Herberman, R.B., and Holden, H. T., Natural cell-mediated immunity. In G. Klein and S.Weinhouse (Eds.), *Advances Cancer Research*, Vol. 27. New York: Academic Press, 1978.
100. Moller, G., and Moller, E., *Transp. Rev.* **29**:3, 1976.
101. Kasai, M., Leclerc, J. C., McVay-Bourdreau, D. L., et al., *J.Exp. Med.* **149**:1260, 1979.
102. Epstein, L.B., The effects of interferons on the immune response *in vitro* and *in vivo*. In W. Stewart, II (Ed.), *Interferons and Their Actions.* Cleveland: CRC Press, 1977.
103. Santoli, D., and Koprowski, H., *Immunol. Reviews* **441**:163, 1979.
104. Good, R. A., Jose, D. C., Cooper, W. C., In B. D. Jankovic and K. Isakovic (Eds.), *Microenvironmental Aspects of Immunity.* Plenum, NY, 1973, p.321.
105. Lotzova, E., and Gutterman, J. U., *J. Immunol.* **123**:607, 1979.

106. Simpson, E., and Cantor, H., *Europ. J. Immunol.* **5**:337, 1975.
107. Reinsch, C. L., Gleiner, N. A., Schlossman, S. F., *Proc. Natl. Acad. Sci. USA* **74**:2989, 1977.
108. Reinisch, C. L., and Andrew, S. L., *J. Exp. Med.* **148**:619, 1978.
109. Suskind, R. M., (Ed.), *Malnutrition and the Immune Response.* New York: Raven Press, 1977.
110. Walford, R. L., Liu, R. K., Gerbase-Delima, M., et al., *Aging Dev.* **2**:447, 1973.
111. Fernandes, G., Yunis, E. J., and Good, R. A., *Proc. Natl. Acad. Sci. USA* **73**:1279, 1976.
112. Dubois, E., and Strain, L., *Biochem. Med.* **7**:336, 1973.
113. Hui, Y. H., DeOme, K. B., and Briggs, G. M., *Cancer Res.* **32**:2086, 1972.
114. Good, R. A., Jose, D. C., and Cooper, W. C., In B. D. Jankovic and K. Isakovic (Eds.), *Microenvironmental Aspects of Immunity.* Plenum, NY, 1973, p. 321.
115. Mertin, J., and Hunt, R., *Proc. Natl. Acad. Sci. USA* **73**:928, 1976.
116. Good, R. A., Fernandes, G., Yunis, E. J., et al., *Am. J. Path.* **84**:599, 1976.
117. Hausen, J. and Thomas, E. D., In HLA Typing: Methodology and clinical aspects, Vol. I., S. Ferrone and B. G. Solheim, eds. CRC Press, Boca Raton, 1982, pp. 158.
118. Hausen, J., Clift, R. A., Beatty, P. G. et al., In UCLA symposium on molecular and cellular biology, New Series: Recent Advances in Bone Marrow Transplantation, UCLA, 1983.
119. Reisner, Y., Kapoor, W., Kirkpatrick, D. D., et al., *Blood* **61**:341, 1983.
120. Reinberz, E. L., Geha, R., Rappaport, J. M., et al., *Proc. Natl. Acad. Sci. USA* **79**:6047, 1982.
121. Paul, L. C., Claas, F. H., Van Es, L. A., et al., *N. Eng. J. Med.* **300**:1258, 1979.
122. Moraes, J. R., and Stastny, P., *J. Clin. Invest.* **60**:449, 1977.
123. Carpenter, C. B., *Kidney Int.* **14**:283, 1978.
124. Terasaki, P. I., Opelz, G., and Mickey, M. R., *Clinical Immunology*, In press.
125. Cochrum, K. C., Perkins, H. A., Payne, R. O., et al., *Transplant Proc.* **5**:391, 1973.
126. Ringden, O., and Berg, B., *Tissue Antigens* **10**:364, 1977.
127. Walker, J., Opelz, G., and Terasaki, P. I., *Transplant. Proc.* **10**:949, 1978.
128. Cullen, P. R., Lester, S., Rouch, J., and Morris, P. J., *Clin. Exp. Immunol.* **28**:218, 1977.
129. Garovoy, M. R., Person, A., and Carpenter, C. B., *Proc. Dial. Transpl. Forum* **9**:208, 1978.
130. Carpenter, C. B., HLA and Renal Transplantation (Editorial) *New Engl. J. Med.* **302**:860, 1980.
131. Opelz, G., and Terasaki, P. I., International histocompatibility workshop study on renal transplantation. In P. I. Terasaki (Ed.), *Histocompatibility Testing*, Los Angeles: UCLA, 592–624, 1980.
132. Dupont, B., Braun, D. W., Yunis, E. J., et al., HLA-D by cellular typing. In P. I. Terasaki (Ed.), *Histocompatibility Testing*, Los Angeles: UCLA, 1980, p. 229.
133. Helderman, H. J., Strom, T. B., and Garovoy, M. R., *J. Clin. Invest.* **67**:509, 1981.
134. Ettenger, R. B., Uittenbogaart, C. H., Pennisi, et al., *Transpl.* **27**:315, 1979.
135. Gailiunas, P., Suthanthiran, M., Busch, G. J., et al., *Kidney International* **17**:638, 1980.
136. Carpenter, C. B., and Morris, P. J., *Transplant. Proc.* **10**:509, 1978.
137. Opelz, G., and Terasaki, P. I., *New Engl. J. Med.* **299**:799, 1978.
138. Cochrum, K., Hanes, D., Potter, et al., *Transplant. Proc.* **13**:190, 1981.
139. Stiller, C. B., Dosetor, J. B., Carpenter, C. B., et al., *Transplant. Proc.* **9**:1245, 1977.
140. Gailiunas, P., Suthanthiran, M., Person, A., et al., *Transplant. Proc.* **10**:609, 1978.

141. Garovoy, M. R., Gailiunas, P., Carpenter, C. B., et al., *Nephron.* **22**:208, 1978.
142. Garovoy, M. R., and Carpenter, C. B., Immunologic monitoring for renal transplantation. In N. R. Rose and H. Friedman (Eds.), *Manual of Clinical Immunology,* Washington, DC: *American Society for Microbiology,* 1980, p. 1042.
143. Gailiunas, P., Busch, G., Person, A., et al., *Transplant. Proc.* **11**:17, 1979.
144. Suthanthiran, M., Gailiunas, P., and Fagan, G., et al., *Transplant. Proc.* **10**:605, 1978.
145. Garovoy, M. R., Suthanthiran, M., Gailiunas, P., et al., *Transplant. Proc.* **10**, 605, 1978.
146. Soulillou, J. P., Peyrat, M. A., and Geunel, J., *Lancet* **1**:354, 1978.
147. Hersch , E. M., Butler, W. T., and Rossen, R. D., et al., *J. Immunol.* **107**:571, 1971.
148. Harris, J., Bagai, R., Rashid, A., et al., *Transplant. Proc.* **4**:659, 1972.
149. Vesella, R. L., Pierce, G. E., Barth, R. F., et al., *Transplantation* **23**:227, 1977.
150. Cosimi, A. B., *Transplant. Proc.* **13**:461, 1981.
151. Thomas, F., Lee. H. M., Wolf, J. S., et al., *Surgery* **79**:408, 1976.
152. Kerman, R. H., Floyd, M., Van Buren, C., et al., *Transplantation* **32**:16, 1981.
153. Cosimi, A. B., Burton, R. C., Kung, P. C., et al., *Transplant. Proc.* **13**:499, 1981.
154. Busch, G. J., Schamberg, J. F., Moretz, R. C., et al., *Lab. Invest.* **35**:272, 1976.

4

Immunobiology of Organ Transplantation

Eduardo A. Santiago-Delpín*

The phenomenon of rejection was discovered by mere chance when clinician-scientists were attempting to use healthy organs from animals or other humans in place of diseased organs and tissues of patients. Obviously, this methodology, albeit quite perfected in the last decades, is only an artifact of present medical therapeutics and, by itself, has affected only a minuscule number of patients. Nonetheless, organ transplantation has brought with it profound changes in our way of thinking in such areas as moral and ethical aspects of donation of living and cadaver organs; legal discussions and controversies regarding the definition of death; sociological disquisitions regarding the social and personal benefits of transplantation to society, to the patient, and to mankind; and perhaps a trifle serendipitously, it has exposed us to the vastness, complexity, and wonders of the immune system. It has recruited, involved, and otherwise interested thousands of scientists from all fields (basic and clinical), who, upon this glimpse of what lies beyond, have dedicated effort, time, money, and their lives to its discovery. Transplantation is responsible for all these activities and changes. Thus, we have managed to get a deeper insight into a system whose paradigm barely existed 20 years ago.

Rejection is quite difficult to define, since this phenomenon varies with the tissues and organs involved, the species involved, and the immune status of the host. It is becoming evident that the fundamental basis of rejection is probably the same in all species and organs, but the manifestations and the effector elements to mount the attack are different. Perhaps an appropriate operational definition should be as follows: Rejection is the process by means of which an organism will recognize and eliminate foreign tissue. This definition is ample enough to include all organisms, and is

* The author is grateful to Drs. David Sutherland and Charles Morrow for contributing part of the sections on blood transfusions, antigen-specific immunosuppression, tissue culture and donor pretreatment.
This work was supported in part by NIH Grant No. RR 08102.

based on the concepts of a recognizing system, specificity, self, and for-eignness.

One important aspect of rejection is the generality with which it is found in other species. Vertebrates present a fairly homogeneous and constant picture, in which the elements involved consist of lymphocyte-mediated damage to the organ. The classical works of Medawar (1) in the forties and subsequently of Brent (2), and Billingham and others (3–5) gradually focused on the importance of lymphatics and lymphocytes as somehow involved in tissue rejection of vertebrates. An important contribution was made in the sixties by Najarian and Feldman when they passively transferred transplan-tation immunity (6, 7) and contact sensitivity (8) with lymphoid cells. This further proved the key role of lymphocytes in rejection in mammals. Sub-sequent studies showed that a humoral component was present too, but further clarification of the respective contributions of cells and antibodies to rejection had to wait several more years.

Rejection phenomena have been observed not only in mammals but in other vertebrates such as birds, reptiles, amphibians, and the bony fishes as well (9). The proportion of cellular to humoral components varies in these species, but the mechanisms are suspected to be similar, although modified during evolution (10).

An area of persistent controversy these days is whether invertebrates have an immune system akin to that of vertebrates (11, 12). Investigators have used transplantation of tissues as a tool to identify these aspects. It has been clear from recent studies that even though the mechanisms may vary, the principle of rejection seems to exist in invertebrates as well. For example, arthropods will *reject* transplanted cells by a mechanism of cell palisading, encapsulation, and necrosis (13). Whether the cells involved are precursors of our lymphoid tissues is not clear, but the end point of the transplantation phenomenon is the same. Annelids reject tissue from different species, but rejection of skin from the same species is weaker and slow to occur. Perhaps the most surprising example of rejection is that found in sponges (14). Sponges will reject tissues from different species of sponges but will readily accept tissues of the same species. Species incompatibility in sponges does not appear to involve any cell damage or killing, perhaps it is just a failure to establish contact. This phenomenon can also be observed in corals in which polyps of the same species readily fuse with each other and form a colony system, whereas different species avoid each other and never establish contact. A discussion of invertebrate immunity is outside the scope of this chapter. It should be remembered, however, that even in invertebrates there are mechanisms of recognition of self and foreignness which are critical in initiating whatever reactions are responsible for the nonacceptance or non-union of foreign tissue (15, 16).

One fascinating discovery of the last 30 years has been the detection of areas in the body which appear to be somehow detached from everyday lymphocyte activity and traffic, in such a way that they appear to be—and have been so called—immunologically privileged sites: areas and tissues that do not elicit rejection, so that tissues implanted onto them will enjoy a prolonged survival. Excellent discussions of immunologically privileged sites which include the brain, testicles, the cheek pouch of the hamster, the cornea and the anterior chamber of the eye, the liver (in part), the uterus, and vascularized skin pedicles, have been published (17–20). It is not clear at this time just what makes a particular tissue invulnerable to the attack by immunocompetent cells but a favorite hypothesis takes into consideration the fact that there are few or no lymphatics draining these tissues, and that antigen is not transported into regional lymph nodes or the circulation, thus preventing sensitization. Nonetheless, a series of recent elegant experiments by Subba Rao (21, 22), using the anterior chamber of the eye, have demonstrated that there is systemic sensitization by grafts inserted into the anterior chamber of the eye, therefore other elements must be involved, and not only the absence of sensitization. It may be possible that this particular anatomical configuration permits a particular set of immunocompetent cells such as suppressor cells to be activated, and not the whole inducer-cytotoxic system.

Finally, we would like to introduce some important operational terms in order to make sure that confusion arising from the application of various names to the same phenomenon is cleared. There are several kinds of grafts. *Free grafts* are those that are transplanted on a suitably prepared tissue bed without the establishment of vascular anastomosis. Examples include skin and cornea. In the first, vascular ingrowth from the edges will nourish the tissue. In the second, nourishment from the aqueous humor of the anterior chamber of the eye will provide nutrition. A second type of graft is the *strut* or *support graft* in which the grafted tissue provides a scaffold for the penetration of autogenous normal tissue. Examples include fascia and bone. Finally, *vascularized grafts* are those in which formal vascular anastomoses are performed in order to provide blood irrigation, oxigenation, and nutrition into the tissues. All of these are solid organs such as the kidney, heart, lungs, pancreas, and liver.

It has been traditional to divide rejection into an *afferent limb* which includes antigen recognition, antigen processing, and antigen presentation; a *central part* which includes the concept of sensitization; and an *efferent limb* in which different mediators mount an offensive attack on the graft. Since so many steps and aspects are involved in each of these limbs, this classification has been abandoned for one in which the different elements of the process are identified.

Another system of classification is based on the rapidity with which the rejection reactions occurs. A *first set rejection* refers to the type of rejection observed when the antigen comes in contact for the first time with the host. It is also called acute rejection. A *second set rejection* involves the presence of immunological memory and is usually seen rapidly after the transplant. It is also called hyperacute rejection. *Chronic rejection* occurs when the rejection phenomenon takes a long time to develop and in which the end point is not well defined. We prefer to use a terminology based on the pathophysiology of rejection, rather than on the time of occurrence.

An *allograft* (allogeneic graft, homograft) is an intraspecies nonidentical graft. An *autograft* is a relocation of organ or tissue in an organism. A *xenograft* (xenogeneic graft, heterograft) is a graft between species: *concordant* if phylogenetically close, *discordant* if phylogenetically distant. An *isograft* (isogeneic graft) is a graft between individuals identical in histocompatibility antigens.

IMMUNOLOGY OF REJECTION

Rejection presupposes recognition of both self and foreignness. The system of recognition must be absolutely perfect in its discrimination and both sensitive and specific. Otherwise, either unnatural, unnecessary, or dangerous autoattack could occur, or the organism would be vulnerable to invasion by potentially dangerous microorganisms. The system must have the inherent ability of recognizing self in such a way that beneficial interactions and communications occur and sensitization-attack reactions are not triggered, while recognizing foreignness as a signal of invasion by noxious agents. All these interactions seem to reside in the cell membrane where couplings and uncouplings necessary for recognition take place. A major system of molecules involved in rejection or acceptance of grafted tissue are those molecular products of the highly polygenic major histocompatibility complex which, at least vertebrates seem to possess as a universal system. These products are present on the surface of all nucleated cells, although sometimes portions of the molecules may be recovered from the circulation and the body fluids. Two classes of molecules have been defined. Class I molecules are present in all nucleated cells (23, 24) and although one is tempted to see their function only as an element for cell-mediated killing of abnormal cells by immunocompetent lymphocytes (25), their biological function seems to be more general and important. It has been suggested that their function is not only that of being a passive receptor for the coupling of abnormal antigens to render the cells susceptible to attack by immunocompetent cells, but perhaps a necessary component involved in self recognition for the formation of tissues and organs, and for cellular communications (26, 27).

Class II molecules are present only in some immunocompetent cells and endothelia, and it has been suggested that their role is very important in the recognition of foreignness, and at the same time in the cell-to-cell interactions which are necessary for precise specific sensitization to take place and for regulation of immune responses (26, 28).

Class I and II molecules are the most important transplantation antigens because, regardless of their true biological function in real life, they are strongly antigenic and are easily recognized by the host as foreign. In addition to histocompatibility antigens, the most important transplantation antigens, there are other groups of antigens which are important in allograft rejection (23, 29–33). These include the ABO groups in man; the vastly polymorphic system of non-MHC histocompatibility antigens found in the rat and in the mouse (these are called *minor* histocompatibility antigens or *minor* transplantation antigens); the Lewis and heterophile antigen systems in man; the vascular endothelium antigens; and the organ-specific antigens found in the different organs. Characteristics of the major and minor histocompatibility complexes are discussed in detail in other chapters.

In recent years the development and maturation of immunocompetent cells has been gradually clarified (34–45) (Fig. 4.1). *Stem* cells apparently give rise to a population of pre-T cells which upon passage and residence inside the fetal thymus, acquire a series of surface markers which are apparently related to stages in their internal maturation. Mature cells spill into the circulation and gradually populate the spleen, lymph nodes, and other peripheral areas. Pre-B cells home into the bone marrow or mammalian

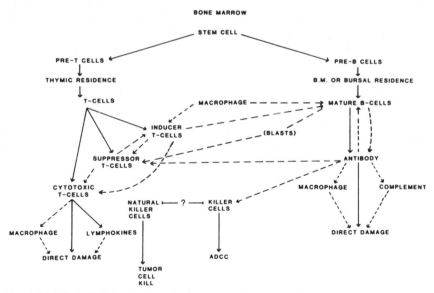

Fig. 4.1. Cell-to-Cell Interactions During An Immune Response. Solid arrows signify *give rise or origin to* →, while broken arrows mean *interrelations or interactions with, or effect upon* - - -→.

liver or, in birds, to the Bursa of Fabricius, and here they acquire their surface markers which are immunoglobulin molecules. Mature B cells then flow into the circulation and home into the peripheral lymphoid tissues. The immunoregulatory role of the spleen and thymus, both during maturation and in the differentiated state, are known (42, 45, 46).

It seems that the key element for initiation of immunological events, sensitization, and rejection is a highly complex but beautifully harmonious series of cell-to-cell interactions (39, 40, 45, 47, 48–51). The macrophage is the initial cell to come in contact with the relevant antigen and by still undefined processes, modifies the antigen in such a way that relevant epitopes or antigenic elements are presented in its surface probably coupled to class II molecules (in the human, the DR system; in mice, the I-a molecules) and interact in close proximity, possibly in contact with the population of T cells which is in charge of initiating cellular and humoral events. This *inducer* T cell has specific surface markers: in the mouse it is the LY-1 positive cell, and in man it is the T134 cell. Close proximity, or even physical contact, is necessary for these cells to receive a specific message (52), although nonspecific messages may be obtained at a distance suggesting the presence of additional cofactors necessary in this initial transaction. The inducer cell, in close proximity to the mature B cell and possibly with the help of the macrophage and/or one of its factors (see interleukin, below), will induce a specific message for antibody production. These cells undergo a series of internal changes including increased synthesis of DNA, the appearance and hectic activity of mitochondria, emergence of smooth and rough endoplastic reticulum, and Golgi apparatus, all for the increased synthesis of proteins which soon will take place (53). Antibodies are produced and they are part of the effector system of rejection. Antibodies have several cybernetic systems for the switching off of antibody production so that antibody does not continue to be produced in excess (54–56). These include the detection of free antibodies by the producing B cell, the production of antiidiotypic antibodies directed against the antibody binding site of the antibody molecule, and the detection of free antibodies by *suppressor* T cells, which apparently trigger a signal directed to the inducer T cell to stop its positive effect on the mature B cell. Suppressor T cell in the mouse pertains to the LY-2,3 subset which is also carried by the cytotoxic-activity cell. In man, the effector-suppressor and cytotoxic cell carry the subtype T5/8 as defined by monoclonal antibodies. It is not clear at this time whether suppressor T cell act directly on mature B cell or by switching off inducer T cell.

A third population of T cell, the effector *cytotoxic* T cell, is the one in charge of mounting a direct offensive attack on the transplanted organ. Again the exact mechanism is not clear, but the action of cytotoxic T cells seems to be mediated by a variety of secreted humoral factors which either

Table 4.1. Lymphokines

I. Attractants (chemotaxis):
  A. For Macrophages
  B. For Lymphocytes
  C. For Eosinophils
  D. For Polymorphonuclears
  E. For Basophils
II. Inhibitors of Movement:
  A. Migration (macrophage) Inhibition Factor (MIF)
  B. Lymphocyte (migration) Inhibitory Factor (LIF)
III. Activators, Instruction Molecules & Effectors:
  A. Macrophage Activating Factor (MAF)
  B. Specific Macrophage Arming Factor (SMAF)
  C. Transfer Factor
  D. Immune RNA
  E. (Interferon)
  F. Blastogenic Factor
  G. Mitogenic Factor
  H. Lymphotoxin (s)
  I. (Immunoglobulins)
  J. Skin Reactive Factor
  K. Helper Factors
  L. Suppressing Factors

do damage directly or recruit other populations of cells to participate in the attack. The substances, called *lymphokines*, are divided into three categories as shown in Table 4.1. There are molecules which, by the generation of a chemotactic gradient, attract other cells into the zone of battle. There are cells that stop the random rapid movement of mononuclear cells and lymphocytes. Finally there are the instructional molecules which order or instruct these immobile cells to grow, multiply, and attack, both specifically and nonspecifically (57–61). Other substances are directly cytotoxic.

More recently, a number of new substances dealing with cell-to-cell interaction have been recognized and baptized as *interleukins*. It is not clear at the time of this writing whether they encompass some of the functions of the lymphokines described above, or whether they are a separate set of molecules which have to deal more with cell-to-cell interaction and the induction of immunity rather than with the final phases of effector damage (62). For example, interleukin I is a substance(s) produced by macrophages which has an effect on fibroblasts, hepatocytes, the brain (as the endogenous pyrogen), polymorphonuclear leukocytes, keratinocytes, LY + 2 cells, and enhances antibody response (63). Interleukin II is the T-cell growth factor which was first observed in preconditioned media. It augments NK-mediated lysis and NK replication. It is needed for B cells to convert into an antibody-secreting cell and is possibly produced in inducer T cells. More recently an Interleukin III is emerging, which apparently originates from activated T cells and induces differentiation of 20 alpha steroid dehydrogenase, a marker of maturation of cytotoxic mature cell lines. The exact role of these elements in the overall strategy of attack by the immune system is not clear. They appear to participate as essential elements of nonspecific biological amplification and cell-to-cell interactions.

Another set of molecules which may have an effect on the final aspects of organ and tissue destruction by rejection are the recently discovered *leukotrienes* (64) and the tromboxanes. These could appear late in rejection, acting in a nonspecific manner, and help to explain the final cell and vascular disruptions which occur in uncontrolled rejection.

The role of *killer* cells is well known in tumor systems. Killer cells are also known as *null* cells because of the sparcity of detectable surface markers on their surface. Specific antibodies bind to them and are responsible for the reaction known as Antibody-Dependent Cell-Mediated Cytotoxicity (ADCC). It appears to be one important mechanism of specific damage to autogeneous tumors. Another population of mononuclear cells known as *natural killer* (NK) cells, which is possibly distinct from the killer cells involved in ADCC, is responsible for tumor cell kill and other aspects of natural immunity (65,66). Their role in kidney transplantation is discussed in a separate chapter.

Thus, once sensitized as shown above, the system amplifies the immune response by several mechanisms. Antibody damage is amplified by the recruitment of cells which produce vasoactive and cytolytic substances. The activation of complement also amplifies some immune rejection phenomena. Cell-mediated damage is amplified through the lymphokines which augment the response both specifically and nonspecifically. The actual damage is brought about by cytotoxins produced by lymphocytes and other recruited cells. Like antibody diversity, heterogeneity has been found to occur in mononuclear cells. Whether this heterogeneity goes parallel and is clonally related as is the heterogeneity of antibody-forming cells is not known and will probably be determined once the appropriate receptors are discovered in T, K, and NK cells. Heterogeneity is suspected because of the variety of markers and responses and receptors to different substances, found in subsets of cells. It is envisioned that these surface differences translate themselves into different functions. The picture that is emerging is one of great complexity in which there is an exquisite control and delicate balance between suppressing and cytotoxic factors.

The discovery of suppressor elements in the control of immunity revolutionized our concepts of immune regulation, tolerance, enhancement, autoimmune disease, pregnancy, cancer, and graft acceptance. The new paradigm is based around the suppressor T cell which probably through specific and nonspecific factors controls antibody and cytotoxic cell activity. It is not clear whether there is a direct effect bearing upon cytotoxic and mature B cells, or whether the loop is only by inactivating inducer cells, or by facilitating the production of blocking factors.

PATHOLOGY OF REJECTION

That there is great resemblance between the cells infiltrating a transplanted organ and the cells found in areas where delayed hypersensitivity reactions are taking place suggests that both are aspects of the single phenomenon of cell-mediated immunity. In both there are mononuclear cells involved although recent studies have shown that monocytes predominate in the delayed hypersensitivity reaction and lymphocytes predominate in the allograft rejection response.

From a pathophysiological point of view, we can divide the rejection phenomenon as occurring under three different circumstances, with three different mechanisms, and with different histological and clinical patterns.

Traditional rejection, also called *first set rejection* or acute rejection, usually occurs early after transplantation (from 7 to 15 days in the unmodified host); the name *acute* stems from the fact that the onset is usually abrupt and sudden. It is usually accompanied by systemic symptoms including fever, cardiovascular changes, and a prompt diminution of organ function. In the case of the skin, there is visible swelling and vascular redistribution. In vascularized organs, of which the kidney has been best studied, one of the earliest changes is the accumulation of mononuclear cells inside the capillaries of the transplanted organ. From that location, we suspect that they are gradually recognizing the foreignness that they have been ordered to attack. Sensitization is presumed to have already occurred by this time. Lymphocytes then traverse the capillary wall and migrate into the interstices around the blood vessels forming the typical perivascular cuffing of lymphocytes. It is suspected that by this stage, lymphokines are released which attract the other elements which eventually results in an explosive multiplication of cells (67–77). In nontreated rejection episodes one will observe a massive accumulation of lymphocytes in the interstices of the organ, with pronounced edema and eventually with perivascular hemorrhages and cellular necrosis. Late changes would include thrombosis of the blood vessels and massive necrosis of the whole organ. Acute rejection is basically a cell-mediated phenomenon but antibodies (29, 76, 78, 79) directed against the class I and class II products (70) basement membrane, endothelia (74), the tubular basement membrane, cryoprecipitins, anti-DNA antibodies, and antismooth muscle antibodies have been identified during these rejections. Deposits of IgG, IgA, C3 and fibrinogen are frequently observed (68, 69).

Second set rejection presupposes presensitization. This may occur by receiving a previous transplant with similar histogenetic characteristics, with previous pregnancies, or with blood transfusions. The mechanism involved encompasses humoral antibodies and specific memory B cells, and it is akin to the anamnestic humoral response. As soon as vascular anastomoses are performed in a vascularized organ, circulating antibodies immediately recognize determinants in the endothelium of the transplanted organ and bind to these determinants. These cytophilic antibodies activate complement (80–82) and the coagulation cascade. There is rapid and massive activation of complement and coagulation. Complement, through factors C3 and C5 induce or produce anaphylotoxin and induce histamine release from PMN cells called by chemotaxis into the area. This produces vasodilatation and increased permeability of the capillary wall with resulting stagnation and edema formation. Stagnation plus activation of coagulation produces minuscule clots in the capillaries, which rapidly propagate to larger vessels. This produces ischemia, hypoxia, and acidosis. Acidosis and ischemia temporarily convert cellular metabolism into anaerobic glycolysis, but since the conditions are unchanged, the cell membrane sodium potassium pump promptly becomes inactive, and there is massive influx of sodium and water into the cell resulting in cell swelling. Ischemia progresses and the acidosis and changes in permeability of membrane induce the release of lysosomal enzymes which are the end point of the process resulting in tissue necrosis (83, 84). Histologically we will observe edema, interstitial hemorrhages, the presence of polymorphonuclear cells, fibrin and red blood cell intravascular clots, and using indirect immunofluorescence, there is a massive deposition of antibody and complement in the vessel wall and of fibrin inside the vessels and in the interstitium (76, 85).

This process is sudden, massive, and irreversible. It usually occurs between 10 minutes and 12 hours after implantation of the organ (85). Occasionally, in a modified immunosuppressed host it may be seen up to 24 hours after implantation. In the clinical situation the only treatment is removal of the organ since localized intravascular coagulation and tissue necrosis will invariably induce a disseminated consumption coagulopathy, as well as release of a variety of toxic vasoactive factors which result in severe cardiovascular instability.

In recent years an *accelerated type of rejection* has been described consisting of rapid loss of function 3 to 5 days after kidney transplantation. Clinical picture is marked by rapid oliguria, fever, systemic toxicity, and rapid loss of kidney function. Examination usually shows a massive infiltration with lymphocytes and polymorphonuclears but repeated testing of the sera to detect preformed antibodies usually yields negative results. This type of accelerated rejection is associated with high pretransplant mixed lymphocyte culture values and there is consensus that it reflects a cellular type of sensitization with resulting *hyperacute* cellular rejection. It is standard practice now to perform pretransplant mixed lymphocyte culture before performing living related transplantation, and either exclude a positive donor, or immunologically modify the recipient who has high stimulation in mixed lymphocyte culture.

Chronic rejection reflects a state of partial acceptance of the graft. In chronic rejection there is the presence of humoral cytotoxic antibodies (86, 87) in small quantities, enough to produce intimal damage but not enough to induce catastrophic hyperacute rejection. It is suspected that these humoral antibodies damage the intima and, as a result, the normal reparative mechanisms of intimal proliferation are put into effect. Nonetheless, since there is constant, repeated reaction, excessive proliferation occurs (71) with damage to blood vessels and glomeruli (69, 87, 88). This results in gradual distal ischemia which in turn produces chronic necrosis and repair with fibroblastic proliferation and collagen deposition. In essence, one is observing damage produced by the normal reparative mechanisms of the organ and a parallelism with liver cirrhosis comes to mind. The end result of this type of rejection is a contracted, scarred organ in which most of the interstitium has been replaced by massive collagen deposition, and the lumina of blood vessels obliterated by unchecked intimal proliferation. The loss of function is gradual and clinical hallmarks include progressive hypertension, proteinuria which in some cases may progress to a nephrotic syndrome, and a gradual but relentless loss of renal function. As in the case of hyperacute rejection, chronic rejection has no treatment and a futile attempt to correct function with increased immunosuppression is dangerous and may be lethal.

MODIFICATION AND PREVENTION OF REJECTION

Antigen Specific Immunosuppression

Antigen specific immunosuppression selectively depresses the action of lymphocyte clones against an allografted organ. This action against the histocompatibility antigens of the donor graft may be active (the recipient is treated with donor histocompatibility antigens) or passive (the recipient is treated with antibodies against the donor antigens). Passive enhancement is reported to have a weak effect in the skin allograft model (89), a stronger effect in rat renal allograft models (90), and overall is considered a relatively weak form of antigen specific immunosuppression (91). Passive enhancement can be achieved by antibodies to either Ia (92) or SD (93) antigens. The mechanisms are postulated to include an arrest of the recipients IgM and especially IgG cytotoxic antibody response directed to graft antigens. F (ab')2 fragments in themselves have been ineffective (94). Besides this humoral effect, a delay in the generation of cytotoxic T cells is also present (95). Currently several problems concerning passive enhancement preclude its wide clinical use. The risk of hyperacute rejection as well as the quantity and type of appropriate anti-serum needed require further study in animal experiments.

Active enhancement, although a stronger form of antigen-specific immunosuppression than passive enhancement, risks sensitization of the host. Nonetheless, the beneficial effects of blood transfusions and successful experimental protocols with ALS and donor marrow (96) as well as TLI and allogeneic marrow (97) demonstrate the efficacy of active enhancement.

Allograft tolerance, as first demonstrated in the classic experiments of Medewar, can be defined as a loss of immunologic response brought about by treatment with antigen. Explanations of immunologic tolerance have included clonal deletion of antigen reactive cells (98), suppression by T cells (T suppressor cells) (99, 100), and antiidiotypic immunization (101, 102). Currently the action of suppressor T cells in all models tested is so everpresent that it must be considered as a most important factor in specific unresponsiveness (103–105). The factors which determine suppressor cell activation are not known with certainty, although the route of administration, the host immune status, and the physical state of the antigens are important (106, 107).

Dizygotic cattle, an example of tolerance found in nature, share placental circulation and develop hematological chimerism (108), tolerating subsequent organ allografts. Induction of tolerance has required different protocols in the neonate and adult. Experimentally, neonatally-induced tolerance is brought about by injecting newborn mice with lymphocytic cells. These same mice when adults accept skin grafts from the tolerance-inducing strain.

Adult immune tolerance has required more stringent experimental designs, with special detail to dose, physical state, and timing of antigens. It has often relied on the simultaneous administration of nonspecific immunosuppressive agents. Tolerance in the adult is more easily produced to weak antigens and may be related to antigen blocking by antibodies.

Antiidiotypic antibodies, by binding to B- or T-cell idiotypes, have been implicated in immunologic tolerance induction (109—111). Antiidiotypic immunization has prolonged rat renal allograft survival (112) and in *in vitro* systems inhibits measurements of cell-mediated immunity (CML and MLC). Nonetheless, their exact role in immunologic tolerance is not clearly defined.

Reduction of Graft Immunogenicity: Tissue Culture

Tissue or organ culture prior to transplantation has been reported to prolong allograft survival of thyroid (113), ovary (114), parathyroid (115), and pancreatic islets (116). It is postulated that donor leukocytes transplanted with the graft are important in recipient sensitization to foreign antigens. Culture is hypothesized to deplete tissue or organ allografts of passenger leukocytes and effect reduced graft immunogenicity. Alternatively, organ culture may reduce the concentration of cell surface antigens. *In vitro* evidence for the reduced passenger leukocyte hypothesis is provided by Terasaki and Opelz (116, 116a) who showed that lymphocytes cultured for more than 40 days (22°C) lost their ability to stimulate lymphocytes in mixed lymphocyte culture (MLC). Similarly, the significant prolongation of thyroid and islet allografts, after culture, is abrogated by the administration of donor leukocytes after transplanation (117).

Reduction of Graft Antigenicity: Donor Pretreatment

Interest in donor pretreatment to prevent subsequent allograft rejection began in 1967 when Guttman (118) reported prolonged survival of rat renal allografts after pretreatment with ATS. Donor pretreatment with cytotoxic drugs led to comparable results (119). Extension of these findings to man has led to conflicting results. Some authors have noted prolonged survival of unmatched cadaver kidney transplants after donor pretreatment with cyclophosphamide and methylprednisolone, while others have noted no effect (120).

The beneficial effect of donor pretreatment has been attributed to several theoretic actions. Transplantation of drugs or drug metabolites in low concentrations thus inhibiting stimulated host lymphocytes may play a role. Also, alteration or depletion of passenger leukocytes may be important: this hypothesis is currently in favor. Finally, donor pretreatment may physically alter the immunogenicity of allografts by action on antigenic determinants.

Antigen Masking or Modification

For a while in vogue, efforts directed at altering transplantation antigens have been partially and inconsistently successful (121). Basically, these techniques consisted of incubating, washing, or otherwise placing certain substances in contact with the graft to be transplanted. It was hoped that a sufficiently permanent coupling would occur with the antigens so as to mask them and render them unavailable for host lymphocyte detection. Typical substances used included ALG (122), phytomitogens (123), Con-A (124), glutaraldehyde (125), chlorphenesin (126), and enzymes (127). The results are variable and the question of organ toxicity must be considered. Some of these methods have been used to achieve the opposite effect, that is, increased antigenicity for the preparation of tumor vaccines (124).

Immunologically Privileged Sites

Besides their potential as protected sites for allotransplantation, immunologists have studied immunoprivileged sites to establish the basic mechanisms of rejection. Naturally occurring privileged sites include the anterior chamber of the eye and the cheek pouch of the hamster. Both of these are characterized by the absence of lymphatic drainage. Similarly intercerebral, prostatic, and testicular tissue have all been studied as areas of poor lymphatic supply and have demonstrated some success in certain experimental allograft models. Privileged sites have also been created by raising alymphatic skin flaps and clearing mammary fat pads. The liver itself, to a lesser extent than the above examples, has been considered as a privileged site. Skin grafts and parathyroid allografts have been shown to have prolonged survival after transplantation to the liver over other sites. Also of interest, liver allografts in man seldom exhibit hyperacute rejection and rarely fail due to chronic rejection.

Blood Transfusions

Although the survival rate of cadaveric renal allografts in patients who have received pretransplant blood transfusions is higher than in those patients who have not (128), the exact mechanism remains unclear. The beneficial effect of random (129) as well as donor specific (130) transfusions in living related renal transplants has been demonstrated. Also of interest, a potentiating effect of blood transfusion and donor-recipient matching on graft survival has been reported in experimental and clinical trials (131). Because of the controversy regarding mechanism, questions remain concerning the optimal type (fresh vs. packed cells vs. HLA donor specific), number, and timing of transfusions. It is generally agreed that peroperative transfusions have no effect although some reports have shown the contrary (132).

The mechanism of pretransplant blood transfusions has been attributed in part to the induction of some degree of unresponsiveness. Since patients who receive just frozen or filtered blood from which the leukocytes have been removed do not seem to benefit, the leukocyte has been implicated in the possible production of enhancing antibodies. Alternatively, transient macrophage blockade by transfused erythrocytes or erythrocyte fragments has been suggested (133). Finally, a nonspecific increase in T suppressor cells has been found in dialysis patients 3 weeks after blood transfusions (134).

Another explanation of the beneficial effects of pretransplantation blood transfusions is selection. Patients who become highly reactive and sensitized after multiple transfusions remain on cadaver kidney recipient lists for prolonged periods due to the inability to find suitable crossmatch negative donors and become virtually untransplantable (135). This selection favors a less reactive population with better prognosis. Sensitization ranges from 3% in random transfused patients (136) to 33% in deliberate donor-specific transfusions for high-MLC recipients (137).

Immunosuppression

In spite of the ingenuity and zest evident from the foregoing comments, clinical success has occurred so far only with immunosuppressive techniques. Unfortunately, we still do not have an ideal (specific and nontoxic) drug, and all drugs and techniques are fraught with multiple biochemical and biological effects (138). Chemical mutagens (139) are the most complex and the most frequently used, in spite of their mutagenicity, carcinogenicity, or even lethality if used injudiciously. A point has been made regarding the multiplicity of effects of these drugs (140). It is convenient to state that drugs and techniques to modify the immune response are given either prophylactically to prevent rejection and/or therapeutically in the treatment of rejection episodes. The evolution of the application and use of these techniques clinically has been lucidly reported by Groth (141).

Radiation was the first technique used in the late 1950s, as *total body irradiation*. Soon it was discovered, however, that the severe bone-marrow toxicity was too high a price to pay and it was abandoned. Rapaport (142) has successfully achieved chimerism by total body irradiation and bone-marrow transplantation in dogs. Use in humans has been limited. Another approach has been the *extracorporeal irradiation* of recipient blood via an external arteriovenous cannula, but this did not gain widespread use. The *irradiation of the transplanted kidney* either prophylactically or during rejection is also used with variable results.

A more recent, and apparently successful, method has been the irradiation of all lymphoid tissue of neck, mediastinum, axillae, retroperitoneaum, and groins, the so-called *Total Lymphoid Irradiation* (TLI). This has met with success in mice, dogs, monkeys, and humans (143–146) and is currently undergoing formal clinical trials (147).

Another approach for pretransplant lymphocyte depletion has been the cannulation and *drainage of the thoracic duct*. Although successful in improving results (148–150) it is cumbersome, uncomfortable, and needs much attention to detail.

Although initially results were variable and skepticism was frequent, the use of *antilymphocyte serum* or more purified globulins has eventually proven successful as an adjuvant in human transplantation, both prophylactically and during rejection treatment (151–160). With the development of *monoclonal antibodies* against lymphocyte subsets, still another approach is possible, and initial limited clinical trials demonstrate promising results.

Steroids are the mainstay of therapy in transplantation. When the general and specific complications of these preparations became evident, every conceivable effort was made to do without them, to no avail. They have multiple immunological and non-immunological effects and it is difficult to define which is *the* main immunosuppressive effect (140). Nonetheless, so far we cannot do without it. A most judicious use is important including the use of the smallest tolerable dose, the use of other adjuvantic drugs, the use of alternate day therapy if possible, the treatment of only two and occasionally three rejection episodes, etc.

Azathioprine is an antimetabolite used by virtually all transplant centers although its value has been questioned. It competes with normal purines in DNA synthesis and forms bizarre DNA in replicating cells which presumably renders them inoperant or nonviable. Although with a different mechanism of action, the alkylating agent *cyclophosphamide* has been successfully used to substitute azathioprine.

Finally, *Cyclosporin-A*, a most interesting drug, has made its appearance in transplantation therapeutics. A fungal metabolite, it is potently immunosuppressive (161, 162) without causing myelosuppression, it may have an element of specificity, its renal toxicity can be controlled, and it has improved transplantation results significantly while at the same time diminishing the effort, energy, and cost of transplant programs. It may act by affecting, killing, or otherwise interfering with the action of inducer T cells (163). Experimental organ transplantation studies in the rat (164), rabbit (165), dog (166), pig (167), and nonhuman primate (168) have demonstrated the potent influence of cyclosporin-A in preventing acute allograft rejection. Calne (167) initiated a clinical trial using cyclosporin-A as the sole immunosuppressive agent in renal transplantation. Rejection prophylaxis did occur. But severe nephrotoxicity was responsible for a high incidence of nonfunctioning grafts. Starzl et al. (169) used a combination of decreased dose of cyclosporin-A followed by corticosteroids and reported a decrease in nephrotoxicity. At the University of Minnesota Hospital, a pilot study of 12 renal allografts was performed using cyclosporin-A combined with prednisone. There were no grafts lost to rejection. In a prospective randomized trial the same group has reported recently (170) that combination of cyclosporin-A plus prednisone provides an excellent alternative immunosuppressive regimen for renal transplants as compared with conventional therapy. With the introduction of cyclosporin-A in transplantation therapeutics, the subject of transplantation has received a new impetus. The initial promise will definitely lead to many more investigations to delineate its exact role in clinical transplantation.

SUMMARY

Rejection does not occur in nature to prevent organ transplantation in humans. Could it be a vestige of earlier systems which prevented fusion of histogenetically disparate organisms, such as occurs in primitive invertebrates? I do not think such is the case because rejection has increased in complexity, sensitivity, discrimination, and magnitude during evolution, where direct fusion of metazoal colonies is not an observable reality anymore. Could it be an ontogenic protective system to destroy and eliminate deviant clones during morphogenesis and differentiation? I think not because, if anything, it would switch off in the adult and be more active in embryonic development, and it is the other way around.

Is rejection just an artifact of organ transplantation? It may well be just a highly magnified state of a normal response to the introduction of foreign cells: a system of defense against microorganisms and abnormal (cancer) cells. But the question of magnitude is still haunting. Rejection is a very strong reaction with a well-coordinated and precisely organized violent attack. It appears to display an excess capability. Perhaps it is related to the mass of tissue transplanted. Perhaps it would be the reaction elicited by tumors if given a chance during tumor growth.

Although the natural counterpart is still unclear, the study of rejection has given us insight and helped clarify one of the most fascinating systems of nature.

REFERENCES

1. Medawar, P. B., *J. Anat.* **78**:176, 1944.
2. Brent, L., *Prog. Allergy* **5**:271, 1958.
3. Billingham, R. E., Brent, L., Medawar, P. B., and Sparrow, E. M., *Proc. R. Soc. London (Biol.)* **143**:43, 1954.
4. Billingham, R. E., Brent, L., and Medawar, P. B. *Proc. R. Soc. London (Biol.)* **143**:58, 1954.
5. Barker, C. F., and Billingham, R. E., *Transplantation* **5**:962, 1967.
6. Najarian, J. S., and Feldman, J. D., *J. Exp. Med.* **115**:1083, 1962.
7. Najarian, J. S., and Feldman, J. D., *J. Exp. Med.* **117**:449, 1963.
8. Najarian, J. S., and Feldman, J. D., *J. Exp. Med.* **117**:775, 1963.
9. Manning, M. J., and Turner, R. J., *Comparative Immunobiology*, p. 62. New York: John Wiley and Sons, 1976.
10. Marchalonis, J. J., *Immunity in Evolution*. Cambridge, MA: Harvard University Press, 1977.
11. Hildemann, W. H., *Life Sci.* **14**:605, 1974.
12. Cooper, E. L. (Ed.), *Contemporary Topics in Immunobiology*. Vol. 4, *Invertebrate Immunology*. New York: Plenum Press, 1974.
13. Manning, M. J., and Turner, R. J., *Comparative Immunobiology*, p. 29. New York: John Wiley and Sons, 1976.
14. Bigger, C. H., Hildemann, W. H., Jokiel, P. I., and Johnston, I. S., *Transplantation* **31**:461, 1981.
15. Chorney, M. J., and Cheng, T. C., Discrimination of self and non self in invertebrates. In J. J. Marchalonis and N. Cohen (Eds.), *Contemporary Topics in Immunobiology*. Vol. 9, *Self/Non-Self Discrimination*, p. 37. New York: Plenum Press, 1980.
16. Hildemann, W. H., *Transplantation* **27**:1, 1979.
17. Ballantyne, D. L., and Converse, J. M., *Experimental Skin Grafts and Transplantation Immunity*. New York: Springer-Verlag, 1979.

18. Peer, L. A. (Ed.), *Transplantation of Tissues*. Baltimore: William and Wilkins Co., 1959.
19. Beer, A. E., and Billingham, R. E., *The Immunobiology of Mammalian Reproduction*. Englewood Cliffs, NJ: Prentice-Hall, 1976.
20. Calne, R. Y., Allografting in the pig. In R. Y. Calne (Ed.), *Immunological Aspects of Transplantation Surgery*, p. 296. New York: John Wiley and Sons, 1973.
21. Subba Rao, D. V., and Grogan, J. B., *Transplantation* **24**:377, 1977.
22. Subba Rao, D. V., and Grogan, J. B., *Cellular Immunol.* **33**:125, 1977.
23. Klein, J., *Biology of the Mouse Histocompatibility-2 Complex*. New York: Springer-Verlag, 1975.
24. Snell, G. D., *Science* **213**:172, 1981.
25. Zinkernagel, R. M., and Doherty, P. C., *J. Exp. Med.* **141**:1427, 1975.
26. Dausset, J., *Science* **213**:1469, 1981.
27. Dausset, J., and Contu, L., *Human Immunology* **1**:5, 1980.
28. Benacerraf, B., *Science* **212**:1229, 1981.
29. Russell, P. S., and Monaco, A. P., *The Biology of Tissue Transplantation*. Boston: Little, Brown and Co., 1964.
30. Krakauer, H., *Transplant. Proc.* **12**:147, 1980.
31. McDonald, J. C., Evans, M. T., and Jacobbi, L. M., *Surgery* **80**:14, 1976.
32. Gonzáles, Z., and Santiago-Delpín, E. A., *Relevant Factors in Skin Graft Survival in Mice*. In preparation.
33. Silvers, W. K., and Wachtel, S. S., *Science* **195**:956, 1978.
34. Owen, J. J. T., The origins and development of lymphocyte populations. In *Ontogeny of Acquired Immunity A Ciba Foundation Symposium*, p.35. New York: Elsevier/North Holland, 1972.
35. Stites, D. P., Wybran, J., Carr, M. C., and Fudenberg, H. H., Development of Cellular Immunocompetence in Man. In *Ontogeny of Acquired Immunity—A Ciba Foundation Symposium*, p. 113. New York: Elsevier/North Holland, 1972.
36. Cooper, M., B. Lymphocyte differentiation. In M. J. Hobart and I. McConnel (Eds.), *The Immune System*, p. 197. London: Blackwell Scientific, 1975.
37. McConnell, I., T & B lymphocytes. In M. J. Hobart and I. McConnell (Eds.), *The Immune System*, p. 98. London: Blackwell Scientific, 1975.
38. Cunningham, A. J., *Understanding Immunology*, p. 127. New York: Academic Press, 1978.
39. Janeway, C. A., Idiotypes, T-cell receptors, and T-B cooperation. In J. J. Marchalonis and N. Cohen (Eds.), *Contemporary Topics in Immunobiology*. Vol. 9, *Self/Non-Self Discrimination*, p. 171. New York: Plenum Press, 1980.
40. Marchalonis, J. J., Molecular interactions and recognition specificity of surface receptors. In J. J. Marchalonis and N. Cohen (Eds.), *Contemporary Topics in Immunobiology*. Vol. 9, *Self/Non-Self Discrimination*, p. 255. New York: Plenum Press, 1980.
41. Stites, D. P., and Caldwell, J. L., Phylogeny and ontogeny of the immune response. In H. H. Fudenberg, D. P. Stites, J. L. Caldwell and J. V. Wells (Eds.), *Basic and Clinical Immunology*, 2nd ed., p. 141. Los Altos, CA: Lange Medical Publications, 1978.
42. Battisto, J. R., Borek, F., and Bucsi, R. A., *Cellular Immunol.* **2**:627, 1977.
43. Brand, A., Gilmour, D. G., and Goldstein, G., *Science* **193**:319, 1976.
44. Perkins, W. D., Robson, L. C., and Schwarz, M. R., *Science* **188**:365, 1975.
45. Cantor, H., *Ann. Rev. Med.* **30**:269, 1979.
46. Llende, M., Santiago-Delpín, E. A., and Lavergne, J., *Immunobiological consequences of splenectomy*. In preparation.
47. Paul, W. E., and Benacerraf, B., *Science* **195**:1293, 1977.
48. Rowley, D. A., Köhler, H., and Cowan, J. D., An immunologic network. In J. J.

Marchalonis and N. Cohen (Eds.), *Contemporary Topics in Immunobiology*. Vol. 9, *Self/Non-Self Discrimination*, p. 205. New York: Plenum Press, 1980.

49. Burnet, F. M., *Immunology, Aging and Cancer*. San Francisco: W. H. Freeman and Co., 1976.
50. Mitchell, G. F., Mishell, R. I., and Herzenberg, L. A., Studies on the influence of T-cells in antibody production. In B. Amos (Ed.), *Progress in Immunology*, Vol. 1, p. 323. New York: Academic Press, 1971.
51. Ruben, L. N., and Edwards, B. F., Phylogeny of the emergence of T-B collaboration in humoral immunity. In J. J. Marchalonis and N. Cohen (Eds.), *Contemporary Topics in Immunobiology*. Vol. 9, *Self/Non-Self Discrimination*, p. 55. New York: Plenum Press, 1980.
52. Rajewsky, K., and Pohlit, H., Specificity of helper function. In B. Amos (Ed.), *Progress in Immunobiology*, Vol. 1, p. 337. New York: Academic Press, 1971.
53. Ford, W. L., Lymphoid cell kinetics in graft-versus-host reactions and allograft rejection. In R. Calne (Ed.), *Immunological Aspects of Transplantation Surgery*, p. 39. New York: John Wiley and Sons, 1973.
54. Bystryn, J. C., Schenkein, I., and Uhr, J. W., A model for the regulation of antibody synthesis by serum antibody. In B. Amos (Ed.), *Progress in Immunology*, Vol. 1, p. 627. New York: Academic Press, 1971.
55. Gershon, R. K., Orbach-Arbouys, S., and Calkins, C., B-cell signals which activate suppressor T-cells. In L. Brent and J. Holborow (Eds.), *Progress in Immunology*, Vol. 2, p. 123. New York: Elsevier/North Holland, 1974.
56. Fitch, F. W., and Sinclair, N. R., Antibody feedback mechanisms. In L. Brent and J. Holborow (Eds.), *Progress in Immunology*, Vol. 2, p. 358. New York: North Holland American Elsevier, 1974.
57. Valdimarsson, H., Effector mechanisms in cellular immunity. In M. J. Hobart and I. McConnell (Eds.), *The Immune System*, p. 179. London: Blackwell Scientific, 1975.
58. Lisafeld, B. A., Minowada, J., Klein, E., and Holterman, O. A., *Int. Archs. Allergy Appl. Immun.* 62:59, 1980.
59. Cohen, M. C., Picciano, P. T., Douglas, W. J., et al., *Science* 215:301, 1982.
60. Friedman, H. (Ed.), Subcellular Factors in Immunity. *Ann. N.Y. Acad. Sci.* 101:332, 1979.
61. Henson, P. M., Mechanisms of tissue injury produced by immunologic reactions. In J. A. Bellanti (Ed.), *Immunology*, Vol. 2, p. 292. Philadelphia: W. B. Saunders, 1978.
62. Watson, J. D., *Transplantation* 31:313, 1981.
63. Butler, R. C., Nowotny, A., and Friedman, H., *Ann. N.Y. Acad. Sci.* 332:564, 1979.
64. Marx, J. L., *Science* 215:1380, 1982.
65. Herberman, R. B., and Ortaldo, J. R., *Science* 214:24, 1981.
66. Herberman, R. B., *Natural Killer (NK) Cells, The Lymphocyte*, p.33. New York: Alan R. Liss, 1981.
67. Herbertson, B. M., The morphology of allograft reactions. In R. Calne (Ed.), *Immunological Aspects of Transplantation Surgery*, p. 4. New York: John Wiley and Sons, 1973.
68. Kries, H., Transplanted kidney: natural history. In J. Hamburger, J. Crosnier, J. F. Bach, and H. Kries (Eds.), *Renal Transplantation Theory and Practice*, p. 177. Baltimore: Williams and Wilkins, 1981.
69. Perez-Tamayo, R., Patología del rechazo. In E. A. Santiago-Delpín, O. Ruiz, and F. Chávez (Eds.), *Transplante de Organos*. Salvat, Mexico, In press.
70. Fabre, J. W., and Ting, A., Immunobiology of transplantation. In P. J. Morris (Ed.), *Kidney Transplantation: Principles and Practice*, p. 1. New York: Academic Press, 1979.

71. Magil, A., Rubin, J., Ladewig, L., et al., *Nephron* **26**:180, 1980.
72. Lafferty, K. J., and Woolnough, J., *Immunological Rev.* **35**:231, 1977.
73. Finkelstein, F. O., Siegel, N. J., Bastl, C., et al., *Kidney Int.* **10**:171, 1976.
74. Cerilli, J., Holliday, J. E., Fesperman, D. P., and Folger, M. R., *Surgery* **81**:132, 1977.
75. Jones, A. L., and Uldall, P. R., *Kidney Int.* **5**:378, 1974.
76. Najarian, J. S., and Foker, J. E., *Transplant. Proc.* **1**:184, 1969.
77. Pauly, J. L., Han, T., Varkarakis, M. J., et al., *J. Surg. Res.* **15**:301, 1973.
78. Najarian, J. S., and Perper, R. J., *Surgery* **62**:213, 1967.
79. Klassen, J., and Milgrom, F., *Transplantation* **8**:566, 1969.
80. Wartenberg, J., and Milgrom, F., *Transplant. Proc.* **11**:1407, 1979.
81. Buckingham, J. M., Geis, W. P., Giacchino, J. L., et al., *J. Surg. Res.* **27**:268, 1979.
82. Katz, J., and Lynne, C. M., *Anethesiology* **37**:440, 1972.
83. Santiago-Delpín, E. A., *Dialysis and Transplantation* **8**:802, 1979.
84. Santiago-Delpín, E. A., Pharmacological principles during organ harvesting. In L. H. Toledo-Pereyra (Ed.), *Organ Procurement and Preservation*. New York: Academic Press, 1982, p. 73.
85. Williams, G. M., *Transplant. Proc.* **6**:71, 1974.
86. Thomas, J. M., Thomas, F. T., Kaplan, A. M., and Lee, H. M., *Transplantation* **22**:94, 1976.
87. Pierce, J. C., Kay, S., and Lee, H. M., *Surgery* **78**:14, 1975.
88. Petersen, V. P., Olsen, T. S., Kissmeyer-Nielsen, F., et al., *Medicine* **54**:45, 1975.
89. Fabre, J. W., Specific immunosuppression. In J. R. Salaman: *Immunosuppressive Therapy*. Toronto: J. B. Lippncot Co., 1981.
90. Fabre, J. W., and Morris, P. J., *Transplantation* **19**:121, 1975.
91. Batchelor, J. R., *Transplantation* **26**:139, 1978.
92. Davies, D. A. L., and Staines, N. A., *Transplant. Rev.* **30**:18, 1976.
93. McKearn, P. J., Weiss, A., Stuart, P., et al., *Transplant. Proc.* **11**:932, 1979.
94. Winearls, C. G., Fabre, J. W., Millard, et al., *Transplantation* **28**:36, 1979.
95. Batchelor, J. R., *Transplant. Proc.* **13**:562, 1981.
96. Monaco, A. P., and Wood, M. L., *Transplant. Proc.* **13**:547, 1981.
97. Strober, S., King, D., Gottlieb, M. S., et al., *Transplant. Proc.* **13**:556, 1981.
98. Billingham, R. E., Brent, L., and Medawar, P.: *Proc. R. Soc. London (Biol.)* **145**:239, 1959.
99. Gruchalla, R.S., and Streilein, J. W., *Transplant Proc.* **13**:574, 1981.
100. Kilshaw, P. J., Brent, L., and Pinto, M., *Nature* **255**:489, 1975.
101. Brent, L., Brooks, O., Medawar, P., and Simpson, E., *Br. Med. Bull.* **32**:101, 1976.
102. Steinmuller, D., *Transplant. Proc.* **11**:1198, 1979
103. Ascher, N. L., Hoffman, R., Chen, S., and Simmons, R. L., *Surgery* **88**:274, 1980.
104. Marquet, R. L., Heystek, G.A., and Borleffs, J. C. C., *Transplant. Proc.* **13**:589, 1981.
105. Tutschka, P. J., Hess, A. D., Berschorner, W. E., and Santos, G.W., *Transplantation* **33**:510, 1982.
106. Golan, D. R., Borel, Y., *J. Exp. Med.* **134**:1046, 1971.
107. Nimelstein, S. H., Hotti, A. R., and Holman, H. R., *J. Exp. Med.* **138**:723, 1973.
108. Owen, R. D., *Science* **102**:400, 1945.
109. Consenza, H., and Kohler, H., *Proc. Natl. Acad. Sci.* **69**:2701, 1972.
110. Binz, H., and Wigzell, H., *Contemp. Top. Immunobiol.* **7**:113, 1977.
111. Binz, H., and Wigzell, H., *Transplant. Proc.* **11**:914, 1979.
112. Stuart, F. P., Scollard, D. M., McKearn, T. J., et al., *Transplantation* **22**:455, 1976.

108   Immunobiology of Transplantation, Cancer and Pregnancy

113. Lafferty, K. J., Bootes, A., Dart, G., and Talmadge, D. W., *Transplantation* **22**:138, 1976.
114. Jacobs, B. B., *Transplantation* **18**:454, 1974.
115. Starling, J. R., Fidler, R., and Corry, R. J., *Surgery* **81**:68, 1977.
116. Lacy, P. E., Davie, J. M., and Finke, E. H., *Science* **204**:312, 1979.
116a. Opelz, G., and Terasaki, P. I., *Science* **184**:464, 1976.
117. Lacy, P. E., Davie, J. M., and Finke, E. H., *Transplantation* **28**:415, 1979.
118. Guttman, R. D., Carpenter, C. B., Lindquist, R. R., et al., *J. Exp. Med.* **126**:1099, 1967.
119. Guttman, R. D., and Lindquist, R., *Transplantation* **8**:490, 1969.
120. Vij, D., and Toledo-Pereyra, L. H., *Dialysis and Transplantation* **9**:105, 1980.
121. Callender, C. O., and Toledo-Pereyra, L. H., *Dialysis and Transplantation* **9**:109, 1980.
122. Callender, C. O., Simmons, R. L., Toledo-Pereyra, L. H., et al., *Transplantation* **16**:377, 1973.
123. Toledo-Pereyra, L. H., Ray, P. K., Callender, C. O., et al., *Surgery* **76**:121, 1974.
124. Simmons, R. L., Rios, A., Toledo-Pereyra, L. H., and Steinmuller, D., *Am. J. Clin. Path.* **63**:714, 1975.
125. Santiago-Delpín, E. A., Yunis, E. J., Callender, C. O., and Najarian, J. S., *Proc. Soc. Exp. Biol. Med.* **141**:996, 1972.
126. Santiago-Delpín, E. A., Yunis, E., Callender, C. O., and Najarian, J.S., *Cell Immunol.* **5**:604, 1972.
127. Ray, P. K., and Simmons, R. L., *Proc. Soc. Exp. Biol. Med.* **142**:846, 1973.
128. Ramírez-Sanchez, J., and Santiago-Delpín, E. A., *Bul. Assoc. Med. P. Rico* **71**:261, 1979.
129. Van Rood, J. J., Balner, H., and Morris, P. J., *Transplantation* **26**:275, 1978.
130. Cochrum, K. C., Haines, D., Potter, D., et al., *Transplant. Proc.* **13**:1657, 1981.
131. Opelz, G., and Terasaki, P. I., *Transplantation* **29**:153, 1980.
132. Williams, K. A., Ting, A., French, M., et al., *Lancet* **1**:1104, 1980.
133. Keown, F.A., and Descamps, B. *Lancet* **1**:20, 1979.
134. Smith, M. D., Williams, J. D., Cole, C. A., et al., *Transplant. Proc.* **13**:181, 1981.
135. Cheigh, J. S., Fotino, M., and Stubenbord, W. T., *JAMA* **246**:135, 1981.
136. Opelz, G., Grauer, B., Mickey, M. R., et al., *Transplantation* **13**:177, 1981.
137. Salvatierra, O., Vincenti, F., and Amend, W., *Ann. Surg.* **192**:543, 1980.
138. Turk, J. L., A comparison of the multiplicity of the effect of immunosuppressive drugs with that of antilymphocytic serum. In A. Bertelli and A. P. Monaco (Eds.), *Pharmacological Treatment in Organ and Tissue Transplantation*, pp. 32–38. Baltimore: Williams and Wilkins Co., 1970.
139. Fishbein, L., Flamm, W. G., and Falk, H. L., *Chemical Mutagens*, Chap. 3. New York: Academic Press, 1970.
140. Santiago-Delpín, E. A., Immunosupressión clínica. In E. A. Santiago-Delpín, O. Ruiz and F. Chavez (Eds.), *Trasplante de Organos*. Salvat, Mexico, In press.
141. Groth, C. G., *Surg. Gynecol. Obstet.* **134**:323, 1972.
142. Rapaport, F. T., Lawrence, H. S., Bachvaroff, R., et al., *Transplant. Proc.* (Suppl. 1) **7**:367, 1975.
143. Slavin, S., Strober, S., Fuks, Z., et al., *J. Exp. Med.* **146**:34, 1977.
144. Strober, S., Gottlieb, M., Slavin, S., et al., *Transplant. Proc.* **12**:477, 1980.
145. Myburgh, J. A., Smit, J. A., Hill, R. R. H., et al., *Transplantation* **29**:405, 1980.
146. Gottlieb, M., Strober, S., Hoppe, R. T., et al., *Transplantation* **29**:487, 1980.
147. Najarian, J. S., Presented at Transplantation Society Congress, Boston, July 1980.
148. Walker, W. E., Niblack, G. D., Richie, R.E., et al., *Surg. Forum* **28**:316, 1977.

149. Richie, R.E., Niblack, G., Johnson, H. K., and Tallent, M. B., *Transplant. Proc.* **12**:483, 1980.
150. Starzl, T. E., Weil, R., Koep, L. J., et al., *Surg. Gynecol. Obstet.* **149**:815, 1979.
151. Starzl, T. E., Marchioro, T. L., Porter, K. A. et al., *Surg. Gynecol. Obstet.* **124**:301, 1967.
152. Monaco, A. P., Campion, J. P., and Kapnick, S. J., *Transplant. Proc.* **9**:1007, 1977.
153. Najarian, J. S., and Simmons, R. L., *New Engl. J. Med.* **285**:158, 1971.
154. Kountz, S. L., Butt, K. H. M., Roa, T. K. S., et al., *Transplant. Proc.* **9**:1023, 1978.
155. Launois, B., Campion, J. P., Fauchet, R., et al., *Transplant. Proc.* **9**:1027, 1977.
156. Mannick, J. A., Nabseth, D. C., Olsson, C. A., et al., *Transplant. Proc.* **4**:497, 1972.
157. Sheil, A. G. R., Mears, D., Kelly, G. E., et al., *Transplant. Proc.* **4**:501, 1972.
158. Simmons, R. L., Condie, R., and Najarian, J. S., *Transplant. Proc.* **4**:487, 1972.
159. Starzl, T. E., Groth, C. G., Kashiwagi, N., et al., *Transplant. Proc.* **4**:491, 1972.
160. Turcotte, J. G., Feduska, N. J., Haines, R. F., et al., *Arch Surg.* **106**:484, 1973.
161. Dunn, D. C., White, D. J. G., and Herbertson, B. M., *Transplantation* **29**:349, 1980.
162. Homan, W. P., Fabre, J. W., Williams, K. A., et al., *Transplantation* **29**:361, 1980.
163. Borel, J. F., *Transplant. Proc.* **12**:233, 1980.
164. Kostakis, A. F., White, D. J. G., and Calne, R. Y., *IRCS Med. Sci.* **5**:280, 1979.
165. Green, C. L., and Allison, A. C., *Lancet* **1**:1182, 1978.
166. Homan, W. P., French, M. E., Fabre, J. W., et al., *Transplant. Proc.* **12**:287, 1980.
167. Calne, R. Y., Rolles, K., White, D. J. G., et al., *Lancet* **2**:1033, 1979.
168. Reitz, B. A., Beiber, C. P., Raney, A. A., et al., *Transplant. Proc.* **13**:393, 1981.
169. Starzl, T. E., Weil, R., Iwatsuki, S., et al., *Surg. Gynecol. Obstet.* **151**:17, 1980.
170. Ferguson, R. M., Rynasiewicz, J. J., Sutherland, D. E. R., et al., *Surgery* **92**:175, 1982.

PART III
Immunobiology of Cancer—
A Phenomenon of Acceptance
of Non-Self

5

Tumor Antigens

Rishab K. Gupta and Donald L. Morton*

By definition the malignant tumor (cancer) cell is the progeny of a normal cell that has lost its cellular mechanisms for controlling proliferation. After malignant transformation, the tumor cell differs from a normal cell in a variety of ways which include: cytology, morphology, proliferative index, biochemistry, antigenic expression, etc. The concept that tumor cells possess specific antigens that are absent on their normal counterpart is the subject to be discussed in this chapter. It has become increasingly evident that these antigens are expressed on a variety of animal and human tumors, and many of these antigens are immunogenic in the individuals in which they arise.

In this chapter we attempt to review the pertinent literature in this area. Also, we attempt to review the characteristics of tumor antigens associated with animal and human tumors and to compare them with transplantation and pregnancy associated antigens. Neoplastic transformation may be viewed as dedifferentiation, that is, reversion of the normal cells to their primitive cell types. These primitive cells produce embryonal substances, such as fetal antigens, ectopic hormones, etc., that are normally absent, or present at low levels in the adult and are expressed by tumor cells. Focus is also directed to the dynamic aspect of the immune response to tumor antigens in the host and their role in surveillance, rejection, and enhancement of tumor growth.

CONCEPT OF TUMOR IMMUNITY

The idea that a tumor elicits an immune response in the host is not a new one. Investigators using randomly bred laboratory mice realized that strong immunity could be induced against transplanted rodent tumors in the early 1900s. As a result, intense laboratory and clinical investigations were un-

* We gratefully acknowledge the critiques and suggestions provided by Dr. Alistair J. Cochran during preparation of this manuscript and the editorial critique and assistance of Dr. P. K. Ray and Ms. E. Jane Shaw. This work was supported by USPHS Grants CA12582 and CA30019-X, by the Cancer Research Coordinating Committee of the University of California, by Armand Hammer Laboratories and John Wayne Clinic of the Division of Surgical Oncology, Jonsson Comprehensive Cancer Center, and by the Medical Research Service of the Veterans Administration.

dertaken anticipating that tumor immunity might lead to the control of malignant disease. It soon became obvious that the immunity against transplantable tumors was not due to tumor-specific antigens, rather it was due to normal transplantation antigens of the tumor. Therefore, interest in tumor-specific immunity subsided until the 1940s.

During the 1940s and 1950s several investigators demonstrated the phenomenon of tumor-specific immunity in chemically-induced tumors. Definitive and critical experiments to document the existence of tumor-specific antigens were performed by Prehn (1). Subsequently, Klein et al. (2) demonstrated tumor immunity in a mouse to its own 3-methylcholanthrene-induced sarcoma. Since these tumor-specific antigens can elicit tumor-specific immunity against tumor transplants in syngeneic animals, they are known as *tumor-specific transplantation antigens* (TSTA).

ANTIGENIC SPECIFICITY OF ANIMAL NEOPLASMS

The antigenic specificities of viral, chemical, and physical carcinogen-induced neoplasms have been found to be quite different.

Chemical-Carcinogen-Induced Neoplasms

It is generally believed that a tumor induced by a chemical carcinogen contains unique TSTA. These TSTA do not cross-react with tumors induced by the same chemical carcinogen in other members of the same syngeneic strain of mice. However, recently several investigators have reported the existence of shared antigens in chemically-induced animal tumors (3–5). Some of these reports were open to the alternative explanation that infection of the animal colony used in such studies by an endemic virus might have caused the appearance of shared antigens in chemically-induced tumors (6). Therefore, any challenge to the thesis that the *TSTA expressed by chemically-induced tumors are individually specific* must be made with *clean* colonies of experimental animals. However, Hellström et al. (4) suggested that chemically-induced tumors do express weak common TSTA in addition to the major strong TSTA. These weak antigens were different from murine leukemia virus (MuLV) antigens. Subsequently, Parker and Rosenberg (7) and Coggin et al. (5) reported that the weak common TSTA could be embryonic or fetal in origin. Induction of transplantation immunity against methylcholanthrene-induced tumors by fetal cells has been shown by Medawar and his co-workers (8).

The possibility of the existence of fetal or embryonic antigens on chemically-induced tumors was further suggested by Brawn (9), who showed inhibition of murine sarcoma colony formation by lymph node cells from multiparous mice. These observations were extended by Baldwin and his co-workers (10) in a microcytotoxicity test and membrane immunofluorescence. Secretion of α-fetoprotein (AFP), a glycoprotein present in normal embryonic serum but not in adult normal serum, by hepatomas induced by chemical carcinogens has been reported by Abelev el al. (11). Immunodiffusion studies revealed an immunologic similarity between the AFP in normal embryonic serum and in adult serum of animals with hepatomas, which suggested that chemical carcinogens caused the derepression of inactive gene coding for the synthesis of AFP that were active during embryogenesis.

Thus, at least two classes of antigens are expressed by chemically-induced animal tumors: one, the TSTA that are strongly immunogenic and that are involved in the rejection of tumor (these TSA are also described as *tumor rejection* (TR) *antigens*), and two, the fetal or embryonic antigens that are only occasionally demonstrable by transplantation techniques but which are readily detected by *in vitro* humoral and cellular reactions (7, 12).

The role of fetal or embryonic antigens in tumor transplant rejection may depend on the type of tumor and the species or strain of animal. Distinct differences in their ability to respond to fetal antigens between various strains of mice have been observed by Ting and Grant (13). Fetal antigens are often associated with rapidly dividing cell populations. Thus, their function in tumor immunity may be due to their role in cell differentiation rather than in the neoplastic process itself. Chemically-induced tumors may express several fetal antigens that are detectable by syngeneic or xenogeneic antisera (12). It has been reported that pregnancy in mice confers a degree of transplantation resistance against a chemically-induced syngeneic tumor and that certain membrane-expressed fetal antigens are operative in resistance against these tumors (14,15).

Several factors appear to affect the strength of the immunogenicity of TSTA on tumors induced by chemical and physical agents. Tumors appearing soon after carcinogen injection express stronger TSTA than those which develop after a longer latency period. It has also been observed that the stronger the dose of the carcinogen, the shorter the latency period for tumor induction (16). Tumors induced by chemical carcinogens express stronger TSTA than those induced by physical agents, such as urethane and cellophane films, and methylcholanthrene tumors induced in guinea pigs possess stronger TSTA than those induced in mice (1).

Viral Carcinogen-Induced Neoplasms

The presence of TSTA on tumor cells induced in mice by the polyoma virus was shown by Sjogren in 1961 (17). In contrast to the non-cross-reacting

TSTA of chemically-induced tumors, the TSTA expressed by oncogenic virus-induced tumors cross-react with any other tumor cells induced by the same virus (17). Subsequent experiments by other investigators confirmed this observation, and further showed that the cross-reacting TSTA on virus-induced tumors were independent of the histologic type of the tumors and of the species, but were dependent on the oncogenic virus (18). Minor cross-reacting TSTA of tumors induced by the Friend, Moloney, and Rauscher groups of RNA-viruses has been reported by Old and Boyse (19).

Richards (20) stated that when a virus induces tumor, the genetic material of the virus is incorporated into the genome of the host cell. This genetic material codes not only for cancer induction, but also for the induction of any immunity against the viral antigens. Some virally-induced tumors express unique *individual* antigens in addition to the common antigens (21). Virally-induced tumors are known to express fetal or embryonic antigens as well (22). Kato (23) observed that the cytotoxicity of an antiserum against SV-40 transformed hamster cells was eliminated by absorption with 11- to 12-day-old hamster embryos, but not by 13- to 15-day-old embryos. This was confirmed by Weppner and Coggin (24).

Three kinds of virus antigens have been described in virally-induced tumors: (a) virus envelop antigens, which may be group, subgroup, or type-specific; (b) virus structural antigens, which are present on the virion and in infected cells; and (c) virus-induced surface antigens, gross cell-surface antigens, TL antigens, etc. The antigenic strength of TSTA on tumors induced by viruses is comparable to that of those expressed by chemically-induced tumors, the spectrum of which ranges from no detectable antigenicity to very strong antigenicity. It has been reported by various investigators (25) that even in the minority of virus-induced tumors that are weakly antigenic, or nonantigenic, immunogenicity can be increased by further infection with oncogenic or nononcogenic viruses.

Spontaneous Neoplasms

Spontaneous or naturally occurring tumors are those that appear sporadically and infrequently in certain animal strains, e.g., leukemia in AKR mice and mammary adenocarcinoma in C3H mice. Those caused by vertical trans-mission of an oncogenic virus are not considered spontaneous tumors. Most artificially-induced tumors are strongly immunogenic, whereas, almost all spontaneous tumors are weakly immunogenic to nonimmunogenic (26). However, it must be realized that a few chemically-induced tumors are nonimmunogenic (1) and a rare spontaneous tumor is strongly immunogenic (27). Weakly antigenic spontaneous tumors do not appear to cross-react with other tumors (28).

Prehn (16) observed that tumors induced by low concentrations of methylcholanthrene possessed little or no immunogenicity. He then proposed that spontaneous tumors might arise because of exposure to low levels of carcinogens present in the environment. This proposition is consistent with the observation that human tumors express weak antigenicity and with the concept that 70 to 90% of cancers in man are induced by environmental factors (29).

EVIDENCE FOR TUMOR IMMUNITY
IN HUMAN NEOPLASMS

A number of clinical observations suggest that tumor immunity might exist in humans. Though alternative explanations, e.g., physiologic, biologic, and endocrinologic, could account for these clinical observations, an immunologic mechanism appears to be most probable (30).

There is a low incidence of successful autotransplants of human tumors even in patients with advanced cancer disease. Resistance was found to be relative rather than absolute, i.e., challenge with greater than 10^8 cells resulted in tumor growth. Similar limitations were observed in animal tumor transplant studies; a challenge with 10^5 tumor cells was rejected by the immune mice, whereas challenge with 10^6 to 10^7 resulted in progressive tumor growth. The immune nature of resistance to autotransplants in human cancer was described by Southam et al. (31), who showed that mixing of autologous leukocytes or plasma with the tumor cells stopped or slowed the growth of autotransplants in about half of the patients.

Spontaneous regression of human tumors, both primary and metastatic, though rare, has been well documented (32). Minor viral and bacterial infections, fever of unknown origin, and changes in hormonal balance appear to play a role in spontaneous regression of neoplasms (30). Complete regression with prolonged postoperative survival in patients with lung carcinoma after incomplete surgical resection has been reported by Abbey Smith (33). Spontaneous regression of small pulmonary metastates following excision of primary tumor has been observed and occurs most frequently in carcinoma of the kidney. Spontaneous regression of chemically-induced (34) and virally-induced (35) tumors has also been observed in laboratory animals.

In some patients, development of metastases histologically and functionally identical to the primary tumor has been noted 10 to 20 years after successful treatment of the primary. When these dormant metastates develop, they often grow rapidly. Delayed recurrence of the disease suggests a host defense which inhibits tumor growth during the disease-free interval.

Microscopic evidence of histiocytic, plasmacytic, lymphocytic, and eosinophillic infiltration of tumor tissues, which appears to be similar to that seen in an organ transplant or tumor transplant that is undergoing rejection, is associated with an improved prognosis. Infiltrates of lymphoid cells have been observed in malignant melanoma, gastric carcinoma, breast carcinoma, neuroblastoma, and Hodgkin's disease.

Griffiths and his colleagues (36) have identified tumor cells in the peripheral blood, lymphatics, pleural cavity, and operative wounds of patients, many of whom subsequently never developed metastases. These reports suggest that highly efficient mechanisms must exist for the destruction and containment of circulating tumor cells. The nature of such mechanisms is speculative, but the host immune defense may be one of them.

The incidence of certain cancers, e.g., neuroblastoma and carcinoma of thyroid and prostate, at postmortem has been found to be unexpectedly higher than would be expected on the basis of clinical incidence (37).

From the foregoing clinical observations it would appear that immune factors in the host play a key role in malignancy in humans. Autotransplant studies performed by Southam (31) provide the most direct evidence that humoral and cellular immunity may be responsible for destruction and containment of tumor in humans.

RECOGNITION OF HUMAN TUMOR ANTIGENS

Since transplantation techniques used in animal models were not applicable to man, the existence of tumor-specific antigens was investigated by skin tests and sensitive *in vitro* immunologic techniques. As a result, tumor-associated antigens (TAA), that are capable of inducing an immune response have now been found in most, if not all, human neoplasms.

In Vivo Cellular Reaction

Evidence for the presence of cellular immunity to TAA has been obtained by delayed cutaneous hypersensitivity reactions to tumor extracts, the skin window technique, and to a limited extent by allo- and autotransplant experiments.

Delayed Cutaneous Hypersensitivity Reaction (DCHR). The skin reaction to an antigen in an individual who has been sensitized to the antigen has been widely accepted as an indication of cell-mediated immunity. Using this method, existence of TAA has been demonstrated in a variety of human neoplasms.

It has been pointed out by Ristow and McKhann (38) that ideal conditions for testing the extracts in the patient who provided the tumor were generally not met, thus raising the possibility of false-positive or false-negative reactions. The results of the skin test depend on the antigenicity of the tumor and also on the capacity of the patient to respond to the tumor antigens.

Skin Window Technique. Black and Leis (39) modified the skin sensitivity test to study tumor-related cellular immunity in breast cancer patients. These investigators applied a cryostat section of autologous tumor tissue or benign breast disease to an abraded area of skin in patients with breast cancer. The tissue section was held in place with a coverslip. After appropriate time the coverslip was removed, fixed, stained, and examined microscopically for cellular exudate that had been evoked by the test tissue. They observed that early tumors caused a greater migration of cellular exudate than advanced tumors. Furthermore, macrophage and basophil reactions to autologous breast tumor sections was much higher than similar reactions to autologous nonmalignant breast tissue.

In Vitro Cellular Reactions

In vitro cellular assays were developed on the assumption that cell-mediated immunity to tumor antigens is the mechanism by which a host rejects its tumor. Some of the most widely used *in vitro* cellular assays are described in this subsection.

Lymphocytotoxicity. Three types of lymphocytotoxicity assays, namely: colony inhibition, long-term (20 to 72 hours) cytotoxicity, and short-term (4 to 8 hours) cytotoxicity, have been used to assess the presence of lymphocytes sensitized to tumor cells in cancer patients, in their close relatives, and in normal individuals.

The discovery of lymphocytes that are cytotoxic to autologous and allogeneic tumor cells of the same histologic type suggested the presence of group-specific tumor antigens. Avis et al. (40) have reported the occurrence of shared antigens between carcinomas and benign tumors. Lymphocytes from cancer patients were found to be cytotoxic to tumor cells of a different kind (41). These results suggest the existence of cross-reactive tumor antigens.

Lymphoblastogenesis. It is well recognized that when lymphocytes are exposed to an antigen or mitogen *in vitro*, they are stimulated to undergo blastogenesis. Autologous intact tumor cells or their extracts (stimulator) have been used to trigger blastogenesis of cancer patients' lymphocytes (responder) to detect the presence of tumor antigens. Lymphoblastogenesis has been shown with a wide variety of autologous tumor cells or their extracts. A good correlation between lymphoblastogenesis by autologous tumor cells or their extracts and DCHR has been observed (42).

It has been reported that lymphocytes from regional lymph nodes of patients with early disease but with no evidence of lymph node metastases respond better to tumor cells than peripheral blood leukocytes; on the other hand, lymphocytes from lymph nodes of patients with advanced disease appear to be unresponsive (42). Furthermore, presence of autologous serum in the assay system has been found to inhibit the lymphoblastogenesis, suggesting a nonspecific or specific blocking of cell-mediated immunity (43).

Leukocyte Migration Inhibition. When sensitized lymphocytes are placed together with specific antigen, certain soluble substances, known as *lymphokines*, are released from these lymphocytes. Some of these lymphokines inhibit migration of macrophages and leukocytes and are designated as MIF (migration inhibitory factor) and LIF (leukocyte inhibitory factor), respectively. The properties of MIF and LIF have been reviewed recently by Rocklin (44).

McCoy (45) reported that leukocyte migration inhibition assays indicated the presence of tumor antigens that were absent in normal adult tissues. Some weak cross-reactions have been observed among sarcomas, melanomas, and carcinomas of breast, colon, and lung (46). Thus, leukocyte migration inhibition assays clearly suggest the expression of tumor-associated antigens by human neoplasms.

Leukocyte Adherence Inhibition. It has been observed by Halliday and his coworkers (47) that blood leukocytes from cancer patients lost their ability to adhere to glass when incubated in the presence of tumor extracts. Using low concentrations of tumor extracts in the leukocyte adherence inhibition assay, several investigators have reported histologic type-specific reactivity in cancer patients (48).

Antibody-Dependent Cellular Cytotoxicity. The antibody-dependent cell mediated cytotoxicity (ADCC) assay was first described by Moller in 1965, who observed that nonimmune lymphoid cells destroyed chemically-induced tumor cells *in vitro* in the presence of specific antiserum (49).

The ADCC assay has been applied to document the presence of tumor-associated antigens that are immunogenic in the host. Various investigators have reported induction of K-cell activity by autologous and allogeneic sera from melanoma patients against biopsied or cultured melanoma cells (50, 51). Hersey et al. observed that several melanoma patients had antibodies to more than one antigen on melanoma cells (52).

Serologic Reactions

Detection and definition of putative tumor antigens in human neoplasms have been achieved by xenoantibody as well as by autologous and allogeneic antibody. These techniques are well described in a recent compendium of methods for serologic analysis of human tumor antigens (53).

Xenoantibody. On the basis of the cytotoxic effect of antisera raised in horses against human tumors on various cultured human tumor cell lines, Bjorklund and his associates (54) claimed that common tumor antigens were expressed by many human neoplasms. Since then, the existence of tumor antigens, such as carcino-embryonic antigen (CEA) and α-fetoprotein (AFP), have been identified.

Using heteroantisera, a number of tumor antigens, other than CEA and AFP, have been detected in various human malignancies, including melanoma (55), sarcoma (56), and carcinomas (57). These antigens are present in tumor cells but not in adult normal cells. However, many of these antigens have been shown to be expressed by fetal tissues as well. Xenoantibodies to human tumor antigens have been produced in a number of species. Though a few investigators have been successful in obtaining specific antimelanoma (58) and antioat cell carcinoma (59) xenoantibodies, to date there is no conclusive report to suggest that the tumor antigens detected by xenoantibody are immunogenic in the cancer host.

Autologous and Allogeneic Antibody. Though detection of humoral antibodies in allogeneic and autologous sera from cancer patients is relatively simple, proving their specificity is an extremely complex task. The specificity of the observed reactions was disclosed by absorption of the sera with normal tissue (autologous and allogeneic). Also, freshly biopsied or autopsied tumor tissues and cultured tumor cells or their extracts have been used as the target antigens. There are many reports in literature regarding the existence of certain components in tumor cells that are immunogenic in the autologous and allogeneic host. Though the biological and chemical characteristics of the majority of these antigenic components are not completely known, they are recognized as tumor-associated antigens (TAA). A recent review summarizes up-to-date findings on humoral immune responses in cancer patients to TAA (60).

Human tumor antigens that are immunogenic in the host have been localized: (a) on the cell surface, (b) in the cytoplasm, and (c) in the nucleus. Of these, TAA expressed on the cell surface are of considerable significance because immune responses elicited against these antigens may influence tumor growth. Cytoplasmic antigens, on the other hand, may not elicit protective immunity in the host. The humoral immune response to these antigens may occur later than to cell-surface antigen. Antinucleolar antibodies have been observed in the sera of patients with malignant melanoma by McBride et al. (61). The nucleolar antigen, apparently a nucleoprotein, is not melanoma specific; however, its presence in tumor cells directly correlates with the clinical status of the patient and indicates a poor prognosis for that individual.

It is conceivable that the serologic reaction observed *in vitro* between sera from cancer patients and their tumor cells could also occur *in vivo*. Surface-bound immunoglobulins on biopsy specimens of various types of human malignancies have been reported (62). Though the immunoglobulins may be bound to the surface of tumor and nontumor cells in various ways (64), there is enough evidence to suggest that at least some immunoglobulins are bound because of antibody-antigen interaction to antigenic determinants on tumor cells. Low pH or high salt eluted material possesses antibody activity against cells of the same or similar tumors (63). We have observed that the antigenic activity of melanoma to autologous serum increased by 32 to 64 fold after elution of immunoglobulins, and the eluted immuno-globulins contained IgG and IgM (63). Thus, tumor-bound immunoglobulins detected in biopsy specimens may be considered as evidence of a humoral immune response to tumor antigens and their immunologic interaction *in vivo*. Witz has reviewed this topic in detail (65).

Monoclonal Antibody. Since the development of somatic cell hybridization technology by Kohler and Milstein (66) to produce monoclonal antibodies, attempts have been made to define human tumor cell surface antigens using these reagents (67a).

In their initial studies, Koprowski and associates (67) obtained monoclonal antimelanoma antibodies that could be grouped into three categories: (a) antibodies which reacted only with a melanoma but not with any other target cells, (b) antibodies which reacted with all melanomas and some colorectal carcinomas, and (c) antibodies which reacted with all melanomas, all human normal cells and all but one of the colorectal carcinomas. Thus, antigens recognized by monoclonal antibodies of categories (a) and (b) were in parallel with those described by Shiku et al. using allogeneic and autologous antibodies (68).

Yeh et al. obtained three hybridomas, using a short term explant of a human melanoma, which secrete antibodies to an antigen that is present on the immunizing cells and which is also expressed by a limited number of other melanomas but not by other tumors and normal cells (69). These investigators observed that melanomas were heterogeneous with respect to expression of the antigen and that the antigen-positive cells could become antigen-negative. Carrel et al. have defined melanoma associated antigen(s) that were expressed by at least 15 different melanoma cell lines (70).

TYPES OF TUMOR ANTIGENS EXPRESSED
BY HUMAN NEOPLASMS

It is now obvious that a wide variety of assay procedures have been employed to discover antigens similar to TSTA on human tumors. Although the data are consistent with the hypothesis that human tumors possess TAA, convincing evidence for the existence of TSTA on human tumors is still lacking. The definition and classification of TAA of human tumors is important from an academic point of view as well as from the practical point of view of developing diagnostic and prognostic tests and immunotherapy. On the basis of serological reactions, TAA of human tumor cells may roughly be grouped into the following three categories: (a) individual TAA for each patient (tumor), (b) common TAA which cross-react with various tumors of the same histologic type, and (c) fetal or embryonic antigens.

Individual Specific

Antigens unique for each tumor obtained from melanoma patients have been detected by complement-dependent antibody-mediated cytotoxicity assay (71) and membrane immunofluorescence test (72). These observations were confirmed by mixed hemadsorption (73), immune adherence (68), and lymphocytotoxicity (74) assays. Expression of individually specific antigen on melanoma cells has also been suggested by the use of monoclonal antibodies (75).

Histologic Type Specific

Human neoplasms of the same histologic type often express common TAA that are different from those of other histologic types. For example, cross-reacting common melanoma membrane antigens that do not react with tumors of other histologic types have been described (76) using allogeneic antibodies. Such common melanoma antigens have also been detected using monoclonal antibodies (67, 70).

Common antigen associated with human sarcomas was first reported by Morton and co-workers (77). Since then several other common sarcoma-associated antigens have been detected by allogeneic antibodies (78).

Embryonic or Fetal

The fact that neoplastic transformation is accompanied by dedifferentiation and reversion of normal adult cells toward an embryonic state is based on the observations that neoplastic cells express antigens usually confined to fetal tissues. Production of these antigens is repressed shortly after birth. However, when adult cells undergo malignant transformation, the production of these primitive embryonic components is resumed. From an immunologic point of view, two types of embryonic antigens have been observed in human malignancies, one recognized by xenoantibodies and not immunogenic in the host and the other recognized by allogeneic antibodies and immunogenic in the host.

Fetal Antigens That Are Not Immunogenic in the Host. These antigens have been recognized by immunizing rabbits with tumor cells or their homogenates. The sera from these animals were absorbed exhaustively with normal adult tissues. The absorbed antisera were then reacted with tumor, fetal, and normal cells or their extracts. Reactions were observed with tumor and fetal preparations, but not with normal preparations. Using this basic methodology, a number of fetal antigens expressed by human neoplasms have now been described in the literature.

Alphafetoprotein (AFP). AFP is one of the most specific immunologic markers of certain tumors, e.g., hepatoma and teratocarcinomas of ovary and testis (79). It is a dominant serum protein during embryonic development and in early life, and its concentration decreases gradually during development of adult life. AFP may act as an albumin substitute in fetal blood. It acts as an estrogen binding receptor in the uterus and fetal brain and as a result may be involved in immunosuppression to ensure escape of the fetus from an immunological rejection by the mother (80). AFP has now been detected in the sera of patients with pancreatic, gastric, and lung carcinomas, and even in patients with leukemia and myeloma (81). Its presence has also been detected in patients with nonmalignant clinical diseases, e.g., viral hepatitis and ataxiatelangiectasia has recently been reported (82).

Carcinoembryonic antigen (CEA). CEA, discovered by Gold and Freedman (83) also occurs in fetal gut, liver, and pancreas during the first two trimesters of gestation. This antigen, originally thought to be specific for adenocarcinomas arising in the gastrointestinal tract and pancreas, was found in a variety of human neoplasms including sarcomas, lymphomas, and other carcinomas (84). Increased levels of CEA also have been observed in patients with ulcerative colitis, pancreatitis, and liver cirrhosis, and in heavy smokers (85).

CEA is a glycoprotein with a molecular weight of about 200,000 daltons and with beta-electrophoretic mobility. It possesses a single polypeptide chain. Materials such as NCA (nonspecific cross-reacting antigen), NGP (normal glycoprotein), CEX (CEA-associated protein), CCEA-2 (Colonic carcinoembryonic antigen-2), CCA-III (Colon carcinoma antigen-III), extracted from various tissues, that cross-react with CEA, have been reviewed by Kleist and Burtin (86).

Though CEA has been shown to be antigenic in animals, its antigenicity in man is controversial. A specific humoral immune response of the IgM class of antibody in humans has been demonstrated by Gold and his co-workers (83). Furthermore, Costanza et al. (87) demonstrated circulating CEA-anti-CEA immune complexes in a patient with colonic carcinoma. They have also demonstrated the deposits of CEA immunoglobulins and complement in the glomerular basement membrane of the kidney. However, LoGerfo et al. were unable to detect any circulating antibodies to CEA in patients with gastrointestinal malignancies (84).

Because the levels of CEA have been found to be elevated in the sera of patients with a variety of neoplastic and nonneoplastic diseases, the CEA determinations have very little diagnostic value. However, monitoring of CEA levels may be useful as a prognostic indicator for colon cancer patients.

Fetal sulfoglycoprotein antigen (FSA). This antigen is found in 96% of patients with gastric cancer (88). FSA is not found in normal colonic mucosa, but exists in the superficial part of the mucosa of fetal stomach and gut. Certain immunological studies suggest that FSA and CEA share some common determinants. FSA production also has been reported as preceding the development of overt carcinoma. The successful removal of gastric cancer is not necessarily followed by a decline in FSA level in gastric juice (88).

Pancreatic oncofetal antigen (POA). POA was found in extracts of human fetal pancreas, in sera from many patients with pancreatic cancer or other cancers and benign conditions. It is a glycoprotein with a molecular weight of 800,000 to 900,000 daltons and beta-electrophoretic mobility. POA is distinct from CEA and AFP. The quantity and incidence are highest in patients with carcinoma of the pancreas (89). The levels of POA in these patients decrease after tumor resection.

Other fetal antigens. Alpha$_2$ H-globulin is present in 81% of sera from children with tumors (90); and beta-oncofetal antigen is associated with carcinoma of various kinds (91).

Fetal Antigens That Are Immunogenic in the Host

Studies in animals. The existence of fetal antigens on tumor cells as demonstrated by an immune reponse in autochthonous animal models has been reviewed by Chism et al. (92). Lymph node cells of pregnant mice have been shown to be cytotoxic for tumors induced by chemical and viral agents, but not for normal fibroblasts. Cells from primiparous animals have been shown to be more cytotoxic than cells from multiparous animals (93). Ray and associates (14,15) observed that immunization of parous animals with fetal antigens during their pregnancies suppressed the growth of challenging tumor transplants. The tumor immunity could also be transferred to virgin animals with spleen cells and sera from primiparous females one day post-partum but not from primiparous females carrying 18-day-old embryos (14). These investigators further reported that emergence of antigens in embryos that confine the antitumor immunity is transient and possibly is not present during the entire period of gestation (15).

Studies in humans. Like other TAAs, the evidence of existence of immu-nogenic fetal antigens in human malignancies, comes largely from *in vitro* studies. The discovery of gammafetoprotein antigen (GFA) was made by use of antibodies present in sera of some tumor-bearing patients. This antigen has been found in 75 to 95% of human carcinomas, sarcomas, and leukemias, and various fetal tissues. GFA was also found in the extracts of 75% benign tumors but not in extracts of 172 normal or non-neoplastic diseased tissues (94). Rosenberg and Brown (95) reported that sera from normal individuals, as well as from sarcoma patients, contained natural antibodies against a determinant expressed on both normal and osteogenic sarcoma cells in tissue culture. These determinants represented fetal antigens that were reexpressed by cells in tissue culture.

Lymphocytes from cancer patients have been shown to be cytotoxic to tumor cells and fetal cells (96). Herberman et al. observed DCHR in patients with colon carcinoma by intradermal injection of extracts of fetal intestine and liver, and pooled allogeneic carcinoma tissues (97). Such a DCHR was not observed by injection of CEA. Thus, it was concluded that the skin reaction was due to fetal antigen(s) different from CEA.

One of the most important discoveries in the field of oncofetal antigens has been made by Irie et al. (98). These investigators showed the existence of a membrane antigen on human tumor cells of various histologic types. This antigen cross-reacted with human fetal brain cells and thus was des-ignated as oncofetal antigen I (OFA-I). OFA-I can be distinguished from CEA and AFP by its distribution in fetal tissues, immunogenic properties, and antigenic specificity on tumor cells (98). Anti-OFA-I antibodies have been detected in 55 to 70% of the cancer patients (99) and in 100% of the women during pregnancy in the third trimester (98). Sidell et al. have found anti-OFA-I to be cytotoxic to tumor cells (100).

Gupta et al. have isolated anti-OFA-I antibodies from sera of melanoma patients and characterized these antibodies by absorption with human fetal brain cells (99). Soluble OFA-I has been separated from other tumor-associated antigens by solvent extraction (101) and it appeared to be glycoprotein. The biological significance of OFA-I in terms of tumor-host relationship has been reviewed recently by Jones et al. (102).

Other Tumor Antigens

A number of antigens that are not fetal by definition but are present in larger quantities in tumors than in normal tissues have been described by various investigators. Xenoantibodies against these antigens have been produced. Such tumor-associated markers include tissue polypeptide antigen (TPA) (103), Kappa casein (104), Ferritin (105), etc.

ORIGIN OF TUMOR ANTIGENS IN HUMAN CANCERS

From the foregoing review it is obvious that most human malignant tissues express tumor antigens. Many of these antigens are capable of inducing immune responses in the host and exhibit cross-reactivity. Fetal antigens may be organ- and tissue-specific, detectable on tumor or fetal cells but not on normal adult cells, and thus could be responsible for the observed cross-reactivity among various tumors.

All animal neoplasms, regardless of their histologic type, induced by a given virus, share a common tumor antigen. This antigen is different from the tumor antigens associated with neoplasms induced by other viruses. By analogy with animal virus-induced tumors, it may be deduced that common cross-reactivity in human neoplasms could be due to common viral etiology. There is no conclusive evidence at this time to prove or disprove this hypothesis; however, the common antigens in Burkitt's lymphoma are induced by the Epstein-Barr virus.

Mechanisms whereby molecules which can act as tumor antigens may appear on the cell surface and make them autoantigenic, have been elegantly illustrated by Cochran (106). He proposed that neoantigens on tumor cells may appear by (a) reexpression of repressed molecules, (b) modification of existing molecules, (c) uncovering of masked molecules, and (d) deletion of existing molecules. The intracellular molecules, which are secluded from the immune system of a host, may not be immunogenic under normal circumstances due to various reasons (106): (a) the number of intracellular molecules released at any one time is very small; (b) released molecules may be destroyed by enzymatic activity or their determinants may be masked; and (c) the healthy individual may have a self-tolerance which deteriorates with age. A progressive increase in autoantibodies has been observed in aging populations (106). In cancer patients antibodies to cytoplasmic antigens appear later than to membrane antigens (107).

TUMOR ANTIGENS IN CIRCULATION
AND IN OTHER BODY FLUIDS

The presence of biologically functional tumor antigens has been observed in the serum and urine of cancer patients (108,109). Tumor antigens in serum may arise as a result of tumor cell lysis or by spontaneous release from living cells. Release of tumor antigens *in vitro* by animal and human malignant cells has been documented (110). The release of tumor antigens into body fluids appears to vary from tumor to tumor. The shed-antigens can react with sensitized lymphocytes or antitumor antibodies and thus may result in blocking the immune defense mechanism of the host (111). Ray and associates (112,113) recently observed that soluble or immobilized tumor antigen could induce humoral and cellular blocking factors both in normal and tumor-bearing animals. The induction was dose-dependent, i.e., low antigen dose caused induction of plasma blocking factors and high dose caused induction of cellular blocking factors. It was suggested that this phenomenon might have a correlation with the immunosuppression caused by the antigen in tumorbearers (112).

Morgan et al. proposed that the shedding of tumor antigens into the culture medium of cultured tumor cells is dependent on glycosylation (114). It was suggested that the mode of glycosylation of tumor antigens differs from that of other proteins synthesized by human tumor cells.

NATURE OF TUMOR ANTIGENS

Reports are now beginning to appear on the biochemical purification and identification of tumor antigens (115). These techniques include gelfiltration, ion exchange and affinity chromatography, isoelectric focusing, and polyacrylamide gel electrophoresis. Solubilization of antigens from tumor cells has been achieved by sonication, salt extraction, detergent, and proteolytic enzyme treatments. In general, tumor antigens are comprised of glycoproteins which are present on plasma membrane and inside the cells.

LeGrue et al. developed a method to extract membrane proteins from viable MAC-F murine sarcoma cells without loss of their viability (116). This procedure involved the use of a single-phase solution of 2.5% n-butanol. The tumor antigens extracted by this method were more potent than those extracted by 3-M KCl.

Bhavanandan et al. isolated a glycoprotein antigen associated with murine B16 melanoma cells by detergent solubilization of the cells followed by gel filtration, ion exchange, and lectin column chromatography (117). These investigators concluded that the antigen contained both complex and simple oligosaccharides which were linked to the protein moiety via N-acetylglu-cosamine to asparagine (117).

Recently attempts have been made to purify tumor antigens from the spent culture media of both animal and human tumor cell lines (118). Gallaway et al. reported that antigens shed into spent culture medium of intrinsically-labeled melanoma cells react with monoclonal and polyclonal antibodies and represent two glycoproteins with molecular weights of 240,000 and 94,000 (119). Tumor antigens also have been isolated from serum of tumor-bearing hosts and from circulating immune complexes in animal models (120).

More recently Woodbury et al. have isolated an antigen from human melanoma cells using immunoprecipitation techniques with monoclonal an-tibodies (121). This antigen is expressed by melanoma cells but not by normal adult human tissues. The p97, a human melanoma-associated antigen is monomeric and probably contains intrachain disulfide bonds. Chemically, it is a sialoglyoprotein (122).

RELATIONSHIP OF TUMOR ANTIGENS WITH HISTOCOMPATIBILITY ANTIGENS

It has been reported that some tumor antigens, especially those of chemically-induced tumors, represent modified histocompatibility antigens or that their expression is governed by genes associated with the major histocompatibility complex. A number of observations reviewed by Curry et al. (123) support this concept: (a) an inverse relationship between the expression of tumor antigens and histocompatibility antigens suggest the involvement of common mechanisms for the synthesis of both antigens; (b) both histocompatibility and tumor antigen systems are pleomorphic and behave as integral parts of membrane molecules; (c) transplantation resistance to syngeneic tumor can be achieved by immunization of a host with normal tissue from an H-2-incompatible strain; (d) the tumor antigens of murine systems appear to be associated with the same molecule as the histocompatibility antigens; (e) growth of a parental tumor in F_1 hybrids has been reported to be better than in the syngeneic parent due to cross-reaction of histocompatibility antigens of the F_1 hybrids with tumor antigens (124); and (f) certain methylcholanthrene-induced sarcomas express H-2 specificities not found on normal cells of the strain of the tumor-bearing animal (125). In recent histogenetic studies Parmiani et al. found that the immunogenicity of either B10 or A minor histocompatibility antigens in eliciting an antisarcoma protective effect was controlled by genes of the D^d region (126).

On the basis of cross-reactions between histocompatibility antigens and tumor antigens of chemically-induced sarcomas of mice, it is suggested that tumor antigens could arise from point mutations resulting in altered antigens having specificities that are shared by other allogeneic strains of mice. Alternatively, tumor antigens may arise by derepression of genes which code for alloantigens that are normally not expressed in the animal strain. However, using a cytogenetically favorable somatic cell hybrid, Klein and Klein (127) established that the genetic determinants of tumor antigens of methylcholanthrene-induced sarcomas of mice were not located on the chromosome 17 that carries the genetic information for H-2 determinants, but that the presence of this chromosome was required for full expression of the immunogenicity of tumor antigens.

Forni and Cavallo have pointed to a relationship between the immunogenicity of tumor cells and the expression of Ia alloantigens (128). The immunization of animals with an Ia negative mutant cell line failed to elicit an effective recognition of tumor antigens, both *in vivo* and *in vitro*.

On the contrary, it has been suggested that tumor antigens and histocompatibility antigens may be physically separable (12) and that these two types of antigens do not cap together (129). Roman and Bonavida observed that there were molecules of 45,000 daltons on SJL tumors that reacted with anti-H-2^d antisera and were not expressed by normal SJL lymphocytes (130). Clementson et al. (131) demonstrated that H-2, TS$_A$, and TS$_X$ antigens of P-815 mastocytoma system bound to *Lens culinaris* lectin; however, only TS$_X$ antigen could also bind to wheat germ agglutinin. Despite similar molecular weight, about 80% TS$_A$ was lost during cell fractionation compared to only 20% of H-2. Furthermore, the TS$_A$ antigen could not be coprecipitated with the H-2 antigen using C3H anti-DBA/2 antibody. The C-1 sarcoma induced by methylcholanthrene expresses tumor antigens that are separable from the alien H-2^k antigens (132). Recently Klein stressed that analysis of tumor antigens and H-2 antigens by serologic techniques can be confused by the occurrence of antimurine leukemia virus antibodies in syngeneic and allogeneic antisera (133).

In the human tumor system, the functional and structural relationship between histocompatibility antigens and tumor antigens was studied by Curry et al. (123). It appeared unlikely that human tumor antigens are modified HLA antigens.

CONSEQUENCES OF IMMUNE RESPONSE TO TUMOR-ASSOCIATED ANTIGENS

It is now obvious that neoplastic cells by virtue of expression of tumor antigens induce both cellular and humoral immune responses. The tumor in the host may be affected by these immune responses in one or more of the following ways: surveillance, rejection, and stimulation.

Immune Rejection of Tumors

The cellular immune response, as in transplantation immunology, is believed to be more important in controlling tumor rejection than the humoral immune response: it has been demonstrated that tumor immunity could be transferred readily in an adoptive manner by lymphocytes and/or macrophages capable of killing tumor cells in the tumor-bearing host. Despite this belief, humoral antibodies in concert with certain lymphocytes may inhibit the growth of tumor cells and destroy them.

Stimulated thymus-derived lymphocytes have receptors on their surface that are specific for tumor antigens expressed on the surface of neoplastic cells. Upon coming in contact with these antigens, the lymphocytes mediate a cytotoxic event, perhaps via a toxic substance called lymphotoxin, that causes disruption of the tumor cell membrane leading to the death of the tumor cell.

Macrophages, both nonspecifically stimulated and specifically armed, play an important role in killing the tumor cells. Macrophages, activated nonspecifically by BCG or its products, have been found to be cytotoxic for tumor cells *in vitro* but not for normal cells. Sensitized lymphocytes that are specifically cytotoxic for a tumor can transmit this specificity to normal macrophages, which, in turn, become specifically cytotoxic to the sensitizing tumor.

Many immune responses are mediated by the products of stimulated macrophages and lymphocytes in the presence of antigen. These products are known as lymphokines and have been shown to be important for the modification and development of cellular immune response. For example, macrophage inhibitory factor (MIF) and macrophage chemotactic factor (MCF) are produced by lymphocytes after antigenic stimulation. These factors control the movement of macrophages or granulocytes in the development of delayed cutaneous hypersensitivity or inflammation. Many other substances, such as macrophage activating factor (MAF), specific macrophage-arming factor (SMAF), mitogenic proteins, etc., that generally contribute to the interactions between different cell types have also been described.

Certain lymphoid cells from normal animals and humans have been shown to be significantly cytotoxic for syngeneic and allogeneic tumors in *in vitro* assays (134). These cells have been termed NK cells. Most NK cells recognize one of two or possibly three targets that are widely distributed on human tumor cells and are called TA1, TA2, and TA3 (135).

Humoral antibodies have been shown in animal models to inhibit tumor growth *in vivo* and destroy tumor cells *in vitro* in the presence of complement. However, antibody must be given prior to or immediately after tumor transplantation in order to be effective. The sensitivity of various types of tumors to cytotoxic antibodies varies considerably. Also, different classes of antibody vary considerably in their ability to reduce tumor cell viability *in vitro* and inhibit tumor growth *in vivo*. Antibodies of IgM class are generally more effective in exerting a cytotoxic effect than antibody of IgG. Thymus-independent lymphocytes, also known as killer or K cells can be potentiated or armed by an antibody specific for tumor antigen to cause tumor cell lysis. This cytotoxic effect (ADCC) is neither complement dependent nor phagocytic. Though both IgA and IgM antibodies can mediate ADCC, it is usually IgG that induces ADCC.

Immune Surveillance

The development and progression of a tumor from a single cell to a clinically detectable cancer requires several steps (136). It is possible that the immune response of the host plays an important role in eradicating and preventing precancerous cells from becoming a blatant neoplasm. Burnett termed this concept immunological surveillance (137).

Evasion of Immune Surveillance. It must be realized that immune surveillance differs from immune response. The immune surveillance presumably operates to eliminate cancer cells as they arise, whereas the immune system may or may not prevent the spread of neoplastic cells from a primary tumor. The development of clinical cancer would represent a failure of mechanisms related to immune surveillance. How it actually happens is not clearly understood; however, a variety of ways by which cancer cells evade the immune surveillance mechanisms have been described.

1. *Insufficient immunogenicity.* Certain tumor cells may have either an extremely weak antigen or an extremely low density of such antigens on the surface. As a result these tumor cells may escape detection and destruction by immune mechanisms.

2. *Antigenic modulation.* Thymus-leukemia (TL) antigen expressed by murine lymphoma cells disappears when the cells are transplanted to an immunized host or carried in tissue culture containing specific antibody. However, this antigen reappears when the cells are transplanted in unimmunized hosts or passed in tissue culture medium without antibody. This phenomenon is known as antigenic modulation. Antigenic shift is also considered as a phenomenon of antigenic modulation and has been observed

in certain animal tumors where lung metastases were antigenically different from the primary tumor.

3. *Immunosuppression*. Factors that cause immunosuppression, such as chemotherapy, neonatal thymectomy, irradiation, steroid or antilymphocytic globulin administration, usually increase the frequency and growth rate, and shorten the latency period, for both virus- and carcinogen-induced tumors in experimental animals. Organ transplant patients, who were kept on immunosuppressive drugs, had a 70-times greater incidence of certain types of spontaneous cancer than the general age-matched population (30).

4. *Immunologic tolerance*. Immunologic tolerance that develops during the fetal or neonatal periods due to exposure to tumor antigens or an oncogenic virus may account for tumor growth in some animals when the immune surveillance system would otherwise afford protection. Mice infected with mammary tumor virus (MTV) as neonates subsequently become tolerant to the tumor antigens of the MTV-induced tumors and as a result could not be immunized against them (138).

Tumor Stimulation

As opposed to the immune surveillance hypothesis, immune reactions may stimulate tumor growth. This has been discussed in some greater detail in other chapters of this volume (see chapters 6, 7, and 8).

Subsequent to demonstration of enhancing or blocking antibody by the Hellströms (111), other serum factors, e.g., circulating free antigen and antigen-antibody complexes have also been implicated as blocking factors (139). Ray has recently reviewed this field and suggested that controlling the suppressor components, humoral and cellular, may be therapeutically beneficial to the tumor host (140). Ray has also indicated that abrogation of the effects of both humoral blocking factor(s) and suppressor cells may potentiate the immune response of the host, which in turn may cause tumor regression (140).

APPLICATIONS OF TUMOR ANTIGENS

It is well recognized that by the time most human cancers are clinically detected, metastates have already occurred. Therefore, extensive efforts have been made to develop diagnostic tests for cancer to detect malignancies before they metastasize (141). Most of the tumor markers that are quantitated are not tumor specific. Furthermore, phenotypic expression of a tumor marker may vary from one neoplasm to another. Theoretically, actual detection of the characteristic tumor antigen in body fluids should provide accurate diagnosis and prognosis of malignancy. This is typified by the quantitation of CEA and AFP; however, their occurrence in nonmalignant conditions has diminished their value as a diagnostic tool. These antigens are now routinely used in monitoring cancer patients and for detection of recurrent disease.

An association of nephrotic syndrome or glomerulonephritis with malignancy and disappearance of proteinuria after surgical ablation of tumor has been reported by various investigators (142). Immune complex deposits in the kidney were demonstrated in many of these patients. In some patients, tumor-related antigen, complement, and IgG antibodies have been detected in the renal glomeruli (143). In view of the association of nephrotic syndrome and occasional proteinuria with malignancy, it is conceivable that the permeability of the basement membrane of the kidney could be drastically altered due to immune complex deposition, and as a result large macromolecules could gain access to the urine. In fact, excretion of tumor antigens into the urine from tumors originating outside the genitourinary tract has been observed by various investigators. John et al. reported a case in which an antigen was excreted into urine of a melanoma patient (144). This antigen reacted with rabbit antibody prepared against cyst fluid from a metastasis of the patient's tumor and showed immunologic similarity to tumor antigen extracted from the cyst fluid. A common melanoma tumor antigen has also been detected at high frequency in the urine of patients with melanotic and nonmelanotic tumors (145). Excretion of tumor antigens is not limited to melanoma only (146).

We have observed tumor antigens in urine from several sarcoma patients and these antigens were immunogenic in the host (147). Analysis of sequential urine samples from these patients revealed that the antigenic activity depended upon the presence of tumor in the host. The antigenic activity disappeared after surgical ablation of the tumor mass. However, the activity reappeared several days before tumor recurrence suggesting that detection of tumor antigens in urine of cancer patients may be potentially helpful to identify the subclinical recurrence of their disease. The significance of the sequential analyses of urinary antigens to monitor the clinical course and in assessing the in vivo effectiveness of tumoricidal chemotherapy and radiation therapy of cancer patients has been reemphasized by the studies of Rote et al. (148). In a preliminary report Huth et al. revealed that a rise in urinary antigen titer during preoperative chemotherapy of sarcomas correlated extremely well with tumor necrosis (149).

It is, thus, obvious that tumor antigens offer great potential in terms of immunologic monitoring of cancer patients undergoing therapy for their malignant disease, as well as for determining the patient's specific immune response which may dictate the choice of further treatment modalities.

Assessment of Cell-Mediated and Humoral Immunity

Sophisticated immunological studies have demonstrated a correlation between the cell-mediated and humoral immune responses and the clinical course of malignancy. Though no systematic studies have yet been performed to correlate serological findings with the clinical parameters in human malignancy, Morton's studies in patients with solid neoplasms suggest a marked correlation between the circulating antibody levels and the clinical course in patients with melanoma and sarcoma (150). Cancer patients with localized disease had higher levels of antitumor antibodies than those with disseminated disease. A similar situation was observed by deKernion et al. in patients with renal cell carcinoma (151).

In addition to correlations of clinical course with humoral antibody, delayed cutaneous hypersensitivity reactions (DCHR) to tumor antigens have been correlated with clinical course. In general, patients with no evidence of disease or minimal disease exhibit DCHR to extracted tumor antigens; whereas, patients with a high tumor burden do not.

Tumor antigens have been used to assess cell-mediated antitumor immunity in *in vitro* assays, such as LMI and LAI, in cancer patients (45). It has been observed that in most cases, the LMI responses have been directed against antigens common to tumors of the same histologic type. Patient's peripheral blood lymphocytes obtained at different times can be tested repeatedly against the same antigen extract. Though LAI using tumor antigens could discriminate between cancer patients and normal subjects on a statistical basis, it did not successfully differentiate early breast cancer patients from those with benign breast disease. A decline in LAI in response to tumor antigens has been observed postsurgery and in cured patients.

The prognostic significance of measuring antibody responses to tumor antigens has been briefly mentioned above in this section. Since these antibodies are also detectable in a majority of close contacts of cancer patients and in some normal donors, their measurement in the general population for cancer diagnostic purposes may not be appropriate. The occurrence of such antibodies at high frequency in close family contacts may suggest the involvement of a transmissible agent in the causation of cancer.

Immune Complexes and Prognosis

Since many tumor antigens have been shown to be immunogenic in the host, the appearance of these antigens in the circulation during subclinical tumor growth should permit them to react with humoral antibodies and circulating immune complexes (CIC). Thus, one would expect to find immune complexes before free antigen could be detected in the circulation. Quan-

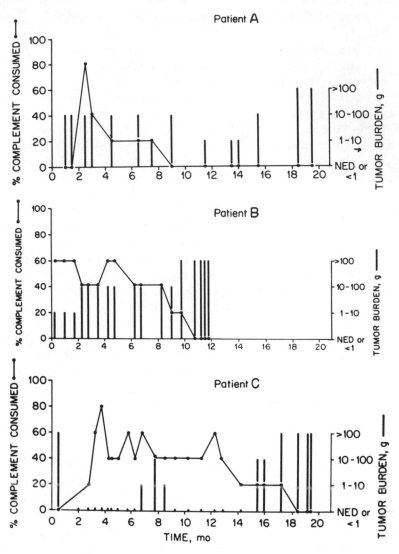

Fig. 5.1. Levels of circulating immune complexes in sequential serum samples of three melanoma patients (A, B, and C). The immune complexes were analyzed by the complement consumption method. The immune complex values of each serum sample is expressed as percent complement consumed by 2 μl of 1:4 diluted test samples. The tumor burden at the time of serum sampling was assessed by determining the number and size of palpable tumor masses, tumor nodules seen on radiological films, scans, and tomograms. A 1 cm³ nodule was arbitrarily considered to weigh approximately 1 gram.

titation and characterization of CIC by sensitive methods may serve as a prognostic indicator of tumor recurrence and a means of evaluating the tumoricidal effectiveness of various treatment modalities (152). During recent years, numerous studies have been perfomed to assess and correlate the levels of circulating immune complexes with clinical course of cancer patients (142).

We have observed that 53% (233 out of 439) of cancer sera contained circulating immune complexes, compared to only 14% (20 out of 140) of normal sera (153). Among cancer patients, the incidence was lowest in melanoma (42%) and highest in lung carcinoma patients (65%). In some patients serum samples were consistently positive even at times when there was no clinical evidence of disease (154). In other patients, circulating immune complexes decreased below detectable level when tumor persisted for several months (Fig. 5.1). In yet other patients, their serum samples became immune complex positive 2 to 4 weeks before clinically detectable tumor recurrence. At the same time complement-fixing antibody levels against

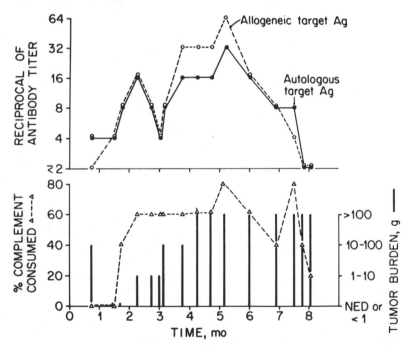

Fig. 5.2. Levels of complement fixing antitumor antibodies against autologous and allogeneic target antigens (Ag), and of immune complexes analyzed by the complement consumption method in serum samples of a melanoma patient taken at various time intervals during clinical course of the disease. The immune complex levels are expressed as percent complement consumed by 2 μl of 1:4 diluted test sample. The body burden of tumor at the time of serum sampling was assessed as mentioned in the legend of Figure 5.1.

autologous and allogeneic tumor cells also increased. After fluctuation the antibodies became undetectable in the serum samples taken at the time when the patient became terminal. The immune complex levels also decreased at this time (Fig. 5.2). This decrease in antitumor antibody concomitant with or prior to decrease in immune complexes during progressive increase in tumor mass suggests that the antigens shed from tumor into circulation complexed with virtually all the circulating antibody, and produced an antigen excess in the circulation.

These antigen-antibody complexes together with the excess free-antigen could, in turn, directly or indirectly produce immunosuppressive serum factors that blocked further production of antibodies. Follow-up of cancer patients with no evidence of disease or minimal tumor burden revealed that 42% (18 out of 43) whose sera were immune complex positive had tumor recurrence within 3 months and 90% (57 out of 63) whose sera were negative had no detectable tumor recurrence up to at least 6 months after the serum analysis (Table 5.1) (155).

Since the currently used assays to detect immune complexes in the circulation of cancer patients are antigen nonspecific, any apparent or inapparent infection at the time of serum sampling might result in false positive circulating immune complex values which in turn would lower the prognostic significance of the immune complex detection assays. Therefore, it is necessary to characterize the detected immune complexes with respect to their antigen portion or develop antigen-specific immune complex detection assays. To overcome this problem, we have isolated antitumor antibodies (99) and tumor-associated antigen from human melanoma (101) and developed a radioimmunoassay (156). The immune complexes were isolated from test and control sera by precipitation with polyethylene glycol, dissociated with potassium isothiocyanate and reassociated in the presence of ^{125}I-labeled

Table 5.1. Incidence of Recurrence of Disease in Cancer Patients with Immune Complex Positive and Negative Serum Samples Taken at the Time of No Evidence of Disease or Minimal Tumor Burden (155).

Diagnosis	Immune Complex	(No. Patient Recurred within 3 Months)/(No. of Patients Follow-up for at least 6 Months)	Percent Recurred within 3 Months	P value
Sarcoma	+	6/9	67	< 0.02
	−	2/12	17	
Carcinomas	+	6/11	55	< 0.01
	−	1/14	7	
Melanoma	+	6/23	26	0.06
	−	3/37	8	
All cancers	+	18/43	42	< 0.001
	−	6/63	10	

Table 5.2. Incorporation of ^{125}I-labeled Melanoma-Associated Antigen into Immune Complexes Isolated from Melanoma and Control Sera* by the Antigenic Competition Method using Protein A Positive *Staphylococcus aureus* Cells

Isolated Immune Complexes from	Sample Size	Percent ^{125}I-Tumor Antigen Sedimented with *S. aureus* Mean ± S.D.	P Value Compared to NSB** by *t*-Test
Control for NSB	—	23 ± 5.1	—
Normal Sera	9	22 ± 3.3	NS***
Sarcoma Sera	8	24 ± 5.4	NS
Melanoma Sera	8	42 ± 13.0	< 0.05

* All serum samples were immune complex positive.
** NSB = nonspecific binding (sedimentation of ^{125}I-tumor antigen with protein A positive *S. aureus* after treatment with potassium isothiocyanate).
*** NS = statistically nonsignificant.

tumor antigen. Using this antigenic competition method we were able to demonstrate that at least part of the immune complexes isolated from cancer sera were composed of tumor antigen and antitumor antibody directed against them (Table 5.2).

Therapeutic Applications

There are many possible applications of tumor antigens to cancer therapy in terms of immunoprevention and immunotherapy. Tumor transplantation experiments in animal models have already demonstrated that immunization with materials expressing tumor antigens prior to tumor challenge is effective in inhibiting tumor growth. Ray and Seshadri reported that immunization of mice with syngeneic embryo cells rendered them partially resistant against chemically-induced fibrosarcoma (14). Spleen cells and sera from embryo cell-immunized animals were capable of killing tumor cells. Though the exact mechanism(s) was not explored by these investigators, it has been suggested that such an immunoprophylactic effect was mediated by the embryonic antigens expressed in common by the syngeneic embryos and the chemically-induced fibrosarcomas. In a subsequent study, Ray and Seshadri demonstrated a similar immunoprotective effect against tumor transplant in multiparous mice (15). Furthermore, spleen cells from pregnant mice showed antitumor effect. The fact that such an antitumor effect in pregnant women may also be operative is suggested from the observed prolonged survival of multiparous patients with malignancy (157). Jones et al. have reported a positive correlation of disease free interval and survival in melanoma patients with high levels of IgM class anti-OFA antibody (102). Therefore, it should, theoretically, be possible to develop a vaccine prepared from purified tumor antigens (embryonic or tumor cells) to prevent certain types of human neoplasms.

A variety of antigenic stimuli including autologous and allogeneic cells both before and after modification with irradiation, mitomycin C, neuraminidase, etc., and their extracts have been tried (158). However, with the exception of an occasional striking regression, the results in most cases have not been impressive or consistent. It seems crucial that immunotherapy, whether with modified tumor cells or purified tumor antigen, be given when the bulk of the tumor mass is removed. This is because the host immune defenses are quite capable of destroying a small number of tumor cells in the range of 1 to 10 million, but not masses of 100 million or more.

During recent years attempts have been made to remove immunosuppressive factors, e.g., immune complexes, by repeated plasmapheresis of cancer patients with metastatic disease (159). Partial regression of tumor was observed in some patients (160). Ray et al. (161), using protein A bearing *Staphylococcus aureus* columns, were able to remove IgG and its complexes from the circulation of tumor-bearing animals and cancer patients. This appeared to have restricted the tumor growth (140). Similar results were reported by Bansal et al. (162) in a patient with colon carcinoma and by Terman et al. (163) in spontaneous canine breast adenocarcinoma after *ex vivo* removal of IgG and immune complexes. The mechanism of the effectiveness of extracorporeal perfusion with protein A is suggested to be removal of immunosuppressive factors which reduce the host immune capacity to interact with tumor antigens expressed on malignant cell surface (140). In this respect, the effect of extracorporeal perfusion is similar to that of surgical removal of tumor which appears to reverse both specific and nonspecific immunosuppression and alter the immune balance in favor of the patient. However, extracorporeal perfusion therapy might be able to take care of micrometastases sufficient to cause immunosuppression but difficult to remove surgically. Thus, immunotherapy, active or passive, in conjunction with surgery and extracorporeal perfusion may be more effective than the techniques that have been tried so far (140). Under these circumstances, passive immunotherapy with cytotoxic (IgM class) monoclonal antitumor antibody obtained from human hybridoma should be particularly useful.

SUMMARY

Despite the controversies that tumor antigens may be altered histocompatibility antigens, the experimental animal models have provided the evidence that TAA unrelated to histocompatibility antigens do exist. Two classes of tumor antigens are expressed by both chemically- and virally-induced animal tumors: the tumor-specific transplantation antigens (TSTA) and the fetal antigens. The role of fetal antigens in tumor transplant rejection is not as well documented as that of TSTA. Recent studies of Ray and Seshadri (14,15) suggest that the fetal antigens provide a degree of resistance against tumor growth. Various strains of an animal species may differ in their ability to respond to fetal antigens.

A number of observations such as spontaneous regressions, delayed recurrences, lymphoid cell infiltration in tumor tissues, etc., suggest that tumor immunity might exist in humans. The existence of tumor antigens in human neoplasms was demonstrated by *in vivo* and *in vitro* cellular reactions and by *in vitro* serologic assays.

Though human tumor antigens may be located in the cytoplasm, in the nucleus, or on the cell surface, the antigens expressed on the cell surface are of importance because the immune response elicited against them may influence tumor growth in the host. The cytoplasmic and nucleolar tumor antigens, though they may not be involved in influencing the tumor growth, may prove to be of prognostic significance. On the basis of serologic reactions human tumor antigens could be categorized as individually specific, histologic type specific, or fetal or embryonic. Old has recognized three classes of human tumor antigens (164). Class 1 antigens are individually specific. Class 2 antigens are expressed by autologous as well as allogeneic tumors of the same histologic type. Class 3 antigens are widely distributed on normal and tumor cells.

Embryonic or fetal antigens are normal embryonic constituents that are repressed shortly after birth. When adult cells undergo malignant transformation, the production of fetal antigens is resumed. Some of these fetal antigens are immunogenic in the host. The immune response elicited against fetal antigens has been shown to be cytotoxic in both cellular and humoral *in vitro* assays. Thus, such antigens may provide a basis for specific immunotherapy of malignant disease in man. For instance, immunization of mice with syngeneic embryo cells provided partial resistance against tumor transplants (14,15). The tumor immunity was transferable to virgin animals with spleen cells and sera from primiparous females (14).

Biologically functional tumor antigens are detectable in body fluids of cancer patients which may arise due to spontaneous release from living tumor cells or due to tumor cell lysis. The shed-antigen can react with sensitized lymphocytes or humoral antibodies and, thus, result in blocking of immune defense mechanism of the host (140). In this respect, the evasion of immune destruction of tumor cells is comparable to the evasion of maternal immune response by the fetal allograft. Experimental data suggest that blocking factors play an important role in enhancement of tumor growth (140). It has been observed that lymphocytes of cancer patients are able to proliferate in a normal manner however, serum samples from any of these patients are capable of inhibiting mitogen-induced lymphocyte proliferation.

Approaches are now being evaluated to remove the blocking factors from circulation of cancer patients by extracorporeal immunoadsorption therapy (140).

Extensive efforts have been made without success to develop diagnostic tests for cancer utilizing both immunologic and nonimmunologic markers. However, at most, the quantitation of tumor markers has been useful for prognostication of cancer recurrence and in evaluation of treatment modalities. In this respect, detection and quantitation of tumor antigens and/or products of cancer patients should provide an insight into the tumor-host relationship.

REFERENCES

1. Prehn, R. T., *Can. Cancer Conf.* **5**:387, 1963.
2. Klein, G., Sjogren, H. O., Klein, E., and Hellström, K. E., *Cancer Res.* **20**:1561, 1960.
3. Economore, G. C., Takeichi, N., and Boone, C. W., *Cancer Res.* **37**:37, 1977.
4. Hellström, K. E., Hellström, I., and Brown, J. P., *Int. J. Cancer* **21**:317, 1978.
5. Coggin, J. H., Adkinson, L., and Anderson, N. G., *Cancer Res.* **40**:1568, 1980.
6. Baldwin, R. W., Immunological aspects of chemical carcinogenesis. In F. F. Becker (Ed.), *Cancer: A Comprehensive Treatise*, Vol. 1, pp. 1. New York: Plenum Press, 1975.
7. Parker, G. C., and Rosenberg, S. A., *J. Immunol.* **118**:1590, 1977.
8. Medawar, P. B., and Hunt, R., *Nature (Lond.)* **271**:164, 1978.
9. Brawn, R. J., *Int. J. Cancer* **6**:245, 1970.
10. Baldwin, R. W., and Glaves, D., *Clin. Exp. Immunol.* **11**:51, 1972.
11. Abelev, G. I., Perova, D. S., Khramkova, N. I., Postnikova, E. A., and Irlin, I. S., *Transplantation* **1**:174, 1963.
12. Ray, P. K., Sengupta, J., Chakraborti, P., and Saha, S., *Ind. J. Exp. Biol.* (Communicated), 1982.
13. Ting, C. C., and Grant, J. P., *J. Natl. Cancer Inst.* **56**:401, 1976.
14. Ray, P. K., and Seshadri, M., *Ind. J. Exp. Biol.* **18**:1027, 1980.
15. Ray, P. K., and Seshadri, M., *Ind. J. Exp. Biol.* **19**:405, 1981.
16. Prehn, R. T., *J. Natl. Cancer Inst.* **55**:189, 1975.
17. Sojgren, H. O., Hellström, I., and Klein, G., *Cancer Res.* **21**:329, 1961.
18. Smith, R. T., *N. Engl. J. Med.* **278**:1207, 1968.
19. Old, L. J.. and Boyse, E. A., *Fed. Proc.* **24**:1009, 1965.
20. Richards, V., *Prog. Exp. Tumor Res.* **25**:1, 1980.
21. Morton, D. L., Miller, G. F., and Wood, D. A., *J. Natl. Cancer Inst.* **42**:289, 1969.
22. Coggin, J. H., Ambrose, K. R., and Anderson, N. G., *J. Immunol.* **105**:524, 1970.
23. Kato, K., *J. Natl. Cancer Inst.* **58**:259, 1977.
24. Weppner, W. A., and Coggin, J. H., Jr., *Cancer Res.* **40**:1380, 1980.
25. Austin, F. C., and Boone, C. W., *Adv. Cancer Res.* **30**:301, 1979.
26. Woodruff, M. F. A., Whitehead, V. L., and Speedy, G., *Br. J. Cancer* **37**:345, 1978.
27. Carswell, E. A., Wanebo, H. J., Old, L. J., and Boyse, E. A., *J. Natl. Cancer Inst.* **44**:1281, 1970.
28. Hammond, W. G., Fischer, F. C., and Rolley, R. T., *Surgery* **62**:124, 1967.

29. Higginson, J., Environment and cancer. In *14th Symp. Fundamental Cancer Res.*, pp. 69. Baltimore: Williams & Wilkins Co., 1972.
30. Morton, D. L., Sparks, F. C., and Haskell, C. M., Oncology. In S. I. Schwartz, C. T. Shires, F. C. Spencer, and E. H. Storer (Eds.), *Principles of Surgery*, 3rd ed. New York: McGraw-Hill Book Co., 1979.
31. Southam, C. M., Brunschwig, W., Levin, A. G., and Dixon, A. S., *Cancer* 19:1743, 1966.
32. Boyd, W., *The Spontaneous Regression of Cancer*. Springfield: Charles C. Thomas, 1966.
33. Abbey Smith, R., *Br. Med. J.* 2:563, 1971.
34. Young, S., and Cowan, D. M., *Br. J. Cancer* 17:85, 1963.
35. Russell, S. W., and McIntosh, A. T., *Nature* 268:69, 1977.
36. White, H., and Griffiths, J. D., *Proc. R. Soc. Med.* 69:467, 1976.
37. Currie, G., *Cancer and the Immune Response*, 2nd ed. Chicago: An Edward Arnold Publication, Year Book Medical Publishers, Inc., 1980.
38. Ristow, S., and McKhann, C. F., Tumor-associated antigens. In I. Green, S. Cohen, and R. T. McClusky (Eds.), *Mechanisms of Tumor Immunity*, pp. 109. New York: John Wiley and Sons, 1977.
39. Black, M. M., and Leis, H. P., *Cancer* 32:384, 1973.
40. Avis, F., Avis, I., Newsome, J. F., and Haughton, G., *J. Natl. Cancer Inst.* 56:17, 1976.
41. Skurzak, H., Steiner, L., Klein, E., and Lamon, E., *Natl. Cancer Inst. Monogr.* 37:93, 1973.
42. Vanky, F. T., and Stjernsward, J., Lymphocyte stimulation (by autologous tumor biopsy cells). In R. B. Herberman and K. R. McIntire (Eds.), *Immunodiagnosis of Cancer*, pp. 998. New York: Marcel Dekker, Inc., 1979.
43. Gainor, B. J., Forbes, J. T., Enneking, W. F., and Smith, R. T., *Clin. Orthop. Rel. Res.* 111:83, 1975.
44. Rocklin, R. E., Leukocyte migration inhibition. In R. B. Herberman and K. R. McIntire (Eds.), *Immunodiagnosis of Cancer*, pp. 964. New York: Marcel Dekker, Inc., 1979.
45. McCoy, J. L., Clinical application of assays of leukocyte migration inhibition. In R. B. Herberman and K. R. McIntire (Eds.), *Immunodiagnosis of Cancer*, pp. 979. New York: Marcel Dekker, Inc., 1979.
46. Cochran, A. J., Mackie, R. M., Ross, C. E., Ogg, L. J., and Jackson, A. M., *Int. J. Cancer* 18:274, 1976.
47. Halliday, W. J., Maluish, A. E., Little, J. H., and Davis, N. C., *Int. J. Cancer* 16:645, 1975.
48. Powell, A. E., Sloss, A. M., Smith, R. N., Makley, J. J., and Hubay, C. A., *Int. J. Cancer* 16:905, 1975.
49. Moller, E., *Science* 147:873, 1965.
50. Saal, J. C., Rieber, E. P., Hadam, M., and Riethmuller, G., *Nature* 265:158, 1977.
51. Kodera, Y., and Bean, M. A., *Int. J. Cancer* 16:579, 1975.
52. Hersey, P., Honeyman, M., Edwards, A., Adams, E., and McCarthy, W. H., *Int. J. Cancer* 18:564, 1976.
53. Rosenberg, S. A., *Serologic Analysis of Human Cancer Antigens*. New York: Academic Press, 1980.
54. Bjorkland, B., Graham, J. B., and Graham, R. M., *Int. Arch. Allergy* 10:56, 1957.
55. Gupta, R. K., Silver, H. K. B., and Morton, D. L., *J. Surg. Oncol.* 13:75, 1980.
56. Singh, I., Tsang, K. T., and Blakemore, W. S., Serologic analysis of tumor-associated surface antigens on human osteosarcoma cells. In S. A. Rosenberg (Ed.), *Serologic Analysis of Human Cancer Antigens*, pp. 161. New York: Academic Press, 1980.

57. Braatz, J. A., Gaffar, S. A., Princler, G. L., and McIntire, K. R., Description of a human lung tumor-associated antigen. In S. A. Rosenberg (Ed.), *Serologic Analysis of Human Cancer Antigens*, pp. 181. New York: Academic Press, 1980.

58. Ghose, T., Novell, S. T., Guclu, A., and MacDonald, A. S., *Eur. J. Cancer* **11**:321, 1975.

59. Bell, C. E., Human lung cancer plasma membrane antigens. In S. A. Rosenberg (Ed.), *Serologic Analysis of Human Cancer Antigens*, pp. 239. New York: Academic Press, 1980.

60. Aryan, S., *Clin. Plastic Surg.* **6**:125, 1979.

61. McBride, C. M., Bowen, J. M., and Dmochowski, L. L., *Surg. Forum* **23**:92, 1972.

62. Seth, P., and Balachandran, N., *Nature* **286**:613, 1980.

63. Gupta, R. K., and Morton, D. L., *Cancer Res.* **35**:58, 1975.

64. Tonder, O., Krishnan, E. C., Jewell, W. R., Morse, P. A., and Humphry, L. J., *Acta Pathol. Microbiol. Scand.* **84**:105, 1976.

65. Witz, I. P., *Adv. Cancer Res.* **25**:95, 1977.

66. Kohler, G., and Milstein, C., *Nature* (London) **256**:495, 1975.

67. Keprowski, H., Steplewski, Z., Herlyn, D., and Herlyn, M., *Proc. Natl. Acad. Sci. USA* **76**:1438, 1978.

67a. Morgan, A. C., Gallaway, D. R., and Reisfield, R. A., *Hybridoma* **1**:27, 1981.

68. Shiku, H., Takahashi, T., Oettgen, H. F., and Old, L. J., *J. Exp. Med.* **144**:873, 1976.

69. Yeh, M-Y., Hellström, I., and Hellström, K. E., *J. Immunol.* **126**:1312, 1981.

70. Carrel, S., Accolla, R. S., Carmgnola, A. L., and Mach, J. P., *Cancer Res.* **40**:2523, 1980.

71. Bodurtha, H. J., Chee, D. P., Lancuis, J. F., Mastrangelo, M. J., and Prehn, R. L., *Cancer Res.* **35**:189, 1975.

72. Lewis, M. G., Ikonopiov, R. L., Nairn, R. C., Phillips, T. M., Hamilton-Fairley, G., Bedenham, D. C., and Alexander, P., *Br. Med. J.* **3**:547, 1969.

73. Carey, T. E., Takahashi, T., Resnick, L. A., Oettgen, H. F., and Old, L. J., *Proc. Natl. Acad. Sci. USA* **73**:3278, 1976.

74. Fossati, G., Colnaghi, M. I., Della Porta, G., Cascinelli, N., and Veronesi, U., *Int. J. Cancer* **9**:567, 1972.

75. Yeh, M-Y., Hellström, I., Brown, J. P., Warner, G. A., Hansen, J. A., and Hellström, K. E., *Proc. Natl. Acad. Sci.* **76**:2927, 1979.

76. Morton, D. L., Malmgren, R. A., Holmes, E. C., and Ketcham, A. S., *Surgery* **64**:233, 1968.

77. Morton, D. L., and Malmgren, R. A., *Science* **162**:1279, 1968.

78. Sethi, J., and Hirshaut, Y., *J. Natl. Cancer Inst.* **57**:489, 1976.

79. Abelev, G. I., and Gamaleya, N. F., Alfa-fetoprotein as a model for studying reexpression of embryonic antigens in neoplasia. In R. B. Herberman and K. R. McIntire (Eds.), *Immunodiagnosis of Cancer*, pp. 76. New York: Marcel Dekker, Inc., 1979.

80. Ruoslahti, E., Engvall, E., and Kessler, M. J., Chemical properties of alfa-fetoprotein. In R. B. Herberman and K. R. McIntire (Eds.), *Immunodiagnosis of Cancer*, pp. 101. New York: Marcel Dekker, Inc., 1979.

81. Sell, S., and Becker, F. F., *J. Natl. Cancer Inst.* **60**:19, 1978.

82. Waldman, T. A., and McIntire, K. R., The use of sensitive assays for alpha-fetoprotein in monitoring the treatment of malignancy. In R. B. Herberman and K. R. McIntire (Eds.), *Immunodiagnosis of Cancer*, pp. 130. New York: Marcel Dekker, Inc., 1979.

83. Gold, P., and Freedman, S. A., Carcinoembryonic antigen; Historical perspective, experimental data. In R. B. Herberman and K. R. McIntire (Eds.), *Immunodiagnosis of Cancer*, pp. 147. New York: Marcel Dekker, Inc., 1979.

84. LoGerfo, D., Herter, F. P., and Bennett, J. S., *Int. J. Cancer* **9**:344, 1972.

85. Williams, R. R., McIntire, K. R., Waldmann, T. A., Feinleib, M., Go, V. L., Kannel, W. B., Dawber, T. R., Casetelli, W. P., and McNamara, P. N., *J. Natl. Cancer Inst.* **58**:1547, 1977.
86. Kleist, S. von, and Burtin, P., Antigens cross-reacting with CEA. In R. B. Herberman and K. R. McIntire (Eds.), *Immunodiagnosis of Cancer*, pp. 322. New York: Marcel Dekker, Inc., 1979.
87. Costanza, M. E., Pinn, V., Schwartz, R. S., and Nathanson, L., *N. Engl. J. Med.* **289**:521, 1973.
88. Häkkinen, I., *Transplant. Rev.* **20**:61, 1974.
89. Gelder, F. B., Reese, C. J., Moossa, A. R., Hall, T., and Hunter, R., *Cancer Res.* **38**:312, 1978.
90. Buffe, D., Rimbant, C., Lemerle, J., Schweisguth, O., and Burtin, P., *Int. J. Cancer* **5**:85, 1970.
91. Fritsche, R., and Mach, J. P., *Nature* **258**:734, 1975.
92. Chism, S. E., Burton, R. C., and Warner, N. L., *Clin. Immunol. Immunopathol.* **11**:346, 1978.
93. Girardi, A. J., Reppucci, P., Dierbman, P., Rutala, W., and Coggin, J. H., Jr., *Proc. Natl. Acad. Sci. USA* **70**:183, 1973.
94. Edynak, E. M., Old, L. J., Vrana, M., and Lardis, M. P., *N. Engl. J. Med.* **286**:1178, 1972.
95. Rosenberg, S. A., Brown, J., Hyatt, C., Shoffner, P., and Tondreau, S., Serologic studies of the antigens on human osteogenic sarcoma. In S. A. Rosenberg, (Ed.), *Serologic Analysis of Human Cancer Antigens*, pp. 93. New York: Academic Press, 1980.
96. Della-Porta, G., Canevari, S., and Fossati, G., *Br. J. Cancer* **28**:103, 1973.
97. Herberman, R. B., Hollinshead, A. C., Alford, T. C., McCoy, J. L., Halterman, R. H., and Leventhal, B. G., *Natl. Cancer Inst. Monogra.* **37**:189, 1973.
98. Irie, R. F., Oncofetal antigen (OFA-I); A human tumor associated fetal antigen immunogenic in man. In S. A. Rosenberg (Ed.), *Serologic Analysis of Human Cancer Antigens*, pp. 493. New York: Academic Press, 1980.
99. Gupta, R. K., Silver, H. K. B., Reisfeld, R. A., and Morton, D. L., *Cancer Res.* **39**:1683, 1979.
100. Sidell, N., Irie, R. F., and Morton, D. L., *Br. J. Cancer* **40**:950, 1979.
101. Gupta, R. K., and Morton, D. L. *J. Natl. Cancer Inst.* **70**:993, 1983.
102. Jones, P. C., Sidell, N., and Irie, R. F., *Cancer Immunol. Immunother.* **8**:211, 1980.
103. Holyoke, D., and Chu, T. M., Tissue polypeptide antigen. In R. B. Herberman and K. R. McIntire (Eds.), *Immunodiagnosis of Cancer*, pp. 513. New York: Marcel Dekker, Inc., 1979.
104. Zangerle, P. F., Hendrick, J. C., Thirion, A., and Franchimont, P., Casè in radioimmunoassay as an index of mammary function and as a tumor marker. In *Cancer-Related Antigens*, pp. 61. Amsterdam: North-Holland, 1976.
105. Marcus, D. M., and Zinberg, N., *J. Natl. Cancer Inst.* **55**:791, 1975.
106. Cochran, A. J., *Man, Cancer and Immunity*. New York: Academic Press, 1978.
107. Lewis, M. G., Hartman, D., and Herry, L. M., *Ann. N.Y. Acad. Sci.* **276**:316, 1976.
108. Cochran, A. J., Mackie, R. M., Grant, R. M., Ross, C. E., Donnell, M. D., Sandilands, G., Whaley, K., Hoyle, D. E., and Jackson, A. M., *Int. J. Cancer* **18**:298, 1976.
109. Gupta, R. K., and Morton, D. L., *J. Surg. Oncol.* **11**:65, 1979.
110. Rahman, A. F. R., Liao, S. K., and Dent, P., *In Vitro* **13**:580, 1977.
111. Hellström, K. E., and Hellström, I., Immunologic enhancement of tumor growth. In I. Green, S. Cohen, and R. T. McCluskey (Eds.), *Mechanisms of Tumor Immunity*, pp. 147. New York: John Wiley and Sons, 1977.

112. Ray, P. K., and Saha, S., *Fed. Proc.* **41**:411, 1982.
113. Raychaudhuri, S., Ray, P. K., Bassett, J. G., and Cooper, D. R., *Fed. Proc.* **39**:696, 1980.
114. Morgan, Jr., A. C., Gallaway, D. R., Imai, K., Ferrone, S., and Reisfeld, R. A., *Fed. Proc.* **39**:351, 1980.
115. Reisfeld, R. A., *Fed. Proc.* **40**:228, 1981.
116. LeGrue, S. J., Kahan, B. D., and Pellis, N. R., *J. Natl. Cancer Inst.* **65**:191, 1980.
117. Bhavanandan, V. P., Kemper, J. G., and Bystryn, J. C., *J. Biol. Chem.* **255**:5145, 1980.
118. McCabe, R. P., Gallaway, D. R., Ferrone, S., and Reisfeld, R. A., Human melanoma associated antigens (MAA): Serologic and structural characterization. In S. Ferrone, S. Gorini, R. B. Herberman, and R. A. Reisfeld (Eds.), *Current Trends in Tumor Immunology*, pp. 269. New York: Garland STPM Press, 1979.
119. Reisfield, R. A., Gallaway, D. R., McCabe, R. P., and Morgan, A. C., Molecular and immunological characterization of human melanoma associated antigens. In R. A. Reisfield and S. Ferrone (Eds.), *Melanoma antigens and antibodies*, pp. 317. New York: Plenum Press, 1982.
120. Thomson, D. M. P., Sellens, V., Eccles, S., and Alexander, P., *Br. J. Cancer* **28**:377, 1973.
121. Woodbury, R. G., Brown, J. P., Yeh, M-Y., Hellström, I., and Hellström, K. E., *Proc. Natl. Acad. Sci. USA* **77**:2183, 1980.
122. Brown, J. P., Nishiyama, K., Hellström, I., and Hellström, K., *J. Immunol.* **127**:539, 1981.
123. Curry, R. A., Quaranta, V., Wilson, B. S., McCabe, R. P., Natali, P. G., Pellegrino, M. A., and Ferrone, S., Expression of HLA antigens on cultured human melanoma cells: Lack of association with melanoma-associated antigens. In S. Ferrone, S. Gorini, R. B. Herberman, and R. A. Reisfeld (Eds.), *Current Trends in Tumor Immunology*, pp. 347. New York: Garland STPM Press, 1979.
124. Pliskin, M. E., and Prehn, R. T., *Transplantation* **26**:19, 1978.
125. Pierotti, M. A., Miotti, S., Invernizzi, G., and Parmiani, G., *Tumori* **65**:295, 1979.
126. Parmiani, G., Ballinari, D., and Sensi, M. L., *J. Immunol.* **124**:662, 1980.
127. Klein, G., and Klein, E., *Int. J. Cancer* **15**:879, 1975.
128. Forni, G., and Cavallo, G., *Prog. Biochem. Pharmacol.* **14**:163, 1978.
129. Yefenof, E., and Klein, G., *Exp. Cell. Res.* **88**:217, 1974.
130. Roman, J. M., and Bonavida, B., *Transplant. Proc.* **11**:1365, 1979.
131. Cementson, K. J., Bertschmann, M., and Widner, S., *Immunochemistry* **13**:383, 1976.
132. Law, L. W., DuBois, G. C., Rogers, M. J., Appella, E., Pierotti, M. A., and Parmiani, G., *Transplant. Proc.* **12**:46, 1980.
133. Klein, P. A., *Transplant. Proc.* **12**:16, 1980.
134. Herberman, R. B., and Holden, H. T., *Adv. Cancer Res.* **27**:305, 1978.
135. Takasugi, M., Akira, D., Takasugi, J., and Mickey, M. R., *J. Natl. Cancer Inst.* **59**:69, 1977.
136. Miller, E. C., *Cancer Res.* **38**:1479, 1978.
137. Burnett, F. M., *Immunological Surveillance.* New York: Pergamon Press, 1970.
138. Morton, D. L. *J. Natl. Cancer Inst.* **42**:311, 1969.
139. Baldwin, R. W., Bowen, J. G., and Price, M. R., *Br. J. Cancer* **28**:16, 1973.
140. Ray, P. K., *Plasma Ther. Trans. Technol.* **3**:101, 1982.
141. Wolf, P. L., Importance of tumor markers. In *Tumor Associated Markers: The Importance of Identification in Clinical Medicine*, pp. 1. New York: Masson Publishing U.S.A., Inc., 1979.
142. Theofilopoulos, A. N., and Dixon, F. J., Immune complexes associated with neoplasia.

In R. B. Herberman and K. R. McIntire (Eds.), *Immunodiagnosis of Cancer*, pp.896. New York: Marcel Dekker, Inc., 1979.

143. Weksler, M. E., *Abstr. Am. Soc. Nephrol.* **99**:19, 1974.

144. Jehn, V. W., Nathenson, L., Schwartz, R. S., and Skinner, M., *N. Engl. J. Med.* **283**:329, 1970.

145. Volkers, C., Cooke, B., Bennett, C., Byrom, N., Campbell, M., Elliott, P., and Whitfield, P., *Aust. N. Z. J. Surg.* **48**:32, 1978.

146. Gupta, R. K., and Morton, D. L., Clinical significance of tumor-associated antigens and antitumor antibodies in human malignant melanoma. In R. A. Reisfeld, (Ed.), *Melanoma Antigens and Antibodies.* New York: Plenum Press, 1981.

147. Gupta, R. K., and Morton, D. L., *Surg. Forum* **26**:158, 1975.

148. Rote, N. S., Gupta, R. K., and Morton, D. L., *Int. J. Cancer* **26**:203, 1980.

149. Huth, J. F., Gupta, R. K., and Morton, D. L., *Surg. Forum* **30**:150, 1979.

150. Morton, D. L., Golub, S. H., Sulit, H. L., Gupta, R. K., Eilber, F. R., Holmes, E. C., and Sparks, F. C., Immunological and clinical responses to active immunotherapy of malignant melanoma. In A. A. Gottlieb, O. J. Plescia, and D. H. L. Bishop (Eds.), *Fundamental Aspects of Neoplasia*, pp. 181. New York: Springer-Verlag, 1975.

151. deKernion, J. B., Ramming, K. P., and Gupta, R. K., *J. Urol.* **122**:300, 1979.

152. Gupta, R. K., and Morton, D. L., Possible clinical significance of circulating immune complexes in melanoma patients. In C. B. Denny (Ed.), *Fundamental Mechanisms in Human Cancer-Immunology.* In press.

153. Gupta, R. K., Theofilopoulos, A. N., Dixon, F. J., and Morton, D. L., *Cancer Immunol. Immunother.* **6**:211, 1979.

154. Gupta, R. K., and Morton, D. L., *Fed. Proc.* **37**:1595, 1978.

155. Gupta, R. K., Golub, S. H., and Morton, D. L., *Cancer Immunol. Immunother.* **6**:63, 1979.

156. Gupta, R. K., and Morton, D. L., Radioimmunoassay for the analysis of tumor-associated antigens with allogeneic antibody. In S. A. Rosenberg, (Ed.), *Serologic Analysis of Human Cancer Antigens*, pp. 645. New York: Academic Press, 1980.

157. Hersey, P., Stone, D. E., Morgan, G., McCarthy, W. H., and Milton, G. W., *Lancet* **1**:451, 1977.

158. Ray, P. K., *Adv. Appl. Microbiol.* **21**:227, 1977.

159. Hersey, P., Isbister, J., Edwards, A., Murray, E., Adams, E., Biggs, J., and Milton, G. W., *Lancet* **1**:825, 1976.

160. Israel, L., Edelstein, R., Mannoni, P., and Radot, E., *Lancet* **2**:642, 1976.

161. Ray, P. K., McLaughlin, D., Mohammed, J., Idiculla, A., Rhoads, J. E., Mark, R., Bassett, J. G., and Cooper, D. R., Ex vivo immunoadsorption of IgG or its complexes – a new modality of cancer treatment. In B. Serrou and C. Rosenfeld, (Eds.), *Immune Complexes and Plasma Exchanges in Cancer Patients*, pp. 197. Amsterdam: Elsevier/ North Holland, 1981.

162. Bansal, S. C., Bansal, B. R., Thomas, H. C., Siegel, P. D., Rhoads, J. E., Cooper, D. R., Terman, D. S., and Mark R., *Cancer* **42**:1, 1978.

163. Terman, D. S., Yamamoto, T., Mattioli, M., Cook, G., Tillquist, R., Henry, J., Poser, R., and Daskal, Y., *J. Immunol.* **124**:795, 1980.

164. Old, L. J., *Cancer Res.* **41**:361, 1981.

6

Ability of Immune Reactivity to Potentiate Tumor Growth

Donna M. Murasko and Richmond T. Prehn

The concept that our immune system is constantly protecting us from cancer by destroying potentially neoplastic cells as they arise is the basis of the theory of immunosurveillance. This theory was readily accepted and seldom challenged by cancer researchers because of its innate appeal. How wonderful it is to have a natural defense system against cancer! And what system could be more appropriate for this task than our immune system which has the capacity to respond to virtually all foreign substances? However, when one considers the high percentage of the population that eventually develops cancer, one reaches the conclusion that our defenses do not always prevent cancer. And if one believes that our immune system has done everything within its power to prevent cancer, then it must be concluded that the immune system is of no more value in further treatment of the cancer and, therefore, the study of *tumor immunology* should be abandoned.

Fortunately, every story has at least two sides. Another view of the role of the immune response during the formation of tumors was proffered by one of us over a decade ago (1, 2) in the theory of immunostimulation. In its simplest form, this theory states that although immune reactivity may sometimes control tumor growth, lesser degrees of immune reactivity may actually promote the growth of tumors. Just as the immunosurveillance theory receives nods of agreement and smiles of contentment, the theory of immunostimulation induces incredulous stares and rejection because the initial impact is so negative—our defense system helping a tumor grow! However, the theory actually gives us encouragement that the immune system may be effective in controlling tumor growth once it becomes clinically apparent: one simply needs to know how to strengthen the antitumor response to an appropriate level in order to achieve immunologic rejection of the tumor.

The purpose of the following presentation is to encourage the reader to ponder the value of the theory of immunostimulation. This will be accomplished by presenting the arguments against the immunosurveillance theory

148

and the data supporting the theory of immunostimulation. Although we will conclude with our evaluation of its importance in neoplasia, the final conclusion is yours whether or not you consider the theory of immunostimulation while designing experimental protocols and evaluating data.

ARGUMENTS AGAINST IMMUNOSURVEILLANCE

The theory of immunosurveillance as formulated by Thomas (3) and elaborated by Burnet (4) is based on the belief that an immune response destroys developing cancer cells in a manner similar to the immune rejection of allografts. The first assumption of this theory is that cancer cells possess antigens different from normal cells (comparable to histocompatibility antigens). The second is that the immune system can respond to these tumor antigens. A corollary of the second assumption is that impaired immunity will increase the incidence of cancer. In this section we will discuss the validity of these points. Since possession of foreign antigens by tumor cells (e.g., as detected by antisera prepared in a heterologous species) is basically irrelevant if a syngeneic host cannot respond to the tumor antigen, points one and two will be considered together. Rather than referring to the *antigenicity* of the tumor (the possession of antigens), we will refer to the *immunogenicity* of the tumor (the ability to induce a specific immune response). Throughout our discussion, immunogenicity will be used to refer to the capacity of a tumor to induce immunity *in vivo* that will restrict to some degree the subsequent growth of implants of that tumor.

Immunogenicity of Tumor Cells

Following the suggestive work of Foley (5), Prehn and Main (6) convincingly demonstrated in 1957 that tumors arising in syngeneic mice possess tumor-specific antigens. Since that time many investigators have shown that most tumors induced in the laboratory by viral, chemical, or physical agents have tumor-specific antigens. These tumor antigens were identified by various procedures, e.g., inhibition of tumor growth by previous immunization with killed tumor cells or virus; reactivity of lymphoid cells or sera from tumor-bearing hosts with tumor cells in *in vitro* assays; and prevention of tumor growth by passive transfer of lymphoid cells or sera from immunized donors to nonimmunized hosts [Stutman, (7) review]. However, so-called spontaneous tumors of rodents, i.e., tumors that arise in low frequency with no overt cause, are seldom immunogenic (8). Also in chemically-induced tumors, immunogenicity tends to be related to the concentration of inducing oncogen; low concentrations that presumably mimic the environmental condition produce tumors of little or no immunogenicity (9). These contrasting groups of tumors (laboratory induced, highly immunogenic vs. spontaneous, weakly immunogenic) raise two questions: (a) why is there such a difference in immunogenicity and (b) which group is more representative of human tumors?

The first question can be posed in an alternate manner: why do weakly immunogenic tumors arise? Proponents of the immunosurveillance theory will respond that weakly-immunogenic or nonimmunogenic tumors arise due to immunoselection in the following manner. A cell is transformed into a tumor cell by some agent. If this tumor cell possesses strong tumor antigens, the immune system recognizes it and eliminates it. If, however, this tumor cell is weakly immunogenic or nonimmunogenic, the immune system cannot respond to it and the tumor grows. Therefore, it is consistent with the theory of immunosurveillance that most tumors that become clinically apparent are weakly immunogenic.

Although it has been shown that some selective forces do occur during tumor induction and progression (10, 11), tumors that arise in immunologically free environments are usually nonimmunogenic, unless a chemical or virus is added to the system (10). These immunologically free environments include tissue culture conditions and diffusion chambers. Cells placed within diffusion chambers are implanted within the peritoneal cavity of a rodent. Although host soluble products can diffuse into the chamber, the cells within the chamber are protected from contact with host cellular components, including lymphocytes. Since nonimmunogenic tumors can and do arise without immunologic intervention, it cannot be concluded that the predominance of nonimmunogenic tumors as spontaneous tumors is dependent on immunoselection. The immunogenicity of the tumor appears to be property conferred by the oncogenic agent, if one is present. Although immunoselection may occur, it need not be the reason for lack of immunogenicity of spontaneous tumors.

The second question is whether human tumors are more related to viral- and chemically-induced tumors or to spontaneous tumors of rodents. In the rodent, the term spontaneous is best equated with tumors that arise infrequently, sporadically, and without known causes. This infrequency, however, is in an inbred rodent population in which all members of the group are at equal risk. In man, where genetically susceptible individuals cannot yet be identified, it is possible that some tumors may actually occur in nearly 100% of the genetically susceptible population. Until the genetic basis of tumor susceptibility in humans is deciphered, one must keep an open mind as to which type of rodent tumor should be used as a model for human tumors.

Another more direct approach to answering the question of whether human tumors are more related to induced or spontaneous tumors of rodents would be to examine the immunogenicity of human tumors. This is actually quite difficult to do. Although reactivity of lymphoid cells and sera from certain cancer patients to their tumor cells can sometimes be demonstrated, it is impossible to establish the specificity and importance of these *in vitro* reactions to rejection of tumors *in vivo*. In laboratory animals, the availability of inbred stains permits transplantation and adoptive transfer studies that establish the existence of tumor antigens that are immunogenic. Similar studies, obviously, cannot be performed in humans.

That the immune system does interact with human tumors has been forcibly argued by Ioachim (12) who pointed out that many human tumors, especially in the early stages of their evolution, are associated with an intense infiltration of lymphocytes and/or related cells. It seems reasonable to assume that this infiltrate is indicative of immunologic recognition of the neoplasm. The presence of this lymphoid infiltrate is usually associated with a better prognosis, as is seen in cases of human breast cancer (13). This apparent association is given as a strong argument in favor of immunosurveillance. However, since this lymphoid infiltrate is primarily concentrated at the periphery of the tumor, the intratumor concentration of lymphoid cells is low and, therefore, may stimulate tumor growth. The prognosis is good because the infiltrate indicates an early, lymphodependent, stage of growth.

The above discussion can be summarized in the following manner: (a) Animal tumors do possess tumor specific antigens. The strength of these antigens as immunogens is primarily dependent on the presence or absence and amount of oncogenic agent. Although immunoselection may occur, it is not a necessary factor for the development of nonimmunogenic tumors. (b) Although human tumors also possess tumor antigens, the immunogenicity of these tumors has not been established. The presence of a lymphoid infiltrate suggests immune response does occur, but its strength cannot be determined. Since these facts allow no firm conclusion concerning the validity of the theory of immunosurveillance, the approach of researchers to prove this theory was to utilize the corollary that an impaired immune system will result in increased neoplasia. The results of these experiments are discussed in the next section.

Effect of Impaired Immunity on the Incidence of Neoplasia

The effect of impaired immunity on the incidence of neoplasia will be considered in three categories: (a) virus-induced tumors, (b) chemically-induced tumors, and (c) spontaneous tumors. In each category the data supporting immunosurveillance will be presented first, followed by the points against the theory.

Virus-Induced Tumors. The incidence of virus-induced tumors is increased when mice are treated with antilymphocyte sera (14), are thymectomized (7), or when virus is given to athymic nude mice (7). In addition, many viruses only induce tumors when given to newborn or immunosuppressed mice and if either of these groups are given injections of lymphocytes from normal mice the neoplasms do not develop. Further, some virus-induced tumors can be prevented by vaccination (7). These results appear to supply strong support for immunosurveillance.

Several questions concerning these results arise, however. First, since these tumors are so highly immunogenic, i.e., they cannot be induced in normal mice, should they be considered artifactual? Second, are there any virus-induced tumor systems that are less immunogenic? If so, what is the effect of immunosuppression on incidence of these tumors? The classic example of a less immunogenic, virus-induced tumor is the murine mammary tumor. This tumor arises spontaneously in mice due to the transmission of murine mammary tumor virus from mother to her progeny in the milk or incorporated in the genetic material. It has been shown by several investigators that neonatal thymectomy reduces the incidence of mammary tumors and the reconstitution of these mice with thymic tissue restores their normal susceptibility to breast cancer (15,16). Finally, is the increased incidence of neoplasia a result of a decrease in an antitumor or an antiviral immunity? It is known that the frequency of viral transformation is directly related to the concentration of virus. If the viral infection is not limited by an antiviral immune response, the number of virus particles increases and the number of transformed cells increases, thus increasing the incidence and/or shortening the latent period of neoplasia. Delineation of the antiviral and antitumor effects is extremely difficult and, to our knowledge, has not been accomplished. Therefore, although an immune response may be important in preventing the induction of some virus-induced tumors, this inhibition may be due to an antiviral response and, therefore, be unrelated to immunosurveillance.

Chemically-Induced Tumors. In tumor induction by chemicals, potentiation of oncogenesis by immunodepression has been difficult to demonstrate, perhaps due to the immunodepression produced by the chemical itself (17). Positive, statistically significant reports exist, but they are usually not overwhelming (18,19). Failures have also been revealed, but one suspects that many negative results have not been reported (20). One interesting study was reported by Stutman who found that although the incidence of polyoma-induced tumors was increased in athymic nude mice compared to heterozygous thymus-containing control mice, the incidence of tumors after treatment with DMBA was virtually the same in both groups (21). Since the number of reports are small, however, the significance of either side of this point remains questionable.

Spontaneous Tumors. The effect of immunosuppression or the lack of an immune response on spontaneous tumors has been studied in both animals and man. In animals the models are immunologically privileged sites and the athymic nude mouse. In man, the models are spontaneous immunodeficiency diseases and recipients of renal allografts, all of whom receive immunosuppressive therapy.

The cheek pouch of the hamster has been used by cancer researchers to determine the oncogenic potential of newly transformed cells or of human tumor material. These grafts are accepted because the cheek pouch lacks any connection with the lymphatic system and is, therefore, an immunologically privileged site (23). If an intact immune system was necessary to prevent neoplasia, as postulated by the immunosurveillance theory, then the cheek pouch should be the site of many neoplasms. However, it is not.

While the cheek pouch is an example of a localized area lacking immunocompetence, the nude mouse is an example of generalized immunodeficiency. Nude mice are genetically deficient of both hair and a thymus (24). The lack of a thymus results in absence of most mature T cells and, therefore, of most immune capabilities. The incidence of spontaneous tumors in this animal is of great interest. However, since they have virtually no immune responsiveness, they are extremely susceptible to infections and die within the first few months of life unless they are kept under strict germ-free conditions. Nude mice have been maintained under these conditions by Outzen, et al. (25) and have been found to have a high incidence of spontaneous neoplasms. However, all of the neoplasms involve the lymphoreticular system. The immunosurveillance theory predicts that such animals should have a high incidence of tumors, but they should be of all cell types, not simply of the lymphoreticular system. Proponents of immunosurveillance could argue that the germ-free environment prevented contact with environmental tumor initiators and promoters which are essential for most tumor induction. However, an alternate explanation is that the defective immune system is lacking the regulatory components necessary to control normal cell growth. Lymphoreticular tumors are developing not because of a lack of surveillance, but due to a defect in cellular interactions and regulation.

Melief and Schwartz reported that cancer develops in about 10% of patients with spontaneous immunodeficiency diseases (26). Of 58 cases of immunodeficiency and cancer, 47 had either a lymphoreticular tumor or acute leukemia. The predominance of lymphoreticular tumors in these patients bears a striking similarity to the incidence of the same tumors in nude mice.

Similar results were reported by these investigators for patients receiving both renal allografts and immunosuppressive therapy. About 5% of these patients develop cancer. Two kinds of neoplasms are particularly frequent: (a) epithelial cancers of the skin, lip, or cervix, and (b) malignant lymphomas. The investigators attributed the increase in the first group of cancers to the more frequent physical examinations of these patients compared to the control population. They also point out that the incidence of lymphomas far exceeds the incidence of other neoplasms. For example, the incidence of reticulum cell sarcoma in women allograft recipients was 700 times greater than expected, but the incidence of breast cancer, the most common neoplasia of women, was not increased in the grafted women. Again, these results are similar to the results from nude mice.

In conclusion, although there is substantial evidence to support the theory of immunosurveillance, these data are not without blemish and, in most cases, alternative interpretations of the data are possible. Having created an atmosphere where alternative explanations are not the exception but the rule, we will describe how the theory of immunostimulation was born and then give the experimental evidence to support the theory.

BASIS FOR IMMUNOSTIMULATION

The theory of immunostimulation was formally presented in 1971 by Prehn and Lappé (2). In this original presentation, the authors assembled evidence that a low level of immune reactivity had the potential to stimulate growth of both normal and neoplastic tissues. We will review in this section some of the material utilized to formulate the theory of immunostimulation. In the following section, more recent evidence to support this theory will be presented.

Evidence from Normal Tissues

One of the principal systems used to demonstrate the stimulatory activity of a weak immune response in the original paper presenting the theory of immunostimulation was maternal-fetal interactions. Since much of this data has become controversial and the system more complex, these experiments will not be presented in detail. For more information concerning this evidence, it is best to consult Prehn and Lappé (2). However, two points regarding this system will be described in order to gain an appreciation for the environment nurturing the formation of the theory of immunostimulation.

Although the first reference to possible immunostimulation was probably made by Metchnikoff in 1899 when he stated that although antiorgan sera were usually inhibitory to their targets, in low dilution they might stimulate their growth (27), the first report to describe a stimulatory effect in a reproductive system was Perlmann (28). He demonstrated that antiserum to unfertilized sea urchin egg was capable of activating the egg nucleus. A more recent and direct investigation of the effect of weak immunization on fetal survival was performed by Lappé and Schalk (29). They showed that maternal immunization with syngeneic male antigen significantly increased the percentage of male progeny. Since the male antigen is only weakly immunogenic and since this increase only occurred if the immunization was performed on splenectomized females, a procedure known to decrease blocking antibody and suppressor cells, this report supports the hypothesis that a weak immune response can stimulate the growth of cells.

In addition to maternal-fetal systems, stimulation of normal tissues can also be observed during graft rejection. Warden and Steinmuller studied survival of thyroid grafts in thyroidectomized rats (30). By assaying thyroxin levels they found that grafts made across a weak histocompatibility barrier temporarily produced more thyroxin (i.e., survived better) than syngeneic grafts. Grafts made across a strong histocompatibility barrier were destroyed almost immediately.

Although the above studies may suggest that stimulation is immunologically specific, it is important to point out that stimulation has also been observed with nonsensitized lymphoid cells or nonspecifically activated lymphoid cells. Admixture of mouse fibroblast cells with nonsensitized syngeneic or xenogeneic spleen cells or with syngeneic spleen cells sensitized to bovine serum albumin enhanced the viability or growth of the fibroblast cells in culture (31). Similarly, lymphotoxin prepared from cultures of cells stimulated with phytohemagglutinin stimulated incorporation of ^{14}C amino acids into cultures of bovine, hamster, rabbit, and mouse cells (32). This stimulation only occurred when small amounts of lymphotoxin were added to the cultures; high quantities inhibited cellular metabolism.

Regardless of the specificity of the reaction, by 1971 there were a number of reports demonstrating that interaction with the immune system could result in increased cellular metabolism of normal tissues. A major criterion for induction of stimulation appeared to be the strength of the reaction—a weak response would be stimulatory, while a stronger response would be inhibitory. Were comparable observations present in tumor systems?

Evidence from Tumor Systems

That prior immunization may result in the enhanced growth of subsequent tumor implants is a well known and common phenomenon. A number of authors have demonstrated that a very low dose of immunogenic tumor cells may survive and grow in an animal, while a slightly larger dose of cells would be inhibited (33–35). This phenomenon, generally referred to as *sneaking through*, was explained by a delay in immunization due to the small number of cells; by the time there are enough cells for immunization, the tumor has already reached a rapid phase and the immune response is ineffective. However, this explanation is not feasible since it can still be observed in previously immunized animals (36, 37). Alternatively, this small inoculum of cells may induce a minimal immune response. This small immune response may actually stimulate cell growth and, therefore, allow the smaller number of cells to develop into a progressive tumor more readily than a larger number of cells. Thus, the theory of immunostimulation can explain the phenomenon of sneaking through.

The most prevalent interpretation at the time when the theory of immunostimulation was developed regarding the increased tumorigenesis observed after immunization was that blocking antibodies inhibited cell-mediated immune reactivity to the tumor (38,39). Interestingly, however, the blocking phenomenon was shown to be dose dependent. Small amounts of antibody protected the tumor, while larger amounts inhibited tumor growth (40), a situation similar to the mechanism postulated for immunostimulation. No definitive experiments were performed that either eliminated or confirmed the possibility that direct stimulation of tumor cells by antibody was the cause of tumor enhancement. A direct stimulatory effect of antibody on tumor cells was not a completely novel idea. In 1958, Gorer (41) wrote concerning the effects of antisera on sarcoma I: "the only direct effect of antibody to be observed upon the neoplastic cells has been the stimulation of mitoses." And in the same paper he wrote in regard to tumor P.B.8, "if conditions are sufficiently favorable to the tumor we may get simple stimulation of mitoses without any damage to the cells. We appear to have two satisfactory factors to account for enhanced growth of P.B.8. If antibody is present in sub-effective amounts we may produce a highly resistant tumor, or the tumor may be so violently stimulated by sub-effective doses of antibody that the host is overwhelmed. Clearly, both factors could act synergistically." Although the immunostimulation hypothesis proposed by Prehn and Lappé in 1971 (2) was not without precedent in the literature, the *in vivo* evidence supporting the hypothesis was far from overwhelming. There was one set of *in vivo* data, however, that was suggestive of a possible role of immunostimulation in tumorigenesis. These data concern mammary tumors in mice.

Spontaneous mammary tumors of C3H mice are induced by an RNA virus transferred from mother to progeny in her milk (42). These virus-induced tumors have very little immunogenicity when grown in C3H mice; in fact, immunization of these mice against the tumor cells can cause enhanced growth of subsequent tumor cell challenge (43). However, these same tumors are very immunogenic when grown in C3Hf mice (syngeneic mice lacking the virus). The effect of treatments designed to alter general immune competence has resulted in opposite effects in C3H and C3Hf mice. Irradiation, which is known to inhibit immune competence and to allow prolonged graft acceptance, increases the incidence of tumors in C3Hf mice as expected (44); however in C3H mice, tumor incidence is decreased (44,45). Similarly, neonatal thymectomy decreases spontaneous mammary tumor formation in C3H mice (15,16,22). Splenectomy, which has been shown to increase the level of cellular immunity and thus inhibit tumor growth (46–49), decreases tumor formation in C3Hf mice (50). This immunopotentiating treatment, however, increases tumor incidences in C3H mice (50,51). These data from the mammary tumor system, specifically the data from the C3H mice in which the mammary tumor is weakly immunogenic, suggest that if the already low level of immune reactivity is further lowered, thus abolishing all immune reactivity, tumor formation is decreased. If the low level of immune reactivity is increased in this system, the tumor incidence is also enhanced. Although it might have been predicted that increasing the immune response would decrease tumor incidence, the level of immune reactivity is probably so low in this system that any increase would still be in the stimulatory range. These observations, therefore, fulfill the predictions of the immunostimulation hypothesis. Alternate explanations of these results based on blocking of cell-mediated immunity, however, still can be envisaged. It was, therefore, necessary to examine systems in which direct stimulation of tumor growth and blocking of cellular cytotoxicity could be differentiated. *In vitro* systems were required for these investigations.

Prior to 1971 very few investigators had reported stimulated growth of tumor cells in the presence of lymphoid cells. Several investigators had shown that normal lymphoid cells could increase cellular metabolism of tumor cells and that this phenomenon was dose dependent: large amounts of lymphoid cells were more likely to inhibit cellular metabolism while smaller numbers of lymphoid cells tended to be stimulatory (31,52). Only two systems, however, demonstrated that sensitized lymphoid cells could stimulate tumor cell growth. Rosenau and Moon (53) immunized BALB/c mice with either C3H or C57BL spleen cells then assayed reactivity of these spleen cells against C3H, C57BL, or DBA/2 tumor cells *in vitro*. When the spleen cells from BALB/c mice immunized with C3H spleen cells were mixed with C3H tumor cells, inhibition of tumor growth was observed as expected, whereas when they were mixed with C57BL tumor cells, no change compared to controls was seen. However, when they were cultured with DBA/2 tumor cells, stimulation of cell growth occurred. This final result can be interpreted as follows: BALB/c immune cells recognize many antigens on the C3H spleen cells as foreign, strong major histocompatibility antigens, as well as many minor antigens. Since BALB/c and DBA/2 mice share the same major histocompatibility antigens, the BALB/c spleen cells cannot respond to any of these strong antigens. However, it is possible that C3H and DBA/2 share certain minor antigens. A BALB/c response against these minor antigens could stimulate the growth of the DBA/2 tumor cells.

The other system demonstrating stimulation of tumor cells by sensitized lymphoid cells *in vitro* is the response of peritoneal cells from animals bearing transplanted tumors. When the tumors were small or several weeks after the tumors were surgically removed, the peritoneal cells demonstrated inhibition of tumor cell growth. However, when these peritoneal cells were obtained from animals with large tumors, the peritoneal cells stimulated the growth of the tumor cells *in vitro* over and above the feeder effect seen in controls treated with normal cells (54,55). These studies are consistent with the theory of immunostimulation and provided the initial basis for its formulation. More recent data supporting this hypothesis will be presented in the next section.

EXPERIMENTAL DATA SUPPORTING IMMUNOSTIMULATION

Although most, if not all, of the data supporting the hypothesis of immunostimulation could be explained by other mechanisms, the arguments against the hypothesis were equally inconclusive and, therefore, insufficient to refute the existence of immunostimulation. During the 10 years since its inception, more systems have been analyzed, more supporting evidence accumulated, and more alternative explanations proffered. The purpose of the present section is to review the more recent data supporting immunostimulation. The following section will attempt to decipher the possible mechanism(s) of the enhancement of tumorigenesis.

Chemically-Induced Tumor Systems

A number of investigators have reported that components of the immune system have the ability to stimulate growth of chemically-induced tumors. These observations have been made in both *in vivo* (56–66) and *in vitro* (67–72) assay systems. Stutman (21) reported that athymic nude (nu/nu) mice develop methylcholanthrene-induced fibrosarcomas at the same frequency and methylcholanthrene-induced lung adenomas at a slightly lower frequency than their heterozygous normal littermates (nu/+). Although not directly supporting immunostimulation, these results suggest that the immune system is not preventing the development of chemically-induced tumors and may actually be enhancing the growth of these tumors. The mice used in this study may represent the two ends of the immunologic spectrum: the nude mice being devoid of T-cell-mediated immune competence; the normal mice being totally immunocompetent, and therefore capable of limiting the development of strongly antigenic methylcholanthrene-induced tumors. Stimulation would be most readily detected in animals that are partially immunocompetent. Nude mice, however, are not totally immunocompetent; they have functional B cells, macrophages, and NK cells. It has been shown that irradiation of nude mice can increase the growth of transplantable, chemically-induced tumors (72). This fact suggests that nude mice do have some form of surveillance against tumors, presumably the NK cells. These data can be interpreted in the following manner: T-cell-mediated reactivity and T-dependent antibody responses are not essential for surveillance against tumors. In fact, low levels of these activities may be responsible for enhanced tumor growth. Using a Winn assay in which lymphoid cells were mixed with tumor cells prior to administration of the mixture to thymectomized, irradiated syngeneic hosts, Prehn (61) directly examined this hypothesis. He found that mixing an intermediate number of spleen cells from mice immunized with a methylcholanthrene-induced tumor with a constant number of cells from the same tumor resulted in enhanced tumor growth compared to either no spleen cells or higher numbers of spleen cells. The stimulation was specific for the tumor since nonimmune spleen cells or spleen cells from mice immunized to an unrelated tumor did not induce comparable enhancement of tumor growth. Similar results were obtained when thymectomized, irradiated mice reconstituted with varying numbers of syngeneic spleen cells were exposed to different amounts of methylcholanthrene (63). Among animals exposed to a high quantity of methylcholanthrene, the sarcoma incidence was significantly higher among animals given intermediate numbers of spleen cells (10^4) compared to animals receiving either no spleen cells or high numbers of spleen cells (10^7). When the dose of chemical carcinogen was low, however, the tumor incidence was the same in all groups. Since the immunogenicity of chemically-induced tumors is directly related to the amount of carcinogen (17), the increased tumor incidence in the group of mice given a high dose of carcinogen and an intermediate amount of spleen cells can be explained by a weak immune response to a highly immunogenic tumor. Although this study did not ascertain that reconstitution with varying amounts of spleen cells actually produced varying degrees of immunocompetence, another investigator performed a similar study with methylcholanthrene-induced papillomas (64). He found that reconstitution with intermediate amounts of spleen cells produced more papillomas than no reconstitution or reconstitution with high amounts of cells. In addition, he demonstrated that rejection of skin allografts was inversely correlated to the amount of reconstitution, i.e., the higher the number of spleen cells, the shorter the time before rejection. These results therefore, are completely consistent with the predictions of the theory of immunostimulation.

Other studies have also shown that cells of the immune system can stimulate growth of chemically-induced tumors *in vivo*. The conditions required to induce increased tumor growth varied among the systems. Giovarelli et al. (6) reported that adoptive transfer of small numbers of normal thymocytes, neutrophils, or splenocytes to newborn mice enhanced the growth of chemically-induced plasmocytomas. Higher numbers of cells either had no effect (splenocytes) or decreased tumor growth (thymocytes and neutrophils). The fact that normal lymphoid cells can either inhibit or enhance tumor growth was not an observation unique to the work by Giovarelli et al. (60). Prehn (61) also demonstrated that normal lymphoid cells could alter growth of chemically-induced tumors; however, the enhancement of tumor growth was greater when specifically immune lymphoid cells were used. It has also been shown that normal lymphoid cells are not the only cells capable of enhancing tumor growth; mixing tumor cells with kidney cells prior to inoculation into a recipient animal also increased tumor growth (62). Therefore, since stimulation of tumor growth can be induced by nonimmunologic procedures, one must set criteria for categorizing observations as possible demonstrations of *immuno*stimulation. Criteria generally used by investigators to ascertain that the reaction they are investigating is immunologic are: (a) the reaction is specific; (b) the reaction is mediated by cells of the lymphoid system; and (c) the reaction occurs after performing procedures known to induce an immunologic reaction detectable either *in vivo* or *in vitro*. Although both criteria a and b are essential to confirm that the observation is immunologic, many investigators consider demonstration of points b and c sufficient, especially since many of the more recent immunologic phenomenon, specifically NK cell and suppresssor cell activities are not specific for a particular antigen or group of antigens.

Most of the *in vivo* observations concerning enhancement of tumor growth either did not examine or did not demonstrate specificity. They are thought to be immunologic primarily because the enhancing activity can be abrogated by depleting specific populations of lymphoid cells. For example, spleen cells from C3H mice bearing a syngeneic methylcholanthrene-induced fibrosarcoma were shown to inhibit tumor growth in a Winn assay if the spleen cells were tested early during tumor growth. Spleen cells from mice bearing larger tumors, however, enhanced tumor growth. Although both reactivities were dependent on the presence of T cells, the inhibitory effect was tumor specific, while the enhancing effects were not (59). Similarly, lymphoid cells sensitized *in vitro* on monolayers of syngeneic fibrosarcoma cells induced by benzpyrene manifested cytotoxicity against the fibrosarcoma cells in an *in vitro* microassay measuring tumor cell detachment. When these same lymphoid cells were injected with fibrosarcoma cells into syngeneic mice, enhanced tumor growth was observed. This enhancement was dependent on the mixing of the tumor cells with the lymphoid cells prior to inoculation. If the tumor cells and lymphoid cells were injected at the same site, but 1 hour apart, there was no effect on tumor growth, while inoculation of the lymphoid cells systemically inhibited tumor growth (58). Although subsequent studies by these investigators demonstrated that both the inhibitory and stimulatory activities of these lymphoid cells were dependent on T cells, the enhancement of tumor growth was not specific since growth of a spontaneously occurring carcinoma (3LL) syngeneic with the benzpyrene fibrosarcoma was enhanced by lymphoid cells cultured on the fibrosarcoma (57). Even though only one of the above studies (61) showed specificity of the stimulation, all the studies (57–61) attributed the increase in tumor growth to immunologic mechanisms, primarily because the enhancement was abrogated by depletion of lymphoid cells.

Although many *in vivo* studies have not investigated the specificity of the stimulation, in *in vitro* systems most investigators have examined not only if stimulation of tumor cells occurs, but also the specificity of the reaction. Four studies performed *in vitro* with chemically-induced tumors all showed enchancement of tumor growth (68–71). The four reports however, demonstrate varying degrees of specificity. In one system, lymph node cells sensitized *in vitro* on methylcholanthrene-induced tumor cells could enhance the growth of the same cells, but not of a Moloney sarcoma virus-induced tumor cell (71). Similarly, spleen cells from mice bearing a syngeneic methylcholanthrene-induced tumor for 6 days enhanced growth of that tumor, but not of syngeneic embryo fibroblast cells or melanoma cells (70). Response to three methylcholanthrene-induced tumors was investigated in the third report (68). In this study peripheral blood lymphocytes, obtained from mice 5 days after tumor cell inoculation when tumors were still not palpable, were stimulatory to tumor growth. One of the three tumors induced lymphoid cells which would only stimulate growth of itself. The other two tumors, although not cross-reactive *in vivo*, induced lymphoid cells which were capable of enhancing growth of both of these tumors. The final report (69) demonstrated that lymphoid cells from mice bearing one methylcholanthrene-induced tumor (1967) could stimulate both the challenge tumor and a non-cross-reacting, methylcholanthrene-induced tumor (1969). If however, lymphoid cells from mice immunized with the non-cross-reacting tumor (1969) were used as control cells rather than normal lymphoid cells, lymphoid cells from 1967 still produced significant stimulation of 1967 tumor cells, indicating that at least part of the stimulation was specific for the immunizing tumor.

Both the *in vitro* and *in vivo* studies described above examined stimulation of tumor growth that was mediated by lymphoid cells and, in the experiments that examined the population involved, these lymphoid cells were usually described as T cells. Two groups of investigators, however, investigated the effect of antiserum on cell growth *in vitro* and *in vivo* (65–67). One group found that antibody produced in rabbits against normal mouse cells would stimulate the growth of syngeneic, DMBA-transformed cells *in vitro* (67). This reaction was *specific*, if one considers that the rabbit antimouse serum did not stimulate normal syngeneic cells and that normal rabbit serum did not stimulate the transformed cells. Further studies by these investigators showed that autoantibodies were produced during promotion of chemically-induced tumors with croton oil or phorbol ester TPA and that mice immunized with syngeneic tissue, but not xenogeneic tissue, demonstrated a higher tumor incidence than control mice (66). They concluded that autoantibodies were induced during promotion of chemically-induced tumors and that these antibodies enhanced tumor growth. The other group found that anti-TNP antibody in low concentrations stimulated a large increase of nucleoside uptake in L cells coupled with TNP, but not in untreated L cells. Higher concentrations of antibody inhibited nucleoside incorporation. The stimulation was augmented by the early components of complement (C1,4,2,3), while the inhibition was increased in the presence of C5-9. Unlike many of the systems examining cell-mediated stimulation in which stimulation *in vitro* rarely correlated to enhanced tumor growth *in vivo*, passive transfer of the anti-TNP antibody to thymectomized, bone-marrow reconstituted mice increased TNP-L cell growth as predicted by the *in vitro* studies: small amounts stimulated growth, while larger amounts did not. This antibody system, therefore, clearly demonstrated that a component of the immune system could specifically and directly stimulate the growth of tumor cells both *in vitro* and *in vivo*.

In summary, there have been a number of studies reporting stimulation of the growth of chemically-induced tumors by components of the immune system both *in vivo* and *in vitro*. The conditions under which stimulation can be observed varied from system to system: early during tumor growth (68,70) or sensitization (71) vs. late during tumor growth (59); source of cells was important—spleen cells (70,60) vs. thymus cells (60), normal lymphoid cells (60) vs. nonspecifically immune cells (69,59) vs. specifically immune cells (61, 70, 71); immune sera (65–67) vs. immune cells (60, 69, 70). One condition that was fairly consistent was that if stimulation displayed a dose dependence, low concentrations were stimulatory, while higher concentrations were inhibitory. Although not all the systems explored the immunologic nature of their systems in the strict sense, most of the observations were attributable to components of the immune system and at least two of the studies (61, 67) not only demonstrated beyond a doubt that their phenomena were immunologic, but also that direct stimulation of the tumor cells by the immune component was the most likely explanation for the increased tumor growth. Therefore, since the formulation of the hypothesis of immunostimulation, there have been a substantial number of reports in which the growth of chemically-induced tumors can be stimulated by an immune response.

Virus-Induced Tumor System

Observations supporting the hypothesis of immunostimulation have not been confined to chemically-induced tumor systems (72). Similar to his work with primary chemically-induced tumors in athymic (nu/nu) nude mice, Stutman (73) examined the development of primary Moloney sarcoma virus-induced tumors in nude mice. He found that although regressison of the tumors occurred in normal (nu/+) mice while they grew progressively in nude (nu/nu) mice, the initial development of tumors was slower in the nude mice than in the normal mice. If the nude mice received thymus grafts, however, the tumors both developed and regressed at the same rate as in the normal mice. These results are consistent with immunostimulation which predicts that although the immune response may inhibit tumor growth at certain times during progression, the initial effect of the immune response on the tumor when the immune response is weak is enhanced tumor growth. Since the nude mice are lacking an effective cell-mediated immune system, they can cause neither the initial stimulation nor later inhibition of the Moloney sarcoma virus-induced tumor.

A number of investigators have shown that immunization can enhance virus-induced tumorigenesis. The route of immunization, material used for immunization, and amount of immunogen were found to be important factors in determining whether the immunization enhanced or inhibited tumor growth. When quail were immunized with avian sarcoma virus (ASV) intravenously, tumorigenesis by subsequent inoculation of ASV was inhibited; however, if the immunization was done intramuscularly, increased tumor incidence was observed (74). Immunization with tumor cell extracts has been shown to increase the incidence of both spontaneous mammary tumors in mice (75) and transplantable, Gross virus-induced tumors in rats (76), while immunization with whole virus preparations inhibited tumorigenesis (75). Similarly, immunization with purified gp52 decreased survival time or increased tumor incidence of transplantable mammary tumors (76). The amount of immunogen used for immunization determined whether stimulation or inhibition of virus-induced tumorigenesis was observed when animals were subsequently challenged with a tumorigenic dose of virus. Inhibition was observed when high amounts of immunogen were used, while stimulation was induced by intermediate amounts of immunogen. Smaller quantities had no effect on tumor induction. This dose response was observed whether the immunogen was purified Friend virus gp85 (78), inactivated Moloney leukemia virus (79), inactivated Friend virus (80), or simian adenovirus 7 (81). Comparable dose dependent effects of immunization were observed when glutaraldehyde-fixed tumor cells were used as immunogens (80). One study reported that immunization with primary mouse mammary carcinomas could either induce protection, enhancement, or no effect on subsequent growth of transplantable mammary tumors (82). There was no obvious reason, however, why certain tumors were inhibitory and others were stimulatory. Many of the authors did not examine the specificity of the stimulation or inhibition of tumor growth observed after immunization (74, 75, 77–79). The studies that did investigate the specificity of the stimulatory effect of immunization suggested that the stimulation was specific: immunization with a non-cross-reacting tumor (76) or a mock virus preparation (80) did not induce comparable enhancement. Although one study (82) reported that protection induced by immunization with mammary carcinomas was specific for the individual carcinoma, while the stimulation was observed against several of the mammary carcinomas, this does not necessarily indicate that the stimulation was nonspecific. The mammary carcinomas were spontaneous tumors of C3H/HeJ mice. These tumors are known to be induced by murine mammary tumor virus and, therefore, share virus-associated antigens..In addition, these tumors have been shown to possess transplantation antigens unique to each tumor, similar to chemically-induced tumors. Therefore, it is possible that the inhibition was due to reaction against the unique antigens, while stimulation was due to interaction with the shared virus-associated antigens. Of the studies that did examine the specificity of the reactions induced by immunization, only the studies that immunized with tumor cells (81, 82) rather than virus or virus components thoroughly investigated the specificity of the stimulation. In order to ascertain that stimulation is truly specific, two tumor systems which have been shown to be susceptible to stimulation after immunization with themselves are required. For example, it has been shown that immunization with inactivated Moloney sarcoma virus can stimulate tumorigenesis by Moloney sarcoma virus. Specificity of the system was investigated by immunizing with SV40 virus. Since it has not been demonstrated that SV40 virus is capable of inducing stimulation of SV40-induced tumorigenesis, a lack of stimulation of Moloney sarcoma virus-induced tumorigenesis may only indicate that SV40 is not a suitable control. Conversely, if immunization with Moloney sarcoma virus does not enhance tumorigenesis by SV40, it is possible that SV40 tumorigenesis is not susceptible to stimulation. Only by using two systems which: (a) are known to be non-cross-reacting by *in vitro* assays and (b) demonstrate stimulated tumorigenesis after immunization with themselves can specificity of the reaction be ascertained. Although the mouse mammary carcinoma study utilized systems that demonstrated stimulation of themselves for

Table 6.1. Specificity of Increased Tumorigenesis in Hamsters after Immunization with Glutaraldehyde-Fixed Tumor Cells

Immunization		Tumor Challenge	Percent Tumor Incidence	Latent Period ± S. E.
Tumor	Dose			
Cx-T#2[a]	10^6	Cx-T#2	100 (10/10)	22.0 ± 0.4
	10^4		83 (29/35)	19.9 ± 0.3
	10^2		91 (32/35)*	16.2 ± 0.3*
	—		72 (26/36)	24.0 ± 0.8
	10^4	14-012	89 (16/18)	14.5 ± 0.8
	10^2		100 (20/20)	12.8 ± 0.6
	—		95 (18/19)	12.2 ± 0.5
14.012[b]	10^6	14-012	100 (10/10)	17.8 ± 0.6
	10^4		90 (18/20)	13.1 ± 0.6
	10^2		100 (20/20)	11.4 ± 0.4*
	—		89 (17/19)	18.6 ± 0.6
	10^4	Cx-T#2	90 (9/10)	25.1 ± 0.2
	10^2		100 (10/10)	26.0 ± 0.3
	—		90 (9/10)	24.2 ± 0.4

[a] LSH embryo fibroblast cells transformed *in vitro* by cytomegalovirus.

[b] LSH embryo fibroblast cells transformed *in vitro* by herpes simplex virus, Type 1.

* Statistical significance as determined by Chi square (Incidence) or Mann Whitney u (Latent Period). All value $p < .05$.

specificity studies, these experiments are difficult to interpret due to the existence of both unique and shared virus-associated antigens on these cells (82). Therefore, only one report demonstrated that stimulation observed after immunization was truly specific (81). A summary of the specificity studies of this study is shown in Table 6.1.

Stimulation of tumor growth *in vivo* has also been reported when reactivity of lymphoid cells from tumor-bearing animals was examined. Blazar et al. (83) examined the lymphoid cells that are found within mammary carcinomas. They found that these intratumor lymphoid cells would stimulate the growth of mammary tumor cells in a Winn assay. Normal lymph node cells or lymph node cells from mice bearing mammary tumors did not significantly alter tumor growth. Adoptive transfer of lymph node cells from mice capable of resisting Rous sarcoma virus transformed cells to neonatal mice given Rous sarcoma virus increased the growth of the tumors in the newborn mice (84). This stimulation did not appear to be specific since adoptive transfer of normal spleen or lymph node cells also increased Rous sarcoma virus tumorigenesis in newborn mice. Another adoptive tranfer study, however, very clearly demonstrated that stimulation of primary Moloney sarcoma virus-induced tumorigenesis is specific (85). Splenocytes and thymocytes from mice whose Moloney sarcoma virus-induced tumor had regressed 2 to 3 months earlier were capable of increasing Moloney sarcoma-virus-induced tumorigenesis in 20-day-old mice. Thymocytes from mice immune to a methylcholanthrene-induced tumor (1460), although capable of stimulating tumor growth of the same methylcholanthrene-induced tumor (1460), had no effect on tumor growth of the Moloney sarcoma virus-induced tumors. The thymocytes from the mice whose Moloney sarcoma-virus-induced tumors had regressed also had no effect on growth of other methylcholanthrene-induced tumors (1315 and 1321). Unfortunately, no information was given on whether or not these latter methylcholanthrene-induced tumors were susceptible to stimulation. Stimulation in these studies was dependent on the presence of thy-1 positive cells.

Results from *in vitro* studies have also indicated that stimulation of tumor cell growth can occur in virus-induced tumor systems. Although lymph node cells from normal mice and from mice bearing mammary carcinomas could sometimes stimulate the growth of mammary carcinoma cells, the enhancement observed with these cells was minimal compared to the stimulation observed with lymphoid cells obtained from within the tumor mass (86). This stimulation was observed not only on the mammary carcinoma cells that induced the tumor, but also on other mammary carcinoma cells. Since all the mammary carcinoma cells were induced by murine mammary tumor virus, it is unknown whether or not this stimulation was specific. The degree of stimulation was directly proportional to the ratio of effector to target cells: the higher the concentration of lymphoid cells the greater the stimulation. Examination of the activity of spleen cells from hamsters either immunized with cytomegalovirus or bearing cytomegalovirus-induced tumors revealed that: (a) stimulation did occur; (b) the stimulation was specific for cytomegalovirus transformed cells; and (c) a biphasic dose response occurred in this system. Low effector to target cell ratios (1:1, 10:1) enhanced tumor growth, while high effector to target cell ratios (500:1, 1000:1) inhibited tumor growth, intermediate ratios caused no significant effect on tumor growth (87). In addition to the ratio of effector to target cells, the time following sensitization was observed to be an important factor in determining whether or not stimulation is observed. *In vitro* sensitization of lymphoid cells for 3 days with Moloney sarcoma cells induced the lymphoid cells to be stimulatory to tumor cell growth, while longer sensitization induced lymphoid cells that were cytotoxic (71). The amount of antigen also was observed to influence the results of immunization. Lymphoid cells from mice immunized with 10^5 polyoma transformed cells stimulated polyoma cell growth, while immunization with 10^6 cells inhibited cell growth *in vitro* (88). In another system, anti-Friend virus antiserum was found to stimulate DNA synthesis of normal cells (89). Although this apppeared to be a nonspecific phenomenon, the investigators observed that purified gp70 but not p30, p15, p12, or p10 from Friend virus could block the stimulatory activity of anti-Friend virus antiserum suggesting that a virus-specific antigen was either the receptor or near the receptor initiating the increased DNA synthesis.

Similar to the data obtained with chemically-induced tumor systems, there have been a substantial number of reports since the formulation of the hypothesis of immunostimulation in which the growth of virus-induced tumors can be stimulated by components of the immune system. An important point to be made concerning these studies is that immunostimulation appears to be a common phenomenon of virus-induced tumor systems since it can be observed with both RNA (74–79, 83–86, 89) and DNA (81, 87, 88) viruses and in mice (75–80, 83–86, 88, 89, 96), hamsters (81, 87), rats (76), and quails (74). The factors that influence the demonstration of stimulation, however, do vary among systems. A number of studies have shown that immunization can cause an increase in primary virus-induced tumorigenesis (74, 75, 78–81) and in growth of transplantable, virus-induced tumors (76, 77, 81). The most prominent factor determining whether or not stimulation would occur was the amount of immunogen used: high doses inhibited growth, lower amounts stimulated growth. The source of lymphoid cells (intratumor or thymus vs. lymph node) appeared to be a critical factor affecting stimulation when adoptive transfers were performed (83, 85). No pattern of factors required for demonstration of stimulation *in vitro* is readily apparent from the studies described. More studies are required before generalizations can be attempted for these systems. A common feature of both the *in vivo* and *in vitro* studies concerning virus-induced tumor systems is that when the systems were examined, specificity was observed. Therefore, although varying conditions are required to induce stimulation in different virus-induced tumor systems, the number and breadth of studies demonstrating stimulation of virus-induced tumorigenesis indicate that the stimulatory potential of the immune system is an important factor to consider when designing prophylactic or therapeutic regimens for tumor control.

Other Transplantable Tumors

Besides chemically- and virus-induced tumors, there is another category of tumors which need to be included in our discussion of immunostimulation. These are the spontaneous tumors of both animals and man, tumors that have arisen without introduction of any known carcinogen or virus. Two of the most extensively studied spontaneous tumors of mice are 3LL Lewis carcinoma and the B16 melanoma. Both of these systems have been used to investigate immunostimulation *in vivo* and *in vitro*. Reactivity against the 3LL tumor in Winn assays has been observed with lymphoid cells sensitized *in vitro* against the 3LL tumor (90) or against syngeneic fibroblasts

(91, 92) or obtained from syngeneic (93,94) or allogeneic (84, 85) mice bearing 3LL tumors. In all cases, stimulation of tumor growth was observed and the effector cell population was determined to be T cells. When *in vitro* sensitized lymphoid cell preparations were assayed against 3LL cells *in vitro*, however, cytotoxicity rather than inhibition was observed (91, 92). Further examination of this paradox showed that while lymphoid cells sensitized *in vitro* on 3LL cells were cytotoxic *in vitro*, lymphoid cells from mice bearing 3LL tumors were stimulatory *in vitro* (96). They also found that lymphoid cells taken early after inoculation of 3LL cells were inhibitory to 3LL cell growth *in vivo*, while cells obtained later during tumor growth were stimulatory (94). The specificity of this system was investigated in some of the studies. One study found that although normal thymocytes could stimulate 3LL growth in a Winn assay, the stimulation was not as pronounced as when thymocytes sensitized against 3LL were used (90). A seemingly apparent conflict was reported in another study which stated that normal lymphoid cells could not stimulate 3LL growth (95). The difference in these two reports could be due to the fact that one study used lymphoid cells syngeneic with 3LL cells (90), while the other utilized allogeneic lymphoid cells (95). Two other reports, however, demonstrated that the stimulation observed in the Winn assay was not specific since lymphoid cells from mice bearing either allogeneic tumors, syngeneic methylcholanthrene fibrosarcomas, or syngeneic B16 melanomas could also stimulate growth of 3LL tumors (94); and lymphoid cells from mice bearing 3LL tumors could stimulate growth of both B16 melanomas and syngeneic methylcholanthrene-induced fibrosarcomas (93). Investigation of the specificity of *in vitro* reactions showed that although *in vivo* sensitized lymphoid cells would only stimulate 3LL cells, *in vitro* sensitized cells would enhance growth of both 3LL and normal fibroblasts (96). Therefore, although the specificity of the stimulation of 3LL cells is ambiguous, there is no doubt that stimulation can occur in this system and that the effector cells are of T-cell lineage.

Not only the local tumor induced by B16 melanoma cells (97), but also the metastases generated by intravenous inoculation of B16 melanoma (98) cells have been shown to be susceptible to the stimulatory activity of lymphoid cells or their products. Mixing lymphoid cells from mice bearing B16 melanomas with B16 melanoma cells prior to intravenous inoculation increased the number of pulmonary metastases (98). If these lymphoid cells were obtained from mice immunized with B16 melanoma cells, inhibition, rather than stimulation of metastases, was seen. The specificity of this system was only investigated *in vitro* (99). Although normal cells were not stimulatory at low lymphoid cell to target cell ratios, both allogeneic and xenogeneic lymphoid cells stimulated with other antigens or mitogens were able to stimulate growth of B16 melanoma cells at low ratios. The stimulation observed *in vitro* was dose dependent: intermediate doses were most stimulatory to B16 melanoma cells, while higher ratios demonstrated either inhibitory or no effect. Stimulated growth of the B16 melanoma can also be observed *in vivo* and *in vitro* after treatment of mice with BCG (97). Both *in vivo* and *in vitro* stimulation were found to be dose dependent: high concentrations (0.5 mg) of BCG stimulated B16 melanoma growth *in vivo* while lower concentrations inhibited tumor growth; *in vitro*, low ratios of effector to target cells stimulated growth, while higher ratios inhibited growth. Specificity of the reaction was not investigated in any of the papers.

The remaining studies, investigating whether or not spontaneous tumors are susceptible to the stimulatory effects of lymphoid cells, were performed *in vitro*. Lymphocytes from mice bearing two different mammary tumor virus-negative spontaneous mammary tumors stimulated the growth of both themselves and each other, but not of mammary tumor virus-positive mammary tumors or Moloney sarcoma virus-induced sarcoma cells (100). The stimulation was observed at ratios of 100 effector cells to 1 target cell, while higher ratios produced variable effects. Similar dose responses were observed when lymphoid cells from dogs bearing spontaneous tumors were cultured with autologous tumor cells (101), low concentrations of lymphoid cells were stimulatory, while higher quantities of lymphoid cells inhibited cell growth.

The effect of macrophages on the growth of human tumor cells *in vitro* was examined by two sets of investigators. Mantovani et al. (102) found that macrophages isolated from ovarian tumors of 11 out of 22 patients were capable of stimulating the growth of at least one of four cultured human and mouse tumors. Eight of the 22 patients had macrophages which were cytotoxic to tumor growth. Although there was no apparent pattern of reactivity that might indicate specificity, the results were reproducible — macrophages from the same subject gave the same pattern of stimulation or inhibition upon repeated testing. Buick et al. (103) approached the investigation of the activity of macrophages from tumor-bearing patients from a different angle. They studied the capacity of tumor cells from malignant effusions to form colonies in agar. In eight of nine cases, removal of macrophages from the effusion decreased the clonogenic capacity of the tumor cells. In reconstitution experiments, they found that the stimulatory effect of macrophages was directly related to the number of macrophages (at least in the quantities studied) in the culture.

The results of these studies with macrophages prompted Salmon, one of the authors of the paper, to present a hypothesis concerning the role of macrophages, more specifically inflammation, in the development of tumors (104). He suggests that inflammatory cells are an integral part of tumor promotion, that a common proliferative factor is required for the growth of antitumor B cells and carcinogen-induced epithelial cells, and that macrophages supply this proliferative factor. Support for this hypothesis comes from the work of Cancro and Potter (105) who observed that adherent peritoneal cells were required for myeloma development and of Namba and Hanaoko (106) who demonstrated that adherent spleen cells were required to adapt a transplantable mouse myeloma to long-term tissue culture.

As in the chemically- and virus-induced tumor systems, dose of the immune component is a critical factor in development of the stimulatory effect. Although specificity was not demonstrated in most systems, the effect appears to be immune in nature. The lack of specificity of the reaction is a major reason why Salmon hypothesized that tumor promotion and clonal proliferation of B cells are affected by a common factor; and that the evolutionary development of a growth promoter, providing positive survival advantage by amplifying the number of clones reactive to a foreign pathogen, would incidentally stimulate the growth of clones of cells that had been tranformed by an oncogenic agent. Whether stimulation of spontaneous tumor cell growth is mediated by T cells or macrophages, the results discussed in this section clearly demonstrate that spontaneous tumors are susceptible to stimulation by components of the immune system.

POSTULATED MECHANISM OF IMMUNOSTIMULATION

The preceding section described the studies that support the hypothesis of immunostimulation which states, that under certain conditions components of the immune system have the capacity to stimulate tumorigenesis. As pointed out in that section, the conditions necessary to observe stimulation vary among systems; the predominant conditions being quantity of the immune component (in general, smaller concentrations are stimulatory, while larger concentrations are inhibitory) and the time after exposure to tumor cells when the lymphoid component is obtained. Although the theory predicts that stimulation would be observed early after exposure to tumor when the immune response to the tumor is limited and weak, some of the studies found that stimulation occurred late during exposure to antigen (59, 93, 95). Another prediction of the hypothesis of immunostimulation is that the stimulatory effect is due to the direct action of the lymphoid component on the tumor target, rather than inhibition of cytotoxic immune response. In this section an attempt will be made to explain the apparent discrepancies between the predictions of the hypothesis and the observed results and to develop a unifying mechanism for immunostimulation.

The first question to be addressed is whether or not the stimulation of tumor growth observed is immunologic. According to the criteria established earlier, a reaction is immune if: (a) it is specific; (b) the reaction is mediated by cells of the lymphoid system, and (c) the reaction occurs after performing procedures known to induce an immunologic reaction detectable either *in vivo* or *in vitro*. Practically all of the studies described fulfill the third criteria. Twenty studies investigated the specificity of the stimulation. Nine of the reports demonstrated specificity (65, 71, 76, 79, 81, 85, 87, 89, 93), while six (59, 62, 93, 94, 98, 104) of them displayed no specificity. Two of the studies were difficult to evaluate since they involved mammary tumors which are known to possess both shared virus-associated and organ-specific antigens and unique tumor antigens (77, 100). The cross-reactivity observed in these studies may reflect reactivity against the shared antigens. The final three studies reported qualified specificity. Although normal lymphoid cells and lymphoid cells from animals bearing non-cross-reactivity tumors did stimulate tumor growth, lymphoid cells from the appropriate tumor demonstrated greater stimulatory activity. Since the stimulatory activity in most of the studies was transferred or observed with spleen cells, lymph node cells, or thymus cells, the second criteria is also fulfilled. The exact nature of the stimulatory component, however, is not known. A number of the studies stated that depletion of T cells abrogates the stimulatory activity (57, 59, 85, 91, 90, 93, 95). It has been reported that a soluble factor produced by T cells is the mediator of the stimulation (94). Macrophages have been implicated as the stimulatory cells in several systems (103, 107), while one study states that macrophages are not responsible for the stimulation (60). Antisera have also been shown to be capable of stimulating tumor cell growth (65, 89). Regardless of identification of the mediator of stimulation, there is sufficient evidence to conclude that stimulation of tumor growth is an immune phenomenon.

What are the major characteristics of this stimulatory activity? The hypothesis of immunostimulation predicts that when an immune response is weak, either due to the strength of the immunogen or to the limited time that elapsed since introduction of the immunogen, stimulation will be observed. Conversely, stronger immune reactivities will be inhibitory. In nine of the ten studies examining the dose dependence of stimulation, low concentrations of immunogens (75, 79–81) or small amounts of lymphoid cells (70, 87, 99–101) were stimulatory to tumor growth, while larger amounts were inhibitory. The tenth report found that *in vivo* high concentrations of BCG were stimulatory, while lower concentrations were inhibitory to tumor growth. *In vitro* investigation of the lymphoid cells from these BCG-treated mice provided the opposite and predicted results (97). An additional study stated that immunization with whole mammary tumor virus was protective, while tumor cell extracts were stimulatory (70). These results are compatible with the hypothesis of immunostimulation since the whole virus preparation is probably more immunogenic than the tumor cell extract.

Studies investigating the temporal aspect of the stimulatory response have not supported this prediction as consistently. Two of five studies have observed the expected temporal appearance of stimulatory activity: lymphoid cells obtained early during tumor growth or after immunization when the level of immune reactivity is low stimulate tumor growth; lymphoid cells from later times either have no effect or are stimulatory to tumor growth (68, 71). The remaining three reports, however, obtained the opposite results (93, 95). These contradictory reports form part of the basis for alternate explanations of the ability of spleen cells to enhance tumorigenesis. These alternative explanations will be discussed below.

In addition to predicting that stimulatory activity of lymphoid components is the result of weak and limited immune reactivity, the hypothesis of immunostimulation also states that this stimulation is not due to the blocking of inhibitory activity of lymphoid cells. Rather, the stimulation is the result of direct interaction between lymphoid cells and target cells. Results from several studies suggest that: (a) direct contact between lymphoid components and target cells is essential for expression of the stimulatory effect and (b) it is not necessary to evoke a blocking mechanism in order to explain the mechanism of immunostimulation. Referring to the former point: four studies have demonstrated that close, if not direct, contact of lymphoid components with target cells is essential for stimulation. First, lymphoid cells can increase the number of metastises (98). This stimulation only occurs if the lymphoid cells and tumor cells are mixed prior to inoculation into an animal. Similar results were observed in tumor growth of 3LL cells (58). Third, if macrophages are removed from contact with tumor cells, the clonogenic capacity of the tumor cells is decreased (103). And finally, if BCG is inoculated prior to challenge with avian sarcoma virus increased tumorigenesis is observed (107). This stimulation only occurs when the BCG is inoculated into the same wing as the subsequent virus challenge. Presumably, the BCG recruits macrophages into the area and the resulting inflammatory response promotes tumor growth (104). The latter point concerning the lack of a need for a blocking or suppressive mechanism to explain stimulation is supported by three studies in which lymphoid cells are transferred into thymectomized, irradiated recipients (61, 91, 98). In all three experiments stimulation of tumor growth is observed. Since the recipient is immuno-suppressed, there is no immune response to block; therefore, the transferred lymphoid cells must be acting directly on the target cells. Opponents of the hypothesis of immunostimulation, however, have a counter explanation of these results. These explanations will be discussed below.

One of the strongest sets of results supporting the ability of components of this immune system to directly stimulate cell growth is the work of Shearer et al. (65) utilizing antibody. These studies utilize *in vitro* assays in which the rate of cell growth is determined by the amount of radioactive nucleosides incorporated. Antitarget cell antibody has been shown to specifically stimulate DNA synthesis of the target cells. Since there are only antibody and target cells in the reaction mixture, there is no component that the antiserum may be blocking and, therefore, the increased target cell growth must be due to direct contact between antibody and target cell. Since *in vitro* assays do not necessarily reflect *in vivo* reactivities (92, 107, 108), it was essential that these antibody studies be extended to *in vivo* experimentation. Passive transfer of antitumor antibody to thymectomized, bone-marrow reconstituted mice stimulated growth of the tumor. Although there were no T cells in the recipient mice, it is possible, however very unlikely, that the antibody was blocking other cellular reactivity that could inhibit the growth of the tumor.

So far only the arguments supporting the hypothesis of immunostimulation have been discussed. Since the hypothesis has not been accepted as fact, there must be interpretations of data that argue against immunostimulation. These counter proposals will now be discussed.

It has been mentioned that three of five studies reported that lymphoid cells obtained early after tumor implantation or immunization were inhibitory to tumor growth, while later lymphoid samples stimulated tumor growth. Opponents of the hypothesis of immunostimulation interpret this in the following manner: the immune system recognizes the tumor as foreign and mounts an inhibitory response. As the tumor grows it releases blocking antigens or induces blocking antibody or suppressor cells which prevent this protective immune response from eliminating the tumor.

Similarly, these investigators will interpret the adoptive transfer experiments to thymectomized irradiated mice as blocking phenomenon. Although the recipient mouse has no immune reactivity to suppress, the lymphoid cell population that is transferred to this animal may contain inhibitory cells that are being inhibited by suppressor cells or blocking antibody. This explanation is even applied to transfer of normal rather than sensitized lymphoid cells. It is reasoned that during the incubation of normal lymphoid cells with the tumor cell, the normal lymphoid cells are recognizing the tumor and responding to it in an inhibitory manner. Stimulation of tumor growth is observed because suppressor cells are blocking this protective immune response.

Further support for the existence of suppressor cells is based on the following observations: (a) The stimulatory cell in many instances is a T cell. The activity of this T cell is radiosensitive (79, 85, 93) and is cortisone-sensitive (94, 109). These are properties of suppressor cells or suppressor activator cells (110). (b) A lymphoid preparation that demonstrates stimulatory activity can be separated into two populations of cells by velocity sedimentation (57) or by a peanut lectin (111). The population of larger, immature cells was shown to be stimulatory to tumor growth, while the population of small lymphocytes inhibited tumor growth (47, 110, 111). Mixture of the two populations of cells resulted in stimulation of tumor growth. Again, the interpretation of these results is that the large cells represent an immature population of cells that function as suppressor cells.

Although it is not possible to refute these arguments, an alternate explanation of these results can be envisaged. It is possible that there are two populations of cells—one that directly stimulates cell growth and another that inhibits cell growth. The population that stimulates cell growth may be immature—their response to the target is not strong, they may be producing low levels of lymphotoxin. The observed growth of the tumor, whether it

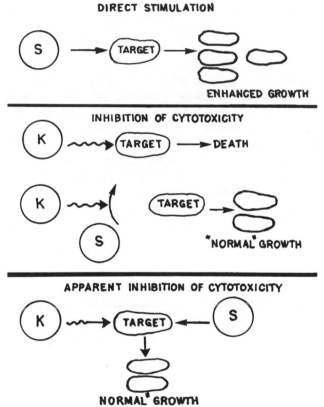

Fig. 6.1. Possible Mechanisms of Observable Enhancement of Tumor Growth by Immune Response. Panel A: Direct Stimulation—In this model stimulatory (S) lymphoid cells directly enhance tumor growth. Panel B: Inhibition of Cytotoxicity—In this model it is assumed that cytotoxic or killer (K) lymphoid cells cause a certain degree of inhibition of growth of all tumors. This cytotoxic activity is prevented by the action of suppressor lymphoid cells (S), which may be identical to stimulatory cells. The result is tumor growth without any host regulation ("normal" growth). Panel C: Apparent Inhibition of Cytotoxicity—In this model the cytotoxic cell (K) and stimulatory cell (S) compete for the same target. The effects of the opposing activities negate each other resulting in tumor growth without any host regulation ("normal" growth).

is stimulation or inhibition, is the sum of the two activities; both of which are reacting directly with the cell. A diagrammatic representation of this scenario is seen in Figure 6.1.

At this time it is not possible to definitively state that the enhanced growth of tumor cells due to interaction with components of the lymphoid system is due soley to suppressor cell activity, blocking factors, or direct stimulation of target cell growth. Data indicate that T cells, macrophages, and antibody may be involved in direct stimulatory activity, that suppressor cells may be responsible for some forms of enhancement of tumor gowth, and that the stimulation may either be specific or nonspecific. Whether all these components interact in every system or that one component is dominant in a particular system is a question that will probably be answered when the mechanism of this phenomenon is deciphered.

SUMMARY

The stated purpose of this review was to present the data supporting the hypothesis that an immune response has the potential to promote the growth of tumors. This enhancing effect of the system is most readily demonstrated when the immune response is weak or limited in scope. Although the mechanism of the stimulatory activity is not known, hopefully the information presented has convinced the reader that this possible deleterious effect should be considered seriously when designing protocols for immunoprophylaxis and immunotherapy.

REFERENCES

1. Prehn, R. T., *J. Reticuloendoth. Soc.* **10**:1, 1971.
2. Prehn, R. T., and Lappé, M. A. *Transpl. Rev.* **7**:26, 1971.
3. Thomas. L., Reactions to homologous tissue antigens in relation to hypersensitivity. In H. S. Lawrence (Ed.), *Cellular and Humoral Aspects of the Hypersensitive States*. New York: Hoeber-Harper, 1959.
4. Burnet, F. M., *Prog. Exp. Tumor Res.* **13**:1, 1970.
5. Foley, E. J., *Cancer Res.* **13**:835, 1953.
6. Prehn, R. T., and Main, J. M. *J. Natl. Cancer Inst.* **18**:769, 1957.
7. Stutman, O., *Adv. Cancer Res.* **22**:261, 1975.
8. Hewitt, H. B., Blake, E. R., and Walder, A. S., *Br. J. Cancer* **33**:241, 1976.
9. Prehn, R. T., *J. Natl. Cancer Inst.* **55**:189, 1975.
10. Bartlett, G. L., *J. Natl. Cancer Inst.* **49**:493, 1972.
11. Bubenik, J., Adamcova, B., and Koldovsky, P., Changes in the antigenicity of tumors passaged against immunoselective pressure. In *Genetic variations in somatic cells*, p. 403. Prague, Czechoslovakia: Academic Publ. House, 1967.
12. Ioachim, H. L., *J. Natl. Cancer Inst.* **57**:465, 1976.
13. Black, M. M., and Leis, H. P., *Cancer* **28**:263, 1971.

14. Hirsch, M. S., and Murphy, P. A., *Nature* **218**:478, 1968.
15. Sakakura, T., and Nishizuka, Y., *Gann* **58**:441, 1967.
16. Yunis, E. J., Martinex, C., Smith, J., Stutman, O., and Good, R. A., *Cancer Res.* **29**:174, 1969.
17. Prehn, R. T., *J. Natl. Cancer Inst.* **31**:791, 1963.
18. Jeejeebhoy, H. F. and Rabbat, A. G., *Transplan.* **9**:164, 1970.
19. Grant, G., Roe, F. J., and Pike, M. C., *Nature* **210**:603, 1966.
20. Haughton, G., and Whitmore, A. C., *Transplan. Rev.* **28**:75, 1976.
21. Stutman, O., *Science* **183**:534, 1974.
22. Martinex, C., *Nature* **203**:1188, 1964.
23. Billingham, R. W., and Silvers, W. K., *The immunobiology of transplantation*, p. 69. Englewood Cliffs, NJ.: Prentice-Hall, 1971.
24. Wortin, H. H., Nehlsen, S., and Owen, J. J., *J. Exp. Med.* **134**:681, 1971.
25. Outzen, H. C., Custer, R. P., and Eaton, G. J., *J. Reticuloendothel. Soc.* **17**:1, 1975.
26. Melief, C. J. M., and Schwartz, R. S., Immunocompetences and malignancy. In *Cancer: A Comprehensive Treatise*, Vol. 1, p. 121. New York: Plenum Press, 1975.
27. Metchnikoff, E., *Ann. Inst. Pasteur* **13**:737, 1899.
28. Perlmann, P., *Exp. Cell Res.* **10**:324, 1956.
29. Lappé, M. A., and Schalk, J., *Transplan.* **33**:491, 1971.
30. Warden, G., and Steinmuller, D., Personal Communication.
31. Taylor, H. E., and Culling, C. F. A., *Lab. Invest.* **12**:884, 1963.
32. Kolb, W. P., and Granger, G. A., *Cell Immunol.* **1**:122, 1970.
33. Humphreys, S. R., Glynn, J. P., Chirigos, M. A., and Golden, A., *J. Natl. Cancer Inst.* **28**:1053, 1962.
34. Old, L. J., Boyse, E. A., Clark, D. A., and Carswell, E. A., *Ann. N.Y. Acad. Sci.* **101**:80, 1962.
35. Potter, C. W., Hoskens, J. M., and Oxford, J. S., *Arch. ges. Virusforsch* **27**:73, 1969.
36. Marchant, J., *Br. J. Cancer* **23**:383, 1969.
37. Bartlett, G. L., Unpublished data, 1969.
38. Takasugi, M., and Hildemann, W. H., *J. Natl. Cancer Inst.* **43**:843, 1969.
39. Bloom, E. T., and Hildemann, W. H., *Transplan.* **10**:321, 1970.
40. Hutchins, P., Amos, D. B., and Preoleau, W. H., Jr., *Transplan.* **5**:68, 1967.
41. Gorer, P. A., *Ann. N.Y. Acad. Sci.* **73**:707, 1958.
42. Bittner, J. J., *Science* **95**:462, 1942.
43. Attia, M. A. M., and Weiss, D. W., *Cancer Res.* **26**:1787, 1966.
44. Prehn, R. T., *J. Natl. Cancer Inst.* **43**:1215, 1969.
45. Spark, J. V., *Acta Path. Microbiol. Scand.* **77**:1, 1969.
46. Prehn, R. T., The immunity-inhibiting role of the spleen and the effect of dosage and route of antigen administration in a homograft rejection. In *International Colloque of Biological Problems of Grafting*, p. 163. Oxford: Blackwell Scientific, 1959.
47. Batcherol, J. R., and Silverman, M. S., Further studies on interactions between sessile and humoral antibodies in homograft reactions. In *Transplan. Ciba Foundation Symp.*, p. 216. London: Churchill, 1962.
48. Ferrer, J. F., *Transplan.* **6**:160, 1968.
49. Ferrer, J. F., *Transplan.* **6**:167, 1968.
50. Dezjulian, M., Zee, T., DeOme, K. B., Blair, P. B., and Weiss, D. W., *Cancer Res.* **28**:1759, 1968.
51. Squartini, F., *Israel J. Med. Sci.* **7**:26, 1971.
52. Chernyakhovskaya, I. J., Kadaghidze, Z. G., Salvina, H. G., Dook, I. L., Svet-Moldavsky, G. J., *Folia Biol.* (Praha) **16**:336, 1970.
53. Rosenau, W., and Moon, H. D., *J. Immunol.* **93**:910, 1964.

54. LeFrancois, D., Youn, J. K., Belehradek, J., Jr., and Barski, G., *J. Natl. Cancer Inst.* **46**:981, 1971.
55. Barski, G., and Youn, J. K., *J. Natl. Cancer Inst.* **43**:111, 1969.
56. Del, T., and Tachivana, T., *J. Natl. Cancer Inst.* **65**:739, 1980.
57. Small, M., and Trainin, N., *J. Immunol.* **117**:292, 1976.
58. Small, M., and Trainin, N., *Int. J. Cancer* **15**:962, 1975.
59. Gabizon, A., Small, M., and Trainin, N., *Int. J. Cancer* **18**:813, 1976.
60. Giovarelli, M., Comoglio, P. M., and Foeni, G., *Int. J. Cancer* **34**:233, 1976.
61. Prehn, R. T., *Science* **176**:170, 1972.
62. Prehn, R. T., *Israel J. Med. Sci.* **9**:375, 1973.
63. Prehn, R. T., *Int. J. Cancer* **20**:918, 1977.
64. Outzen, H. C., *Int. J. Cancer* **26**:87, 1980.
65. Shearer, W. T., and Parker, C. W., *Fed. Proc.* **37**:2385, 1978.
66. Ryan, W. L., Curtis, G. L., Heidrick, M. L., and Steinbeck, F., *Proc. Soc. Exp. Biol. Med.* **163**:212, 1980.
67. Heidrick, M. L., Ryan, W. L., and Curtis, G. L., *J. Natl. Cancer Inst.* **60**:1419, 1978.
68. Jeejeebhoy, H. D., *Int. J. Cancer* **13**:665, 1974.
69. Prehn, R. T., *J. Natl. Cancer Inst.* **56**:833, 1976.
70. Norbury, K. C., *Cancer Res.* **37**:1408, 1977.
71. Kall, M. A., and Hellström, I., *J. Immunol.* **114**:1083, 1975.
72. Prehn, R. T., and Outzen, H. C., *Int. J. Cancer* **19**:688, 1977.
73. Stutman, O., *Nature* **253**:142, 1975.
74. Bauer, H., Hayami, M., and Stephen-Gervinus, J. C., *J. Immunol.* **122**:806, 1979.
75. Stutman, O., *Cancer Res.* **36**:739, 1976.
76. Rao, V. S., and Bonavida, B., *Cancer Res.* **36**:1384, 1976.
77. Creemers, P., Ouwehand, J., and Bentvelzen, P., *J. Natl. Cancer Inst.* **59**:895, 1977.
78. Hunsmann, G., Moenning, V., and Schafer, W., *Virology* **66**:327, 1975.
79. Murasko, D. M., and Prehn, R. T., *J. Natl. Cancer Inst.* **61**:1323, 1978.
80. Murasko, D. M. *Effect of amount of virus and strain of mouse used for immunization against Friend-virus induced leukemogenesis.* Manuscript submitted.
81. Murasko, D. M., *Tumor formation in hamsters immunized with virus or virus-transformed cells: Inhibition, enhancement, specificity.* Manuscript submitted.
82. Vaage, J., *Cancer Res.* **38**:331, 1978.
83. Blazar, B. A., Laing, C. A., Miller, F. R., and Heppner, G. H., *J. Natl. Cancer Inst.* **65**:405, 1980.
84. Banks, R. A., Babcock, G. F., Whitmore, A. C., and Haughton, G., *J. Natl. Cancer Inst.* **63**:1423, 1979.
85. Hellström, I., Hellström, K. E., and Bernstein, I. D., *Proc. Natl. Acad. Sci.* **76**:5294, 1979.
86. Blazar, B. A., Miller, F. R., and Heppner, G. H., *J. Immunol.* **120**:1887, 1978.
87. Murasko, D. M., and Lausch, R. N., *J. Natl. Cancer Inst.* **56**:1083, 1976.
88. Walia, A. S., and Lamon, E. W., *J. Natl. Cancer Inst.* **58**:1671, 1977.
89. Moroni, C., Forni, L., Hunsmann, G., and Schumann, G., *Proc. Natl. Acad. Sci. USA* **77**:1486, 1980.
90. Small, M., *J. Immunol.* **118**:1517, 1977.
91. Carnaud, C., Ilfeld, D., Levo, Y., and Trainin, N., *Int. J. Cancer* **14**:168, 1974.
92. Ilfeld, D., Carnaud, C., Cohen, I. R., and Trainin, N., *Int. J. Cancer* **12**:213, 1973.
93. Treves, A. J., Cohen, I. R., and Feldman, M., *Israel J. Med. Sci.* **12**:369, 1976.
94. Treves, A. J., Cohen, I. R., and Feldman, M., *J. Natl. Cancer Inst.* **57**:409, 1976.
95. Manor, Y., Treves, A. J., Cohen, I. R., and Feldman, M., *Transplan.* **22**:360, 1976.
96. Schecter, B., Treves, A. J., and Feldman, M., *J. Natl. Cancer Inst.* **14**:137, 1974.

97.   Chee, D. O., and Bodurtha, A. J., *Int. J. Cancer* **14**:137. 1974.
98.   Fidler, I. J., *Cancer Res.* **34**:494, 1974.
99.   Fidler, I. J., *J. Natl. Cancer Inst.* **50**:1307, 1973.
100. Medina, D., and Heppner, G., *Nature* **242**:329, 1973.
101. Fidler, I. J., Brodey, R. S., and Beck-Nielsen, S., *J. Immunol.* **112**:1054, 1974.
102. Mantovani, A., Peri, G., Polentaruth, N., Bolis, G., Mangioni, C., and Spreafico, F., *Int. J. Cancer* **23**:457, 1979.
103. Buick, R. N., Fry, S. E., and Salmon, S. E., *Br. J. Cancer* **41**:342, 1980.
104. Salmon, S. E. and Hamburger, A. W., *Lancet* 1289, 1978.
105. Cancro, M., and Potter, M., *J. Exp. Med.* **144**:1–54, 1976.
106. Namba, Y., and Hanaoka, M., *J. Immunol.* **109**:1193, 1972.
107. Wainberg, M. A., and Israel, E., *Infec. Immun.* **22**:328, 1978.
108. Howell, S. B., Dean, J. H., Esker, E. C., and Law, L. W., *Int. J. Cancer* **14**:662, 1974.
109. Small, M., *J. Immunol.* **121**:1467, 1978.
110. Gershon, R. K., Makyr, M. B., and Mitchell, M. S., *Nature* (London) **250**:594, 1974.
111. Umiel, T., Lenker-Israeli, M., Itzchaki, M., Trainin, N., Reisner, Y., and Sharon, N., *Cell Immunol.* **37**:134, 1978.

7

Specific and Nonspecific Immunologic Tumor Growth Facilitation

Hisakazu Yamagishi, Neal R. Pellis,
and Barry D. Kahan

The bulwarks of host defense against neoplastic disease are lymphocytes which recognize malignant cell surface antigens as foreign, and mount an immune response with the capacity to inhibit tumor growth. However, the immune response seldom protects the host from progressive neoplastic disease. Indeed, primary tumor growth is generally observed in cancer patients and in experimental animals, and may even be augmented by a defective immune response enabling *escape* from host *immune surveillance* with accelerated neoplastic growth in the face of concomitant immunity (1–3). Two tumor escape mechanisms may participate in this phenomenon: First, cell-mediated tumor facilitation (4–11) may be mediated by the suppressive action of T lymphocytes (12–17), B lymphocytes (18–20), and/or macrophages (21–30). Second, tumor growth facilitation may be due to humoral factors, both nonspecific materials produced by neoplastic cells (31–33) or by lymphoid cells (34–36), and specific substances including antibodies (37–39), circulating tumor antigens, and antigen-antibody complexes (40). These factors ostensibly inhibit cytotoxic T lymphocytes and/or block antigenic sites on neoplastic cell surfaces, thereby potentiating outgrowth *in vivo* by shielding the neoplasm from host resistance. Figure 7.1 schematically depicts the components of tumor growth facilitation. Neoplastic growth releases antigen which may induce blocking antibody and/or directly generate facilitating cells (active, lymphocyte-mediated, tumor facilitation). In addition, suppressive effects occur due to soluble factors produced by tumor cells or lymphoid cells (T cells, B cells, and macrophages), which misdirect antigen recognition. The vectorial outcome of the biological activities of tumor-facilitating and tumor-protective immune responses usually eventuates in relentless progression of neoplastic disease. Thus a critical dissection of

179

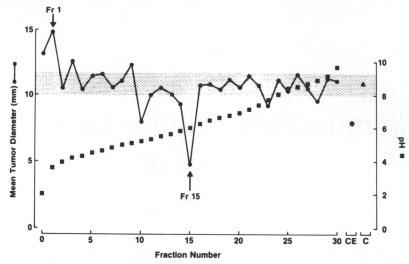

Fig. 7.1. Biological activity of fractions of MCA-F extracts eluted from pIEF Sephadex gel slab. Crude extract and 31 individual fractions of MCA-F were injected subcutaneously into ten syngeneic mice. Ten days later fraction- (●), crude extract- (◗), and saline- (▲) treated mice were challenged subcutaneously with 10^4 viable MCA-F cells. Tumor size at day 25 was assessed by caliper measurements of the diameter of the neoplastic mass. The shaded area depicts the mean tumor diameter ± standard error in control, saline-treated mice.

the components which facilitate tumor growth may provide a basis for the design of specific immunotherapeutic protocols which favor the host, rather than tumor progression.

SPECIFIC TUMOR GROWTH FACILITATION

Facilitation of tumor growth may result from diverse biologic effects. In addition to the host response to bioactive substances released from dividing tumor cells: therapeutic intervention with irradiation, immunosuppressive drugs, surgery, or antigenic tumor extracts may facilitate tumor growth. Potentiation of tumor growth may be triggered by (a) antigens associated with the cell surface or cytosol and (b) bioregulatory substances found in both normal and neoplastic cells. The former substances often engender tumor-specific immune responses, while the latter do not.

Tumor Facilitating Antigen

Tumor growth facilitation may result from interference with protective immune responses induced by tumor-associated antigens as manifest in (a) arrest of lymphoproliferation or blocking responses by lymphocytes or antibodies and (b) activation of suppressor T (Ts) lymphocytes. Many investigators have reported that inactivated tumor cells or extracts containing tumor-specific transplantation antigens (TSTA) induce specific resistance in autochthonous or syngeneic hosts against challenge with supralethal numbers of neoplastic cells (10, 11, 41–57). Although tumor extracts may induce immunoprotection in syngeneic hosts, soluble fractions also promote rather than inhibit tumor growth *in vivo*. Tumor extracts depress lymphocyte proliferation and inhibit *in vitro* cell-mediated cytotoxicity (58–67). For example, Stevens et al. (66) demonstrated that a 3M KCl extract of an X-irradiation-induced small bowel adenocarcinoma in Holzman rats blocked *in vitro*, tumor-bearing, lymphocyte-mediated cytolysis of cultured allogeneic, adenocarcinoma cells. The fraction which was soluble in 50% ammonium sulfate blocked lymphoid cell-mediated cytotoxicity, whereas the insoluble material had a greater effect upon target tumor cells. Furthermore, tumor cell extracts facilitate neoplastic outgrowth *in vivo* (68–70). Vaage (68) reported that administration of tumor antigen extracts specifically facilitated outgrowth in both immunized and unimmunized mice. Rao et al. (69) demonstrated specific enhancement of tumor growth in Wistar-Furth rats by 3M KCl tumor extracts. The mechanism by which specific tumor growth facilitation occurs involves the activation of radiosensitive lymphocytes.

Hellström and Hellström (70) demonstrated that the growth of a small number of cells (1 × 10⁴) from either of two chemically-induced Balb/c sarcomas was specifically facilitated when X-irradiated (15,000 rads) cells of the same sarcoma were mixed with the tumor inoculum. Tumor enhancement did not occur in recipients given 450 rads total body X-irradiation. Tumor neutralization tests revealed that enhanced tumor growth occurred only in the presence of radiosensitive (450 rads) splenic cells present in both nonimmune and tumor-bearing mice.

The dicotomy of host response to extracted tumor antigens was addressed in the biochemical fractionation of crude extracts from murine tumor cells. Tumor antigens were released from cell surfaces by the hypertonic salt (3M KCl) extraction procedure (48, 71) from two antigenically distinct neoplasms, MCA-F and MCA-D. Following treatment of tumor cells with 10 volumes of 3M KCl for 16 hours at 4°C, and sedimentation at 165,000 g, the supernate was concentrated and dialyzed against 200 volumes of 0.15 M phosphate buffered saline (pH 7.2). Insoluble nucleoproteins were removed by 165,000 g centrifugation, yielding a final crude *solubilized* antigen (CSA). Fractionation of crude extracts was performed by preparative isoelectric focusing (pIEF) in a slab of Sephadex G-75 using a 2% ampholyte gradient (72–74), pH range 3.5 to 10.0 (40% Ampholine solution, LKB Instruments, Inc., Sweden). The resultant 31 fractions were eluted, concentrated, dialyzed, and the protein content estimated by the Bradford (75) method. Crude extract and pIEF fractions (Fr) were assayed for TSTA activity by subcutaneous (s.c.) injection of 0.5 mg CSA or an equivalent concentration of one of the pIEF fractions. Control mice were treated with saline. Ten days later, all subjects were challenged s.c. with 10^4 viable MCA-F cells. Tumor growth was monitored by serial caliper measurements of tumor. Pretreatment with 22 μg of Fr 15 (pI 6.00) of MCA-F evoked significant reduction in tumor growth (60%, p < 0.001) when compared with saline-treated controls (Fig. 7.1). In contrast, treatment of mice with the acidic fractions, (pI 2.0 and 3.6), facilitated tumor growth by 22% (p < 0.005) and 36% (p < 0.001), respectively. None of the other pIEF fractions significantly altered tumor growth.

Reduction of tumor growth by the pIEF fraction significantly prolonged host survival. Antigen-induced changes in tumor growth were reflected in the survival of challenged hosts (72). The 50% survival times (ST_{50}) of challenged mice correlated with the reduction or facilitation of tumor growth

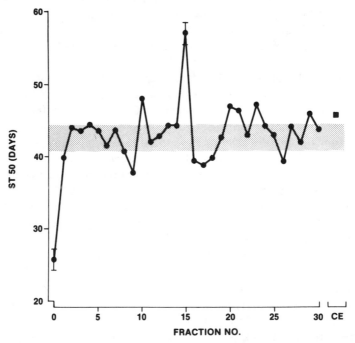

Fig. 7.2. Fifty percent survival time of hosts pretreated with pIEF fractions and challenged 10 days later with 10^4 MCA-F cells. Serial determinations of percent survivors were converted to probit values and regressed against the $\log_{10}$ day of observation. ST_{50} was derived from the intersection of probit 5 with the regressed survival line. The $ST_{50} \pm$ SE of control mice is shown by the shaded area.

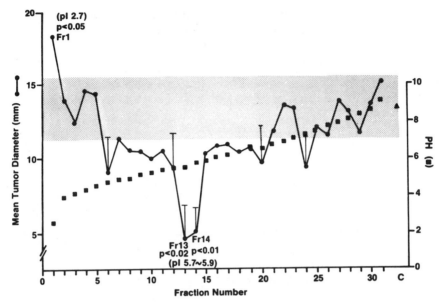

Fig. 7.3. Biological activity of fractions of MCA-D extracts eluted from pIEF Sephadex gel slab. The 31 individual fractions of MCA-D were injected subcutaneously into 10 syngeneic mice. Ten days later fraction- (●), and saline- (▲) treated mice were challenged subcutaneously with 10^4 viable MCA-F cells. Tumor size at day 39 was assessed by caliper measurements of the diameter of the tumor. Control mean tumor diameter ± standard error is depicted by the shaded area.

(Fig. 7.2). Control mice displayed an ST_{50} of 56.6 ± 1.5 days. All control mice were dead by 59 days after challenge, while 50% of hosts treated with Fr 15 were alive at 59 days, and 20% survived 100 days after challenge. On the other hand, all Fr 1-treated mice were dead by 46 days (p < 0.001).

Two opposing immunobiological activities were also present in the antigenically distinct MCA-D tumor cell extracts. The acidic Fr 1 (pI 2.7) significantly facilitated (p < 0.05) the growth of MCA-D, while isoelectrically focused Fr 13 and 14 (pI 5.7 and 5.9, respectively) reduced tumor growth (p < 0.02 and < 0.01, respectively) when compared to saline-treated controls (Fig. 7.3).

Carrier ampholytes potentially present in the fraction did not participate in these effects. Ampholytes were electrofocused in the absence of 3M KCl crude extracts. Groups of 10 mice pretreated with sham Fr 1 and with Fr 15 were compared with nontreated mice for neoplastic outgrowth after challenge with 10^4 viable MCA-F, MCA-D, and MCA-C tumor cells. Tables 7.1 and 7.2 show that administration of focused ampholytes (pI 3.5 and pI 5.7) had no effect on the growth of MCA-F, MCA-D, and MCA-C tumor cells. Thus residual ampholytes contained in pIEF fractions of crude extracts do not

Table 7.1. Specificity of Tumor Facilitation Induced by pIEF Isolated Antigen (Fr 1)[a]

Mice Pre-treated with	Challenged Tumor Cells	Mean Tumor Diameter (mm)[b] ± SE at Day 25	"p"[c]
Fr 1 (pI 3.6)[d]	MCA-F	10.9 ± 0.5	<0.001
Ampholytes[e]		6.0 ± 1.0	NS[f]
None		5.6 ± 0.8	—
Fr 1 (pI 3.6)	MCA-D	6.8 ± 1.7	NS
Ampholytes		5.4 ± 1.4	NS
None		6.3 ± 1.8	—
Fr 1 (pI 3.6)	MCA-C	3.9 ± 1.1	NS
Ampholytes		3.1 ± 1.3	NS
None		3.6 ± 1.0	—

[a] Specificity of tumor-facilitating fraction Fr 1 was assessed by immunoprotection test. Fr 1 (pI 3.6) from MCA-F extract and ampholyte fraction (pI 3.5) were administered s.c. into groups of 10 mice; 10 days later 10^4 MCA-F, MCA-D, and MCA-C cells were challenged s.c. into right flank.

[b] Mean tumor diameter was calculated from the measurement of two diameters (10 mice/group).

[c] Significance as determined by Student's t-test.

[d] pIEF fraction of MCA-F crude extracts.

[e] pIEF fraction of ampholyte (pI 3.5) without extract.

[f] NS: not significant.

contribute to either the immunoprotective (pI 5.7–6.0) or the tumor-facilitating (pI 2.0–3.6) activity.

The immunological specificity of the response to Fr 1 and to Fr 15 was investigated by a cross-immunoprotection test protocol using two antigenically distinct MCA tumors (Tables 7.1–7.4). Parallel groups of 10 mice treated with either 14 µg of Fr 1 or 22 µg of Fr 15 purified from crude 3M KCl MCA-F extracts were challenged 10 days later either with MCA-F cells or with antigenically distinct fibrosarcoma MCA-D or MCA-C cells. Table

Table 7.2. Specificity of Tumor Protection Induced by pIEF Isolated Antigen (Fr 15)[a]

Mice Pre-treated with	Challenged Tumor Cells	Mean Tumor Volume (cm^3)[b] ± SE at Day 28	"p"[c]
Fr 1 (pI 6.0)[d]	MCA-F	0.55 ± 0.14	<0.001
Ampholytes[e]		1.86 ± 0.17	NS[f]
None		1.78 ± 0.23	—
Fr 1 (pI 6.0)	MCA-D	1.54 ± 0.45	NS
Ampholytes		1.32 ± 0.25	NS
None		1.23 ± 0.38	—

[a] Specificity of tumor-protective fraction Fr 15 (pI 6.0) from MCA-F extracts was assessed by immunoprotection test. Fr 15 (pI 6.0) and ampholyte fraction (pI 5.7) were administered s.c. into groups of 10 mice; 10 days later 10^4 MCA-F and MCA-D were challenged s.c. into right flank.

[b] Mean tumor volume was calculated from the mean tumor diameter.

[c] Significance as determined by Student's t-test.

[d] pIEF fraction of MCA-F extracts.

[e] pIEF fraction of ampholytes (pI 5.7) without extract.

[f] NS: not significant.

Table 7.3 Specificity of Tumor-Facilitating Fraction (pI 2.7) and Tumor-Protective Fraction (pI 5.7 ~ 5.9) from MCA-D Extracts[a]

Host Pretreatment	Mean Tumor Diameter (mm)[b] ± SEM at day 39			
	MCA-D	"p"[c]	MCA-F	"p"[c]
None	13.3 ± 2.2	—	20.0 ± 1.3	—
Fr 1 (pI 2.7)	21.3 ± 1.2	< 0.05	18.8 ± 0.9	NS
Fr 13 (pI 5.7)	4.6 ± 2.6	< 0.02	ND[e]	
Fr 14 (pI 5.9)	5.1 ± 1.7	< 0.01	19.6 ± 1.6	NS[d]

[a] Specificity of tumor-facilitating fraction Fr 1 (pI 2.7) and tumor-protective fraction Fr 13 (pI 5.7), Fr 14 (pI 5.9) was assessed by immunoprotection test. Fr 1, Fr 13, and Fr 14 from MCA-D extracts were administered s.c. to groups of 10 mice that were challenged 10 days later with 10^4 MCA-D and MCA-F cells.

[b] Mean tumor diameter was calculated from mean value of two diameters of 10 mice/group.

[c] Significance as determined by Student's t-test.

[d] NS: not significant.

[e] ND: not done.

7.1 shows that pretreatment with MCA-F Fr 1 facilitated the growth of the homologous inoculum by 96% (p < 0.005), but had no effect upon MCA-D or MCA-C. In contrast, pretreatment with MCA-F Fr 15 reduced the growth of the homotypic inoculum by 69% (p < 0.001), but afforded no protection against MCA-D cells (Table 7.2). Assessment of the specificity of the fractions obtained from MCA-D extracts revealed a similar relationship between the two qualitatively different antigens (Table 7.3). Pretreatment of hosts with 10 μg MCA-D Fr 1 (pI 2.7) facilitated homotypic, MCA-D tumor growth, while immunoprotective Fr 13 (pI 5.7) and 14 (pI 5.9) evoked significant reduction of outgrowth (p < 0.02 and p < 0.01, respectively).

Table 7.4. Specificity of Antigen Extract Induced Spleen-Cell-Mediated Tumor Facilitation[a]

Target Tumor Cells	Spleen Cells from Donors Pretreated with	Mean Tumor Diameter (mm)[b]	"p"[c]
MCA-F	CSA[d]	11.0 ± 1.8	< 0.025
	None	5.2 ± 1.9	—
MCA-D	CSA	6.8 ± 0.9	NS[e]
	None	7.5 ± 0.7	—
MCA-C	CSA	8.2 ± 1.6	NS
	None	7.6 ± 1.0	—

[a] Spleen cells (10^7) from donors treated 6 days prior with MCA-F CSA were admixed with 10^4 MCA-F, MCA-D, or MCA-C target tumor cells and inoculated subcutaneously into three groups of 10 mice.

[b] Mean diameter was calculated by measurement of tumor diameters in groups of 10 mice 26 days after LATA.

[c] Significance as determined by Student's t-test.

[d] Crude 3M KCl antigen of MCA-F.

[e] NS: not significant.

Neither the tumor-facilitating fraction nor the immunizing fraction from MCA-D influenced the *in vivo* outgrowth of MCA-F cells. Thus crude 3M KCl extracts of MCA-F and MCA-D tumors contain at least two antigenic components resulting in immune responses with antagonistic effects on neoplastic outgrowth.

In vitro experiments performed by others suggest that substances with antagonistic actions may be present in tumor cells and crude extracts. Brandchaft et al. (63) reported that 3M KCl extracts of Moloney virus-induced leukemia cells contain both immunogenic and immunosuppressive components. Immunogenic components were demonstrated by their ability to (a) combine with antibody and thereby inhibit complement-mediated cytotoxicity or (b) stimulate blastogenesis in normal syngeneic lymphocytes. In contrast, immunosuppressive components inhibited DNA synthesis by normal syngeneic lymphocytes responding in a mixed lymphocyte culture reaction. Blackstock et al. (64) fractionated crude 3M KCl extracts of meth-ylcholanthrene-induced fibrosarcomas by ultrafiltration. Both high molecular weight ($> 300,000$) and low molecular weight ($< 30,000$) components non-specifically inhibited ^{3}H-thymidine incorporation by lymphoid cells taken from tumor-bearing animals, while the intermediate material (molecular weight 30,000 to 100,000 daltons) stimulated proliferation. Paranjpe et al. (58) demonstrated specific depression of cell-mediated immune responses to autologous tumor cells by a homogenate of an SV 40-transformed fibro-sarcoma (E_4 tumor) of mice. Tumor specificity of the immunodepression was shown in three ways. (a) The serum of E_4 tumor-immune mice, but not of normal mice given injections of the E_4 tumor homogenate 24 hours pre-viously, suppressed antitumor immunity *in vitro*, as measured by the release of ^{51}Cr from labeled E_4 tumor cells incubated with immune spleen cells. (b) The intraperitoneal (ip) inoculation of E_4 tumor homogenate did not alter the cellular response of BCG-sensitized mice to tuberculin. (c) The ip injection of a homogenate of an antigenically unrelated tumor did not depress the cellular immune response of E_4 tumor-immune mice to E_4 tumor cells.

Thus the cell extracts from chemically-induced (64, 70, 72), virus-induced (58, 63), and X-irradiation-induced (66) tumors have components which may facilitate tumor growth *in vivo*. The extract used to induce immuno-protection, upon multiple injections at weekly intervals, enhanced tumor growth (54, 55, 69, 76). The mechanism by which the facilitating antigens described herein accerlerate the outgrowth of tumor inocula is uncertain. Indeed, the lymphoid system is a critical intermediary (vide infra). Tumor-facilitating antigens may act by (a) generating suppressor T cells, (b) directly blocking cell-mediated immunity, (c) eliciting specific blocking antibody, or (d) possibly altering antigen processing cells, thereby not only *preventing* immunization, but also activating the production of soluble, systemically-distributed tumor-enhancing substances.

Specific Tumor-Facilitating Cells

Antigen-induced facilitation of tumor growth *in vivo* and *in vitro* may result from the interaction of neoplastic cells directly with immune cells or indirectly with antibodies capable of binding to tumor cell surface antigens. The lymphocyte-mediated stimulation of tumor growth, originally described by Prehn (4), showed that low numbers of putatively tumor immune lymphocytes facilitated rather than abated neoplastic outgrowth in the adoptive transfer assay. Subsequently Fidler (77), Jeejeebhoy (78), Kall and Hellström (79), and Fujimoto et al. (12, 13) showed that murine lymphocytes from tumor-bearing or tumor-immune hosts facilitated tumor growth *in vivo* and *in vitro*. Suppressor lymphocytes which specifically promote tumor growth were demonstrated by Rotter and Trainin (80), and Fujimoto et al. (12, 13). A few reports (5–8) demonstrated that nonspecific tumor facilitation occurred *in vivo*. The suppressor cells are not necessarily the same population as the tumor-facilitating cells. Treves et al. (5) and Umiel and Trainin (6) reported that transfer of an admixture of spleen cells from donor C57BL mice bearing Lewis lung carcinoma for 10 days and neoplastic cells resulted in enhanced tumor growth and increased incidence in normal secondary recipients. Lymphocytes may promote tumor outgrowth, since depletion of the spleen cell population with antitheta serum plus complement ablated tumor growth facilitation. Small and Trainin (7) and Small (8) reported that tumor growth was facilitated by thymocytes, whether or not they were sensitized to tumor antigen. The population of thymocytes mediating the effect was eliminated by treatment with thymic humoral factor, suggesting that they were immature T cells. Thus mature T cells may inhibit tumor growth, whereas precursor lymphocytes may be responsible for tumor facilitation.

Similar conclusions were reached by Pellis et al. (11) by analysis of the progression of the immune response to tumor antigens. Lymphocytes obtained 6 days after immunization with crude 3M KCl extracts facilitated neoplastic growth, while those harvested at 9 days neutralized tumor growth. Since the opposing biological activities of tumor facilitation and tumor protection induced by the pIEF fractions of 3M KCl fractions are mediated by lymphocytes (73), this system afforded a model to dissect cellular mediation of immune and escape mechanisms. Spleen cells from mice pretreated with 0.5 mg MCA-F crude soluble antigen (CSA) 2, 6, 9, 12, or 15 days prior to harvest were admixed with homologous tumor cells prior to s.c. inoculation into groups of 10 syngeneic normal mice. The spleen cells obtained at these times displayed a sinusoidal progression of tumor-facilitating and neutralizing activities (Fig. 7.4). Spleen cells from mice treated 6 days previously with MCA-F CSA facilitated tumor outgrowth by 118% (p < 0.001). On the other hand, spleen cells from mice treated 9 or 12 days previously with CSA reduced tumor growth by 62% (p < 0.01) and 44% (p < 0.02), re-

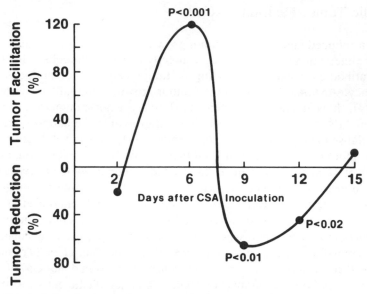

Fig. 7.4. Activity of spleen cells from hosts treated with crude soluble antigen at various intervals before LATA. Spleen cells obtained 2, 6, 9, 12, and 15 days after subcutaneous inoculation of 0.5 mg crude 3M KCl extract from MCA-F tumor were assayed by local adoptive transfer. At each interval, 10^7 normal or immune spleen cells were admixed with 10^4 viable tumor cells and then inoculated s.c. into 10 normal syngeneic recipients. Tumor growth was monitored by serial measurement (Pellis and Kahan, 1978).

spectively. There was no significant change in tumor growth at 2 or at 15 days after sensitization with CSA. Unlike the tumor facilitation mediated by thymocytes (8), that mediated by spleen cells following treatment with extracted tumor antigens displayed antigen specificity as documented by local adoptive transfer assays (LATA) using the antigenically distinct MCA-F, MCA-D, and MCA-C target cells. Table 7.4 shows that the facilitating spleen cells induced by CSA acted specifically on the outgrowth of the homotypic MCA-F tumor ($p < 0.025$), but not on the outgrowth of the antigenically distinct MCA-D or MCA-C neoplasms. Recent evidence suggests that Fr 15 does not induce tumor-facilitating lymphocytes at any time from day 2 to day 15 after antigen treatment (unpublished data). The potential relationship between the tumor facilitation observed early in the course of sensitization with crude antigen and that following treatment with Fr 1 was investigated by LATA. Spleen cells from mice treated with $14 < g$ Fr 1 were admixed with MCA-F cells and then injected into normal secondary recipients (Fig. 7.5). Spleen cells from Fr 1-treated mice significantly facilitated MCA-F tumor outgrowth ($p < 0.002$) when compared to recipients of age-matched normal spleen cells, suggesting that Fr 1 activity is mediated

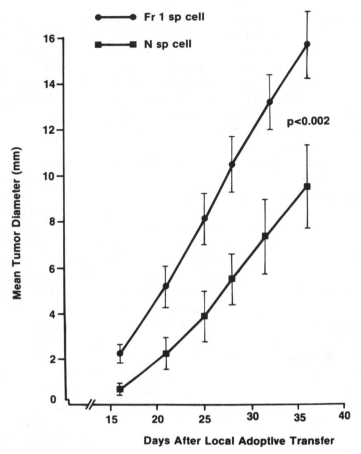

Fig. 7.5. Tumor facilitation by spleen cells obtained from mice pretreated with Fr 1. Spleen cell activity from normal donors (■———■) and from mice pretreated with 14 μg Fr 1 (●———●) of MCA-F was assessed by LATA.

by tumor-facilitating lymphoid cells. Thus the facilitation of tumor growth induced by antigenic constituents of tumor cells results from interaction of antigen modified lymphocytes with tumor cells. The tumor-facilitating lymphocyte may thus represent an unfortunate overregulation of the immune response to tumors by suppressor lymphocytes.

Suppressor Cells

Tumor-specific and nonspecific suppressor cells may regulate host resistance, thereby determining the fate of neoplastic cells. Specific suppression may be associated with T lymphocytes while nonspecific suppression is directed by phagocytic cells. Elgert and Farrar (81) showed that two populations of suppressor cells coexisted in the spleens of Balb/c mice bearing a transplantable fibrosarcoma. Suppression of *in vitro* lymphoproliferation by low numbers of spleen cells was mediated by T cells while greater numbers of macrophages were required to achieve similar suppression. The importance of both populations in host anergy is apparent especially since tumor progression was attended by a dramatic increase in the number of splenic macrophages. Antigen specific, suppressor T cells are generated in tumor-bearing hosts (12–15), in animals treated with 3M KCl extracts (9, 16, 76), or during mixed lymphocyte culture (MLC) *in vitro* (17). Fujimoto et al. (12, 13) reported that intravenous transfer of 10^7 to 10^8 washed thymocytes or spleen cells from tumor-bearing animals into secondary hosts significantly inhibited tumor rejection. Ablation of tumor immunity was not observed in recipients of lymphoid cells derived from normal or from allogeneic tumor-bearing animals. These tumor-specific suppressor cells were resistant to hydrocortisone (2.5 mg per mouse), but sensitive to treatment with antitheta serum and complement. Specific suppressor cell activity was demonstrable as early as 24 hours after tumor transplantation. Takei et al. (14, 15) reported that suppressor T cells generated in tumor-bearing hosts specifically inhibited the induction of cytotoxic T cells. Yamauchi et al. (16) noted that 3M KCl extracts of the methylcholanthrene-induced sarcoma, S1509a, predominantly activated specific, suppressor T cells which expressed surface markers controlled by genes in the I-J subregion of the mouse H-2 complex. The participation of I-J bearing cells in the progression of neoplastic disease was previously noted in the work of Green et al. (82) who showed that treatment of tumor-bearing Balb/c mice with I-J antisera significantly reduced tumor outgrowth.

The activation of suppressor cells by tumor antigen may be the common mechanism by which tumor cells are perpetuated in otherwise immune hosts. Activation must be ultimately controlled by the molecular structure of the antigen, and its route of entry to or emergence within the host. The ease of induction of tumor-specific suppressor lymphocytes by tumor extracts (10, 54, 55, 69, 73, 76, 83, 84) suggests that cell-bound tumor antigen may be considerably less efficient in the induction of T_s compared to tumor-neutralizing mechanisms. In the MCA-F model, tumor-enhancing lymphocytes could not be demonstrated in the spleens of hosts immunized with irradiated tumor cells (11). In contrast, the spleen of 3M KCl extract-treated mice possessed lymphocytes with potent tumor-facilitating activity (10). In addition to the distinction between *soluble* and *cell-bound* antigen, the immune response is also controlled by molecules modifying the immunogen, namely, more acidic tumor antigens induce facilitation, while those closer to neutrality induce protection (73, 85). Since both enhancing and immunoprotective antigens are tumor specific, both materials may bear the same tumor-specific epitope, the action of which is profoundly affected by substituent groups accounting for differing isoelectric as well as immunobiological properties. Thus, suppressor cells evoked by intact MCA-F cells or their subcellular antigens influence the balance between the generation of cytotoxic lymphocytes and unrestrained tumor growth (30).

Suppressive Factors Produced by Lymphoid Cells

Soluble mediators produced by lymphocytes in peripheral lymphoid organs regulate immune responses. Tada et al. (86) reported the presence of a specific suppressor T-cell factor in lymphoid cell extracts of rats and mice following immunization with hapten-carrier antigens. The active moiety which was sensitive to treatment with trypsin had an apparent molecular weight of 35,000 to 55,000 daltons. Furthermore, Taniguchi et al. (87) demonstrated that the T-cell factor specifically suppressed the secondary IgG responses of primed spleen cells. The factor was not released from primed T cells upon short-term culture with antigen; it remained bound to the membranes of residual cultured cells. Only physical disruption of the plasma membrane released the T-cell factor responsible for specific modulation of the IgG response. The suppressor activity was completely adsorbed with alloantisera specific for products of the I region of the H-2 complex; various anti-immunoglobulin antisera had no effect. Analysis of the specificity of the alloantisera capable of binding the suppressor molecule indicated that it was an I region product, probably coded by genes in the I-J subregion.

Waksman and Tada (88) found that the specific suppressor T-cell factor derived from thymocytes of mice immunized with a relatively high dose of protein inhibited the development of specific antibody-forming cells *in vitro* and suppressed cell-mediated immunity to the homologous tumor antigen. A nonspecific factor which inhibited DNA synthesis by proliferating cells was obtained from cells stimulated *in vitro* with mitogen or exposed *in vivo* to a single large dose of antigen a day or two earlier. The thymocyte producing the antigen specific factor bore the Ly-1 − , 2+ , 3+ phenotype, carried determinants of the I-region of the H-2 complex, and acted only on T cells bearing the same I-region genes, but expressing Ly-1+ , 2+ , and 3+ .

The soluble suppressor T-cell factor described by Green et al. (82) was immunologically specific, less than 70,000 daltons in weight, and was destroyed by pronase, but not RNase, treatment. The factor shared antigenic determinants with products of the K end of the murine major histocompatibility complex; although most likely, the suppressive factor was from the closely linked I-region, probably related to I-J rather than the I-A genes.

Perry et al. (89) demonstrated retardation of tumor outgrowth in mice pre-treated with anti-I-J alloantiserum.

A nonspecific, soluble, suppressor T-cell factor was reported by Thomas et al. (90). The addition of spleen cells immune to ovalbumin (Ova ISC) to spleen cells immune to sheep erythrocyte (SRBC ISC) in Mishell-Dutton cultures dramatically reduced the PFC response to SRBC. The cells mediating this suppression were radiosensitive, depleted by antitheta antiserum and complement, and nonadherent to glass bead columns. Ova ISC-induced inhibition also occurred in dual culture chambers separated by a cell im-permeable membrane. The suppressor factor was sensitive to trypsin treatment and to heating at 80°C, but not at 70°C, for 30 minutes. The molecular weight by sucrose gradient analysis was between 55,000 and 60,000 daltons. The suppressor factor appeared to be distinct from a T-cell *helper* factor which was sensitive to heating at 70°C for 30 minutes. It was proposed that the nonspecific suppressor factor may have a significant role in the phenomenon of *antigenic competition*. The available data suggest that nonspecific and specific suppressor materials have similar molecular characteristics.

Soluble Tumor Facilitating Factors

The serum from tumor-bearing animals blocks lymphocyte cytotoxicity against cultured tumor cells (37, 91). The blocking factors in tumor-bearer serum exhibit properties of 7S immunoglobulins, suggesting tumor-specific antibody. Baldwin et al. (40) reported that tumor-specific antigen-antibody complexes block lymphocyte-mediated cytotoxicity against rat hepatoma cells. *In vitro* analysis of specific serum-mediated blocking of lymphocyte responses suggested that these factors facilitated neoplastic growth *in vivo*. Indeed, early work on the mechanism of enhancement of allograft survival by treatment of graft recipients with alloantiserum suggested that antitumor antibodies *protect* neoplastic cells from destruction by cytotoxic lymphocytes *in vivo*. Pierce (38) found that sera from mice bearing Moloney virus-induced sarcoma cells facilitated tumor *in vivo* growth. Ran and Witz (31) showed that the eluate prepared from the surface of a chemically-induced mouse sarcoma growing *in vivo* facilitated tumor growth. Subsequently, the eluate was shown to contain tumor bound Ig which is ostensibly tumor-specific (92), an observation confirmed in a Polyoma virus-induced sarcoma by Bansal et al. (32). The relative participation in neoplastic growth regulation *in vivo* by tumor-specific antibody and/or by antigen-antibody complexes (93) versus activtion of T_s or suppressor macrophages remains controversial.

Hollander et al. (34) and Isakov et al. (35, 36) found supernates of spleen cell cultures from tumor-bearing mice to facilitate neoplastic growth. This factor, produced by the tumor cells, directly affects the antigenic triggering of antibody-producing B lymphocytes. Hellström and Hellström (33) described specific and nonspecific tumor facilitation by cell-free *tumor fluid* (TF) obtained when culture medium of 3-methylcholanthrene-induced sarcoma cells was centrifuged at 5,000 g and passed through 0.45 μm pore size Millipore filters. TF specifically inhibited cell-mediated cytotoxicity to tumor targets *in vitro*. Also, subcutaneous inoculation of TF with the tumor cells facilitated tumor outgrowth *in vivo* due to both specific and nonspecific components. The *in vivo* tumor facilitation was best demonstrated when sarcoma cells and TF were inoculated together, suggesting the importance of the local milieu within a growing tumor. Tumor-specific facilitation was also demonstrated in one of two experiments when TF was given intraperitoneally, suggesting that it also generated systemic immune effects. The authors suggest that TF includes both specific tumor-facilitating antigen and facilitating factors which carry no antigenic discrimination.

The Role of Spleen in Specific Tumor Growth Facilitation

In addition to the classic role of the spleen in the orchestration of antibody and cell-mediated immune responses, it plays a critical role in the regulation of tumor immunity and neoplastic growth facilitation. Investigating the antibody response to type III pneumococcal polysaccharide (SSS-III), Amsbaugh et al. (94) reported that splenectomy of an adult mouse alters suppressor and amplifier T-cell activity. Seven days after splenectomy amplifier T-cell activity was diminished, suggesting that the spleen is an important site for the generation and/or maintenance of amplifier T-cell activity. Enomoto and Lucas (95) reported that the spleen was essential for the induction of both active and passive enhancement of kidney graft survival in rats. However, Kilshaw et al. (96) found that splenectomy did not affect the induction of active enhancement of the less vascularized skin grafts. Critical investigation of the role of splenic tissue in the tumorigenesis of MCA-F revealed that splenectomy only affected the initial stages (0 to 3 days after tumor inoculation) of neoplastic progression. Splenectomy, three days after tumor initiation, resulted in significant reduction of tumor outgrowth (97), suggesting that splenic suppressor cells participate in the promotion of tumor growth.

Although some reports document the role of spleen cells in the facilitation of tumor growth *in vivo*, splenectomized hosts respond to tumor-facilitating antigens to the same extent as parallel, sham-operated controls. Induction of accelerated tumor outgrowth by pretreatment with the acidic Fr 1, tumor-enhancing antigen occurs in hosts with or without splenic tissue (98). Fraction

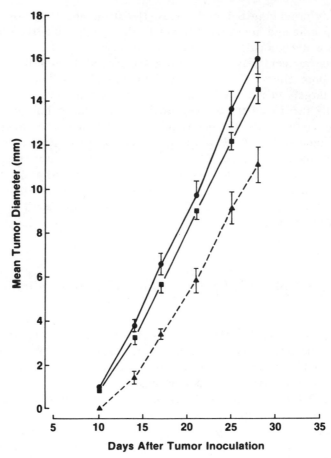

Fig. 7.6. Effect of splenectomy upon active tumor facilitation. Groups of 10 mice were inoculated subcutaneously with 14 μg Fr 1 of MCA-F 3 weeks after splenectomy (■) or sham-operation (●———●). Ten days later all hosts and age-matched nonoperated control mice (▲) were inoculated s.c. with 10^4 viable MCA-F cells. Mean tumor diameter was monitored by serial caliper measurements.

1 from the methylcholanthrene-induced fibrosarcoma, MCA-F, was inoculated into three groups of 10 syngeneic C3H/HeJ mice: splenectomized, sham-splenectomized, and nonoperated. Ten days later each animal was challenged subcutaneously with MCA-F cells. Figure 7.6 shows that both splenectomized and sham-operated mice display similar facilitation of MCA-F tumor out-growth ($p < 0.001$ and $p < 0.002$, respectively) compared to nonoperated controls, suggesting that the spleen is not essential for active specific tumor facilitation.

NONSPECIFIC TUMOR GROWTH FACILITATION

Nonspecific Tumor-Facilitating Cells in Tumor-Bearing Mice

In addition to the specific tumor-facilitating cells found in the spleens of mice pretreated with either crude 3M KCl extracts or pIEF fractionated, acidic antigen (Fr 1), nonspecific tumor-facilitating cells can be demonstrated in tumor-bearing mice (Fig. 7.7). Spleen cells from mice bearing MCA-F tumors for 3, 6, 9, 15, or 30 days were admixed with MCA-F cells and inoculated subcutaneously into normal syngeneic mice as a local adoptive transfer assay (LATA). Immunological specificity of the spleen cell activity was assessed by admixing MCA-F tumor-bearer spleen cells with either MCA-F or the antigenically distinct MCA-D or MCA-C cells. In the early stages of tumorigenesis (Figs. 7.8 and 7.9), namely 3 days after MCA-F inoculation, spleen cells from tumor-bearing mice indiscriminantly facilitated the outgrowth of MCA-F, MCA-C, and MCA-D tumors ($p < 0.001$), compared to spleen cells from normal donors and to the control tumor growth curve. Thus the tumor-facilitating cells generated in the early stage of tumor

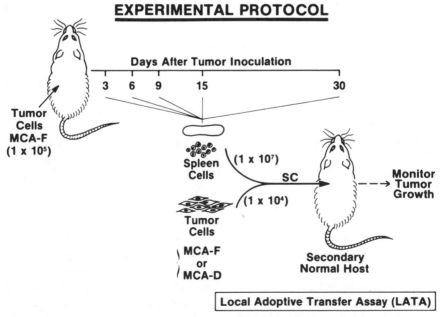

Fig. 7.7. Experimental protocol of the assessment of spleen cell activity during tumor progression by local adoptive transfer assay.

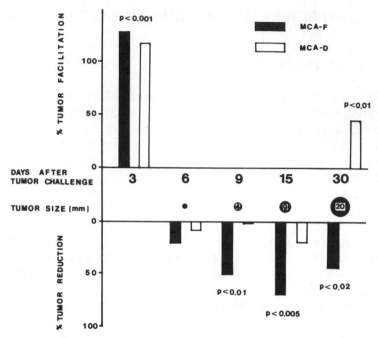

Fig. 7.8. Progression of the immune response in spleen cells at various times after tumor inoculation. Unfractionated tumor-bearer and normal spleen-cell populations were assessed for their effect upon tumor growth in the LATA. Spleen cells from MCA-F inoculated hosts were admixed with 10^4 MCA-F cells and with 10^4 MCA-D cells (1000:1) and the mixtures injected subcutaneously into 10 syngeneic recipients.

growth were nonspecific. However, 9 to 15 days after MCA-F inoculation, tumor-bearing spleen cells neutralized MCA-F tumor growth ($p < 0.01$, $p < 0.005$ respectively), but not MCA-D, suggesting the emergence of a specific cell-mediated immune response. Finally, in late stages of tumor growth (namely 30 days after MCA-F inoculation), spleen cells neutralized MCA-F ($p < 0.02$), but facilitated MCA-D ($p < 0.01$) growth, suggesting the presence of both specific tumor-neutralizing cells and nonspecific tumor-facilitating cells.

The nonspecific tumor-facilitating cells present in the early stages of tumorigenesis were resistant to 700 R irradiation, suggesting that facilitation was effected by preformed substances in cells which need not undergo DNA replication to promote tumor growth (Table 7.5). Depletion of phagocytic, adherent cells using the carbonyl-iron/magnet procedure followed by adherence to plastic petri dishes prior to LATA abrogated the tumor-facilitating activity (Fig. 7.10). Thus nonspecific, tumor-facilitating activity appears to be due to a radioresistant, phagocytic, adherent cell population, presumably macrophages. In parallel experiments MCA-F-bearing mice were shown to

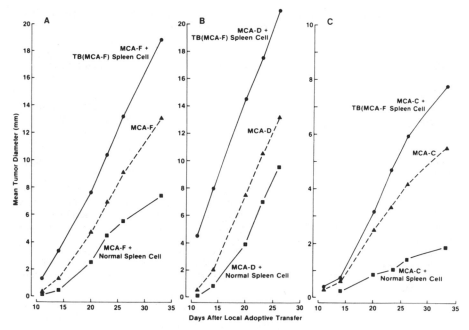

Fig. 7.9. Specificity of splenic tumor-enhancing cells from mice bearing MCA-F tumor for 3 days. Spleen-cell activity was assessed by LATA. 10^4 antigenically distinct tumor MCA-F (Panel A), MCA-D (Panel B), and MCA-C (Panel C) cells were admixed with 10^7 spleen cells from 3 days tumor-bearing (●——●) or age-matched and sex-matched normal untreated (■) mice donor and inoculated s.c. into normal syngeneic secondary hosts. 10^4 MCA-F, D and C cells only (▲) were inoculated as control group.

possess splenic macrophages which suppressed the evocation of delayed hypersensitivity to the chemical sensitizer dinitrochlorobenzene (DNCB) (99–101). Possibly the same macrophages are responsible for the nonspecific facilitation of MCA-F and MCA-D fibrosarcoma (9, 30, 98).

The properties of tumor-neutralizing cells obtained from nine-day tumor bearers contrast sharply with those of the apparent macrophage-mediated enhancement prior to that time. The tumor-bearing spleen cell (TBsp) population which specifically neutralized neoplastic outgrowth was radiosensitive (Table 7.6), and ablated by treatment with anti-Thy-1.2 serum and complement (Table 7.7). Thus the neutralizing activity of TBsp is probably mediated by a tumor-specific, radiosensitive T-lymphocyte subpopulation. In the late stages of tumor growth, 30 days after MCA-F inoculation, the two cell populations are both active (Table 7.8). Irradiation of TBsp cells abrogated the specific tumor-neutralizing effect, but did not alter the nonspecific tumor-facilitating activity. Furthermore, when a spleen cell population which neutralized MCA-F ($p < 0.005$), but facilitated MCA-D

Table 7.5. Effect of Irradiation Upon the Tumor-Facilitating Activity of Spleen Cells from Three-Day Tumor Bearers

Spleen-Cell Donor	LATA Tumor Target	Tumor Diameter (mm ± SEM) at 26 Days after LATA[a]
None	MCA-F	8.0 ± 1.2
Normal		6.5 ± 1.2
TBsp		13.1 ± 1.0 (p < 0.001)[b]
Tbsp-x[c]		13.8 ± 1.1 (NS)
None	MCA-D	8.4 ± 1.4
Normal		6.4 ± 0.6
TBsp		14.5 ± 0.5 (p < 0.001)[b]
TBsp-x[c]		15.8 ± 1.0[d] (NS)

[a] Three days after inoculation of 1×10^5 MCA-F cells into each of 20 C3H/HeJ mice, spleen cells were harvested. Normal and tumor-bearer spleen cells were individually mixed with 10^4 MCA-F or with 10^4 MCA-D cells and inoculated subcutaneously into groups of 10 syngeneic hosts. The average of the mean tumor diameters ± the standard error at the stipulated day after transfer are shown.

[b] Significance of Student's t-test comparison with recipients of normal spleen cells.

[c] Spleen cells were exposed to 700 rads of gamma irradiation prior to use in the LATA.

[d] Significance of difference between untreated tumor bearer and X-irradiated tumor-bearer spleen cells.

(p < 0.01), was depleted of adherent, phagocytic elements, there was a significant increase in neutralizing activity against the MCA-F tumor (p < 0.005) with attendant loss of the facilitating activity against MCA-D (p < 0.005) (Table 7.9). Depletion of adherent, phagocytic cells from the normal spleen cell population did not alter the outgrowth of MCA-F or MCA-D. Thus tumor-facilitating cells present in the TBsp popultion may either suppress the activity of T-cell-mediated, tumor-neutralizing elements or act directly on tumor cells to promote neoplastic progression. In summary, the spleens of mice bearing MCA-F neoplasms contain cell populations that mediate both tumor facilitation and tumor neutralization. Nonspecific tumor-facilitating cells, probably macrophages, are present during the early and late stages of tumorigenesis. Specific tumor-neutralizing cells, probably T cells, are detected during intermediate and late stages of tumor growth. The presence of tumor-neutralizing cells may signify a mature immune response to the tumor antigen. However, these cells may not interact with the tumor if they are unable to leave the spleen, or possibly are dampened by suppressor lymphocytes/macrophages or by noncytolytic antibody. In the MCA-F model, macrophages consistently appear to antagonize host resistance to neoplastic outgrowth. For example, depletion of adherent, phagocytic elements potentiated the neutralizing activity of spleen cells from late stage tumor bearers, which already displayed predominant tumor neutralization.

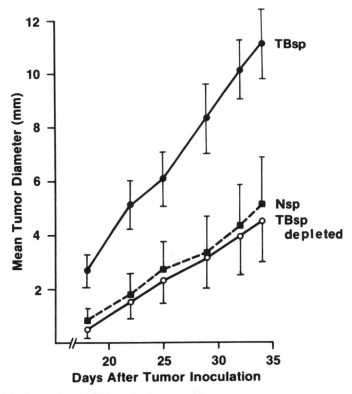

Fig.7.10 Activity of adherent spleen cells from 3-day tumor-bearing hosts. Tumor-bearer spleen cells were incubated in petri dishes for 1 hour, and the nonadherent fraction replated and incubated for an additional hour. Nonadherent tumor-bearer spleen cells (●——●), un-fractionated normal (■– – –■) and unfractionated tumor-bearer (○——○) spleen cells were admixed with 10^4 MCA-F cells (1000:1 effector:target) and injected subcutaneously into 10 syngeneic hosts.

The tumor-facilitating macrophages documented herein may represent an *in vivo* correlate of the *in vitro* suppressive activity previously reported by others. Poupon et al. (102) noted a nonspecific, adherent, non-T-cell splenic population from C3H mice bearing a MCA-induced fibrosarcoma that sup-pressed *in vitro* lymphoid cell proliferation following mitogen stimulation. Pope et al. (24) reported that the suppressive cells from DBA/2J mice bearing MCA-induced neoplastic lymphocytes were depleted from the spleen by passage through nylon wool, by treatment with carbonyl iron, or by adherence to plastic, but not by exposure to anti-Thy-1.2. Oehler et al. (25) described a population of adherent, phagocytic spleen cells, which suppressed the

Table 7.6. Effect of Irradiation Upon the Tumor-Neutralizing Activity of Spleen Cells from Nine-Day Tumor Bearers

Spleen-Cell Donor	LATA Cell Target	Tumor Diameter (mm ± SEM) at 22 Days after LATA[a]
None	MCA-F	10.2 ± 1.0
Nsp		9.5 ± 1.2
TBsp		4.7 ± 1.0[b] (p < 0.01)
TBsp-x		8.1 ± 1.2[c] (p < 0.05)
None	MCA-D	6.0 ± 0.8
Nsp		5.3 ± 0.7
TBsp		5.8 ± 0.7 (NS)
TBsp-x		6.7 ± 1.2 (NS)

[a] Three days after inoculation of 1×10^5 MCA-F cells into each of 20 C3H/HeJ mice, spleen cells were harvested. Normal and tumor-bearer spleen cells were individually mixed with 10^4 MCA-F or with 10^4 MCA-D cells and inoculated subcutaneously into groups of 10 syngeneic hosts. The average of the mean tumor diameters ± the standard error at the stipulated day after transfer are shown.
[b] Comparison with normal spleen cells.
[c] Comparison with nonirradiated tumor-bearer spleen cells.

mixed lymphocyte culture reaction that was resistant to treatment with antithymocyte serum (ATS) and complement and to treatment with radiation. Eggers et al. (22) reported that tumor-bearing mice contained nonspecific suppressor cells against alloantigens. Finally, Kirchner et al. (21) suggested that antagonists of T lymphocytes belonged to the monocyte/macrophage series. In comparison to the tumor growth promotion induced by Fr 1, the nonspecific, macrophage-mediated facilitation may be crital to the early establishment of nascent, polyclonal tumors.

Table 7.7. Effect of Anti-Θ Treatment of TBsp from Nine-Day Tumor Bearers Upon Tumor-Neutralizing Activity[a]

Spleen-Cell Donor	Treatment[a]	Mean Tumor Diameter (mm ± SEM) at 27 Days after LATA	"p"[b]
None	None	12.8 ± 1.2	—
Nsp	None	12.9 ± 1.0	—
	C'	10.0 ± 1.2	NS
	Anti-Θ + C'	11.9 ± 1.4	NS
TBsp	None	3.3 ± 1.5	< 0.001
	C'	3.2 ± 1.0	< 0.001
	Anti-Θ + C'	9.2 ± 1.8	NS

[a] Spleen cells obtained from either normal animals or from hosts 9 days after MCA-F tumor inoculation were treated in vitro with monoclonal anti-Thy-1.2 antiserum and rabbit complement prior to LATA in syngeneic normal hosts.
[b] Significance as determined by Student's t-test.

Table 7.8. Specificity and Radiosensitivity of Spleen-Cell Activity from Mice Bearing MCA-F Tumor for 30 Days[a]

LATA Target Cell	Spleen-Cell Donor	Mean Tumor Diameter (mm ± SEM) at 30 Days after LATA[a]
MCA-F	None	12.2 ± 1.4
	Nsp	11.6 ± 1.3
	Nsp-x	10.4 ± 1.2 (NS)
	TBsp	6.8 ± 0.8[b] (p < 0.002)
	TBsp-x	9.7 ± 0.9[c] (p < 0.05)
MCA-D	None	8.7 ± 1.0
	Nsp	8.7 ± 0.8
	Nsp-x	9.0 ± 0.9 (NS)
	Tbsp	12.0 ± 0.7[b] (p < 0.005)
	TBsp-x	11.5 ± 0.3[c] (NS)

[a] Three days after inoculation of 1×10^5 MCA-F cells into each of 20 C3H/HeJ mice, spleen cells were harvested. Normal and tumor-bearer spleen cells were individually mixed with 10^4 MCA-F or with 10^4 MCA-D cells and inoculated subcutaneously into groups of 10 syngeneic hosts. The average of the mean tumor diameters ± the standard error at the stipulated day after transfer are shown.

[b] Significance of difference between Nsp and TBsp.

[c] Significance of difference between TBsp and TBsp-x.

Nonspecific Suppressor Cells

In addition to antigen-specific, T-lymphocyte, suppressor cells, other immunoregulatory pathways often dampen the immune response to antigens other than those on the tumor cell. Hodes et al. (17) reported antigen indiscriminant suppression mediated by a radiosensitive (1000 rads) T-cell population. Small (8) suggested that nonspecific suppressor cells mediating

Table 7.9. Effect of Depletion of Adherent and Phagocytic Cells from Spleen-Cell Populations at 30 Days after MCA-F Inoculation

LATA Target Cell	Spleen Cell	Mean Tumor Diameter (mm ± SEM) at 27 Days after LATA[a]	"p"[b]
MCA-F	None	10.0 ± 1.1	NS
	Nsp	10.1 ± 1.1	—
	Nsp (depleted)	10.1 ± 1.2	NS
	TBsp	4.8 ± 0.9	< 0.001
	TBsp (depleted)	1.9 ± 0.0 (p < 0.005)[c]	< 0.001
MCA-D	None	8.7 ± 1.0	NS
	Nsp	8.7 ± 0.8	—
	Nsp (depleted)	9.0 ± 0.9	NS
	TBsp	12.0 ± 0.7	< 0.01
	TBsp (depleted)	7.7 ± 0.6 (p < 0.005)[c]	NS

[a] Three days after inoculation of 1×10^5 MCA-F cells into each of 20 C3H/HeJ mice, spleen cells were harvested. Normal and tumor-bearer spleen cells were individually mixed with 10^4 MCA-F or with 10^4 MCA-D cells and inoculated subcutaneously into groups of 10 syngeneic hosts. The average of the mean tumor diameters ± the standard error at the stipulated day after transfer are shown.

[b] Significance by Student's t-test comparison with Nsp.

[c] Significance of difference between TBsp and TBsp (depleted).

tumor growth facilitation may be immature cells of the T image. Other investigators found nonspecific suppressor cells to be macrophages (21–23, 26–29, 102) or B cells (18–20). Spleen cells from Moloney sarcoma virus tumor-bearing mice suppressed PHA responses. The suppressor activity of tumor-bearing spleen cells was not depleted by antitheta plus complement (20). Suppression was removed from the spleen cell population by adherence to nylon wool columns and by magnetic attraction of cells which had phagocytized carbonyl iron. Their results suggest that cells in the monocytes/macrophages series possess the capacity to inhibit DNA synthesis by T lymphocytes. The role of macrophages in this immunosuppression was confirmed by Glaser et al. (23), who demonstrated spleen cells from mice bearing primary tumors induced by the Moloney strain of murine sarcoma virus strongly inhibited the *in vitro* generation of the specific, secondary, cell-mediated cytotoxicity response of spleen cells from M-MuSV regressor mice. The suppressor cells were resistant both to treatment with antitheta serum and complement and to irradiation (2500 rads).

Nonspecific suppressor cells have also been observed with chemically-induced tumors. Eggers et al. (22) reported that spleen cells from mice bearing methylcholanthrene-induced tumors, displayed less cytotoxicity when challenged *in vitro* with alloantigens than did spleen cells from normal mice. Since the suppressor activity was removed by nylon column passage, but not by antitheta treatment, it was presumed to be due to macrophages. Poupon et al. (102) reported that antigen-nonspecific, suppressor cells detected in spleens from mice bearing methylcholanthrene-induced tumors were adherent, non-T cells bearing surface immunoglobulin. Similarly Pope et al. (24) reported that spleen cells from mice bearing methylcholanthrene-induced sarcomas or a mammary adenocarcinoma suppressed the mitogen responses of normal spleen cell and lymph node cells. While the suppressor cells were removed by passage through nylon wool or by carbonyl iron treatment, they were not affected by antitheta nor by anti-IgG serum and complement. Padarathsingh et al. (29) attributed the suppression of proliferative responses to T- and B-cell mitogens to esterase-positive adherent cells.

Recently, Jessup et al. (99–101) demonstrated that C3H/HeJ mice bearing the MCA-F fibrosarcoma fail to respond to sensitizing doses of the allergen dinitrochlorobenzene. Inability to mount a cutaneous response was related to the activation of suppressor microphages. These suppressors did not prevent the initiation (proliferative stage) of the immune response to DNCB, but rather interfered with effector cell function in the elicitation of delayed hypersensitivity.

Normal spleen cells or spleen cells from mice treated with immunomodulators contain nonspecific suppressor macrophages (25–27). Normal rat spleens contain suppressor cells which (a) inhibit proliferative and cytotoxic

responses of lymphocytes to alloantigens *in vitro*, (b) adhere to plastic, and
(c) are phagocytic (25). Suppressor activity resisted treatment with (a) anti
rat thymocyte serum and complement, (b) 2500 rads of irradiation, and (c)
mitomycin C. Suppression was apparently absent from the thymus, but
found in high concentrations in peritoneal exudates, suggesting a macrophage
origin. Baird et al. (26, 27) reported that mouse macrophages isolated from
the peritoneal exudates or spleens of normal or immunomodulator-treated
mice inhibited the proliferation of spleen cells stimulated with B- or T-cell
mitogens. Thus suboptimally activated macrophages may suppress the initiation and the performance of tumor immune responses either by direct
interaction with potentially cytotoxic lymphocytes or by elaboration of immunoregulatory substances.

Not only experimental animals but also cancer patients bear nonspecific
suppressor cells. Patients with a variety of solid tumors may have impaired
cellular immunity, as assessed by delayed cutaneous hypersensitivity reactions
to such antigens as streptokinase, streptodornase, and *Candida*. Particularly
in the presence of large total body tumor burdens, patients may display
impaired contact sensitivity to 2, 4-dinitro-4-chlorobenzene (DNCB). Con-
currently, *in vitro* lymphoproliferative responses to nonspecific mitogens
or to specific antigens may be significantly depressed. Zembala et al. (28)
described nonspecific inhibition of T-cell function by circulating suppressor
monocytes. Broder (103) analyzed the role of suppressor cells in the pathogenesis of immunodeficiency using an *in vitro* immunoglobulin biosynthesis
assay to analyze the peripheral blood lymphocytes from multiple myeloma
patients. Lymphocytes from myeloma patients depressed *in vitro* production
of polyclonal immunoglobulin. In addition, peripheral blood mononuclear
cells from greater than 50% of the myeloma patients tested suppressed
polyclonal immunoglobulin production when cocultured with normal lymphocytes. The suppressor cells were radioresistant and phagocytic, suggesting
a monocyte/macrophage cell.

Finally, nonspecific suppression has been attributed to B lymphocytes.
Gorczynski (19) and Kilburn et al. (20) reported that the depressed immune
response of Moloney sarcoma virus-infected spleens was due to the presence
of suppressor cells, which were sensitive to antimouse immunoglobulin
serum and complement, but resistant to antitheta serum and complement,
suggesting a B lymphocyte origin. There remains the possibility that antibody-
armed macrophages were the target of selection by anti-Ig and complement.

Nonspecific Immunosuppressive Humoral Factors

The immune responses of tumor-bearing hosts may also be regulated by
nonspecific, humoral immunosuppressive factors. Factors capable of inhibiting normal lymphoid responses to mitogenic stimuli were described in the

sera of tumor-bearing patients (104–107) and mice (108–110). Glasgow et al. (104) reported an immunosuppressive polypeptide in the serum of cancer patients. In a more detailed study of this peptide Nimberg et al. (105) fractionated sera from cancer patients upon DEAE-cellulose chromatography using a linear gradient of 0.005–0.3 M sodium acetate, pH 5.0, into six discrete fractions. The fraction containing albumin and γ-globulins displayed the strongest immunosuppressive activity. Similar fractions from normal sera were inactive. Fractions from cancer-bearing patients were subjected to ultrafiltration using P-10 Diaflo membranes, displaying a 10,000 MW exclusion. A dose of 0.1 to 0.3 mg/ml dialysate (presumably < 10,000 daltons) significantly suppressed lymphocyte proliferation to PHA, as well as the number of plaques of lysed SRBC produced by hemolytic antibody. The *in vivo* role of this peptide has not been elucidated; however, the observations in experimental animals suggest that it may contribute to tumor progression.

Brooks et al. (106) described an antibody-like molecule found in the sera of patients with intracranial tumors. This *antibody-like* substance suppressed lymphocyte activation either by altering the cell surface or by directly blocking a membrane receptor. Whitney and Levy (108, 109) reported the presence of an immunosuppressive factor in the sera of mice with a methylcholanthrene-induced rhabdomyosarcoma. Also Palmer et al. (110) observed a unique serum protein in mice bearing different tumors, including fibrosarcomas, mammary adenocarcinomas, lymphomas, and anaplastic carcinomas, but not in the normal fetus or in pregnant, hepatectomized, granuloma-bearing mice.

Molecular characterization of the factors isolated from serous fluids of tumor-bearing animals suggests that some may be similar to those reported in humans with neoplastic disease. Yamazaki et al. (111) found three immunosuppressive factors in the Ehrlich ascites fluid of tumor-bearing animals using Diaflo membranes: UM-10R (MW 100,000–10,000), UM-2R (MW 10,000–1,000), and UM-05R (MW 1,000–500). The fraction termed UM-2R inhibited hemolytic antibody plaque responses to SRBC most effectively when administered 1 to 2 days before immunization with SRBC. The low molecular weight fraction (UM-05R) was markedly immunosuppressive when as little as 0.5 μg was injected 1 to 2 days before administration of antigen. Similarly, ascitic and culture fluids from Ehrlich tumor cells suppressed *in vitro* lymphocyte responses to PHA and delayed the rejection of skin allografts (112). Soluble suppressor activity resisted sedimentation at 100,000 g for 1 hour and treatment with trypsin, but was sensitive to incubation at 60°C for 30 minutes. Kamo et al. (113) reported that a mastocytoma factor was resistant to ultraviolet radiation and to sedimentation at 100,000 g for 90 minutes, but was sensitive to heating at 56°C for 30 minutes. Differences in the molecular characteristics of the suppressor substances may reflect different tissue sources.

Nelson (114) has postulated that macrophages are the source of the several serum immunoregulatory factors. Also, Opitz et al. (115, 116) suggested that one immunoregulatory factor released from macrophages is thymidine, which, in excessive amounts, inhibits DNA synthesis by feedback regulation. Thymidine is probably a degradation product from the DNA of cells phagocytosed and digested by macrophages. Prostaglandins also have a wide variety of biologic activities, including immunosuppressive effects. Plescia et al. (61) reported that aspirin and indomethacin, which are prostaglandin synthesis inhibitors, block the *in vitro* immune suppression induced by the methylcholanthrene-induced tumor cells. Addition of prostaglandin E_2 to cultures also suppressed *in vitro* immune antibody formation, suggesting that either induction of synthesis or release of prostaglandins may mediate tumor-induced immunosuppression. Their role in the regulation of macrophage activity may represent a common second signal to many different stimuli. For instance, macrophage activation by lymphokines results in reverse regulation or prostaglandin E_2. Similar observations have been reported in patients with neoplastic disease. A number of the factors putatively mediating tumor-induced immunosuppression in humans are low molecular weight products such as thymidine and prostaglandins. The hyporesponsiveness of lymphocytes from patients with Hodgkins's disease is probably due to the excessive production of prostaglandin E_2 *in vitro* by glass adherent, mononuclear suppressor cells (117).

Immunosuppressive factors originating in the tumor may not only defuse local immune responses, but also may effect systemic anergy to both tumor-related and unrelated antigens. Werner et al. (59) reported that freshly harvested tumor cells release a peptide (500–2,000 MW) which inhibits protein and DNA synthesis in normal lymphocytes. Viable tumor cells or their cell-free culture supernates nonspecifically suppress the *in vitro* plaque-forming cell response to SRBC (60, 61, 118, 119). Similar suppressive factors have been identified in 3M KCl extracts prepared from various virus-induced tumors (63). Materials released from human colonic carcinomas nonspecifically suppress and induce stasis in a wide variety of proliferating cells, including stimulated lymphocytes (67, 120). Inhibition is not restricted exclusively to lymphocyte functions. Tumor cells produce substances which inhibit various macrophage functions such as migration, activation, and phagocytosis (24, 59–63, 65, 67, 118, 119, 121). Therefore, essentially two classes of humoral immunosuppressive factors have been identified in neoplastic disease: (a) those produced and exported by the tumor and (b) regulatory substances released by host lymphoid cells, including macrophages.

SUMMARY

1. Under experimental and clinical situations, solubilized tumor cell extracts evoke specific tumor growth facilitation. Our results in a murine solid tumor model suggest that tumor facilitation is induced by an acidic antigen (pI 2.0–3.6) which activates lymphoid cells to promote rather than abate tumor growth. Both facilitation and immunoprotection appear to have tumor-specific transplantation epitopes. The tumor-facilitating antigen may generate suppressor cells from the thymus-derived lymphoid series or possibly from macrophages, which produce potent antilymphoproliferative agents. In our experimental model, the tumor-facilitating cell suppressed cytotoxic activity in LATA, suggesting that the tumor-facilitating cell has the suppressor activity. The relationship of tumor-facilitating cells to classical suppressor T lymphocytes is not known.

2. Concurrent with tumor progression, specific or nonspecific suppressor cells, tumor-facilitating cells, and/or cytotoxic cells generated in tumor-bearing hosts interact with each other; the predominant activity usually is neoplastic progression. In early, middle, and late stages of tumorigenesis, the relative role of each of the cellular participants changes but the vectorial outcome is relentless growth of tumor.

3. Specific or nonspecific soluble factors produced by tumor cells or lymphoid cells (T cells or macrophages) may cause tumor facilitation by interaction with (a) the tumor cell directly and/or (b) the surface of lymphoid cell. Elucidation of the various factors, whether derived from the tumor cells or from the host, on a variety of immunologic responses may provide insight into new metabolic targets for innovative therapeutic protocols which attempt to shift the homeostatic balance to favor the host.

REFERENCES

1. Deckers, P. J., Davis, R. C., Parker, G.A., et al., *Cancer Res.* **33**:33, 1973.
2. Lamon, E. W., Skurzak, H. M., and Klein, E., *Int. J. Cancer* **10**:581, 1972.
3. Vaage, J., *Cancer Res.* **31**:1655, 1971.
4. Prehn, R. T., *Science* **176**:170, 1972.
5. Treves, A. J., Carnaud, C., Trainin, N., et al., *Eur. J. Immunol.* **4**:722, 1974.
6. Umiel, T., and Trainin, N., *Transplantation* **18**:244, 1974.
7. Small, M., and Trainin, N., *J. Immunol.* **117**:292, 1976.
8. Small, M., *J. Immunol.* **118**:1517, 1977.
9. Yamagishi, H., Pellis, N. R., Mokyr, M. B., et al., *Cancer* **45**:2929, 1980.
10. Pellis, N. R., and Kahan, B. D., *Meth. Cancer Res.* **14**:29, 1978.
11. Pellis, N. R., Mokyr, M. B., Babcock, J. R., et al., *Immunol. Commun.* **7**:431, 1978.
12. Fujimoto, S., Green, M. I., and Sehon, A. H., *J. Immunol.* **116**:791, 1976.
13. Fujimoto, S., Green, M. I., and Sehon, A. H., *J. Immunol.* **116**:800, 1976.

14. Takei, F., Levy, J. G., and Kilburn, D. G., *J. Immunol.* **116**:288, 1976.
15. Takei, F., Levy, J. G., and Kilburn, D. G., *J. Immunol.* **118**:412, 1977.
16. Yamauchi, K., Fujimoto, S., and Tada, T., *J. Immunol.* **123**:1653, 1979.
17. Hodes, R. J., Nadler, L. M., and Hathcock, K. S., *J. Immunol.* **119**:961, 1977.
18. Turk, J. L., Parker, D., and Poulter, L. W., *Immunology* **23**:493, 1972.
19. Gorczynski, R. M., *J. Immunol.* **112**:1826, 1974.
20. Kilburn, D.G., Smith, J. B., and Gorczynski, R. M., *Eur. J. Immunol.* **4**:784, 1974.
21. Kirchner, H., Chused, T. M., Herberman, R. B., et al., *J. Exp. Med.* **139**:1473, 1974.
22. Eggers, A. E., and Wunderlich, J. R., **114**:1554, 1975.
23. Glaser, M., Kirchner, H., Holden, H. T., et al., *J. Natl. Cancer Inst.* **56**:865, 1976.
24. Pope, B. L., Whitney, R. B., Levy, J. G., et al., *J. Immunol.* **116**:1342, 1976.
25. Oehler, J. R., Herberman, R. B., Campbell, D. A. J., et al., *Cell. Immunol.* **29**:238, 1977.
26. Baird, L. G., and Kaplan, A. M., *Cell. Immunol.* **28**:22, 1977.
27. Baird, L. G., and Kaplan, A. M., *Cell. Immunol.* **28**:36, 1977.
28. Zembala, M., Mytar, B., Popiela, T., et al., *Int. J. Cancer* **19**:605, 1977.
29. Padarathsingh, M. L., Dean, J. H., Jerrells, T. R., et al., *J. Natl. Cancer Inst.* **62**:1235, 1979.
30. Yamagishi, H., Pellis, N. R., Macek, C. M., et al., *Eur. J. Cancer* **16**:1417, 1980.
31. Ran, M., and Witz, I. P., *Int. J. Cancer* **9**:242, 1972.
32. Bansal, S. C., Hargreaves, R., and Sjogren, H. O., *Int. J. Cancer* **9**:97, 1972.
33. Hellström, K. E., and Hellström, I. H., *Int. J. Cancer* **23**:366, 1979.
34. Hollander, N., Isakov, N., Segal, S., et al., *Int. J. Cancer* **22**:471, 1978.
35. Isakov, N., Segal, S., Hollander, N., et al., *Int. J. Cancer* **22**:465, 1978.
36. Isakov, N., Hollander, N., Segal, S., et al., *Int. J. Cancer* **23**:410, 1979.
37. Hellström, I. H., and Hellström, K. E., *Int. J. Cancer* **4**:587, 1969.
38. Pierce, G. E., *Int. J. Cancer* **8**:22, 1971.
39. Hellström, K. E., Hellström, I. H., and Nepom, T., *Biochim. Biophys. Acta* **473**:121, 1977.
40. Baldwin, R. W., Price, M. R., and Robbins, R. A., *Nature* (New Biol) **238**:185, 1972.
41. Forbes, J. T., Nakao, Y., and Smith, R. T., *J. Exp. Med.* **141**:1181, 1975.
42. Rogers, M. J., and Law, L. W., *Int. J. Cancer* **23**:89, 1979.
43. Baldwin, R. W., and Price, M. R. In F. F. Becker (Ed.), *Cancer 1: A Comprehensive Treatise*, pp. 353. New York: Plenum Press, 1975.
44. Klein, G., Sjogren, H. O., Klein, E., et al., *Cancer Res.* **20**:1561, 1960.
45. Kahan, B.D., and Pellis, N. R., *J. Surg. Res.* **18**:263, 1975.
46. Law, L. W., and Appella, E. In F. F. Becker (Ed.), *Cancer: A Comprehensive Treatise*, pp. 135. New York: Plenum Press, 1975.
47. Meltzer, M. S., Leonard, E. J., and Rapp, H. J., *J. Natl. Cancer Inst.* **54**:1349, 1975.
48. Pellis, N. R., Tom, B. H., and Kahan, B. D., *J. Immunol.* **113**:708, 1974.
49. Pellis, N. R., Shulan, D. J., and Kahan, B. D., *Biochem. Biophys. Res. Commun.* **71**:1251, 1976.
50. Prehn, R. T., and Main, J. M., *J. Natl. Cancer Inst.* **18**:759, 1957.
51. Pasternak, L., Pasternak, G., and Karsten, U., *Cancer Immunol. Immunother.* **3**:273, 1978.
52. Pasternak, G., Milleck, J., Pasternak, L., et al., *Folia Biol.* (Praha) **26**:1, 1980.
53. Bubenik, J., Indrova, M., Nemeckova, S., et al., *J. Int. J. Cancer* **21**(3):348, 1978.
54. Coggin, J. H., *Cancer Res.* **39**:2952, 1979.
55. Simkovic, D., Chorvath, B., Duraj, J., et al., *Neoplasma* **25**:647, 1978.
56. Barra, Y., Astier, A-M., and Meyer, G., *J. Natl. Cancer Inst.* **58**:721, 1977.

57. Prager, M. D., Hollingshead, A. C., Ribble, R. J., et al., *J. Natl. Cancer Inst.* **51**:1603, 1973.
58. Paranjpe, M. S., and Boone, C. W., *Cancer Res.* **35**:1205, 1975.
59. Werner, D., Maier, G., and Lommel, R., *Eur. J. Cancer* **9**:819, 1973.
60. Wong, A. R., Mankovitz, R., and Kennedy, J. C., *Int. J. Cancer* **13**:530, 1974.
61. Plescia, O. J., Smith, A. H., and Grinwich, K., *Proc. Natl. Acad. Sci. USA* **72**:1848, 1975.
62. Delustro, F., and Argyris, B. F., *Cell. Immunol.* **21**:177, 1976.
63. Brandchaft, P. B., Aoki, T., and Silverman, T. N., *Int. J. Cancer* **17**:678, 1976.
64. Blackstock, R., Schimpff, R. D., and Smith, R. T., *Proc. Soc. Exp. Biol. Med.* **157**:354, 1978.
65. Pike, M. C., and Snyderman, R., *J. Immunol.* **117**:1243, 1976.
66. Stevens, R. H., Brooks, G. P., Osborne, J. W., et al., *J. Immunol.* **120**:335, 1978.
67. Remacle-Bonnet, M. M., Pommier, G. J., Luc, C., et al., *J. Immunol.* **121**:44, 1978.
68. Vaage, J., *Cancer Res.* **32**:193, 1972.
69. Rao, V. S., Bagai, R., and Bonavida, B., *Cancer Res.* **36**:1384, 1976.
70. Hellström, K. E., and Hellström, I. H., *Proc. Natl. Acad. Sci. USA* **75**:436, 1978.
71. Reisfeld, R.A., and Kahan, B. D., *Fed. Proc. Fed. Amer. Soc. Exp. Biol.* **29**:2034, 1970.
72. Yamagishi, H., Pellis, N. R., and Kahan, B.D., *J. Surg. Res.* **29**:295, 1979.
73. Pellis, N. R., Yamagishi, H., Macek, C. M., et al., *Int. J. Cancer* **26**:443, 1980.
74. Pellis, N. R., Yamagishi, H., Shulan, D. J., et al., *Cancer Immunol. Immunother.* **11**:53, 1981.
75. Bradford, M., *Anal. Biochem.* **72**:248, 1976.
76. Minami, A., Mizushima, Y., Takeichi, N., et al., *Int. J. Cancer* **23**:358, 1979.
77. Fidler, I., *J. Natl. Cancer Inst.* **50**:1307, 1973.
78. Jeejeebhoy, H. F., *Int. J. Cancer* **13**:665, 1974.
79. Kall, M. A., and Hellström, I., *J. Immunol.* **114**:1083, 1975.
80. Rotter, V. R., and Trainin, N., *Transplantation* **20**:68, 1975.
81. Elgert, K. D., and Farrar, W. L., *J. Immunol.* **120**:1345, 1978.
82. Green, M. I., Fujimoto, S., and Sehon, A. H., *J. Immunol.* **119**:757, 1977.
83. Nordlund, J. J., Ackles, A., and Gershon, R. K., *Cell. Immunol.* **56**:258, 1980.
84. Nordlund, J. J., Cone, R. E., Ackles, A., et al., *Cell. Immunol.* **56**:273, 1980.
85. LeGrue, S. J., Kahan, B. D., and Pellis, N. R., *J. Nat. Cancer Inst.* **65**:191, 1980.
86. Tada, T., Taniguchi, M., and Takemori, T., *Transplant. Rev.* **26**:106, 1975.
87. Taniguchi, M., Hayakawa, K., and Tada, T., *J. Immunol.* **116**:542, 1976.
88. Waksman, B. H., and Tada, T., *Cell. Immunol.* **30**:189, 1977.
89. Perry, L. L., Benacerraf, B., and Greene, M. I., *J. Immunol.* **121**:2144, 1978.
90. Thomas, D.W., Roberts, W. K., and Talmage, D. W., *J. Immunol.* **114**:1616, 1975.
91. Hellström, I.H., Hellström, K. E., and Sjogren, H. O., *Cell. Immunol.* **1**:18, 1970.
92. Witz, I. P., *Adv. Cancer Res.* **25**:95, 1977.
93. Thomson, D. M. P., *Int. J. Cancer* **15**:1016, 1976.
94. Amsbaugh, D. F., Prescott, B., and Baker, P. J., *J. Immunol.* **121**:1483, 1978.
95. Enomoto, K., and Lucas, Z. J., *Transplantation* **15**:8, 1973.
96. Kilshaw, P. J., Brent, L., and Thomas, A. V., *Transplantation* **17**:57, 1974.
97. Yamagishi, H., Kahan, B. D., and Pellis, N. R., *Fed. Proc.* **38**:1104, 1979.
98. Yamagishi, H., Pellis, N. R., and Kahan, B. D., *Surgery* **87**:655, 1980.
99. Jessup, J. M., Pellis, N. R., and Kahan, B. D., *J. Surg. Res.* **28**:460, 1980.
100. Jessup, J. M., Kahan, B. D., and Pellis, N. R., *J. Immunol.* **127**:2183, 1981.
101. Jessup, J. M., Kahan, B. D., and Pellis, N. R., *Cancer* **49**:1158, 1982.
102. Poupon, M. F., Kolb, J. P., and Lespinats, G., *J. Natl. Cancer Inst.* **57**:1241, 1976.

103. Broder, S., Disorders of Suppressor Immunoregulatory Cells in the Pathogenesis of Immunodeficiency and Autoimmunity. In T. A. Waldman (Moderator), *Ann. Intern. Med.* **88**:226, 1978.
104. Glasgow, A. H., Nimberg, R. B., Menzoian, J. O., et al., *N. Engl. J. Med.* **291**:1263, 1974.
105. Nimberg, R. B., Glasgow, A. H., Menzoian, J. O., et al., *Cancer Res.* **35**:1489, 1975.
106. Brooks, W. H., Netsky, M. G., Normansell, D. E., et al., *J. Exp. Med.* **136**:1631, 1972.
107. Sucui-Foca, N., Buda, J., McManus, J., et al., *Cancer Res.* **33**:2373, 1973.
108. Whitney, R. B., and Levy, J. G., *Eur. J. Cancer* **10**:739, 1974.
109. Whitney, R. B., and Levy, J. G., *J. Natl. Cancer Inst.* **54**:733, 1975.
110. Palmer, W. G., Orme, T. W., and Boone, C.W., *J. Natl. Cancer Inst.* **52**:279, 1974.
111. Yamazaki, H., Nitta, K., and Umezawa, H., *Gann* **64**:83, 1973.
112. Gresser, I., Vignaux, F., Maury, C., et al., *Proc. Soc. Exp. Biol. Med.* **149**:83, 1975.
113. Kamo, I., Patel, C., Kateley, J., et al., *J. Immunol.* **114**:1749, 1975.
114. Nelson, D. S., *Nature* (London) **246**:306, 1973.
115. Opitz, H. G., Neithammer, D., Lemke, H., et al., *Cell. Immunol.* **16**:379, 1975.
116. Opitz, H. G., Neithammer, D., Jackson, R. C., et al., *Cell. Immunol.* **18**:70, 1975.
117. Goodwin, J. S., Messner, R. P., Bankhurst, A. D., et al., *N. Engl. J. Med.* **297**:963, 1977.
118. Anderson, R. J., McBride, C. M., and Hersch, E. M., *Cancer Res.* **32**:988, 1972.
119. Rodey, G. E., Sprader, J. C., and Bortin, M. M., *Cancer Res.* **34**:1289, 1974.
120. Remacle-Bonnet, M. M., Pommier, G. J., Kaplanski, S., et al., *J. Immunol.* **117**:1145, 1976.
121. Bonnard, G.D., and Herberman, R. B. In A. Rosenthal (Ed.), *Immune Recognition*, p. 819. New York: Academic Press, 1975.

8

Immunotherapy of Cancer— Present Status and Future Trends

Prasanta K. Ray and Syamal Raychaudhuri

The concept of immunologic intervention in the treatment of cancer dates back to the late nineteenth (1, 2) and early twentieth centuries (3). Progress in this area, however, has been far from satisfactory. The idea of immunologic manipulation as a modality of cancer treatment developed when it was reported that some, but not all, spontaneously occurring animal and human tumors have tumor-associated antigens (TAA) (4, 5, 6) which are not normally found in the host, at least at the detectable level. Different types of antigens have been detected on tumors (consult the chapter by Gupta and Morton) which can elicit immunologic reactions in the host.

The concept that in spite of being antigenic in nature, a tumor can grow by a *sneaking-through* mechanism has not received much support because it has been reported that the immune system can mount an attack against autochthonous and syngeneic tumors (7–9), in a variety of ways (10, 11). This will be discussed in greater detail later.

The term immunotherapy means immunological manipulation of the host such that the host can mount both cellular and humoral immune responses against the tumor. This manipulation consists of various approaches including counteraction of the blocking activity existing in the tumor-bearing host. In general, tumors may thrive and survive by counteracting and/or destroying two opposing forces —immunocompetent factors and normal cells. The outcome is usually in favor of the tumor cells. The rapid turn-over and increasing mass of tumor cells are important advantages favoring a tumor growth. Another mechanism involved is the induction of blocking phenomena (cellular and humoral) by the tumor cells. A third mechanism may involve a direct attack on immunocompetent cells by releasing some factors like lymphotoxin. It is also possible that the tumor may deplete the host nutritionally and make it immunocompromised. The immunotherapeutic attempts might be more successful if adequate attention is given to the monitoring of these factors.

Surgery and radiotherapy have shown much success in the treatment of certain neoplasms, but both have their own limitations (12). Chemotherapy has also been used successfully with some tumors, but its general applicability is limited because of its nonspecificity.

It is known that tumor-bearing hosts can exhibit immune reactions against their tumors, and that the operation of this immunity depends on the tumor size, tissue location, and microenvironment in which the tumor is growing. Various attempts have been made at modifying this host immunity for therapeutic benefit. The experimental data obtained from animal research have indicated that immunotherapy is worth investigating in humans. In the following section, we will discuss various approaches of passive immunotherapy in both animal and human models.

Immunotherapeutic attempts at treating cancer are still in the experimental stage. Improper design, dosage and scheduling, and lack of knowledge regarding parameters to be studied have brought frustration or at best partial success so far. Although cure rates with conventional cancer therapies have, in general, not been too high, immunotherapy is still not widely recommended, even though in some types of cancer, it has shown some success clinically. Another pressing problem besetting the immunotherapist is that he has to deal mostly with the failures of conventional treatment modalities. Naturally, these patients have far-advanced disease and a poor immunologic profile, sometimes as a result of high-dose chemo- and radiation therapy (6, 13). The tumor load itself may also contribute to the immunosuppressed status of the patient. It is possible that immunotherapy may not find use as a treatment of choice in far-advanced cancer patients because of its limitation for handling a large tumor load. Immunotherapy, however, may find proper usage either as a treatment for very early forms of cancer, or as an adjunct for the treatment of minimal residual disease (see chapter 13). Reports from a number of laboratories on their experiences using immunotherapeutic approaches in the treatment of cancer have shown some promise, enough to encourage further investigation in the proper use of the immune system of the host to combat cancer.

In this monograph we will (a) review the different approaches of immunotherapy of cancer, both in animals and in humans; (b) try to evaluate the progress made so far; and (c) highlight the areas which are at a developmental stage and worth investigating further.

PASSIVE IMMUNOTHERAPY OF CANCER

General Considerations

Passive immunotherapy means immunological intervention in a tumor-bearing host by passive transfer of immunocompetent sera or cells. Immunocompetent cells or sera can be prepared in syngeneic, allogeneic, or heterologous systems. The cells or sera may be specific or nonspecific. It has been described that passively transferred cells or sera may react with the tumor using different mechanisms. The committed effector cell might react with tumor cells directly, causing lysis (7–9, 13). The tumor cells might also be killed by sensitized lymphocytes in the presence of cytophilic antibody with receptor sites for both tumor cells and lymphocytes (14). The lymphocytes can be made committed by *in vitro* sensitization against tumor cells in one-way mixed lymphocyte tumor-cell (MLTC) culture (15–18). Recent studies have shown that the committed lymphocytes are directed towards both H-2 antigens and TAA, and might elicit graft-vs.-host (GVH) reaction (19). It has been demonstrated that *in vitro*-sensitized lymphocytes consist mainly of T lymphocytes (6), although the role of macrophages (20) and natural killer (NK) cells (21) has not been excluded.

Immune sera may interfere with the host immune system by evoking complement-mediated cytotoxicity (22) or may initiate antibody-dependent tumor-cell lysis by lymphocytes (22). Serum factors may also help arm macrophages, or by attaching to tumor cells make them vulnerable to destruction by macrophages. The demonstration of *blocking and unblocking* sera (23) necessitates careful screening during serotherapy so that *blocking serum factors* are not transferred along with cytotoxic serum factors.

Serum Transfer in Animals

Most of the early approaches to passive immunotherapy centered around using antisera against corresponding tumor cells. The antisera were raised in syngeneic, allogeneic, and xenogeneic systems and transferred to the tumor host. The therapeutic effect was dependent on the route and time of inoculation of the tumor and sera (Table 8.1). Many of these studies have been done with serotherapy given before the tumor inoculation, which is obviously not applicable in human situations. The tumor-growth inhibitory or stimulatory effect of serotherapy seems to be dependent on various factors—relative ratio of number of specific antibodies to tumor cells, type of

Table 8.1. Passive Immunotherapy with Various Agents

Name of Author	Date	Immunotherapeutic Agent	Efect of Immunotherapy
Hericourt & Richet (24)	1895	Antisera against human tumorous material in animals	Subjective and objective improvement claimed
Gorer & Amos (25)	1956	Antisera against EL-4 Lymphoma	Little effect
Moore et al. (26)	1957	Normal human γ-globulin	No effect
McCredie et al. (27)	1959	Antiserum against autologous primary breast cancer in sheep	No effect
Sumner & Foraker (28)	1960	Whole blood from regressor melanoma patient	50% showed complete regression
Teimourian & McCune 1963	(29)	Whole blood from surgically cured melanoma patient	25% showed *almost* total regression of pulmonary metastases
Attia & Weiss (30)	1966	Antisera to spontaneous mammary cancer; methylcholanthrene-induced sarcoma	Contradictory effect
Alexander et al. (31)	1967	Lymphoid cells nucleic acids	Effectiveness depended on the route and day of inoculation
Laszlo et al. (32)	1968	Plasma raised against normal lymphocytes	Leukocyte count dropped temporarily in CLL patients
Skurkovich et al. (33)	1969	Autotransfusion of cells and remission sera from the same patient	Few positive effects in ALL patients
Herberman et al. (34)	1969	Alloantigen	Leukocyte count dropped temporarily in CLL patients
Fass (35)	1970	Plasma from Burkitt's lymphoma patient who underwent remission	No effect
Horn & Horn (36)	1971	Plasma from surgically cured renal-cell carcinoma patient	One patient remained disease-free
Hellstrom et al. (37)	1970	Sera of regressed animal or unblocking serum	Regression of established tumor
Reif & Kim (38)	1971	Antisera against L-1210 leukemia	Prolongation of survival of mice
Bansal & Sjogren (39)	1973	Unblocking serum	Total tumor regression
Negroni & Hunter (40)	1973	Syngeneic antisera and complement	Increased resistance to polyoma virus-induced tumor
Kassel et al. (41)·	1973	Complement	Spontaneous leukemia regression
Yutoku et al. (42)	1974	Antisera against BALB/C myeloma tumor	Prolongation of survival
Order et al. (43)	1974	Antisera against partially purified cell-free supernatant of ovarian cancer cells	Prolongation of survival

(Table continued on p. 214.)

Table 8.1. (*Continued*)

Name of Author	Date	Immunotherapeutic Agent	Efect of Immunotherapy
Mizejewski & Allen (44)	1974	Antisera against α-fetoprotein from hepatoma	Partial inhibition of tumor growth
Motta (45)	1974	Antisera raised against tumor in presence of antisera against normal cell component	Inhibition of growth of Gardner lymphosarcoma
Levi et al. (46)	1963	Antisera raised against Ehrlich ascites tumor and AKR-leukemia cells.	Growth inhibition
Schlager & Dray (47)	1975	Intralesional therapy with antisera to fibrin	Regression of hepatoma
Collins et al. (48)	1978	Antisera against friend leukemia virus (FLV) or Flvgp 71	Protection against FLV-induced disease and viremia
Reif et al. (49)	1977	Antisera against leukemia cells with directed specificity plus cytoxan.	Significant prolongation of life
Lozzio et al. (50)	1977	Antisera against human chronic myelogenous leukemia cell line	Suppression of growth of human myelosarcoma in nude mice
Wright et al. (51)	1975	Unblocking plasma	No effect
Albo et al. (52)	1978	Effect of plasma of patient's parent was compared with plasma of unrelated normal individual.	No effect in ALL patients
O'Neill (53)	1980	Antisera against spontaneous mouse tumor plus cytosine arabinoside	Increased mean survival of tumor-bearing mice

antibody, antigenicity of tumors, presence of other auxiliary factors (complement), presence of blocking factors in the passively transfused sera, etc. Except for a few findings, most of the results observed in animals were promising. The same kind of serotherapeutic approach was followed by many clinicians in treating human cancer, but results were not as promising.

Human Studies Involving Serum Transfer

One of the early attempts at human tumor immunotherapy occurred in 1895 when Hericourt and Richet (24) treated 50 cancer patients with antiserum produced against tumorous material. Subjective and objective improvements were observed in many of the patients. Sumner and Foraker (28) reported long-term regression of a malignant melanoma patient after transfusion with blood from a regressed melanoma patient. Laszlo et al. (32) treated chronic lymphocytic leukemia (CLL) patients with isoantibodies produced in humans against normal lymphocytes. A transient fall in the number of lymphocytes and a reduction in the size of lymph nodes were observed. Skurokvich et al. (33) took a new immunotherapeutic approach when they treated an acute leukemia patient by transfusion of his plasma and cells collected during remission. An increased duration of remission was observed when compared to historical control. Fass (35) treated Burkitt's lymphoma patients with passive transfer of plasma from a Burkitt's lymphoma patient in remission. Horn and Horn (36) treated hypernephroma patients with plasma from a surgically cured hypernephroma patient. Sumner and Foraker (28) and Teimourian and McCune (29) demonstrated that regressor sera can alter the course of growing tumors.

Wright et al. (51) compared the therapeutic benefit of conventional therapy with BCG scarification plus unblocking plasma or BCG scarification plus normal plasma. No significant difference of tumor-growth pattern was observed with the BCG scarification and unblocking plasma as compared to other therapy.

Passive immunotherapy of human cancer with serum would be more feasible if heterologous serum could be used. However, complications are usually observed, such as anaphylaxis, serum sickness, thrombocytopenia, and antilymphocytic activity. Various laboratories have engaged in raising more specific heterologous sera by a number of procedures. Some of the studies shown in Table 8.1 include those investigations.

Cell Transfer in Animals

The importance of cellular components in fighting the growth of tumors has been advocated by many researchers. There are also other reports (54, 55) demonstrating inhibition of growth of tumors after passive transfer of tumor-sensitized lymphocytes. Such information led investigators to use *in vivo* and *in vitro* tumor-sensitized lymphocytes experimentally and clinically. Much of the work suggests high cytotoxic reactivity of tumor-sensitized lymphocytes against tumor (56).

Baker et al. (19) have recently reported that during the *in vitro* sensitization of lymphocytes by tumor cells, two distinct subpopulations can be activated, one specific for alloantigens and the other for tumor-specific transplantation antigens (TSTA). It has also been reported that these two subpopulations can be separated (6,19). Even though there are differences of opinion as to whether the cells are effectors or suppressors, most available evidence indicates that these sensitized cells are predominantly T lymphocytes (56).

The other cell types which are involved in tumor-killing are NK cells (may be immature T cells), K cells, and macrophages (56, 57). These cell types may act either alone or together (38) in effective passive immunotherapy.

Table 8.2A. Passive Immunotherapy with Cells or Adoptive Immunotherapy (Animal Study)

Name of Author	Date	Immunotherapy Given	Therapeutic Effect
Woodruff et al. (58)	1963	Lymphocytes from normal and tumor-sensitized rats to mice-bearing tumor	Increased survival although many mice died due to GVH reaction
Delmore & Alexander (59)	1964	Sensitized syngeneic, allogenic, and xenogeneic lymphocytes were transferred to treat carcinogen-induced sarcoma	In many animals retardation or regression of growth was observed
Alexander et al. (31, 60, 61)	1966 1967 1971	Sensitized sheep lymphocytes were used to treat autochthonous rat sarcoma	Depending on the size of tumor, temporary reduction was observed
Bordberg et al. (62)	1972	Mice with subcutaneous tumor were treated with splenic or lymph-node lymphocytes from syngeneic mice immunized against tumor	Many animals underwent complete regression of tumor
Fass and Fefer (63)	1972	Treated mice with Friend lymphoma with cytoxan and immune lymphocytes	Prolongation of life of tumor-bearing mice
Putman (64)	1978	K36 leukemia was treated with (a) allogeneic H-2 compatible splenocyte sensitized against leukemia cells and cytoxan; (b) allogeneic H-2 incompatible cells plus cytoxan; and (c) splenocytes from allogeneic H-2 compatible mice sensitized against gross-virus-induced lymphoma	Maximum effect was using #C protocol
Rollinghoff & Wagner (65)	1973	*In vitro* sensitized lymphocytes were mixed with plasma cell tumor and transferred to mouse	Inhibition of growth was observed
Treves et al. (66)	1975	*In vitro* sensitized spleen cells against tumor were inoculated in mice having established tumor	Some effect
Cohen et al. (67, 68)	1971 1973	Treated tumor with lymphocytes sensitized to tumor antigen *in vitro*	1. Enhancement of tumor growth 2. Elicitation of autoimmune reaction
Latin & Lozzlo (69)	1974	Rauscher leukemia virus inoculated mice were treated with mouse lymphocytes stimulated with PHA	Increased survival time

Table 8.2A. (*Continued*)

Name of Author	Date	Immunotherapy Given	Therapeutic Effect
Van Loveren & DenOtter (70)	1974	Murine lymphoma (SL-2) was treated with macrophages armed and activated *in vitro*	Prolonged the life span of SL-2 lymphoma when armed and activated macrophages were mixed together and inoculated in mice
Kedar et al. (71)	1978	*In vitro* sensitized lymphocytes against tumor cells and cyclophosphamide	Prolongation of survival of leukemic mice

Since the original attempts of Ehrlich and Burnett, many others have tried to develop successful adoptive immunotherapy schemes. Some of the experimental and clinical efforts are summarized in Table 8.2A.

Human Studies Involving Cell Transfer

Many of the immunotherapeutic approaches which were tried in animals have also been used on human cancer patients with mixed effects (Table 8.2B).

Woodruff and Nolan (72) attempted to treat human advanced cancer with a high dose of spleen cells (50-480 x 10^8) from noncancer patients undergoing splenectomy. A partial positive effect was reported. Nadler and Moore (73) took a different approach. Malignant melanoma patients were immunized against another patient's tumor. Then, sensitized lymphocytes were transferred to the patient carrying the immunizing tumor. An occasional therapeutic effect was observed. Schwarzenberg et al. (74) treated leukemia patients with leukocytes from patients with chronic granulocytic leukemia. Temporary remissions were obtained in 9 of 21 patients. Andrews et al. (75) used thoracic-duct lymphocytes from a normal relative of the patient sensitized against the tumor for the treatment of acute lymphocytic leukemia and melanoma. No therapeutic effect was seen. Moore and Gerner (76) treated 28 patients with large numbers of allogeneic *in vitro*-cultured lymphocytes with no therapeutic effect. Yonemoto and Terasaki (77) treated 14 patients with lymphocytes from histocompatible donors in different ways. Eight patients were treated with whole blood or HL-A matched leukocytes from HL-A identical donor or siblings with no therapeutic effect. The rest of the patients were treated with thoracic-duct lymphocytes. Two of these patients showed an objective improvement but one of these two patients was also given chemotherapy. A very novel approach reported by Feneley et al. (78) was also described by Powels (79). Chorionepithelioma patients were treated

Table 8.2B. Passive Immunotherapy with Cells or Adoptive Immunotherapy
(Human Study)

Name of Author	Date	Immunotherapy Given	Therapeutic Effect
Woodruff & Nolan (72)	1963	Treated patients with advanced malignant disease with lymphocytes from unrelated donors	Subjective and objective improvements were observed
Nadler & Moore (73)	1969	Two patients with cancer cross immunized with tumor of each other and subsequent reciprocal transfusion of peripheral blood lymphocytes	Occasional regression was reported
Schwarzenberg et al. (74)	1966	Acute leukemia patient was treated with leukocytes from patient with chronic granulocytic leukemia	Transient remission was observed
Andrews et al. (75)	1967	Malignant melanoma patient was treated with thoracic-duct lymphocytes from normal relative immunized against patient's tumor	No effect
Moore & Gerner (76)	1970	Allogeneic and autologous lymphocytes were cultured *in vitro* and used to treat patient with advanced cancer	No therapeutic effect was observed in case of allogeneic transfusion and very temporary objective improvement was observed in 1 out of 6 patients
Yonemoto & Terasaki (77)	1972	a. Infusion of HLA-matched lymphocytes from sibling by plasmapheresis	No effect
Feneley et al. (78)	1974	b. Infusion of thoracic-duct lymphocytes from sibling	Objective response was observed in 2 out of 6 patients

with adoptive immunotherapy. Two husbands of two patients were immunized against normal tissue of each other. As this tumor has normal transplantation antigens, patients were treated with corresponding hyperimmune lymphocytes. A *transient but definite neoplastic regression* was observed.

Transfer of Immune RNA

Since the time of Gravey and Campbell (80) many attempts have been made to use immune RNA, experimentally and prophylactically, to manage immunodeficiencies in neoplastic disease. These researchers showed that an RNA fraction isolated from lymphoid tissue, as well as macrophages of immunized animals, could transfer immunity to nonimmune animals. Friedman (81) demonstrated that immunity-transfer ability of the RNA fraction can be abrogated by both RNase and antisera against the antigen used for the preparation of the sensitized RNA, suggesting the possibility of RNA-antigen complex in immune reactions. Immune RNA has the ability to synthesize specific antibody and induce blastogenic transformation of lymphocytes, migration inhibitory factor, allogeneic graft rejection, and also rejection of tumor cells.

Alexander (82) showed that the RNA fraction of sheep lymphocytes sensitized against a rat sarcoma could retard the growth of the rat sarcoma.

Pilch et al. (83) showed that xenogeneic immune RNA can kill metastatic tumor. Kern and Pilch (84) collected immune RNA from the spleens of Fisher rats bearing the MC3-R tumor. This immune RNA could potentiate killing of MC3-R tumor cells by syngeneic spleen cells *in vitro*. That immune RNA can be used immunotherapeutically in man was seen in the work of Praque and Drag (85) and Pilch et al. (83). They showed that after incubation of normal human blood lymphocytes with xenogeneic RNA fraction immunized with human tumor, the lymphocytes showed more cytotoxicity *in vitro*. Kern and Pilch (84) demonstrated the effect of immune RNA on cultured cell lines (both tumor and fibroblast).

Immunotherapy with Transfer Factor

In 1949, Lawrence (86) showed that ruptured and nonviable leukocytes could passively transfer cutaneous hypersensitivity. He also showed that a dialyzable material from cell lysate could do the same thing. Various attempts have been made to determine the nature of transfer factor. The exact nature of the molecule has not yet been well worked out, but it appears that both peptides and nucleotides are important for its activity (87).

Spitler (88) has recently shown that transfer factor can abrogate tolerizing activity and suggested that this abrogation is mediated by the ability of transfer factor to inhibit the production of a suppressor cell. The fact that certain preparations of transfer factor are active while others are not led to the question of whether there is any direct relationship between *in vitro* and *in vivo* activity (89).

Neidhart and Logublio (90), and Price et al. (91) treated osteogenic sarcoma and melanoma with transfer factor. In both cases, transfer factor was prepared from another individual who had the same tumor but was cured of disease; no effect was observed.

Spitler et al. (92) demonstrated regression of metastatic melanoma in 2 of 6 patients with minimal disease at the time of therapy. Blume et al. (93) reported the effectiveness of transfer factor as an adjunct to surgery in the treatment of stage 1 melanoma.

ACTIVE IMMUNOTHERAPY OF CANCER

General Considerations

Active immunotherapy is defined as immunization of a patient with an immunomodulating agent which will activate the patient's immune system, nonspecifically or specifically, depending on the immunomodulating agent used. Nonspecific immunomodulating agents, such as bacteria and bacterial toxin, activate the lymphoid system by the accumlation of leukocytes and their products in their vicinity. Although the leukocytes and released lymphokines are directed towards the stimulatory antigens and will react with the specific cells carrying the antigens, they will also destroy other cells in the vicinity of such a hypersensitive reaction. The immunomodulating agent might attach to the cell surface, exerting haptenic reaction (6), or might help to change the macromolecular configuration of the surface membrane (6).

Ray et al. (94) have observed that bacteria are able to adhere to the surface of tumor cells, and that this interaction may be necessary for bacteria-induced tumor-growth inhibition. The immunogen can also influence the maturation of a particular type of immunocyte (95). For example, mycobacteria can influence the formation of antibody synthesis, cytotoxic lymphocytes, and activation of macrophage function (95).

There are some immunomodulating agents which can activate NK cell activity, and also antibody-dependent cellular cytotoxicity (6). In contrast to nonspecific immunomodulation, specific active immunotherapy can be achieved by directing specificity only against tumor-associated transplantation antigen. In the following section, we will describe both nonspecific and specific active immunotherapy.

Nonspecific Active Immunotherapy with Microbes and Their Products

Microorganisms and their products have long been conceived as possible therapeutic agents in the treatment of cancer. This concept can be traced back as early as the latter part of the nineteenth century. The early history of the role of bacteria and bacterial products in the treatment of malignant disease has been exhaustively reviewed (96).

Heat-treated mixtures of streptococci and *Serratia marcescens*, also known as *Coley's toxins* (97) were used clinically for the treatment of cancer for many years, although their effectiveness was not clearly established. Parker et al. (98) reported prolongation of life span of animals carrying a rapidly growing transplanted fibrosarcoma by direct intratumor injection of spores of *Clostridium histolyticum*. They also reported marked regression of both sarcoma and carcinoma using Clostridium histolyticum toxin.

Calmette in 1936 (99) observed that BCG had paraspecific action against some secondary and heterologous infections. More recently, this nonspecific activity of BCG has been used in cancer therapy, appearing to lend support to the long-held belief of clinicians and epidemiologists that there is an antagonism between tuberculosis and cancer. Old et al. (100, 101) and Weiss et al. (102) reported that BCG acted by stimulation of the reticuloendothelial system against the growth of various transplantable tumors. Similar observations were made by Lemonde and Clode-Hyde (103) using a spontaneous murine leukemia. Weiss et al. (104) reported that MER of BCG caused growth inhibition of tumors. Zbar et al. (105) studied the action of cell-wall bacillary components in cancer immunotherapy with encouraging success. Turcotte and Quevillion (106) identified two phenotypes of BCG—one stimulating neoplastic growth and the other suppressing it.

Ray et al. (107) showed that BCG was effective in suppressing the growth of DBDN-induced fibrosarcoma in mice in a dose-dependent manner, when administered along with tumor cells. The BCG-induced antitumor activity required close contact between the BCG and the tumor.

In recent years the cellular and molecular basis of BCG-mediated tumor regression has gained much attention. The striking preponderance of macrophages at the site of tumor rejection elicited by BCG appears to indicate that macrophages are the effector cells. Furthermore, the available data suggest that the augmentation of cell-mediated immunity after treatment with BCG can be ascribed to the stimulation of T cells via the macrophages. The important question not yet resolved is whether there is any selectivity of BCG for tumor. Complications of BCG cancer therapy are more severe than those seen with BCG tuberculosis therapy. BCG administration can cause fever, hypertension, bacteremia, and, rarely, death due to hypersensitivity reaction (108). Even so, there have been some positive reports about BCG therapy in humans. Mathe et al. (109) reported prolonged remission in clinical leukemia. Morton et al. (110) observed spectacular results in cases of melanoma. Mathe et al. (111) recently emphasized the importance of active immunotherapy in cancer treatment. Mathe suggested that an agent should satisfy the following criteria to be a systemic immune adjuvant:

1. It should be well defined or well characterized.
2. It should stimulate a distinct cell population.
3. It should not stimulate suppressor cells.
4. It should not have any side effects.

Since Coley's work on the tumorilytic effect of "mixed bacterial toxins," a number of microbial products have been studied for their effects on host resistance to spontaneous tumors (112) or to allogeneic or syngeneic tumor grafts in experimental animals.

Intratumor injection of *Corynebacterium parvum* into the solid tumor mastocytoma p815 caused marked inhibition of tumor growth, increased survival time, and resulted in complete tumor regresssion in 44% of animals (113). The protective effect of intratumor *C. parvum* injection was entirely T-cell dependent; cured mice were immune to tumor-cell rechallenge. Millas et al. (114) investigated the effect of *C. granulosum* inoculation on the growth in mice of a transplantable methylcholanthrene-induced fibrosarcoma. Tumor growth was inhibited when the tumor was transplanted subcutaneously and C. granulosum was inoculated shortly after.

Other bacteria besides BCG and Corynebacteria have been tested for antitumor activity. Unfortunately, the bacteria which appear to have antitumor potential are mostly pathogenic; e.g., *Listeria monocytogenes* (115), *Brucella abortus* (116), *Streptococcus pyogenes* (117), and *Bordetella pertussis* (118).

Ray et al. (119, 120) observed that *Streptococcus faecalis* can inhibit the growth of sarcoma-180 ascites tumor cells transplanted in A/J mice. *S. faecalis* inhibited the growth of the S-180 ascites tumor when it was inoculated with the tumor after *in vitro* incubation. Immunization of animals with S. faecalis resulted in a strong antitumor response.

Ray et al. (121) showed that heat-killed and formalin-fixed *Straphylococcus aureus* Cowan I could inhibit the growth of MC-2 fibrosarcomas in C3H/Hej mice, and also 7, 12 dimethylbenz-anthracene-induced primary mammary adenocarcinomas in Sprague-Dawley rats.

The effectiveness of active nonspecific immunotherapy has also been investigated in association with chemotherapy or surgery in human patients with lung carcinoma, malignant melanoma, breast carcinoma, colorectal carcinoma, sarcoma, and head and neck cancer with mixed results.

Use of Nonspecific Immunomodulators

Immunomodulation of Host by Poly (A): Poly (U). Polyadenylic acid-polyuridylic acid [poly (A): poly (U)] is a double-stranded synthetic poly-nucleotide which can affect a variety of cellular and humoral immune functions. It can stimulate phagocytic activity of macrophages (122), stimulate primary and secondary response to an antigen, potentiate delayed-type hypersensitivity reaction and graft-vs.-host reaction, restore T-cell function and induce T-cell differentiation in athymic nude mice. Poly (A):poly (U) is not only able to enhance antibody production, but also to restore antibody production in low-responding animals.

Lacour et al. (123) investigated whether poly (A):poly (U) inoculation of new born C3H/Hej female mice could protect them from subsequent development of mammary tumors caused by mammary tumor virus.

It was suggested that poly (A):poly (U) exerted its antitumor effect by inducing the production of interferon. In another experiment, Drake et al. (124) showed that poly (A):poly (U) could inhibit growth of AKR spontaneous leukemia. It was also observed that poly (A):poly (U) could also inhibit postsurgical metastatic spread of tumor.

Wanebo et al. (125) studied the effect of intravenous inoculation of poly (A):poly (U) over a dose range. They observed that the polynucleotide elicited paradoxical immune responses. While it activated the responses of T cells to certain antigens it diminished their response to some mitogens, and also depressed the number of circulating lymphocytes.

Immunomodulation of Host with Levamisole. Levamisole is an antihelminthic drug capable of amplifying immune responses of both animals and humans. It can stimulate phagocytosis and lymphocyte function when these functions are depressed (126). However, it cannot stimulate immune function to levels greater than normal.

Levamisole has also been found to have antiviral activity. In the field of cancer immunotherapy, levamisole has been used alone and in conjunction with immunomodulators and chemotherapeutic agents (127).

Sampson (128) studied the effect of levamisole on breast cancer in rats. He observed dose-dependent tumor-growth inhibition, but only at low doses of levamisole. Higher doses had no effect.

Olkowski et al. (129) explored the effect of combined immunotherapy with levamisole and BCG on the immunocompetency of patients with squamous cell carcinoma of the cervix, head, and neck, after radiation therapy. Their findings indicated that BCG and levamisole had a negative effect on several immunological parameters as compared to a control group where no immunotherapy was given.

Wanebo et al. (130) compared levamisole with surgical adjuvant treatment of squamous cell carcinoma of the head and neck in a randomized double-blind study. Although the sample size was small, a significantly decreased recurrence rate was observed in stage II patients with oral cancer treated with levamisole.

Hortobagyi et al. (131) treated 114 patients with measurable metastatic breast cancer with fluorouracil, adriamycin, cyclophosphamide, and levamisole. Another group of 117 patients was treated with the same drugs plus BCG given by scarification. Chemoimmunotherapy with levamisole or with BCG plus levamisole prolonged remission of the responding patients.

Immunomodulation of Host with Thymosin. Thymosin (extracted from fetal calf thymus) is a hormone produced by thymic epithelia cells which influences cellular and humoral responses in both animal and human systems (132, 133). Thymosin treatment has been used to correct suppressed cell-mediated immunity in cancer patients. It has been observed that the *in vitro* effect of thymosin could be correlated with the *in vivo* effect due to therapy (133). Costanzi et al. (134) treated 10 patients with advanced metastatic disease with bovine thymosin fraction V. Thymosin increased cell-mediated immunity as judged by increased rosette formation and skin reactivity. However, an objective response was seen in only one patient. Cohen et al. (135) studied the effect of thymosin V in patients with small-cell bronchogenic carcinoma who received remission induction chemotherapy. Prolonged survival was observed in patients receiving thymosin 60 ng per square meter, as compared to the other groups.

Immunomodulation of Host with Interferon. Interferon is a substance produced by vertebrate cells in response to virus. It has been shown that interferon can inhibit the growth of oncogenic viruses both *in vitro* and *in vivo* in experimental animals. It has also been shown that interferon can inhibit the growth of transplantable tumors (136). Interferon may inhibit growth of tumor cells by interfering with their multiplication both *in vivo* and *in vitro* in cell culture (137). Various laboratories have demonstrated that tumor inhibitory activity of interferon is due to its ability to activate nonsensitized host lymphoid cells and to enhance the phagocytic activity of macrophages (137). It has been suggested that interferon might induce the production of some factor in the host which can inhibit tumor growth. It is now known that various agents including bacteria and the synthetic polymer polyinosinic-polycytidylic acid, poly (I)-poly (C), can induce the production of interferon (137).

Gresser et al. (138) treated AKR mice with spontaneous leukemia with mouse-brain interferon and showed increased survival and cure rate. Male mice responded to the interferon more than females. It was suggested that this might be explained by the greater susceptibility of female mice to leukemia. Liberman et al. (139) have shown that in C57/BL mice, which are very susceptible to X-ray-induced viral leukemia, exogenous interferon could suppress the development of lymphosarcoma. In contrast, endogenous interferon had no effect.

Salerno et al. (140) studied the effect of interferon on development of carcinogen-induced tumors in mice. It was suggested that the interferon might have inhibited the growth of tumors in mice.

Gresser and Bourali-Maury (141) reported that mouse-brain interferon protected mice from tumor growth and development of pulmonary metastases from Lewis lung tumor (3LL) implanted subcutaneously.

The earliest attempt at treating human malignancy with interferon was made by Falcoff et al. (142). They treated 18 acute leukemia patients with amnion-produced human interferon. Though the results were impressive, the therapeutic effect of the interferon could not be evaluated since there were no suitable controls.

Strander et al. (143) treated 11 malignant tumor patients with systemic intramuscular inoculation of interferon isolated from human leukocyte cultures. No definite antitumor effect was observed, but it was suggested that high-dose, long-term interferon treatment might be valuable.

Strander and Einhorn (144) described the effect of interferon on the growth pattern of osteosarcoma cell lines. They observed that inhibition of tumor growth was related to the dose of interferon used.

Horoszewicz et al. (145) demonstrated that human fibroblast interferon can inhibit the growth of human malignant cell *in vitro* and *in vivo*. Two patients with metastatic melanoma were injected with fibroblast interferon intralesionally. In one patient, after 14 treatments, no tumor was found at the tumor site. In the other patient the treated lesions decreased drastically in size, while the tumor in the control site continued to grow.

Immunomodulation with Protein A. Ray and colleagues (215, 219, 220) described for the first time that purified protein A of *Staphylococcus aureus* Cowan I, a powerful immunopotentiating agent, caused regression of primary mammary adenocarcinomas in rats. Plasma of treated animals showed increased antitumor antibody activity and also potentiated the peripheral blood mononuclear cell mediated cytotoxicity against tumor targets.

ACTIVE SPECIFIC IMMUNOTHERAPY OF CANCER

General Consideration

Active specific immunotherapy means active immunization of host with altered (either irradiated or enzyme-treated) tumor cells so as to develop immunity against tumor-specific transplantation antigens (TSTA). The tumor cells might be autochthonous, syngeneic, or allogeneic. During the early years of active immunotherapy, clinicians used autologous tumor cell suspension of macerated tumor cells or even extract of tumor cells as immunogen.

Immunotherapy with Altered Tumor Cells

Czajkowski et al. (146) treated human cancer patients by immunizing them with tumor cells coupled to globulin raised against the tumor. Of 42 cancer patients treated, 1 showed an objective response.

Hughes et al. (147) used an isolated subcellular tumor fraction therapeutically by mixing it with adjuvants. Thirteen out of 20 patients treated did not respond to the treatment. Out of the 7 improved patients, 2 showed a slight subjective response and 1 showed an objective response.

Humphrey et al. (148) treated two cancer patients by immunizing each one with crude tumor vaccine from the other and subsequently passively transferring plasma and cells from one to the other.

It was shown by Sanford (149), Currie and Bagashawe (150), Simmons et al. (151), and Ray and colleagues (152, 154, 155) that if tumor cells are treated with neuraminidase the transplantability of the tumor is decreased. Simmons et al. (211) also showed that the growth of already established tumor could be inhibited if the tumor-bearing mice were challenged with neuraminidase-treated syngeneic tumor cells. In further work Simmons et al. (153) showed that the immunopotentiating effect of neuraminidase-treated tumor cells could be augmented by the nonspecific immunomodulant BCG. The effect of bacterial neuraminidase on the immunogenicity of tumor cells has been reviewed by Ray (154).

Dore et al. (156) reported comparative effect of irradiated tumor cells either alone or with *Vibrio cholera* neuraminidase-treated tumor cells. The growth of isogeneic AKR leukemia cells survived more in the group that received irradiated tumor cells (5×10^6) s.c. on day 1, 5, 9, 13, and 17. The enzyme-treated tumor cell group served as control. It was suggested that in spite of the presence of cellular cytotoxic activity, it was blocked due to the presence of blocking antibody perhaps induced by the enzyme-treated cells.

Godrick et al. (157) investigated the development of lung metastasis in mice with methylcholanthrene-induced fibrosarcoma. The mice could be protected from developing lung metastases if syngeneic tumor cells were inoculated at the time of amputation.

Rios and Simmons (158) studied the effect of surgery and neuraminidase-treated tumor cells as active specific immunotherapy. They first surgically reduced the size of the tumor and followed this with active immunotherapy. They observed that excision of tumor in conjunction with immunotherapy was very effective in halting tumor growth. Seigler et al. (159) treated 719 patients with malignant melanoma at different Clark's level with 2.5×10^7 X-irradiated and neuraminidase-treated tumor cells along with BCG as immunostimulant and observed encouraging results. Currie et al. (160) studied the immunotherapeutic effect of irradiated tumor cells along with chemotherapy in malignant melanoma patients. Although they did not have appropriate controls for comparison, an objective response was observed in 17 of 30 patients. The objective response correlated well with the presence or absence of blocking activity of serum as demonstrated *in vitro*.

Wallace et al. (161) took a novel approach by preparing autochthonous tumor cells and lysing them with vaccinia virus. Tumor cell vaccine prepared this way had immunopotentiating effects in mice. Decreased tumor mass was observed in two out of seven patients with this treatment.

Juliard et al. (162) studied intralymphatic immunization of patients with $10-120 \times 10^6$ irradiated autochthonous or allogeneic tumor cells. Many patients developed sensitivity to recall antigens. An objective response was seen in five out of nineteen patients, and no disease progression in six out of nineteen.

In a recent report Bartlett et al. (163) showed that mixed systemic inoculation of LSTRA tumor vaccine (intraperitoneal and intravenous) could cause prolongation of lifespan of tumor-bearing host.

In another report, Bartlett and Kreider (164) demonstrated that the immunotherapeutic effect of irradiated LSTRA tumor cells could be augmented by a nonspecific stimulant like C. parvum.

Immunotherapy with Purified Tumor Antigen

Yamagishi et al. (165) observed that 3M KCl-eluted tumor antigen could be separated into tumor-enhancing and tumor-protecting fractions. After preparative isoelectrofocusing, they found the protecting factor in Fraction 15, pI 6.0, and the enhancing factor in Fraction 1, pI 2.6.

Kahan et al. (166) have used purified antigen prepared by isoelectric focusing (Fraction 15) in immunotherapy. When the minimum tumorigenic dose (MTD) of cells was given 1 day after immunotherapy, both the incidence of tumor and the rate of tumor growth were decreased.

IMMUNOTHERAPY INVOLVING SUPPRESSOR CONTROL

General Considerations

From the foregoing discussion it appears that the immunopotentiating factors utilized for augmenting the immune response of the host, and attempts at both specific and nonspecific immunotherapy, have had mixed successes. Occasional successes with minimal residual tumors have been claimed, but most of the attempts showed either partial or no response. Unfortunately, reports sometimes indicate facilitation of tumor growth following immunotherapeutic attempts. Immunotherapy, especially with active specific agents, can have disastrous results if not properly regulated. Passive transfer of cells or serum can also introduce cellular and humoral suppressor components to the host system, with deleterious effects. Thus, because of cellular and humoral suppressor components, immunotherapeutic attempts have so far had only partial success (215).

Specific and Nonspecific Tumor-Growth-Enhancing Factors

It is known that antigenic tumors can grow *in vivo* in spite of the presence of specifically sensitized lymphocytes in the host. The lymphocytes show antitumor cytotoxicity *in vitro*, but they cannot function internally because of the presence of immunosuppressive factors (167–170). In general, two types of mechanisms, cellular and humoral, are responsible for the immunosuppressive effects. Cell-mediated facilitation of tumor growth (171, 172) may be mediated by suppressor cells. These cells may be T lymphocytes (173), B lymphocytes, (174), and/or macrophages (175). The humoral factors may be both specific and nonspecific. Specific humoral factors having the ability to facilitate tumor growth are antigen (168), antibody (176), and antigen-antibody complex (177). Nonspecific humoral factors which facilitate tumor growth can be soluble substances produced by tumor cells (178) or by lymphoid cells (179). Several plasma proteins can also nonspecifically act as immunosuppressive factors in cancer patients (180).

Ex Vivo Removal of Humoral Blocking and/or Immunosuppressive Factors as a Modality of Cancer Treatment

It is believed that immune processes in tumor-bearing hosts remain mostly inactive *in vivo*, perhaps because of specific and nonspecific blocking factors discussed above. Of the three specific blocking factors, antigen-antibody complexes have been suspected of playing a role in the induction of allograft tolerance and in the maintenance of that tolerance and, also, of being a contributing factor to immunosuppression in cancer. The exact mechanism of immune-complex-induced suppression of the immune response is not fully understood. Several reports indicate that immune complexes may bind to the F_c receptors on (a) target tumor cells, masking their antigenic sites (181); (b) effector lymphocytes, abrogating their reactivities against the tumor cells (181); or (c) suppressor cells, activating their suppressor effects (182). Immune complexes have also been suspected of having the ability to inhibit natural killer cell activity (183) and antibody-dependent, cell-mediated cytotoxicity (183).

In addition to the wide-spread blocking activity of immune complexes, antibody can also facilitate tumor growth. In studies involving animal tumor models, immunologic enhancement was documented in all general classes of tumors, including sarcomas, carcinomas, lymphomas, and leukemias (184). It was also observed that the sarcomas and carcinomas can be very easily potentiated by antibody while lymphomas and leukemias are usually suppressed by antibody (185). The basis of sensitivity is not known. An interesting recent report by Rubenstein and colleagues (186) suggests that IgM, IgG, and IgG_2, in comparable amounts by weight, are individually capable of enhancing the growth of sarcoma I. These results are contradictory to an earlier hypothesis that tumor enhancement and suppression are mediated by different immunoglobulin subclasses. However, another important aspect which should be taken into consideration is that tumor-growth suppression and enhancement are dependent on the dosage of antiserum; low or intermediate doses usually enhance, while larger doses frequently suppress (186–188).

In some *in vitro* tumor models, *unblocking* or deblocking activity was first demonstrated in the sera of animals showing spontaneous regression of Moloney virus-induced sarcoma (189). Hellström *et al.* (190) have also demonstrated unblocking activity in the sera of tumor-free human cancer patients. The effect of *unblocking sera* on counteracting tumor growth may be due to either (a) its ability to deactivate the serum blocking activity or (b) its ability to mediate antibody and complement-dependent cytotoxicity.

Combination therapy involving splenectomy, BCG immunization, and-unblocking sera was utilized in a rat polyoma tumor model (191) with partial effect. It is clear that while unblocking sera can counteract the blocking effect to some extent, their clinical usage is questionable because of its limitations: (a) Purification and identification of specific tumor-associated antigen for each individual tumor is a difficult proposition. Therefore, immunization of the host with specific tumor antigen does not yet appear to be a practical possibility. (b) The optimal method of production of unblocking serum factor by immunization of the host with tumor antigen is not well standardized. However, careless use of antigen for immunization may produce enhancing factors, both humoral and cellular, instead of unblocking factors (170). (c) A large amount of unblocking factors may be needed to unblock the serum blocking activity and affect tumor growth. This has been difficult to obtain to date. Of course, if unblocking factor is always a cytotoxic antibody, then recent techniques with monoclonal antibodies might offer a cautiously optimistic solution. (d) Tumor-free individuals are not always available as a source of unblocking sera. Thus, it appears that this approach may provide therapeutic benefit only if methods are developed to (i) produce large amounts of specific unblocking sera, (ii) isolate specific tumor-associated antigen, (iii) abrogate serum-blocking activity, and (iv) elicit autogenous production of unblocking factors and suppression of blocking factors.

Various approaches have touched on some of these needs. Noonan et al. (192) investigated the role of thoracic-duct drainage in controlling the growth of tumors in mice by attempting to remove blocking factors from the lymph. While they reported some beneficial effect, a harmful effect of such an approach has also been reported (193). However, all these methods remove beneficial serum factors, immune components, enzymes, and biochemical components (194). An attempt to remove plasma blocking factors by plasmapheresis (180) also had the above limitations (194).

Steele et al. (195) observed that plasma from polyoma and carcinoma-bearing rats lost its blocking activity when adsorbed *in vitro* with protein A-containing *Staphylococcus aureus* (SA) Cowan I. An extracorporeal method of adsorbing plasma IgG using SA as the adsorbent has been described (196, 200). This method has been refined and modified by Ray and colleagues (197–204), who utilized it to adsorb plasma blocking factors in human colon cancer patients. These patients showed augmented immune reactivity, both specific and nonspecific, resulting in subjective and objective changes. Ray et al. (202, 203) also utilized their extracorporeal procedure to treat dogs with transmissible veneral tumors and observed tumor regression in these animals.

To study plasma adsorption effects on tumor growth, Ray and colleagues (199, 202, 203, 205) have developed a rat tumor model using a dimethyl-benzanthracene-induced primary mammary adenocarcinoma. A protocol has been developed which gave a maximum of 80% tumor regression (range 30 to 80%) within only 5 days of treatment (218). The regressor animals showed augmented antibody and complement-mediated cytotoxicity, as well as antibody-dependent cell-mediated cytotoxicity (205).

Thus, the removal of humoral blocking factors, particularly the blocking immune complexes, may remove the block from the effector lymphocytes, enabling them to function against tumors. Several other observations suggest that such reactions can actually be induced by plasma adsorption over SA (197–205).

Diener and Feldman (206) suggested that immune complexes may be involved in the regulatory mechanism in the body and that they can act by delivery of a signal to induce tolerance. If this is true, then removal of immune complexes by the extracorporeal method we described (197–205) may break the tolerance of the host to its tumor, allowing the autochthonous immune components to function against tumors causing tumor regression.

Gershon and colleagues (207) have suggested that tumor-antigen-antibody complexes may activate suppressor T cells, which then inhibit the antitumor activity of macrophages. Therefore, removal of immune complexes by extracorporeal adsorption may become beneficial to reduce both humoral and cellular blocking effect in a tumor host (205).

So far, Ray et al. have successfully induced tumor regression in a number of tumor models: (a) primary mammary tumor-bearing rats (199, 202, 203,

205, 218); (b) dogs with both transmissible veneral tumors (202, 203) and spontaneously occurring canine lymphosarcoma, fibrosarcoma, and rectal carcinoma (Ray et al., unpublished observation); and (c) patients with metastatic colon carcinoma (197–204), brain and kidney tumors (Ray et al. unpublished observation). These observations have been confirmed by Terman et al. (208) and Holohan et al. (209) in dogs with spontaneously occurring breast tumors. These authors later used a protein A-collodion charcoal for plasma perfusion and simultaneous cytosine arabinoside infusion to show tumor necrolytic reactions in spontaneous dog tumors (210) and in human breast tumors (211). Jones and colleagues (212) have described reversal of feline leukemia following plasma adsorption over SA and radiation treatment. However, the role of removal of blocking factors in these studies (208–211) is not entirely clear for lack of proper controls.

Immunotherapy by Controlling the Suppressor Cell Function

One of the major advances in the field of tumor immunology during the past few years has been the tremendous increase in knowledge regarding the role of suppressor cells on tumor growth (171, 172). Suppressor cells have been found in both tumor-bearing animals and humans and have been described to be T cells, B cells, and macrophages or monocytes (173–175). Suppressor cells have been observed to have the ability to act as permitters and promoters of malignancy. A detailed review of work in this area has been published by David Naor (213). It is now becoming clear that suppressor cells can block the immune activity of both the arcs of the immune system. Thus, selective abrogation of suppressor cell activity should be beneficial in cancer therapy. Ray and Raychaudhuri (214) have described that an immunostimulatory dose of cyclophosphamide, which provided anti-suppressor cell activity, caused regression of methylcholanthrene fibrosarcomas in mice.

A number of drugs have been reported to have the ability to kill suppressor cells or abrogate their effects. These are shown in Table 8.3. It appears that various approaches can lead to abrogation of suppressor cell activity. These include irradiation, thymectomy, splenectomy, treatment with hydrocortisone, cyclophosphamide, antithymocyte serum, anti-I-J-serum, and indomethacin. However, these approaches must be used cautiously, since complete loss of suppressor cells may lead to an autoimmune response. A number of questions about suppressor cells still remain unanswered: (a) how these cells are induced, (b) how they act, (c) whether they always release immunosuppressive factors, (d) where their specificity lies, and (e) how the target cell is recognized. As soon as these questions are answered, a more definitive approach to control the suppressor cell activity will be available and should provide a major leap forward in the area of suppressor control as a modaity of cancer treatment (215). In a recent publication

Table 8.3. Sensitivity of Suppressor Cells from Tumor Bearing Host to Various Agents

Tumor Type	Host	Type of Suppressor Cell	Sensitive to	References
3 LL spontaneous tumor	C57 BL/6 mice	T cell	HC BUdR X-irradiation	Treves et al. (221) Carnaud et al. (222) Treves et al. (223) Rotter and Trainin (224) Small (225)
MSV-induced tumor	C57 BL/6 mice	Macrophage	BUdR	Kirchner et al. (226, 227)
Friend Leukemia	Balb/C	T cell	HC	Kumar and Bennett (228)
ALL	Man	T cell	X-irradiation	Broder et al. (229)
MCA-induced sarcoma	A/J mice	T cell	ATS treatment	Fujimoto et al. (230, 231)
DMBA-induced mammary tumor	Fisher rat	Not known	HC	Kumar et al. (232)
B-16 melanoma	C57 BL/6 mice	Not known	X-irradiation	Stelzer and Wallace (233)
SV-40 transformed fibroblasts	Balb/C mice	Not known	HC	Blasecki and Tevethia (234)
Murine tumor	C57 BL/6	Not known	Cimetidine	Gifford et al. (235)
Cancer of stomach, lung	Man	Nylon wool nonadherent cell	OK-432	Uchida and Hoshino (236)
KMT-17 tumor	WKA rats	T cell	Busulfan	Mizushima et al. (237)
Methylcholanthrene induced tumor	Mice	Not known	Indomethacin	Fulton and Levy (238)
Tumor bearing mice and cancer patients	Mice and patients	T cell	Thymosin	Serrou et al. (239)
P 815	DBA/2 mice	T cell	Radiation	Tilkin et al. (240)
Methylcholanthrene fibrosarcoma	C3H/Hej mice	Not known	Cyclophosphamide	Ray and Raychaudhuri (214)
S1509a methylcholanthrene induced fibrosarcoma	A/J $(H-2^a, I-J^k)$	T cell	Monoclonal anti-I-J antibody	Drebin et al. (241)

Drebin, Benaceraff and colleagues (216) have described that intravenous administration of monoclonal anti-suppressor cell antibody (anti-I-J antibodies) inhibits tumor growth in syngeneic and semisyngeneic hosts.

Immunotherapy by Controlling Both the Arcs of the Suppressor Mechanism (Humoral and Cellular)

From the foregoing discussion it appears quite logical that Ray's concept of controlling both the arcs of suppressor mechanisms (215) should provide an impressive inhibition of tumor growth. Ray and Raychaudhuri (214) have described that a relatively low dose of Cyclophosphamide which augments the host immunity, can inhibit the growth of methylcholanthrene fibrosarcomas. The effect was ascribed to the ability of cyclophosphamide to destroy the suppressor cells. Ray and colleagues (217) have observed in rats with dimethylbenz-anthracene-induced mammary adenocarcinomas that plasma adsorption with SA to remove the soluble blocking factors and low dose cyclophosphamide infusion to destroy the suppressor cells can result in appreciable tumor regression. Cyclophosphamide treatment alone did not result in any tumor regression, while animals receiving plasma adsorption therapy alone showed some moderate tumor regression. In dogs with spontaneously occurring lymphosarcoma, plasma adsorption therapy and low dose hydrocortisone treatment resulted in significant tumor remission (Ray et al. unpublished observation), whereas the same tumor showed progressive growth when it was treated with hydrocortisone alone.

Thus, Ray's hypothesis (215) of 'suppressor control as a modality of cancer treatment' may prove to be a valuable tool in the management of cancer, particularly for minimal residual disease following reduction of the primary tumor volume by conventional means.

It should be mentioned that the data discussed above are preliminary. Extensive investigations are required to understand various parameters associated with this type (215) of treatment. Continuing research in this area is needed to develop a concerted strategy for the control of malignancy, involving a pharmacoimmunologic approach which will decrease the blocking effect (humoral and cellular) on one hand, and provide specific immune augmentation on the other (215).

SUMMARY

Immunologic approach in cancer prevention and control shows much promise today, after several years of frustrating trial and error. While knowledge has been gathered about a variety of means to augment both specific and nonspecific immune reactivity in a tumor host, it has become apparent that hypersensitization may become deleterious and can actually facilitate tumor growth. Such a facilitation can be due to the generation of suppressor factors. Thus, overenthusiasm in the area of immunotherapy of cancer, after the first few years of its prospective beginning, led to a frustrating silence for a considerable period of time.

During the past few years new techniques for the isolation and purification of tumor-associated antigens have been developed; technology for producing large amounts of monoclonal antibodies is now known; the role of suppressor cells in tumor-bearing hosts has been recognized; and a new concept in immunotherapy involving the control of suppressor mechanisms (215) is evolving. All these show much promise for the future in developing successful immunotherapy regimens. However, it may be that the best use of immunotherapy will be in treating early cancer, minimal residual tumors, and in the prevention of metastases or recurrence, when the major portion of primary tumor has been taken care of by conventional modalities of treatment (215).

REFERENCES

1   Coley, W. B., *Ann. Surg.* **14**:199, 1891.
2. Coley, W. B., *Med. Res.* **43**:60, 1893.
3. Coca, A. F., and Gilman, P. K., *Phillip J. Sci.* (Med. Sci) **4**:391, 1909.
4. Weiss, D. W., *Immunotherapy of Cancer*. W. D. Terry and D. Windhorst (Eds.), p. 101. New York: Raven Press, 1978.
5. Herberman, R. B., *Mechanisms of tumor immunity* I. Green, S. Cohen, and R. T. McCluskey (Eds.), p. 175. New York: Wiley, 1977.
6. Weiss, D. W., *Current topics in microbiology and immunology*, p. 21. Berlin and Heidelberg: Springer-Verlag, 1980.
7. Hellström, I., Warner, G. A., Hellström, K. E., et al., *Int. J. Cancer* **11**:280, 1973.
8. Herberman, R. B., *Adv. Cancer Res.* **19**:207, 1974.
9. Raychaudhuri, S., Ray, P. K., Bassett, J. G., and Cooper, D. R., *Fed. Proc.* **39**(3):696, 1980.
10. Benjamini, E., Theilen, G. H., Torten, M., Fong, S., et al., *Ann. NY Acad. Sci.* **277**:305, 1976.
11. Kamo, I., and Friedman, H., *Adv. Cancer Res.* **25**:271, 1977.
12. Woodruff, M. F. A., *Transplantation Proc.* **11**(1):1077, 1979.
13. Whitney, R. B., Levy, J. G., and Smith, A. G., *J. Natl. Cancer Inst.* **53**:111, 1974.
14. Berkin, A., *New York State Journal of Med.* 849, 1979.
15. Globerson, A., *Curr. Topp. Microbiol. Immunol.* **75**:1, 1976.
16. Kedar, E., Raanan, Z., Kafka, I., et al, *J. Immunol. Methods* **28**:303, 1979.
17. Mokyr, M. B., Braun, D. P., Usher, D., et al, *Cancer Immunol. Immunother.* **4**:143, 1978.
18. Vose, B. M., Vanky, F., Foopp, M., and Dlein, E., *Int. J. Cancer* **20**:895, 1978.
19. Baker, P. E., Gills, S., and Smith, K. A., *J. Exp. Med.* **149**:275, 1979.
20. Wagner, H., Feldman, M., Boyle, W., and Schrader, J. W., *J. Exp. Med.* **136**:331, 1972.
21. Gerson, J. M., Viresio, L., and Herberman, R. B., *Int. J. Cancer* **27**:243, 1981.
22. Rosenberg, S. A., and Terry, W. D., *Adv. Cancer Res.* **25**:323, 1977.
23. Hellström, K. E., and Hellström, I., *Adv. Cancer Res.* **12**:167, 1969.
24. Hericourt, J., and Richet, C., *c.r. hebd. Scand. Acad. Sci.*, (Paris) **121**:567, 1895.
25. Gorer, P. A., and Amos, D. B., *Cancer Res.* **16**:338, 1956.
26. Moore, G., Scandberg, A., and Amos, D. B., *Surgery* **41**:972, 1957.
27. McCredie, J. A., Brown, E. R., and Cole, W. H., *Proc. Soc. Exp. Biol. Med.* **100**:31, 1959.
28. Sumner, W. C., and Foraker, A. G., *Cancer* **13**:179, 1960.
29. Teimourian, B., and McCune, W. S., *Am. Sur.* **29**:515, 1969.
30. Attlia, M. A. M., and Weiss, D. W., *Cancer Res.* **26**:1787, 1966.
31. Alexander, P., Delorme, E. J., Hamilton, L. D. G., and Hall, J. G., *Nature* (London) **213**:569, 1967.
32. Laszlo, J., Buckley, C. E., and Amos, D. B., *Blood* **31**:104, 1968.
33. Skurkovich, S. V., Makhonova, F. M., Reznchenko, F. M., et al., *Blood* **33**:186, 1969.
34. Herberman, R., Rogentine, G. N., Oren, M. E., *Clin. Res.* **17**:328, 1969.
35. Fass, L., *J. Natl. Cancer Inst.* **44**:145, 1970.

36. Horn, L., Horn, H. L., *Lancet* **2**:466, 1971.
37. Hellström, I., and Hellström, K. E., *Int. J. Cancer* **5**:195, 1970.
38. Reif, A. E., and Kim, C. H., *Cancer Res.* **31**:1606, 1971.
39. Bansal, S. C., and Sjogren, H. O., *Int. J. Cancer* **11**:162, 1973.
40. Negroni, G., and Hunter, E., *J. Natl. Cancer Inst.* **51**:265, 1973.
41. Kassel, R. L., Old, L. J., Carswell, E. A., et al., *J. Exp. Med.* **138**:925, 1973.
42. Yotoku, M., Grossberg, A. L., and Pressman, D., *J. Natl. Cancer Inst.* **53**:201, 1974.
43. Order, S. E., Kirkman, R., and Knapp, R., *Cancer* **34**:175, 1974.
44. Mizejewski, G. J., and Allen, R. P., *Nature* (London) **250**:50, 1974.
45. Motta, R. *Adv. Cancer Res.* **14**:161, 1974.
46. Levi, E., *Nature* (London) **199**:501, 1963.
47. Schlager, S. I., and Dray, S., *Proc. Natl. Acad. Sci. USA* **72**:3680, 1975.
48. Collins, J. J., Sanfillippo, F., Tsony Chou, L., et al., *Therapy* **21**:51, 1978.
49. Reif, A. E., Li, R. W., and Robinson, C. M., *Cancer Treatment Reports* **61**:1499, 1977.
50. Lozzio, B. B., Machado, E. A., Lair, S. V., and Lozzio, C. B., *Cancer Treatment Reports* **61**:1679, 1977.
51. Wright, P. W., Hellström, K. E., Hellström, I., et al., *Med. Clinics of North America* **60**:607, 1976.
52. Albo, V., Krivit, W., and Hartmann, J., *Proc. Am. Assoc. Cancer Res.* **9**:104, 1978.
53. O'Neill, G. J., *Br. J. Cancer* **41**:839, 1980.
54. Old, L. J., Boyse, E. A., Clarke, D. A., and Carswell, E. A., *Ann. Acad. Sci.* **101**:80, 1962.
55. Law, L. W., *Transplant Proc.* **2**:117, 1970.
56. Herberman, R. B., and Holden, H. T., *Adv. Cancer Res.* **27**:305, 1978.
57. Gershon, J. M., Holden, H. T., and Herberman, R. B., *J. Natl. Cancer Inst.* **65**:905, 1980.
58. Woodruff, M. F. A., and Nolan, B., *Lancet* **2**:426, 1963.
59. Delmore, E. J., and Alexander, P., *Lancet* **2**:117, 1964.
60. Alexander, P., Connell, D. I., and Mikulska, Z., *Cancer Res.* **26**:1508, 1966.
61. Alexander, P., and Delmore, E. J., *Isr. J. Med. Sci.* **7**:239, 1971.
62. Bordberg, H., Oettgen, H. F., Choudy, K., and Beattie, E. J., Jr., *Int. J. Cancer* **10**:539, 1972.
63. Fass, L., and Fefer, A., *Cancer Res.* **32**:2427, 1972.
64. Putman, D. L., Kind, P. D., Goldin, A., and Kenda, M., *Int. J. Cancer* **23**:230, 1978.
65. Rollinghoff, M., and Wagner, H., *J. Natl. Cancer Inst.* **51**:1317, 1973.
66. Treves, A. J., Cohen, I. R., and Feldman, M., *J. Natl. Cancer Inst.* **54**:777, 1975.
67. Cohen, R. R., Crloberson, A., and Feldman, M., *Transplant. Proc.* **3**:891, 1971.
68. Cohen, I. R., *Cell Immunol.* **8**:209, 1973.
69. Lain, S. V., and Lozzio, B. B., *J. Natl. Cancer Inst.* **53**:1165, 1974.
70. Van Loveren, H., and Denotter, W., *J. Natl. Cancer Inst.* **52**:1917, 1974.
71. Kedar, E., Raanan, Z., and Schwartzbach, M., *Cancer Immunol. Immunother.* **4**:161, 1978.
72. Woodruff, M. F. A., and Nolan, B., *Lancet* **11**:426, 1963.
73. Nadler, S. H., and Moore, G. E., *Arch. Surg.* **99**:376, 1969.
74. Schwarzenberg, L., Mathe, G., Chneider, M., et al., *Lancet* **2**:365, 1966.
75. Andrews, G. A., Congdon, C. C., Edwards, C. L., et al., *Cancer Res.* **27**:2535, 1967.
76. Moore, A. E., and Gerner, R. E., *Ann. Surg.* **172**:733, 1970.
77. Yonemoto, R. H., and Terasaki, P. I., *Cancer* **30**:1438, 1972.
78. Feneley, R. C. I., Eckert, H., Ridell, A. G., et al., *Br. J. Surg.* **61**:825, 1974.
79. Powels, R. L., *Pharmac. Ther.* **4**:281, 1979.
80. Gravey, J. S., and Campbell, B. H., *J. Exp. Med.* **105**:361, 1957.
81. Friedman, H., *Ann. N.Y. Acad. Sci.* **332**:187, 1979.

82. Alexander, P., *Cancer Res.* **27**:2521, 1967.
83. Pilch, Y. H., Meyers, G. H., Jr., Sparks, F. C., et al., *Curr. Probl. Surg.* **1**:1, 1975.
84. Kern, D. H., and Pilch, Y. H., *Ann. N.Y. Acad. Sci.***332**:196, 1979.
85. Praque, R. E., and Drag, S., *Cell. Immunol.* **5**:30, 1972.
86. Lawrence, H. S., *Proc. Soc. Exp. Biol. Med.* **71**:516, 1949.
87. Peterson, E. A., and Kirkpatric, C. H., *Ann. N.Y. Acad. Sci.* **332**:216, 1979.
88. Spliter, L. E., *Ann. N.Y. Acad. Sci.* **332**:228, 1979.
89. Sutcliffe, S. B., Maziarz, G., and Gottlieb, A. A., *Ann. N.Y. Acad. Sci.* **332**:184, 1979.
90. Neidhart, J. A., and Lo Gublio, A. F., *Seminars in Oncology* **1**:379, 1974.
91. Price, B., Hewlett, J. S., Deodhar, S. D., and Barna, B., *Cleveland Clin Q* **41**:1, 1974.
92. Spitler, L. E., Wybran, J., Fudenberg, H. H., and Levin, A. S., *Clin. Res.* **21**:22, 1973.
93. Blume, M. R., Rosenbaum, E. H., Cohen, R. J., et al., *Cancer* **47**:882, 1981.
94. Ray, P. K., Raychaudhuri, S., and Chakravortry, N., *Ind. J. Exp. Biol.* **18**:783, 1980.
95. Weiss, B., and Sachs, L., *Proc. Natl. Acad. Sci. USA* **75**:1374, 1978.
96. Nauts, H. C., Swift, W. E., and Coley, B. L., *Cancer Research* **6**:205, 1946.
97. Nauts, H. C., Fowler, G. A., and Bogatko, F. H., *Acta Med. Scand.* (Suppl. 276), **145**:1, 1953.
98. Parker, R. C., Plummer, H. C., Siebermann, C. O., and Chapman, M. G., *Proc. Soc. Exper. Biol. Med.* **66**:461, 1947.
99. Calmette, A., In Massor and Co., *L'infection bacillaire et la tubcreulose chez I' home et chez les animaux*, p. 752, 1936.
100. Old, L. J., Clarke, D. A., and Benacerraf, B., *Nature* **184**:291, 1959.
101. Old, L. J., Benacerraf, B., Clarke, D. A., et al., *Cancer Research* **21**:1281, 1961.
102. Weiss, D. W., Rose, S., Bonhag, R. S., et al., *Nature* **190**:889, 1961.
103. Lemonde, P., and Clode-Hyde, M., *Proc. Soc. Exp. Biol. Med.* **3**:739, 1962.
104. Weiss, D. N., Bonhag, R., and Leslie, P., *J. Exp. Med.* **124**:1039, 1966.
105. Zbar, B., Rapp, H. R., and Ribi, E., *J. Natl. Cancer Inst.* **48**:831, 1972.
106. Turcotte, R., and Quevillion, M., *J. Natl. Cancer Inst.* **52**:215, 1974.
107. Ray, P. K., Poduval, T. B., and Sundaram, K., *J. Natl. Cancer Inst.* **58**:763, 1977.
108. McKhann, C. F., and Gunnarson, A., *Cancer* **34**:1521, 1974.
109. Mathe, G., Amiel, J. L., and Schwarzenberg, L., *Lancet* **1**:697, 1969.
110. Morton, D. L., Eilber, F. R., and Malmgren, R. A., *Surgery* **68**:158, 1978.
111. Mathe, G., Florentin, I., Olsson, L., et al., *Prog. Exp. Tumor Res.* **25**:242, 1980.
112. Lemonde, P., *Natl. Cancer Inst.* **39**:21,1973.
113. Scott, M. T., *J. Natl. Cancer Inst.* **53**:861, 1974.
114. Millas, L., Hunter, N., Basie, I., Mason, K., et al., *J. Natl. Cancer Inst.* **54**:895, 1975.
115. Blast, R. Cl Jr., Zbar, B., Mackaness, C. B., and Spo, H. J., *J. Natl. Cancer Inst.* **54**:749, 1975.
116. Tatiana, K., Veskova Korneyly, L., et al., *J. Natl. Cancer Inst.* **52**:1651, 1974.
117. Ikuro, K., Taisuke, O., Shozoyasuhara, et al., *Cancer* **37**:2201, 1976.
118. Purvell, D. M., Kreider, J. W., and Baitlett, G. L., *J. Natl. Cancer Inst.* **55**:123, 1975.
119. Ray, P. K., and Raychaudhuri, S., *Ind. J. Exp. Biol.* **16**:1198, 1978.
120. Ray, P. K., Raychaudhuri, S., and Chakabarty, N., *Ind. J. Exp. Biol.* **18**:337, 1980.
121. Ray, P. K., Cooper, D. R., Bassett, J. G., and Mark, R., *Fed. Proc. Fed. Am. Soc. Exp. Biol.* **38**(3):4558, 1979.
122. Braun, W., *Regulatory factors in the immune response: Analysis and perspective in cyclic AMP cell growth and the immune response* W. Braun, L. M. Lichtenstein, and C. W. Parker, (Eds.), pp. 4–23. New York: Springer-Verlag, 1979.
123. Lacour, F., Delage, G., and Chianale, C., *Science* **187**:256, 1975.
124. Darke, W. P., Cimino, E. F., Mardiney, M. R., Jr., and Sutherland, J. C., *J. Natl.*

Cancer Inst. **52**:941, 1969.
125. Wanebo, H. J., Kemeny, M., Pinsky, C. M., et al., *J. Immunol.* **277**:288, 1976.
126. Vershaegen,H., Decree, J., DeCock, W., et al., Levamisole and the immune response. *New Eng. J. Med.* **289**:1148, 1973.
127. Amery, W. K., Spreafico, F., Rojas, A. F., et al., *Cancer Treat. Rep.* **4**:167, 1977.
128. Sampson, D., *Cancer Treat. Rep.* **62**:1627, 1978.
129. Olkowski, Z. L., McLaren, J. R., and Skeen, M. J., *Cancer Treat. Rep.* **62**:1651, 1977.
130. Wanebo, H. J., Hilal, E. Y., Pinsky, C. M., et al., *Cancer Treat. Rep.* **62**:1663, 1978.
131. Hortobagyi, C. N., Yap, H. Y., Blumenschein, G. R., et al., *Cancer Treat. Rep.* **62**:1685, 1978.
132. Schafer, L. A., Goldstein, A. L., Gutterman, J. U., et al., *Ann. N.Y. Acad. Sci.* **277**:609, 1976.
133. Saki, H., Costanzi, J. J., Loukas, D. F., et al., *Cancer* **36**:974, 1975.
134. Costanzi, J. J., Gagliano, R. G., Delaney, F., et al., *Cancer* **40**:14, 1977.
135. Cohen, M. H., Chretien, P. B., Ihde, D. C., et al., *JAMA* **241**:1813, 1979.
136. Gresser, I., Berman, I., Dethe, G., et al., *J. Natl. Cancer Inst.* **41**:505, 1968.
137. Gresser, I., *Adv. Cancer. Res.* **16**:97, 1972.
138. Gresser, I., and Bourali, C., *J. Natl. Cancer Inst.* **45**:365, 1970.
139. Lieberman, M., Merigan, T. C., and Kaplan, H. S., *Proc. Soc. Exp. Biol. Med.* **138**:575, 1971.
140. Salerno, R. A., Whitmire, C. E., and Garcia, I. M., *Nature* (New Biol.) **239**:31, 1972.
141. Gresser, I., and Bourali-Maury, C., *Nature* (New Biol.) **236**:78, 1972.
142. Falcoff, E., Falcoff, R., Fournier, F., et al., *Ann. Inst. Pasteur* (Paris) **3**:562, 1966.
143. Strander, H., Cantell, K., Carlstrom, G., et al., *J. Natl. Cancer Inst.* **51**:733, 1973.
144. Strander, H., and Einhorn, S., *Int. J. Cancer* **19**:468, 1977.
145. Horoszewicz, J. S., Leong, S. C., and Ito, M., *Cancer Treat. Rep.* **62**:1899, 1978.
146. Czajkowski, N. P., Rosenblatt, M., Wolf, P. K., and Vasquez, J., *Lancet* **2**:905, 1967.
147. Hughes, L. F., Kearney, R., and Tully, M., *Cancer* **26**:269, 1970.
148. Humphrey, L. J., Jewell, W. R., Murray, R., and Frieffen, W. A., *Ann. Surg.* **173**:47, 1971.
149. Sanford, B. H., *Transplantation* **5**:1273, 1967.
150. Currie, G. A., and Bagshawe, K. D., *Br. J. Cancer* **22**:843, 1968.
151. Simmons, R. L., Rios, A., Lundgren, G., and Ray, P. K., *Surgery* **70**:38, 1971.
152. Ray, P. K., Thakur, V. S., and Sundaram, K., *J. Natl. Cancer Inst.* **56**(1), 83, 1976.
153. Simmons, R. L., and Rios, A., *Science* **174**:591, 1971.
154. Ray, P. K., *Adv. Appl. Microbiol.* **21**:227, 1977.
155. Ray, P. K., and Seshadri, M., *Indian J. Exp. Biol.* **17**(1):36, 1979.
156. Dore, J. F., Hadjlyannakis, M. J., Goudert, A., et al., *Lancet* **1**:600, 1973.
157. Godrick, E. A., Michaelson, J. S., Vanwijck, R., and Wilson, R. E., *Ann. Surg.* **176**(A):544, 1972.
158. Rios. A., and Simmons, R. L., *Int. J. Cancer* **13**:71, 1974.
159. Seigler, H. E., Cox, I., Mutzner, P., et al., *Ann. Surg.* **190**(3):366, 1979.
160. Currie, G. A., and Mcelwain, T. J., *Br. J. Cancer* **31**:143, 1975.
161. Wallace, M. K., Steplewski, Z., Koprowski, H., et al., *Cancer* **39**:560, 1977.
162. Juliard, G. G. L., Boyer, P. J. J., and Yamashiro, C. H. Y., *Cancer* **41**:2215, 1978.
163. Bartlett, G. L., Kreider, J. W., Purnell, D. M., et al., *Int. J. Cancer* **24**:629, 1979.
164. Bartlett, G. L., and Kreider, J. W., *Int. J. Cancer* **24**:636, 1979.
165. Yamagishi, H., Pellis, N. R., and Kahan, B. D., *J. Surg. Res.* **26**:392, 1979.
166. Kahan, B. D., Tanaka, T., and Pellis, N. R., *J. Natl. Cancer Inst.* **65**:1001, 1980.
167. Hellström, I., and Hellström, E. K., *Int. J. Cancer* **4**:587, 1969.
168. Alexander, P., *Cancer Res.* **34**:2077, 1974.
169. Kirchner, H., Chused, T. M., Herberman, R. B., et al., *J. Exp. Med.* **139**:1473, 1974.

170. Raychaudhuri, S., Ray, P. K., Bassett, J. G., and Cooper, D. R., *Fed. Proc.* **39**(3):696, 1980.
171. Prehn, R. T., *Science* **176**:170, 1972.
172. Yamagishi, H., Pellis, N. R., Mokyr, M. B., and Kahan, B. D., *Cancer* **45**:2929, 1980.
173. Yamauchi, K., Fujimoto, S., and Tada, T., *J. Immunol.* **123**:1653, 1979.
174. Kilburn, D. G., Smith, J. B., and Gorxzynski, R. M., *Eur. J. Immunol.* **4**:784, 1974.
175. Gelaser, M., Kirchner, H., Holden, H. T., and Herberman, R. B., *J. Natl. Cancer Inst.* **56**:865, 1976.
176. Hellström, K. E., Hellström, I., and Nepom, T., *Biochim. Biophys. Acta* **473**:121, 1977.
177. Baldwin, R. W., Price, M. R., and Robbins, R. A., *Nature* **238**:185, 1972.
178. Hellström, K. E., and Hellström, I., *Int. J. Cancer* **23**:366, 1979.
179. Isakov, N., Hollander, N., Segal, S., and Feldman, M., *Int. J. Cancer* **23**:410, 1979.
180. Israel, L., Edelstein, R., and Mannoni, P., *Cancer* **40**:3146, 1977.
181. Kerbel, R. S., and Daires, A. J. S., *Cell* **3**:105, 1974.
182. Gershon, R. K., Mokyr, M. B., and Mitchell, M. S., *Nature* **250**:594, 1974.
183. Cowan, F. M., Klein, D. L., Armstrong, G. R., and Pearson, J. W., *Biomed.* **30**:23, 1979.
184. Moller, G., *Nature* **204**:846, 1964.
185. Moller, G., *J. Natl. Cancer Inst.* **30**:1177, 1963.
186. Rubenstein, P., Decary, F., and Streun, E. W., *J. Exp. Med.* **140**:591, 1974.
187. Rosenberg, S. A., and Terry, W. D., *Adv. Cancer Res.* **25**:323, 1977.
188. Bansal, S. C., and Sjogren, H., *Nature* **233**:76, 1971.
189. Hellström, I., and Hellström, K. E., *Int. J. Cancer* **5**:195, 1970.
190. Hellström, I., Hellström, K. E., Sjogren, H. O., and Warner, G. A., *Int. J. Cancer* **7**:1, 1971.
191. Bansal, S. C., and Sjogren, H. O., *Int. J. Cancer* **12**:179, 1973.
192. Noonan, P. F., Gasdren, M. A. H., Clunie, G. J. A., et al., *Int. J. Cancer* **13**:640, 1974.
193. Proctor, J. W., Rudenstam, C. M., and Alexander, P., *Nature* **242**:29, 1973.
194. Ray, P. K., *Med. et Hyg.* **39**:1737, 1981.
195. Steele, G., Ankerest, J., and Sjogren, H. O., *Int. J. Cancer* **14**:83, 1974.
196. Bansal, S. C., Bansal, B. R., Thomas, H. L., et al., *Cancer* **42**:1, 1978.
197. Ray, P. K., Idiculla, A., Rhoads, J. E., Jr., et al., Extracorporeal immunoadsorption of pathologic plasma immunoglobulin G or its complexes. A novel approach for their selective removal from the plasma. In "First Annual Apheresis Symposium. Current concepts and future trends." American Red Cross Blood Services, Chicago, October 1979, pp. 203–215.
198. Ray, P. K., In *Proceedings of the Workshop on Therapeutic Plasmapheresis and Cytopheresis*, Rochester, Mayo Clinic, April 25, 26, 1979, U.S. Department of Health and Human Services, NIH, Bethesda. October 1981, pp. 334–339.
199. Ray, P. K., Cooper, D. R., Bassett, J. G., and Mark, P. *Fed. Proc.* **38**(3):4558, 1979.
200. Ray, P. K., Besa, E., Idiculla, A., et al., *Cancer* **45**:2633, 1980.
201. Ray, P. K., Idiculla, A., Mark, R., et al., *Cancer* **49**:1800, 1982.
202. Ray, P. K., Idiculla, A., and Rhoads, J. E., Jr., Extracorporeal immunoadsorption using protein A—containing *Staphylococcus aureus* column. A method for the quick removal of abnormal IgGs and/or its complexes from the plasma. In H. Borberg and P. Reuther (Eds.), *Plasma Exchange Therapy. International Symposium Weisbaden 1980*, pp. 150–154. New York: Thieme-Stratton, 1980.
203. Ray, P. K., McLaughlin, D., Mohammed, J., et al., *Ex vivo* immunoadsorption of IgG

or its complexes—A new modality of cancer treatment. In B. Serrou and C. Rosenfeld (Eds.) *Immune Complexes and Plasma Exchanges in Cancer Patients* Vol. 1, p. 1970. Amsterdam: Elsevier/North Holland, 1981.

204. Ray, P. K., Clarke, L., McLaughlin, D., et al., Immunotherapy of Cancer. Extracorporeal adsorption of plasma-blocking factors using non-viable *Staphylococcus aureus* Cowan I. In J. H. Beyer, H. Borberg, C. W. Fuchs, and G. A. Nagel, (Eds.), *Plasmapheresis in Immunology and Oncology*, pp. 102–113. Basel: S. Karger, 1982.

205. Ray, P. K., Raychaudhuri, S., and Allen, P., *Cancer Res.* **42**:4970, 1982.

206. Diener, E., and Feldman, M., *Transplant. Rev.* **8**:76, 1972.

207. Gershon, R. K., Birnbaum-Mokyr, M., and Mitchell, M. S., *Nature* **250**:594, 1974.

208. Terman, D. S., Yamamoto, T., Mattioli, M., et al., *J. Immunol.* **124**:795, 1980.

209. Holohan, T. V., Phillips, T. M., Bowles, C., et al., *Cancer Res.* **42**:3663, 1982.

210. Terman, D. S., Yamamoto, T., Tillquist, R. L., et al., *Science* **209**:1257, 1980.

211. Terman, D. S., Young, J. B., Shearer, W. T., et al., *N. Engl. J. Med.* **305**(20): 1195, 1981.

212. Jones, F. R., Yoshida, L. H., Ladiges, W. C., and Kenny, M. A., *Cancer* **46**:675, 1980.

213. Noar, D., *Adv. Cancer Res.* **29**:45, 1979.

214. Ray, P. K., and Raychaurhuri, S., *J. Natl. Cancer Inst.* **67**:1341, 1981.

215. Ray, P. K., *Plasma Ther. Transfus. Technol.* **3**:101, 1982.

216. Drebin, J. A., Waltenbough, C., Schatten, S., et al., *J. Immunol.* **130**:506, 1983.

217. Ray, P. K., Mohammed, J., Raychaudhuri, S., In *Fourth International Congress of Immunology*, Paris, July 21–26, 1980.

218. Ray, P. K., Mohammed, J., Allen, P., et al., *J. Biol. Resp. Modif.* **2**(6), 1983.

219. Bandyopadhyay, S., Mobini, J., and Ray, P. K., *Fed. Proc.* **42**(3):2270, 1983.

220. Ray, P. K., and Bandyopadhyay, S., *Immunol. Commun.*, in press, 1983.

221. Treaves, A. J., Cohen, I. R., and Feldman, M. J., *Natl. Cancer Inst.* **57**:409, 1976.

222. Carnaud, O., Markoni, C. Z., and Trainin, N., *Cell. Immunol.* **14**:87, 1974.

223. Treaves, A. J., Carnard, C., and Trainin, N., *Eur. J. Immunol.* **4**:722, 1974.

224. Rotter, V., and Trainin, N., *Transplantation* **20**:68, 1975.

225. Small, M., *J. Immunol.* **118**:1517, 1975.

226. Kirchner, H., Chused, T. M., Herberman, R. B. *et al.*, *J. Exp. Med.* **139**:1473, 1974.

227. Kirchner, H., Howard, G. Z., and Trainin, N., *J. Natl. Cancer Inst.* **55**:971, 1975.

228. Kumar, V., and Bennett, M., *Nature* **265**:345, 1977.

229. Broder, S., Poplack, D., Whang-Peng, J. *et al.*, *N. Eng. J. Med.* **298**:66, 1978.

230. Fujimoto, M. I., Greene, A. H., and Sehon, A. H., *J. Immunol.* **116**:791, 1976.

231. Fujimoto, M. I., Greene, M. I., and Sehon, A. H., *J. Immunol.* **116**:791, 1976.

232. Kumar, V., Caruso, T., and Bennett, M., *J. Exp. Med.* **143**:728, 1976.

233. Stelzer, V., and Wallace, K., *Proc. Am. Assocn. Cancer Res.* **18**:66, 1977.

234. Blasecki, J. W., and Tevethia, S., *J. Immunol.* **114**:244, 1975.

235. Gifford, R. R., Voss, B. V., and Ferguson, R. M., *Surgery* **90**:344, 1981.

236. Uchida, A., and Hoshino, T., *Int. J. Cancer* **26**:401, 1980.

237. Mizushima, Y., Sendo, F., Takelchi, N. *et al.*, *Cancer Res.* **41**:2917, 1981.

238. Fulton, A. M., and Levy, J. G., *Int. J. Cancer* **26**:669, 1980.

239. Serrou, B., Cupissd, D., Thierry, C. *et al.*, *Recent Results in Cancer Res.* **75**:110, 1980.

240. Tilkin, A. F., Schaaf-Lafontaine, N., Van Acter, A. *et al.*, *Proc. Natl. Acad. Sci.* **78**:1809, 1981.

241. Drebin, J. A., Waltenbaugh, C., Schatten *et al.*, *J. Immunol.* **130**:506, 1983.

9

Immunomodulation and Cancer Therapy

P. Reizenstein, L. Olsson, and G. Mathé

Immune reactivity may be modulated nonspecifically by a variety of components known as immune adjuvants (1–4).

Specific modulation presupposes reactivity against a defined antigen, whereas nonspecific modulation is assumed to affect the immune response against a variety of antigens. The modulation may result both in an increased immunological response, as for instance after a vaccination, and in a decreased one, as for instance after desensitization.

In 1893, Coley (5) reported regression of human malignant neoplasms after treating the patients with erysipelas products. Coley's report was soon forgotten and first revived 66 years later, when Old et al. (6) demonstrated that BCG had tumoricidal properties against transplantable murine tumors. Most investigations carried out later have confirmed and extended these early observations (3, 7, 8). The data on the antineoplastic effect of bacterial immune adjuvants were rapidly adapted to the immune-surveillance hypothesis, proposed by McFarlane-Burnett (9). This hypothesis suggests that T cells can recognize as *non self* and destroy tumor cells which are assumed to have tumor-specific surface neoantigens. In planning experiments with specific immunotherapy it is frequently also assumed that those antigens are cross-reactive from one individual to another.

The effects of nonspecific adjuvants were originally ascribed to an assumed general increase in antitumoral immune-surveillance activity. The validity of this interpretation must be questioned today because of the apparent complexity of the immune system. Adjuvant treatment does not always lead to an increase in the activity of immune cells, and such a possible increase does not necessarily increase the activity of the cytotoxic immune mechanisms. The effect of adjuvants on the suppressor and helper activity of T cells and macrophages modulates the activity of the immune cells (10).

EFFECTS OF NONSPECIFIC IMMUNE ADJUVANTS
IN HEALTHY ANIMALS

Studies on the effects of nonspecific immune adjuvants like bacterial products (11–14) and polynucleotides (15, 16) have almost exclusively been carried out in healthy, non-tumor-bearing animals. In such animals, nonspecific immune adjuvants may stimulate cytotoxic T lymphocytes, lymphocyte reactivity to mitogens (15–20), and mononuclear phagocytes as regards their phagocytic capacity (21) and cytotoxic effect (22–24). Some of the cell types mentioned may be subdivided into several subpopulations: T5 and T8 antigen-bearing suppressive and possibly cytotoxic lymphocytes (10, 25–29), T4-bearing *helper* lymphocytes (30–32) and the T6 bearing early lymphocytes. The suppressor cells may inhibit B lymphocyte response to foreign antigens, T-lymphocyte reactivity to mitogens, and perhaps the T-lymphocyte-mediated cytotoxic reactions. Cell functions, however, do not always parallel the cell markers. Since increased activity of both suppressor T-cell and suppressor macrophage activity may be induced by immune adjuvants, it is obvious that immune adjuvants cannot always be expected to induce an increased immune response or increased cytotoxic activity. In some unpublished experiments on the effect of intravenous injections of various doses of BCG on suppressor T-lymphocyte activity in animals, we found that BCG doses of 3 mg (about 21×10^6 viable units) or more induce a suppressor T-cell activity that inhibits the T-lymphocyte response to phytohaemagglutinin. The immune response is dependent on the BCG dose (33–35).

EFFECTS OF NONSPECIFIC IMMUNE ADJUVANTS
IN TUMOR-BEARING ANIMALS

The relevance of the studies reported so far is limited because they were performed on healthy mice. Immune reactions in healthy mice are not representative of immune reactions in tumor-bearing mice, since tumors themselves influence the reactivity of the immune system (36, 37). In leukemic AKR mice, BCG (38) stimulates neither the mitogen response of B and T lymphocytes nor the number of spleen cells capable of producing antibodies against sheep red blood cells in a modified Jerne plaque forming assay, and these assays had no value as prognostic tests.

RELEVANCE OF *IN VITRO* STUDIES
OF THE IMMUNOLOGICAL RESPONSE

What must be required of *in vitro* assays of tumor antigenicity and cytotoxicity before such studies are claimed to be relevant for malignant tumor growth *in vivo*? The complexity of the immune system indicates that the activity of an immune function measured *in vitro* may not be the same *in vivo*, since *in vitro* systems in general may be considered as simplifications of the *in vivo* condition. Moreover, many steps in the preparation procedure probably eliminate important immune reactive cells (31, 39, 40). A close correlation between the activity of an *in vitro* parameter and its corresponding *in vivo* phenomenon is required in order to claim *in vivo* significance of an *in vitro* assay. For instance, in acute myeloid leukemia, results obtained with the *in vitro* mitogen reaction seem to agree reasonably well with those obtained with the delayed hypersensitivity reaction *in vivo* (50).

With regard to malignant tumors, however, it is not sufficient to demonstrate the correlation between *in vitro* parameters and tumor growth *in vivo*, since a growing tumor may affect many normal and non-tumor-related functions of the tumor-bearing organism. The lymphocyte response to mitogens, for example, has often been studied in relation to *in vivo* growth of malignant tumors (41–43). However, lymphocyte stimulation by mitogens seems to be an artificial *in vitro* event, since many more lymphocytes are stimulated by mitogens than by most other antigens. This explains why cytotoxic activity is found against tumor cells by mitogen-stimulated cells *in vitro* (49).

It has been shown that some malignant cells contrary to other kinds of foreign cells, are able to secrete substances that may suppress the immune system (44–48). Therefore, the lack of a detectable immune reactivity against a tumor cell does not rule out the possibility that the cell is antigenic. Caution is therefore required when *in vitro* results are interpreted.

IMMUNOPROPHYLAXIS OF EXPERIMENTAL
TUMORS WITH BCG

Almost 40 years elapsed between the isolation of attenuated BCG in 1921 by Calmette and Guerin (51) and the first experimental attempts to control malignant cell growth by BCG (6). The antineoplastic effects of BCG may conveniently be divided into prevention of establishment of malignant tumors and inhibition of growth of established malignant tumors.

Old et al. (6) studied the BCG effect on growth of a number of chemically-induced malignant cell types. It was found that BCG pretreatment inhibited the take of 45% of the tumors, did not affect 45%, and probably facilitated take on the remaining 10%. Subsequent studies on tumor takes in BCG-treated mice (52, 53), rats (34), and guinea pigs (54, 55) using grafts of tumors that arose spontaneously or were induced by virus or chemicals confirmed and extended the observation of Old et al. (6). These studies showed that systemic BCG treatment prior to a tumor graft may exert generally an inhibitory, sometimes a neutral, and rarely a stimulatory effect on tumor takes. The experimental proof that BCG prophylaxis may inhibit tumor takes is thus rather convincing.

THE MECHANISM OF THE IMMUNOPROPHYLACTIC EFFECT OF BCG

To identify the mechanism of the BCG-effect is important (56, 57). The immunological reactions stimulated by BCG may be divided into specific immunity to BCG and an adjuvant effect.

BCG vaccination induces immunity to a subsequent challenge with virulent Mycobacteria in man (58) and in several animal species (59). Antibodies to Mycobacteria have been demonstrated in vaccinated individuals, but the antibodies have no bactericidal effect and after transfer to healthy animals do not protect against tuberculosis (60). In contrast, immunity may be transferred by immunocompetent cells. Delayed hypersensitivity reactions induced by tuberculin are easily demonstrated in BCG-immunized humans and, to variable degrees, in animals (45, 61). The antigen of BCG that confers immunity against tuberculosis is not yet identified (62).

The cross-reactivity between BCG and some malignant cell types is of particular interest. Borsos and Rapp (63) found cross-reactivity between BCG and a guinea pig hepatoma cell line. It was initially suspected that this was due to a similarity between BCG antigens and tumor antigens on the hepatoma cell line (line 10), but Bucana and Hanna (64) showed that the antigen common to BCG and hepatoma line-10 cells was different from line-10 tumor-specific antigens.

Cross-reactivity has also been shown between BCG and human malignant melanoma (65). Antibodies against melanoma cells were raised in rabbits, and it was demonstrated that such antibodies bound significantly higher amounts of radiolabeled BCG than radiolabeled antigens of three other bacterial sources (Listeria, Brucella, and Salmonella).

BCG also has an adjuvant effect on various components of the immune system. Intravenous injections of BCG in mice cause hyperplasia of thymic epithelium and systemic granulomatous histiocytic reactions in liver, spleen, and lymph nodes (66, 67), whereas subcutaneous injections produce a histiocytic reaction at the site of injection and in the regional lymph nodes, but not in the liver and spleen. The changes in lymphoid organs after BCG injection may in part be explained by the influence of BCG on lymphocytes. Intravenous BCG enhances splenic trapping of lymphocytes, and subcutaneous BCG the lymph node trapping of lymphocytes (11, 68).

Lymphoid cells may also be directly activated by BCG . The uptake of ^{3}H-thymidine was increased in both splenic and thymic lymphoid cells after BCG injection. However, maximal stimulation was seen only if a sufficient number of macrophages were stimulated (69, 70). In the regional lymph nodes draining the footpad after BCG injection, blast transformation and cell proliferation were observed and the changes seemed positively correlated to the virulence of the BCG strain. A similar model was used by Miller et al. (71) to test the influence of BCG on the proliferative response of the popliteal node to foodpad injection of sheep red blood cells. BCG significantly increased the number of red cell antibody producing cells, but it is notable that a BCG injection did not influence the immune reactivity of the opposite footpad. These results indicate an enhancing effect of BCG on antibody production. However, other studies have indicated that BCG in some doses and by some routes of administration may depress the antibody response (72, 73).

BCG may also stimulate natural killer (NK) cell activity (74, 75) and the macrophage cell system. BCG activates macrophages as shown by increased metabolism, phagocytic ability (76, 77), cytotoxicity to malignant cells (78, 79), and secretion of extracellular enzymes (80).

IMMUNOTHERAPY OF EXPERIMENTAL TUMORS WITH BCG

It has been firmly established that BCG treatment after tumor cell grafting may inhibit tumor growth. However, many of these studies have been performed with serially transplanted malignant tumors, which in fact reduces their relevance.

In the serially-transplanted murine E (AKR) leukemia, an antileukemic effect was only obtained by one BCG dose, whereas other doses had no effect or, in some cases, even enhanced leukemia growth (35). The effect of BCG depends on the tumor load at the start of BCG administration and the dose of BCG. Leukemia cell-growth inhibition was only obtained with a leukemia graft of 10^2 or 10^3 cells. BCG had no effect on higher leukemia graft doses. An interesting point was that mice cured by BCG became resistant to malignant cell loads that were 10–20 times higher than the primary tumor graft from which they were cured. This dose-dependency of the BCG effect has also been shown in several other tumor-host systems, but due to the use of different strains of BCG in the various experiments, direct comparison becomes difficult. The immune-modulating effect of BCG varies according to the strain of BCG (81). The dose-dependency of the effect by BCG on malignant cell growth has also been demonstrated with intratumoral BCG injections. The guinea pig line-10 tumor, a serially transplanted hepatoma, has been studied particularly (54).

In this system it is especially notable that intratumoral BCG injections may induce regression of both primary tumors and local metastases (82). Regression of naturally occurring bovine eye carcinoma by intralesional BCG treatment has also been reported (83). Therefore, intratumoral BCG application may prove to be relevant for some solid tumors.

The optimal number of BCG injections and the optimal time between these injections to obtain maximal tumor regression is not established. Some reports claim that one BCG injection is insufficient (12), while others state that a more prolonged exposure is necessary to obtain a maximal antitumoral effect (52, 84). In some systems (35) eight injections with weekly intervals seemed to be optimal.

Many experiments concerning BCG effects on experimental tumors with distinct neoantigens have conclusively shown that the T-lymphocyte activity is correlated to the antineoplastic effect of BCG against such tumors (85–88). However, other immune mechanisms may be involved, since T cells have frequently been the only ones that have been studied. For instance, Prehn (89) suggests that the antitumoral effect of BCG may be an *innocent bystander* of BCG adjuvant effects on the immune system. A similar antineoplastic bystander effect has been proposed in relation to graft-versus-host reactions (90).

Is tumor regression correlated to any immune parameters? In E (AKR) mouse leukemia, the antibody-dependent lymphocyte-mediated cytotoxicity (ADLMC) was not well correlated to tumor regression (91). However, a close relationship between natural killer cells (NK) and K cells and tumor regression has been suggested in recent reviews (92, 93).

COMBINATION OF SPECIFIC AND NONSPECIFIC IMMUNIZATION IN EXPERIMENTAL SYSTEMS

Antineoplastic treatment with BCG has often, in both clinical trials and animal experiments (3, 4), been combined with simultaneous injections of rather high numbers of tumor cells. The rationale has been that the organism is specifically immunized against a supposed tumor antigen by the tumor cells, and that the concomitant BCG stimulation nonspecifically enhances the immunological reactions against this antigen. However, the results of experiments combining BCG with tumor cells are conflicting. Some results show beneficial effects of the combination as compared to the effect of only one of the adjuvants (52, 55), while others suggest that the addition of cells did not increase the antitumoral effect of BCG alone (91). In some studies there is even enhancement of tumor growth. In E(AKR) leukemia, we found that the antileukemic effect of BCG was eliminated by concomitant administration of irradiated E(AKR) leukemia cells (91). However, no systematic studies on combining doses have been performed, and it is possible that the conflicting results are due to dose variations.

If BCG has any effect, it is only on small tumor loads. In the clinical situation, it is therefore expected that BCG in most cases will be given as an adjunct to a chemotherapeutic regimen. BCG has been combined with cytostatics with variable success in both animals and humans (94–97). Most cytostatics attack cells in S phase and/or mitosis (98) whereas malignant cells in G_0–G_1 phase are barely affected. Therefore, a cytostatic treatment lasting only weeks can not be expected to destroy dormant malignant cells with a long transit time in the G_1-phase (99, 100) and such cells may induce a clinical relapse of the disease.

BCG, however, seems to kill E(AKR) leukemic cells (101), cells mainly in the G_1 phase. This G_1-phase preference may possibly be explained by the fact that most cells seem to have a maximal antigen expression during the G_1 phase (102, 103) and/or by the fact the G_1 cells are more sensitive to cytotoxic attack than cells in other cell cycle phases (104). However, the antitumoral mechanisms activated by BCG are complex, and the effects of various cytostatics on these mechanisms have scarcely been investigated. Cytostatics may depress immune functions for a time, but a rebound effect is seen later (105–107). Studies on the effects of cytostatics on the different subpopulations of the immune system, and the time schedule to restore the normal function of these subpopulations are necessary before it is possible to design rational protocols that combine BCG and cytostatics.

IN VITRO EFFECTS IN MAN OF NONSPECIFIC ADJUVANTS

Long-term treatment with adjuvants like C. parvum, or BCG results in a confirmed increase in NK activity (108, 109). Other findings such as the maintenance of high production by macrophages of colony-stimulatory activity (57), and the activation of the macrophage helper cell function still have to be confirmed (106). Still other results such as the increase in the null-cell proportion (108) or the increase in the blastogenic response to PHA (50, 109, 110) are controversial. The controversy is perhaps explained by the duration of adjuvant therapy. Over 3 months of weekly treatment seems to reduce the PHA response (110).

CLINICAL EFFECTS OF NONSPECIFIC ADJUVANTS

The most well documented clinical effect has been described in acute myeloid leukemia (111–115), where a significant increase of the duration of the first remission, the frequency of the second remission (116), and survival was seen. However, the effect seems to be temporary and permanent cures are rare (117). Moreover, there seem to be subgroups of patients which do not respond to immune manipulation. This will be discussed below (114, 118, Table 9.1).

In skin cancer, 80% of the lesions regress after intralesional BCG (119).

In non-Hodgkin lymphoma, effects of BCG have been described (119, 120), but again, there are subgroups of patients which do not respond (Table 9.1).

In bronchial carcinoma, in general, results are nonconclusive (122–125). Of 10 published studies involving patients given or not given specific adjuvants, the patients were benefited significantly in four and harmed in two (126). However, these results become more interesting when the subgroups are considered (Table 9.1). It is not yet possible to identify the subgroup characteristic which determines the possible sensitivity to nonspecific adjuvant administration, but it could be genetically determined and, also, related to the tendency of the tumor to relapse.

In melanoma, 11 of 13 reviewed studies (126) gave nonsignificant results, and the value of immunoadjuvants in stage I or II melanoma has not yet

Table 9.1. Subgroups of Patients and the Response to Nonspecific Adjuvant Therapy

Diagnosis	Patient Group with a Significant Effect	Reference	Patient Group with No Significant Effect	Reference
Acute Myelogenous Leukemia	A group with 35% remissions	114	A group with 65% remissions	114
Non-Hodgkin Lymphoma	Young, or stage I, or women, or in the initial phase of the disease	120, 121	Old, or stage II–IV, or men, or in the relapse phase	120, 121
Bronchial Carcinoma	Non-small cell carcinoma, or blood groups A, B, AB, Rh+	124, 138, 139	Small cell carcinoma, or blood groups O, Rh–	124, 137, 138
Acute Lymphatic Leukemia	Appr. median remission duration 60 days, after end of chemptherapy, no neuroprophylaxis, or with HLA BW17 & AW 33 phenotype	134, 135, 136	Long remissions with neuroprophylaxis	136, 139, 140, 141

been demonstrated (127, 128). The same is still true for other solid tumors, like advanced cancer (131) and bladder cancer (132). Some of these studies have yielded hopeful results (126, 129, 130, 132), but as yet they are either controversial, or not yet confirmed. Effects of cytokines and of medicamental biological response modifiers in man have been in part discussed by P. K. Ray (Chapter 8) in this volume and have also been reviewed elsewhere (133).

SUMMARY

Effect of BCG and Specific Immunization in Animals

Depending on the dose and the time after administration, BCG may stimulate cytotoxic or suppressor T cells and macrophages, which can inhibit the T-cell response to PHA in healthy animals. In tumor-bearing animals, the tumor itself can modify the immune reaction. Some tumor cells secrete immunosuppressors.

BCG can inhibit tumor takes in animals, probably by stimulating NK and macrophage activity.

BCG can also inhibit the growth of small numbers of established experimental tumor cells, both after local and after systemic administration. In experimental tumors with distinct neoantigens, the effect seems to be mediated by T cells and NK cells, which may, in contrast to cytostatics, be able to attack tumor cells in G_0–G_1 phases, as are suppressor T cells in regard to their targets.

Specific immunization of animals against transplantable tumors is possible in some situations, whereas tumor enhancement can result in others (33, 34).

Effect of BCG and Specific Immunization in Man

Depending on the time of administration, BCG in man results in a maintained NK activity and probably in a stimulation of certain macrophage functions.

In man, it is possible to produce both a humoral and a cellular immunologic reaction by injecting tumor cells, but neither cross-reactions between individuals nor the beneficial effects of these specific immunologic reactions have been demonstrated.

Clinically, BCG seems to have a temporary and limited effect in subgroups of patients with acute myeloid leukemia and non-Hodgkin lymphoma, a controversial effect in acute lymphatic leukemia and nonsmall cell carcinomas of the lung, and nonconfirmed or controversial effects in advanced breast cancer or stomach cancer. In other solid tumors, mostly negative results have been reported. No confirmed clinical effects of specific immuno-modulation have been reported, but experiments with removal of supposedly blocking antibodies and administration of monoclonal ones are in progress.

Immunomodulators other than BCG, such as levamizole, azimexon, tuftsin, retinoid acids, and cytokines, are becoming a new family of drugs of increasing interest. This aspect has been discussed in another chapter of this volume (see chapter 8).

In summary, although some human tumors have weak, private neoantigens, the specific T-cell response to neoantigens which can protect animals against experimental tumors has not yet been demonstrated to play a clinical role in man. However, on-going experiments trying to use the cytotoxic effect of possibly virus-associated, tissue-specific, or differentiation monoclonal antibodies are of interest. In addition, nonspecific modulation of the NK-cell and macrophage activity with BCG or interferon has temporary clinical effects in subgroups of patients with certain, but not all types of tumors.

REFERENCES

1. Freund, J., *Adv. Tuberc. Res.* **10**:130, 1956.
2. Wolstenholme, G. E. W., and Knight, J. (Eds.), *Immunopotentiation, Ciba Found. Symp. 18*. Amsterdam: Elsevier/North Holland, 1973.
3. Mathe, G., *Cancer active immunotherapy. Its immunoprophylaxis and immunorestoration. Recent Results in Cancer Research*, Springer Verlag, New York Vol. 55, 1976.
4. Shearer, W. T., and Fink, M. P., *Prog. Hematol.* **10**:247, 1977.
5. Coley, W. B., *Med. Rec.* **43**:60, 1893.
6. Old, L. J., Clarke, D. A., and Benacerraf, B., *Nature* (London) **184**:291, 1959
7. Bast, R. C., Zbar, B., Borsos, T., and Rapp, H. J., *N. Engl. J. Med.*, **290**:1413–1420 and 1458–1469, 1974.
8. Baldwin, R. W., and Pimm, M. V., *Adv. Cancer Res.* **28**:91, 1978.
9. Burnet, F. M., *Prog. Exp. Tumor Res.* **13**:1, 1970.
10. Broder, S., and Waldman, T. A., *N. Engl. J. Med.* **299**:1281–1284 and 1335–1341, 1978.
11. Florentin, I., Huchet, R., Bruley-Rosset, M., et al., *Cancer Immunol. Immunoth.* **1**:31, 1976.
12. Halle-Pannenko, O., Bourut, C., and Kamel, M., *Cancer Immunol. Immunoth.* **1**:17, 1976.
13. Renoux, G., and Renoux, M., *C. R. Acad. Sci.* (D) **274**:3034, 1972.
14. Merluzzi, V. J., Badger, A. M., Kaiser, C. W., et al., Effect of levamisole on murine lymphoid populations. In M. A. Chirigos (Ed.), *Control of neoplasia by modulation of the immune system*, p. 25. New York: Raven Press, 1977.
15. Cone, R. E., and Johnson, A. G., *J. Exp. Med.* **133**:665, 1971.
16. Jacobs, M. E., Steinberg, A. D., Gordon, J. K., et al., *Arthritis and Rheumatism* **15**:201, 1972.
17. Anderson, J., Sjoberg, O., and Moller, G., *Transpl. Rev.* **11**:131, 1979.

18. Mitchell, M. A., Kirkpatrick, D., Mokyr, M. B., et al., *Nature New Biol.* **243**:216, 1973.
19. Moller, G., Anderson, J., and Sjoberg, O., *Cell.Immunol.* **4**:416, 1972.
20. Howard, J.G., Christie, G. H., and Scott, M.T., *Cell. Immunol.* **7**:290, 1973.
21. Spitznagel, J., and Allison, A. C., *J. Immunol.* **104**:128, 1970.
22. Unaue, E. R., Askonas, B. A., and Allison, A. C., *J. Immunol.* **103**:71, 1969.
23. Bruley-Rosset, M., Florentin, I., Khalil, A. M., et al., *Int. Arch. Allerg. Appl. Immunol.* **51**:594, 1976.
24. Meltzer, M. S., and Stevenson, M. M., *J. Immunol.* **118**:2176, 1977.
25. Miller, J. F. A. P., and Mitchell, G. F., *Transpl. Rev.* **1**:3, 1969.
26. Gershon, R. K., *Transpl. Rev.* **26**:170, 1976.
27. Hodes, R. J., and Hathcock, K. S., *J. Immunol.* **116**:167, 1976.
28. Davies, A. J.S., *Transpl. Rev.* **1**:43, 1969.
29. Cerottini, J. C., Nordin, A. A., and Brunner, K. T., *Nature* (London) **227**:72, 1970.
30. Claman, H., Chaperon, E. A., and Triplett, R. F., *Proc. Soc. Exp. Biol.* (N.Y.) **122**:1167, 1966.
31. Claesson, M. H., *Acta Morphol. Nealand. Scand.* **9**:1, 1971.
32. Waldmann, H., *Immunol. Rev.* **42**:202, 1978.
33. Ray, P. K., Poduval, T. B., and Sundaram, K., *J. Natl. Cancer Inst.* **58**:763, 1977.
34. Ray, P. K., De, B. K., Guha, S., et al., *Ind. J. Exp. Biol.* **18**:123, 1980.
35. Olsson, L., Ebbesen, P., Kiger, N., et al., *Europ. J. Cancer* **14**:355, 1978.
36. Wislow, O. S., and Wheelock, E. F., *J. Immunol* **114**:211, 1975.
37. Roman, J. M., and Golub, E. S., *J. Exp. Med.* **143**:482, 1976.
38. Olsson, L., and Ebbesen, P., *J. Immunol.* **122**:772, 1979.
39. Yust, I., Smith, R. W., Wunderlich, J. R., et al., *J. Immunol.* **116**:1170, 1976.
40. Kay, H. D., Bonnard, G. D., West, W. H., et al., *J. Immunol.* **118**:2058, 1977.
41. Mathe, G., and Weiner, R. (Eds.), *Investigation and stimulation of immunity in cancer patients. Recent Results in Cancer Research*, Springer Verlag, New York Vol. 47, 1974.
42. Hersh, E. M., and Oppenheim, J. J., *N. Engl. J. Med.* **173**:1006, 1965.
43. Sutherland, R. M., Rodger, I. W., and McRedie, J. A., *Cancer* **27**:574, 1971.
44. Levy, J. G., Smith, A. G., Whitney, R. B., et al., *Immunology* **30**:565, 1976.
45. Pike, M. C., and Snyderman, R. J., *Immunol.* **117**:1243, 1976.
46. McMaster, R., Buchler, K., Whitney, R., et al., *J. Immunol.* **118**:218, 1977.
47. Broder, S., Poplack, D., Whang-Peng, J., et. al., *New Engl. J. Med.* **298**:66, 1978.
48. Ogier, C., Sjogren, A. M., and Reizenstein, P., *Cancer Immunol. Immunother.* **12**:241, 1982.
49. Waterfield, J. D., Waterfield, E. M., Anaclerio, A., et al., *Transplant Rev.* **29**:277, 1976.
50. Uden, A. M., Lindemalm, C., Pauli, C., et al., *Cancer Immunol. Immunother.* **4**:239, 1978.
51. Guerin, C., The history of BCG. In S. R. Rosenthal (Ed.), *BCG vaccination against tuberculosis*, p. 48. Boston: Little Brown, 1957.
52. Mathe, G., Pouillart, P., and Lapeyraque, F., *Br. J. Cancer* **23**:814, 1969.
53. Parr, I., *Br. J. Cancer* **26**:174, 1972.
54. Rapp, H. J., *Israel J. Med. Sci.* **9**:366, 1973.
55. Zbar, B., Bernstein, I. D., and Rapp, H. J., *J. Natl. Cancer Inst.* **46**:831, 1971.
56. Bast, R. C., and Bast, B. S., *Ann. N.Y. Acad. Sci.* **277**:60, 1976.
57. Reizenstein, P., Andersson, B., and Beran, M., Possible mechanism of action of immunotherapy of acute non-lymphatic leukemia. Macrophage production of colony stimulating activity. EORTC Plenary Session, Paris, June 23–27, 1980. To be published in *Rec. Res. Cancer Res.*

58. Eickhoff, T. C., *Ann. Rev. Med.* **28**:411, 1977.
59. Arnasson, B. G., and Waksman, B. H., *Bibl. Tuberc.* **19**:1, 1964:
60. Lefford, M. J., McGregor, D. D., and Mackaness, G. B., *Infect. Immunol.* **8**:182, 1973.
61. Chung, E. B., Zbar, B., and Rapp, H. J., *J. Natl. Cancer Inst.* **51**:241, 1973.
62. Nassau, E., and Nelstrop, A. D., *Tubercle* **57**:197, 1976.
63. Borsos, T., and Rapp, H. J., *J. Natl. Cancer Inst.* **51**:1085, 1973.
64. Bucana, C., and Hanna, M. G., *J. Natl. Cancer Inst.* **53**:1313, 1974.
65. Minden, P., Sharpton, T. R., and McClatchy, J. K., *J. Immunol.* **116**:1407, 1976.
66. Rosenthal, S. R., *BCG vaccination against tuberculosis.* Boston: Little, 1957.
67. Rappaport, H., and Khalil, A., *Cancer Immunol. Immunoth.* **1**:45, 1976.
68. Zatz, M., *J. Immunol.* **116**:1587, 1976.
69. Mitchell, M. S., Mokyr, M. D., and Kahane, I., *J. Natl. Cancer Inst.* **55**:1337, 1975.
70. Mokyr, M. B., and Mitchell, M. S., *Cell Immunol.* **15**:264, 1975.
71. Miller, T. E., Mackaness, G. B., and Lagrange, P. H., *J. Natl. Cancer Inst.* **41**:1669, 1973.
72. Neveu, P. J., *Clin. Exp. Immunol.* **26**:169, 1976.
73. Peters, L. C., Hanna, M. G., Gutterman, J. U., et al., *Proc. Soc. Exp. Biol. Med.* **147**:344, 1974.
74. Wolfe, S. A., Tracey, D. E., and Henney, C. S., *Nature* (London) **262**:584, 1976.
75. Herberman, R. B., Nunn, M. E., Holden, H. T., et al., *Int. J. Cancer* **19**:555, 1977.
76. Werb, Z., and Gordon, S., *J. Exp. Med.* **142**:361, 1975.
77. Werb, Z., and Gordon, S., *J. Exp. Med.* **142**:346, 1975.
78. Eccles, S. A., Macrophages and cancer. In J. E. Castro (Ed.), *Immunological aspects of cancer*, p. 123. England: MIP Press, 1978.
79. Keller, R., Cytostatic and cytocidal effects of activated macrophages. In D. S. Nelson (Ed.), *Immunobiology of the macrophage*, p. 487. New York: Academic Press, 1976.
80. Gordon, S., and Cohn, Z. A., *J. Exp. Med.* **147**:1175, 1978.
81. Mathe, G., Attempts at using systemic immunity adjuvants in experimental and human cancer therapy. In G. E. V. Wolstenholme and J. Knight (Eds.), *Immunopotentiation*, p. 305. Ciba Found. Symp. 18, Elsevier/North Holland, 1973.
82. Zbar, B., Hunter, J. T., Rapp, H. J., et al., *J. Natl. Cancer Inst.* **60**:1163, 1978.
83. Kleinschuster, S. J., Rapp, H. J., Lueker, D. C., et al, *J. Natl. Cancer Inst.* **58**:1807, 1978.
84. Tanaka, T., *Gann* **65**:145, 1974.
85. Bansal, S. C., and Sjogren, H. O., *Int. J. Cancer* **11**:162, 1973.
86. Hanna, M. G., Snodgrass, M. J., Zbar, B., et al., *J. Natl. Cancer Inst.* **51**:1897, 1973.
87. Hawrylko, E., and Mackaness, G. B., *J. Natl. Cancer Inst.* **51**:1683, 1973.
88. Parr, I., Wheeler, E., and Alexander, P., *J. Natl. Cancer Inst.* **59**:1659, 1977.
89. Prehn, R. T., *Israel J. Med.* **9**:375, 1973.
90. Johnson, P. R., and Hersey, P., *Brit. J. Cancer* **33**:370, 1976.
91. Olsson, L., Florentin, I., Kiger, N., et al., *J. Natl. Cancer Inst.* **59**:1297, 1977.
92. Herberman, R. B., and Holden, H. T., *Adv. Cancer Res.* **27**:305, 1978.
93. Welsch, R. M., *J. Immunol.* **121**:1631, 1978.
94. Amiel, J. L., and Berardet, M., *Europ. J. Cancer* **10**:89, 1972.
95. Pearson, J. W., and Chaparas, S. D., *Chirigos, M. A. Cancer Res.* **33**:1845, 1973.
96. Tagliabue, A., Polentarutti, N., Vecchi, A., et al., *Europ. J. Cancer* **13**:657, 1977.
97. Terry, W. D., and Whindhorst, D. (Eds.), *Immunotherapy of cancer: present status of trials in man.* New York: Raven, 1977.
98. Rajewsky, M. F., *Proliferative parameters relevant to cancer therapy. Recent results cancer research* **52**:156, 1975.
99. Fisher, B., and Fisher, E., *Science* **130**:918, 1958.

100. Weinhold, K. F., Goldstein, L. T., and Whelock, E. F., *Nature* **270**:59, 1977.
101. Olsson, L., and Mathe, G., *Cancer Res.* **37**:1743, 1977.
102. Cikes, M., *J. Natl., Cancer Inst.* **45**:979, 1970.
103. Lerner, R. A., Oldstone, M. B., and Cooper, N. R., *Proc. Natl. Acad. Sci. USA* **68**:2584, 1971.
104. Pellegrino, M. A., Ferrone, S., and Cooper, N. R., *J. Exp. Med.* **140**:578, 1974.
105. Arends-Merino, A., Sjogren, A. M., and Reizenstein, P., *Anticancer Res.*, **3**: 1983.
106. Arends-Merino, A., Giscombe, R., Ogier, C., et al., *Cancer Immunol. Immunoth.* **14**:32, 1982.
107. Ray, P. K., and Raychudhury, S., *J. Natl. Cancer Inst.* **67**:1341, 1981.
108. Thatcher, N., Lamb, B., and Swindell, R., *Cancer* **47**:285, 1981.
109. Haghbin, M., Cunningham-Rundels, S., Thaler, H. T., et al., *Cancer* **46**:2577, 1980.
110. Reizenstein, P., Ogier, C., and Sjogren, A. M., *Immunotherapy versus chemotherapy: Response to PHA, allogeneic lymphocytes, and leukemic myeloblasts of remission lymphocytes. Recent Results Cancer Research* **75**:29, 1980.
111. Powles, R. L., Russel, J., Lister, T. A, et al., *Brit. J. Cancer* **25**:265, 1977.
112. Bekesi, J. G., Holland, J. F., and Roboz, J. P., *Clin. North Am.* **61**:1083, 1977.
113. Reizenstein, P., Effect of immunotherapy on survival and remission duration in acute nonlymphocytic leukemia. In W. D. Terry and D. Windhorst, (Eds.), *Immunotherapy of cancer: present status of trials in man*, p. 329. New York: Raven Press, 1977.
114. Reizenstein, P., Andersson, B., Bjorkholm, M., et al., BCG plus leukemic cell therapy in patients with acute non lymphoblastic leukemia: effect in groups with high and low remission rates. In W. D. Terry and D. Windhorst (Eds.), *Immunotherapy of Cancer*, p. 17. New York: Raven Press, 1982.
115. Reizenstein, P., and Miale, T. D., Concluding remarks: immunotherapy of acute myeloid leukemia in man. In H. Rainer (Ed.), *Immunotherapy of malignant diseases*, p.441. Stuttgart: F. K. Schattauer Verlag, 1978.
116. Kay, H. E. M., Acute lymphoblastic leukemia. 5-year-follow-up of the *Concorde* trial of ALL immunotherapy. In *Immunotherapy of cancer: present status of trials in man.* New York: Raven Press, 1977.
117. Whittaker, J. A., Reizenstein, P., Callender, S. T., et al, *Brit. Med. J.* **282**:872, 1981.
118. Anthony, H., *Cancer Immunol. Immunoth.* **11**:287, 1981.
119. Whittaker, J., Bailey-Wood, R., and Hutchins, S., *Brit. J. Haematol.* **45**:389, 1980.
120. Hoerni, B., Chauvergne, J., Hoerni-Simon, G., et al., *Cancer Immunol. Immunoth.* **19**:57, 1977.
121. Hoerni, B., Durand, M., Richaud, P., et al., *Brit. J. Haematol.* **42**:507, 1979.
122. McKneally, M. F., Maver, C. M., and Kansell, H. W., *Lancet* **1**:593, 1977.
123. Pines, A., *Lancet* **1**:380, 1976.
124. Moayeri, H., Takita, H., and Sokal, J. E., *Cancer Immunol. Immunoth.* **6**:223, 1979.
125. Solan, A. J., Vogl, S. E., Zaravinos, T., et al., *Cancer Immunol. Immunoth.* **8**:263, 1980.
126. Belpomme D., Marty, M., and Gisselbretch, C., et al., *Path. Biol.* **29**:179, 1981.
127. Terry, W. D., *New Eng. J. Med.* **303**:1174, 1980.
128. Presant, C. A., Bartolucci, A. A., Smaller, R. V., et al., Effect of Corynebacterium parvum on combination chemotherapy of disseminated malignant melanoma. In W. D. Terry and D. Windhorst (Eds.), *Immunotherapy of Cancer: present status of trials in man*, p. 113. New York: Raven Press, 1978.
129. Pinsky, C. M., De Jager, R. L., Wittes, R. E., et al., Corynebacterium parvum as adjuvant to combination chemotherapy in patients with advanced breast cancer: preliminary results of a prospective randomized trial. In W. D. Terry and D. Windhorst,

(Eds.), *Immunotherapy of cancer: present status of trials in man*, p. 647. New York: Raven Press, 1978.

130. Yasue, M., Murakami, M., Nakazato, H., et al., *Cancer Chemoth. Pharmacol.* **7**:5, 1981.

131. Bancewicz, J., Calman, K. L., Macpherson, S. G., et al., *J. Royal Soc. Med.* **73**:197, 1980.

132. Morales, A., *Cancer Immunol. Immunoth.* **9**:69, 1980.

133. Reizenstein, P., Mathe, G., Immunomodulating agents. In M. A. Chirigos, (Ed.), *Mechanisms of immune modulation*. New York: Marcel Dekker, (in press).

134. Mathe, G., Amiel, J. L., Schwarzenberg, L., et al., *Lancet* **2**:697, 1969.

135. Pauli, C., Vanky, F., Lindemalm, C., et al., *Cancer Immunol. Immunoth.* **5**:1, 1978.

136. Tursz, T., Hors, J., Lipinski, M., et al., *Brit. Med. J.* **1**:1250, 1978.

137. Mikulski, M. S., McGuire, W. P., Louie, A. C., et al., *Cancer Treat. Rev.* **6**:177, 1979.

138. Mikulski, M. S., McGuire, W.P., Louis, A. C., et al., *Cancer Treat. Rev.* **6**:125, 1979.

139. Heyn, R., Joo, P., Karon, M., et al., BCG in the treatment ot acute lymphocytic leukemia. In W. D. Terry and D. Windhorst, (Eds.), *Immunotherapy of cancer: present status of trials in man*. New York: Raven Press, 1977.

140. Leventhal, B. G., Immunotherapy of acute lymphoid leukemia. In W. D. Terry and D. Windhorst, (Eds.), *Immunotherapy of cancer: present status of trials in man*. New York: Raven Press, 1977.

141. Medical Research Council, *Brit. Med. J.* **4**:189, 1971.

PART IV
IMMUNOBIOLOGY OF PREGNANCY—A PHENOMENON OF LIMITED ACCEPTANCE OF NON-SELF

10

Unique and Modified Concepts of the Survival of the Fetus in an Immunologically Privileged Site

Rajgopal Raghupathy and G. P. Talwar*

At the turn of this century, tumor biologists observed a variability in the survival of tumors; while some tumors enjoyed extended survival in animals, some disappeared rapidly from others. Gradually the importance of animal strains in tumor susceptibility was realized and a genetic control of tumor transplantation was suggested. In 1938, Peter Gorer (1) stated that "iso-antigenic factors present in the grafted tissue and absent in the host are capable of eliciting a response which results in the destruction of the graft." This was followed by elegant transplantation studies of Peter Medawar (2) who for the first time, presented evidence for the immunologic nature of the rejection of tissue transplants by allogeneic hosts.

The fact that rejection is mediated by an immunological reaction caused by an antigenic disparity between the host and the graft formed the basis of the laws of transplantation. This states that syngeneic grafts succeed, while allogeneic grafts fail. The apparent exception to this rule is the enigma of pregnancy, which has often been alluded to as Nature's allograft. The fetuses of outbred animals present to the mother an array of paternal transplantation antigens and are, therefore, alien to the mother. But fetuses are mysteriously protected by the mother and are not rejected. This paradox has continued to mystify biologists for a long time. An understanding of this phenomenon might serve to supplement our knowledge about cancer and allograft rejection (3).

It would be pretentious for us to state that we are attempting to prepare a comprehensive review of this field. For detailed reviews, the reader is referred to several of the articles available in the literature (4–7).

* We wish to thank Dr. Tom Wegmann and Dr. Phil Gambel for helpful suggestions and discussions, and Ms. Carla Cumming for expert secretarial assistance.

Medawar (8) pioneered the field when he observed that the conceptus was analogous to an allografted tissue and he extended some ingenious explanations for the success of the fetal allograft. (a) The uterus is an immunologically privileged site, protecting the fetus by bringing about a delay in either the recognition of the fetus as foreign or preventing the entry of maternal antibodies and sensitized cells into the fetus. (b) A maternal antifetal immune response is not triggered, because the conceptus is non-immunogenic. (c) The phenomenon of pregnancy involves an alteration in the maternal immune system, whereby maternal antifetal reactions are either weak or are absent. (d) The placenta is an immunologic barrier.

Some of these theories are not valid now as evinced by experimentations; but they do provide an excellent framework for elucidating the mechanisms preventing fetal rejection.

THE UTERUS AS AN IMMUNOLOGICALLY PRIVILEGED SITE

Tissues transplanted into a number of specialized sites in the body, such as the brain and the anterior chamber of the eye, survive for extended periods of time. This immunological privilege is due to a lack of vascular supply or drainage which prevents an immediate recognition of the foreign antigens in the grafted tissue by the immune system of the host (9). The privileged status of the hamster's cheek pouch, for example, is attributed to a lack of lymphatics connecting this site to the regional lymph nodes. It has been suggested that the fetal allograft might enjoy a similar privilege in the uterus, wherein the afferent or the efferent limb of the immune response is obstructed (10).

It has been demonstrated that tumor allografts transplanted into the uterine horn of pregnant, nonpregnant, and pseudopregnant female rats are promptly rejected (11). Transplantation immunity can be elicited by the intrauterine route; skin grafting and the transfer of leukocytes or lymph-node cells into the uterus sensitizes the host into rejecting a subsequent skin graft (12). Thus the nonpregnant uterus when exposed to allogeneic cells or skin allografts, is just as efficient a site for the elicitation and expression of an immune response, as the other sites in the body (13). It is clear that allogeneic embryos appear to be protected when transplanted into the uterus, while they are rejected when transplanted into ectopic sites in experimentally immunized female mice (14). Blastocysts from C57B1 matings transplanted to the kidney of specifically hyperimmunized C3H mice, were rejected. Autologous blastocysts similarly transferred developed properly. However C57B1 blastocysts transplanted to the uterus of hyperimmunized C3H mice developed successfully to term. Kirby (14) suggested that decidual tissue surrounding the embryonic graft protects the embryos from immunological attack, while those eggs transplanted to the extrauterine site are not afforded similar protection. In addition, lymphocytes injected into the uterus of nonpregnant mice can elicit systemic responses leading to an accelerated rejection of skin grafts; however, female mice are not sensitized by intrauterine injections during pregnancy. This suggests that physiologic or immunologic modifications occurring in the uterus during pregnancy could result in some sort of protection being afforded to the fetus (15).

A few other studies also suggest that decidual tissue in the uterus could form an immunologic or anatomic barrier during the early stages of gestation, before the placenta is established (7). Decidual tissue forms the maternal component of the placenta and it consists of large stromal cells. Interestingly there is evidence that decidual cells originate from the bone marrow of the mother (16), and this finding could have interesting implication in attributing an immunological function to the decidual cells in the uterus. Skin allografts placed on a decidualized uterine bed enjoy extended survival; however, the difference between this artificial allograft and pregnancy, is that adoptive immunization with sensitized lymphoid cells results in an accelerated rejection of the skin grafts, while similar treatments do not compromise pregnancy (17).

Therefore the maternal immune system can be sensitized via the intrauterine route, but the induction of a graft rejection reaction in this site is probably modified by anatomic, physiologic, endocrinologic, and/or immunologic components. The argument for an involvement of decidual cells in protecting the conceptus by rendering the uterus refractory to immunologic attack is strong. But this question has not yet been resolved satisfactorily (6). The uterus is clearly not a immunologically privileged site in the classical sense of the term as it was initially proposed by Medawar. Decidual tissue is vascularized and lymphatic vessels do permeate this tissue. Thus the uterus is unlike the anterior chamber of the brain or the eye lens. However, with evidence accumulating in favor of the placenta serving as an immunologic barrier (see below), it seems likely that the placenta might indeed confer a sort of immunologic privilege to the fetus.

ANTIGENICITY OF THE EMBRYO AND PLACENTA

Research in the field of fetal-maternal immunology has centered around the antigenic characteristics of the embryo, the nature of immune responses to the fetoplacental unit, the effect of these reactions on pregnancy, and the trafficking of cells and macromolecules across the placenta. The central issue is the antigenicity of the embryo and placenta.

After the ovum is fertilized by sperm, it is quarantined within the zona pellucida, and the fertilized egg undergoes a series of developmental changes before the blastocyst is ready for implantation. The blastocyst consists of an outer trophectoderm layer, an inner cluster of cells called the inner cell mass, and the blastocoele cavity. The trophectoderm differentiates into the trophoblastic elements of the placenta after the blastocyst implants itself on the uterine wall. The trophoblast and the maternal decidua together comprise the definitive placenta and the major interface between mother and fetus is located at the junction of the maternal decidua and the fetal placenta. At no time during gestation is the fetus directly in contact with either maternal blood or maternal tissue.

A proportion of primiparous females and a much higher proportion of multiparous females in a variety of species manifest immune responses directed against fetal and placental antigens, indicating the presence of antigens, foreign to the mother in the conceptus. Direct investigations into the antigenicity of embryonic tissues have resulted in a firm consensus that the embryo is antigenically mature and does express antigens that are foreign to the mother. The study of the cell surface markers on embryonic tissue is significant not only in understanding the fetal-maternal relationship, but it may also be crucial to the processes of early differentiation, embryonic development, and the oncogenetic aspects of biology (19). Antigens of interest could be categorized into (a) paternal histocompatibility antigens (b) tissue-specific antigens of the placenta, and (c) oncofetal antigens.

Histocompatibility Antigens

Simmons and Russell (20) demonstrated that 7-day mouse embryos were rapidly rejected when transplanted to the kidney capsule of sensitized animals. They inferred the presence of alloantigens on the embryo. Since then many investigators have examined the expression of paternal H-2, minor H-2, and non-H-2 transplantation antigens by the embryo and placenta at different stages during ontogeny. The surface of the two-cell stage embryo is devoid of both major and nonmajor histocompatibility antigens. Heyner et al. (21, 22) suggested that this lack of antigenicity might serve to explain how the embryo eludes recognition by the maternal immune system. Paternal H-2 antigens appear first around day 4 in the inner cell mass of preimplantation blastocysts as demonstrated by indirect immunofluorescence (23) and transplantation studies (24) and these antigens were reported as being absent from the surface of the preimplantation embryo (23, 24). Webb et al. (25) observed that only the inner cell mass is capable of synthesizing H-2 antigens in the late blastocyst. Major histocompatibility antigens on the preimplantation stage blastocyst disappear at the onset of implantation (26). Even though

MHC antigens constitute the major antigenic system with regard to graft rejection, other alloantigenic systems have been elucidated, which are capable of provoking potentially harmful responses in allograft experiments. Muggleton-Harris and Johnson (27) have demonstrated the presence of minor histocompatibility alloantigens on both the inner cell mass and the trophectoderm. Non-H-2 antigens are consistently demonstrable during early embryogenesis; paternal non-H-2 antigens appear first at the six to eight cell stage (28).

The placenta and the outermost fetal membranes, and not the embryo itself, are juxtaposed in intimate and continuous contact with the potentially hostile maternal environment and, therefore, the antigenic status of the definitive placenta, of the trophoblast in particular, is perhaps of supreme importance. The ectoplacental cone (EPC) of the postimplantation murine embryo continues to proliferate and differentiate into the definitive trophoblast, which consists of three components: the labyrinthine trophoblast in contact with maternal blood, the spongiotrophoblast in contact with maternal decidua, and the trophoblastic giant cells.

H-2 and non-H-2 antigens were expressed on 13-day placental cells as demonstrated by the mixed hemadsorption assay (20), and the trophoblast cells were identified as being H-2 positive by microscopic examination of the cell types involved. Using an *in-vivo* model, Wegmann et al. (30) demonstrated that the allogeneic murine placenta does express paternally derived H-2 antigens in a manner accessible to the maternal circulation and this was confirmed using a monoclonal antipaternal H-2K antibody (31), in order to represent alloantigen expression in quantitative terms. Wegmann et al. (32) performed quantitative binding studies *in vivo* to estimate the density of paternal H-2K antigens per gram placenta from day 10 until day 17 of gestation (33). Recent experiments have also provided evidence for the presence of paternally derived H-2D antigens on the allogeneic placenta (34). Radioautographic analyses of placentas after the injection of the radiolabeled anti-H-2K antibody into the tail veins of target and control pregnant mice revealed the presence of paternal antigen-bearing cells in the spongy zone of the trophoblast and in the parietal endoderm in the yolk sac plexus (35). These results correlate with those obtained by the *in vitro* studies of Jenkinson and Owen (36) suggesting that it is the spongiotrophoblast cell population, and not the labyrinthine cell population that is primarily responsible for the antigenic characteristics of the placenta. Chatterjee-Hasrouni and Lala (37) have demonstrated the expression of paternal H-2 antigens by the trophoblast cell component of the placenta by employing a quantitative radioautographic technique on placental cell suspensions. These three major studies serve to establish the presence of paternally-derived H-2 antigens on the placenta, and particularly in the trophoblast at the fetal-maternal interface.

In contrast to the expression of paternal H-2K and H-2D antigens, the placenta appears to be devoid of I-region coded determinants. Delovitch et al. (38) carried out sensitive immunoprecipitation techniques which indicated that Ia antigens appeared only around day 11 of gestation and, furthermore, appeared to be limited to the liver until day 16. Studies conducted by Jenkinson and Searle (39) revealed that Ia antigens are absent from selected preimplantation and postimplantation embryonic and trophoblastic tissues. Recent studies performed by Chatterjee-Hasrouni and Lala (40, 41) demonstrate the absence of paternal I-region defined antigens despite the presence of H-2K and H-2D antigens, on mouse trophoblast cells *in vitro*. Employing an *in vivo* model Reghupathy et al. (33) were unable to detect paternal I-A antigens on the placenta.

The configuration of paternal alloantigenic determinants on the placenta at the fetal-maternal interface has been suggested to be of great significance with regard to maternal immunorecognition of her *alien conceptus* (42). We shall deal with the possible involvement of these alloantigens in manipulating maternal immune responses in a later section of this chapter.

The situation in the human is more complicated. The syncytiotrophoblast in humans forms the boundary of the maternal-fetal interface and it is at this junction that the fetal and maternal tissues are in actual contact. Goodfellow et al. (43) examined purified preparations of placental plasma membranes and were able to demonstrate paternally-derived HLA-A and HLA-B antigens, albeit at lower levels than on splenic lymphocytes. They suggested that the syncytiotrophoblast probably lacks these antigens. Ia antigens were not demonstrable. Using a mixed agglutination assay and antibody absorption techniques, Seigler and Metzgar (44) observed that human trophoblast syncytium was devoid of HLA antigens, but demonstrated that fetal tissues possess HLA antigens at 6 weeks of gestation. Immunofluorescent and immunoperoxidase studies by Faulk and his co-workers (45, 46) demonstrated that while cells of the chorionic villi do express HLA antigens, the trophoblast lacks these antigens. Thus it is possible that only the nontrophoblastic components of the human placenta express paternal HLA antigens; while the outer syncytiotrophoblast cells are devoid of HLA alloantigens. Two studies, however, have resulted in positive findings. Loke at al. (47) reported the presence of HLA antigens on the trophoblast villi. Montgomery and Lala (48) have recently performed sensitive radioautographic analyses which revealed weak but positive specific labeling for HLA-A, -B, and -C antigens on 7 to 8 week old trophoblast cells. However, the possibility of contamination of nontrophoblastic placental cells cannot be ruled out. It appears that the human placenta does express paternal HLA antigens, but it remains to be unequivocally established that the human trophoblast is not deficient in HLA alloantigens.

When the question of homograft rejection of the conceptus is considered, the antigenic status of the placenta is most relevant because the placental tissues constitute the initial and major focus of any immunologic interaction. Though early studies did report an apparent deficiency of foreign antigens on the placenta, it is now clear that paternal histocompatibility antigens and other antigenic components are expressed on the placenta disproving the early model of placental antigenic anonymity. The human situation awaits clarification and there may well be a species difference insofar as antigenicity of the placenta is concerned.

Organ/Tissue-Specific Antigens

Tissues like the testis, brain, and eye lens express tissue-specific antigens that are normally sequestered from the immune system, and to which the system can respond immunologically, if the barriers are breached. The placental organ or tissue-specific antigens form another antigenic system of interest in elucidating maternal-fetal interactions.

Wiley and Calarco (49) raised antibodies to the mouse placenta, and those antibodies bound specifically to the blastocyst trophectoderm and not to the embryonic ectoderm of the inner cell mass. These studies indicated the existence of trophectoderm/trophoblast-specific antigens even during the early stages of gestation. The presence of tissue-specific antigens on the trophoblast, during the later stages of gestation has been reviewed extensively by Beer and Billingham (50). Faulk et al. (51) generated heterologeous antitrophoblast antibodies to purified human trophoblast membranes, and these antibodies reacted specifically with trophoblastic tissues and not with adult tissues.

A variety of placenta-associated and placenta-specific substances have been described (52), but most of these proteins await proper characterization. A series of proteins, Placental Proteins (PPI-6) and a few other minor proteins has been identified, but the relationship between the antigenicity of these proteins and the fetal-maternal relationship is unknown at present (6). Faulk et al. (53) serologically defined two trophoblast antigens in the human placenta. Antigen TA_1 cross-reacts with antigens on some human cell lines (eg., HeLa, Human amnion) and TA_2 is shared with lymphocytes. TA_1 and anti-TA_1 antibodies inhibit mixed leukocyte reactions (MLR) *in vitro*. Whether pregnant women recognize these antigens as foreign and react immunologically to these proteins, is not known.

Oncofetal Antigens

In addition to its invasive properties, the trophoblast seems to share some other characteristics with malignant tissues, such as common antigenic determinants and presence of several hormones (4, 19, 54–56). These hormones and antigens also termed as *neogen* (19) pose yet another potentially antigenic stimulus to the mother.

Rabbit antiserum raised against teratoma 402X cells, after appropriate absorptions to eliminate antimouse reactivity, could react with mouse embryos (57). Similarly, antibodies directed against a teratocarcinoma line could bind to the inner cell mass and trophectoderm of blastocysts, demonstrating the presence of neogens on the early embryo (58). The F9 antigen (or the F9 group of antigens) is the prototypical neogen and it is expressed by a number of species (59). The F9 antigen is expressed on the 2-cell mouse embryo and is present on the ICM until day 10 of gestation, while it disappears from the trophectoderm after day 4 (60). This antigen is only one example of a neogen, but a variety of other embryonic antigens exist, which cross-react with tumor-associated antigens, and are perhaps not expressed by normal, adult somatic cells (61). Ray and Seshadri (62) have demonstrated that immunization of animals with 14 to 15-day-old embryos induces the development of an antitumor response in syngeneic animals. Immunized animals were able to inhibit the growth of dimethylbenz-dithionaphthene-induced fibrosarcomas in tumor-transplant studies, while spleen cells and sera from immunized animals manifested tumor-killing capabilities in adoptive transfer experiments. Ray et al. (63) have also demonstrated that Swiss mice embryos and sarcoma-180 ascites tumors share two types of antigens; histocompatibility antigens and a common oncofetal antigen. Tumor-associated antifetal antibody activity has been demonstrated in normal human pregnancy (64).

Thus the placenta confronts the maternal immune system with an array of antigens. What then protects the placenta from being attacked by the maternal immune surveillance mechanisms? The trophoblast would be expected to be endowed with unique immunological properties and perhaps diverse immunoregulatory capabilities in order to help avoid rejection by the mother. The ingenious mechanisms by which the placenta could do this will be discussed.

MATERNAL IMMUNE RESPONSES AGAINST HER CONCEPTUS

Medawar implied that maternal immunocompetence was decreased during pregnancy, but it now seems clear that there is no alteration in the intrinsic reactivity and function of lymphocytes (4, 5) even though a few studies have reported a decreased immunoreactivity during pregnancy.

The fetoplacental unit confronts the mother with a variety of antigens throughout gestation and there is some evidence for the transfer of fetal cells across the placenta into the mother. Hence, the maternal immune system is provoked into making antibodies and cellular responses directed at fetal and placental antigens.

The antigens most immunogenic to the mother appear to be the paternally inherited MHC antigens and red blood cell antigens of the fetus. Antipaternal HLA-A and HLA-B antibodies are detectable at about the same levels. The incidence and titers of these antibodies increase with parity. These antibodies are of the leucoagglutinating and/or cytotoxic variety (65, 66) and are capable of inhibiting mixed leukocyte reactions (MLR) *in vitro* indicating the possible influence of these antibodies in preventing stimulation between maternal lymphocytes and paternal antigens on fetal lymphoid cells (65). Cytotoxic antipaternal HLA-DR antibodies (66) and antihuman Ia-like antibodies (67) have also been identified. Cytotoxic and hemagglutinating antibodies directed against H-2 alloantigens are detectable in pregnant mice (68, 69) and these responses appear to be strain dependent (70). Antibodies directed at the A, B, and H blood group antigens have been described in human pregnancies (71), and erythroblastosis fetalis caused by the passage of anti-Rh antibodies into an RH-positive fetus is a well known phenomenon (72). These anti-RBC antibodies are cytotoxic in most cases, but it is possible that these antibodies could mediate an attack on fetal red cells by opsonization or by antibody-dependent cell-mediated cytotoxicity (ADCC). Apparently, spontaneous abortions and fetal wastage syndromes often involve only the RBC antigens (73) and not the HLA antigens even though there have been a few isolated studies implicating anti-HLA antibodies as the etiologic agents in congenital abnormalities of the newborn (74). Therefore it is not possible to draw unequivocal conclusions regarding the relationship between anti-HLA antibodies and fetal abnormalities. The presence of cytotoxic and agglutinating anti-H-Y antibodies has been shown in multiparous female mice (75) and rats (76).

In the previous section we have discussed the expression of placental tissue-specific and tissue-associated antigens. That some of these antigens are immunogenic to the mother has been evinced by studies demonstrating the presence of antibodies to trophoblast antigens (77, 78).

Cell-mediated responses against fetoplacental antigens appear to be infrequent and are not demonstrable with ease. Cellular antifetal responses in human pregnancies are manifested as cytotoxic T lymphocytes directed against fetal antigens (79) and placental antigens (80), and they have also been demonstrated by MLR assays (81, 82, 83) and by leukocyte migration inhibition tests (84). Youtananukorn and Matangkasombut (85) have demonstrated that pregnant women are regularly sensitized to placental antigens. In mice, cellular responses towards paternal H-2 antigens have been measured by cytotoxicity assays (86), graft-versus-host reactions (87), and MLR, and it is clear that maternal cells are weakly reactive against paternal antigens. Specific reactivity between maternal lymphocytes and fetal antigens in mice has been demonstrated using a colony inhibition assay. Chaouat et al. (89) have reported the existence of immune cells specific to paternal alloantigens in the spleens of pregnant mice.

If indeed the maternal immune system responds to the genetically alien conceptus by making antibodies and cellular reactions, what are the mechanisms preventing these humoral and cellular effectors from mediating an attack on the placenta and the fetus? A variety of hypotheses have been proposed: (a) The trophoblast appears to be somewhat inert and refractory to the attack by maternal immune components. (b) The capacity of the trophoblast to elude maternal immune effectors, in spite of its antigenicity could be partly attributable to the fibrinoid-like mucoprotein which is intimately associated with the trophoblast cell surface. Human trophoblast cells possess a membrane-bound mucoprotein coat (91). (c) An acid mucopolysaccharide has been described as covering the placental microvilli (92). The suggestion of a siolomucoprotein layer posing an impermeable barrier, has been contradicted by the studies of Simmons et al. (93) who demonstrated that trophoblast cells incubated in neuraminidase, do not sensitize all allogeneic mice to donor histocompatibility antigens. Furthermore, pretreatment of trophoblast implants with neuraminidase did not interfere with proliferation and growth in highly immunized allogeneic recipients. High doses of neuraminidase (500 units/ml) could inhibit trophoblast growth even in syngeneic recipients, while lower doses (125 to 250 units/ml) which are sufficient to increase the immunogenicity of mouse lymphoid cells do not affect trophoblast immunogenicity. These authors speculate that since neuraminidase does not appear to expose any paternal antigens, the trophoblast does not express adequate quantities of histocompatibility antigens on its surface. Recent studies (see above) however have clearly demonstrated the presence of paternal antigens on the placenta. Taylor et al. (94) have shown that while normal mouse ectoplacental cone trophoblast cells are capable of eliciting some degree of transplantation immunity, treatment with neuraminidase increased this to a level comparable to that induced by spleen cells, presumably by disruption of cell-surface sialomucoprotein masking the transplantation antigens. These studies were performed using 500 units/ml of neuarminidase, as this concentration preserved trophoblast viability as judged by the exclusion of trypan blue. This mucoprotein layer has been postulated to inhibit not the recognition event, but the effector limb of the immune response arc, by rendering the trophoblast cells negatively charged and thereby repulsing the negatively charged lymphocytes.

Transferrin receptors have been identified on the syncytial surface of human trophoblasts and it has been postulated that these receptors may be involved in the immunoregulation of the maternal immune system by inhibiting maternal immune reactions (95).

Hellström and Hellström (96) ascribed a shielding role for blocking antibodies in protecting antigenic tumor cells from sensitized lymphoid cells of the host. Similarly, the presence of blocking or enhancing antibodies to trophoblast or placental antigens has been suggested as being immunologically protective for the placenta. Blocking antibodies have been identified in multiparous mice (97) and in pregnant women (98). In the antioncofetal immune response system of Ray et al. (63) spleen cells from pregnant mice injected into tumor-bearing animals could cause a decrease in the growth rate of the tumor, but sera from these pregnant mice also contained blocking activity against the corresponding spleen cells. Bell and Billington (99) have reported that the majority of the antipaternal antibodies in pregnant mice are of the noncytotoxic IgG subclass and, therefore, these antibodies might mediate efferent enhancement after binding to the antigens on the placenta, thereby preventing injurious attack by cytotoxic antibodies and sensitized cells.

Furthermore, it has been clearly demonstrated that IgG antibodies constitute one of the factors responsible for the inhibition of mixed lymphocyte reactions observed with maternal serum (100). Immunoglobulins of maternal origin have been immunochemically eluted from the placenta (101) and these immunoglobulins have been shown to be potent inhibitors of mixed lymphocyte reactions (102). Immune complexes have been reported as probably being protective agents in the sera of tumor-bearing hosts (103) and they have also been identified in pregnancy (104, 105) and a role similar to that performed by blocking antibodies has been postulated.

While most of these hypotheses have yet to be substantiated by relevant experiments, it is conceivable that one or more of these suggested mechanisms may actually contribute to the success of the fetal allograft.

ROLE OF THE PLACENTA IN FETAL MATERNAL INTERACTIONS

Fetal-Maternal Trafficking, Placental Antigens, and Maternal Immunostimulation

It is relevant at this stage to address the crucial question: what are the agents responsible for stimulating the maternal immune system into making immune responses directed against fetal antigens? The likely candidates are fetal cells and soluble antigens and the placenta itself. It is the placenta, particularly components of the fetally-derived trophoblast, which are actually juxtaposed with maternal tissue and are bathed in maternal blood. Hence the placenta is likely to be the major immunogenic component of the conceptus.

In addition, it is important to ascertain whether fetal lymphoid cells and macromolecules can traverse the placenta, in adequate quantities to provide sufficient immunogenic stimulus. Obviously, fetal RBC do cross the placenta during pregnancy as evinced by the phonomenon of Rh disease, where fetal Rh-positive red cells sensitize Rh-negative mothers into making an anti-Rh(D) antibody response which is detrimental to subsequent Rh-positive fetuses. Though the proportion of women receiving fetal RBC during pregnancy is not high (5 to 20%), the frequency is higher at delivery (5 to 50%). Small amounts of fetal blood containing lymphocytes (106) and RBC have been reported to find their way into maternal blood before parturition (107–109). A number of studies have employed the procedure of scanning maternal blood samples for putative male fetal cells detectable by quinacrine staining of the F. body and the results have been confusing and contradictory, and as such have not permitted unequivocal conclusions to be drawn from them. Herzenberg et al. (110) employed elegant immunogenic and cell-sorting techniques to examine maternal blood for the presence of fetal cells. Using immunogenic and cytogenetic criteria they established the existence of fetal cells in human maternal blood during pregnancy. However, one cannot rule out the remote possibility that these fetal cells originated from a previous pregnancy at parturition, when fetal blood is often disseminated into maternal circulation. It needs to be emphasized that the amount of immunogenic material i.e., the number of antigen-bearing fetal cells entering maternal circulation is far more important than the mere presence of fetal cells in the pregnant female. It has not been possible as yet to ascertain whether the fetal cells coming into contact with maternal blood do indeed constitute an adequate immunogenic stimulus.

Lawler et al. (111) have demonstrated the presence of anti-HLA antibodies in sera after molar pregnancies. This suggests that the mother need not be exposed to allogeneic fetal cells in order to mount a response against fetal antigens and it is, therefore, likely that the placenta provides the major immunogenic stimulus to the mother. The unique antigenic characteristics of the placenta could conceivably play a highly important role in maternal immunostimulation. The type and intensity of immune responses engendered in the mother are far more important than the mere presence or absence of an immune response in pregnancy. Cell-mediated reactions are crucial in allograft rejection and cell-mediated antifetal responses in pregnancy do not appear to be strong, nor are these responses frequent. Hence, it would be to the advantage of the fetus for the placenta to be able to manipulate the type of immune responses elicited in the mother. In mice it is clear that the placenta expresses class I paternal MHC antigens and is devoid of paternal class II MHC antigens and this peculiar configuration could play an important role by eliciting enhancing antibodies in preference to a detrimental cytotoxic cellular reaction. I-region determined antigenic differences between stimulator and responder cells appear to be essential in the MLR, as a difference in only the K or the D region stimulates very weak or no reactions (112). Billington (113) suggests that a prolonged low dose release of relatively weak antigen would serve to induce immunological enhancement. The placenta and the fetus would seem likely to offer this form of stimulus. Low density expression of paternal H-2 antigens has been demonstrated in the studies of Chatterjee-Hasrouni and Lala (37). Therefore it seems quite possible that the dual criteria of a low level expression of H-2K and H-2D antigens and a lack of I-region determinants are satisfied in this case with the result that only a humoral response is elicited in pregnancy, while strong cellular antifetal responses are avoided. Furthermore, these antigens on the placenta might preferentially induce an enhancing antibody response versus a potentially harmful cytotoxic antibody response. A dominance of enhancing antibodies would not only ensure the inaccessibility of cytotoxic antibodies to the antigen-bearing cells in the placenta, but would also mask the antigens and render them inaccessible to cytotoxic cells in case cell-mediated antifetal/ antiplacental responses are generated. In any case, there appears to be a failsafe mechanism, since it seems likely that the placenta might serve as an immunologic barrier (if not an anatomic barrier) to the entry of the maternal cells and this is discussed below.

The Placenta as an Antibody Filter

Even though enhancing antibodies could constitute the major alloantibody response in pregnancy, one cannot overlook the fact that cytotoxic antibodies are generated in pregnancy, as evinced by human and animal experiments. Cytotoxic T cells are not seen consistently during allogeneic pregnancy, but are generated in a proportion of the pregnancies. In a previous section we have discussed possible mechanisms which the placenta might employ to elude these effector mechanisms. It is now pertinent to question whether these effectors can traverse the placenta and gain access to the fetus.

   A number of studies have focused on the transplacental passage of macromolecules and cells from the mother to the fetus. Molecules are transported across the placenta in a selective manner and the transplacental transfer of beneficial maternal antibodies to the fetus is essential for conferring immunity to the fetus, against a variety of infections. Since maternal IgG antibodies can traverse the placenta, it is conceivable that potentially lethal antibodies may enter fetal circulation too. There have been sporadic reports implicating transplacentally transferred antibodies in neutropenia in humans (114, 115, 116) and anti-HLA antibodies have been reported to cause congenital abnormalities (74). These studies are isolated and more convincing data are required before any conclusions can be drawn regarding the transplacental passage of antifetal (antipaternal) antibodies to the fetus. Swinburne (117) postulated that paternal alloantigens on the placenta could confer on the placenta an immunoabsorbent capacity, by virtue of which the placenta could function as a specific immunologic filter, obstructing the passage of potentially deleterious antibodies to the fetus, while allowing beneficial maternal antibodies to get through. In humans, antipaternal HLA antibodies found in maternal circulation are not found in the fetal blood, if the fetus bears the same haplotype; these antibodies can be eluted off the placenta. However, if the fetus lacks the appropriate antigens, these antibodies are not found in placental eluates, but are detectable in cord blood (118, 119). These and other studies suggest that cytotoxic antifetal antibodies are absent in the neonatal blood perhaps because of sequestration in the placenta (121). Raghupathy et al. (33) have demonstrated that radiolabeled monoclonal antipaternal H-2K antibody injected into allogeneically and syngeneically pregnant mice are dealt with differently by the allogeneic and syngeneic placentas. These antibodies reach the fetuses of the nontarget control pregnancies in much higher concentrations than the fetuses bearing the target antigens, i.e., the allogeneic fetuses. The allogeneic target placentas take up dramatically higher levels of the radiolabeled antipaternal antibody than do the syngeneic control placentas. This study provides formal evidence that the placenta serves as a specific immunoabsorbent barrier to the entry of antifetal antibodies. In the human placenta, paternal HLA antigen-bearing cells in the chorionic villi could serve to absorb anti-HLA antigens. In any case, after binding the antibody the antigen-bearing cells could pinocytose the antibodies which are then conceivably digested. The alternative fate of this antibody could be released from the cells in the form of antigen-antibody complexes, and macrophages within the villous core bearing Fc and C3 receptors may function as scavengers by eliminating these complexes. The net result would be to prevent these antibodies from gaining access to the fetal circulation. Fetal Gm antigens are expressed within the chorionic villi of human placenta (122) and Faulk (123) speculates that the chorionic villi could serve as an immunoabsorbent barrier for a variety of antibodies. It thus seems likely that the placenta might render a sort of immunologic privilege or sanctuary to the fetus for survival until parturition.

Maternal-Fetal Trafficking

After having dealt with the passage of immunoglobulins across the placenta, we can now address the question, can maternal cells traverse the placenta and enter fetal circulation? Maternal XX lymphocytes have been identified in XY male offspring (125, 126), but it is difficult to conclude from these experiments that these cells did enter the fetus by traversing the placenta and that they were not transferred to the fetus via the colostrum. Desai and Creger (106), however, provide evidence for the passage of maternal lymphocytes and platelets across the placenta, but it has been reported that the passage of maternal leukocytes to the fetus is lower than claimed (127). In mice there are conflicting results, some investigators claim that maternal cells do traverse the placenta to enter the fetus (128), while Billington et al. (129) were unable to substantiate these findings. Beer and Billingham (130) reported the runting of neonates by provoking a graft-versus-host reaction in the pregnant mother and suggested that the runting observed in the 2-week-old neonates implied a transplacental passage of maternal effector lymphocytes. Actually it is possible that these effector cells were transferred to the suckling neonate via the colostrum and not via the placenta. Further, there is no evidence in this study to clearly show that maternal lymphocytes had indeed gained access to the neonates. In fact, a number of studies clearly demonstrate that the fetuses develop normally in spite of the mother being strongly sensitized to fetal antigens by paternal skin grafting (131, 132, 133).

Thus maternal leukocytes do not appear to gain access to the fetal circulation in large numbers and it is highly likely that the placental barrier prevents the access of all but a few maternal lymphocytes into the fetus. In fact, it is tempting to conceive of a situation wherein the placenta could serve as an efficient antifetal alloreactive cell-trapping mechanism much as it serves as an antibody filter.

In retrospect it would appear that the placenta, by virtue of its remarkable immunologic characteristics, could render the uterus an immunologically privileged site, even though as mentioned earlier, the classic immunologically privileged site model is not valid.

Immunoregulation and Immunosuppression in Pregnancy

One of the simplest explanations extended for the success of the fetal allograft is that the immune system of the pregnant female is systemically suppressed, as a consequence of which she is supposedly rendered incapable of generating deleterious antifetal immune reactions. Such a generalized nonspecific immunosuppression might be conducive to fatal infections, but there is no evidence for increased susceptibility to diseases during pregnancy. Pavia and Stites (134) clearly demonstrated a lack of systemic immunosuppression in pregnancy. Pregnancy does not prolong allograft survival in mice (135).

A multitude of protein and steroid hormones are elaborated by the conceptus during pregnancy and conceivably any of these factors could exercise a modulating influence on the activity of the immune cells during pregnancy. The manner in which these factors probably suppress deleterious reactions is by bringing about an effector blockade of sensitized maternal cells, because maternal cellular effectors can be and are stimulated during pregnancy. Immunosuppressive and immunoregulatory capabilities have been ascribed to hCG, human placental lactogen, glucocorticosteroids, alphafetoprotein, and progesterone (136, 137). Most of these factors have been scrutinized only in *in vitro* systems; caution must be exercised in extrapolating *in vitro* experimental findings to the all-important *in vivo* situation, and until these factors are experimentally shown to have *in vivo* capabilities, they have to be viewed with suspicion. Recent evidence suggests that the immunosuppressant activity reported to hCG is actually due to contaminating proteins, either immunoglobulins (138), nonimmunoglobulin factors (139), or of undetermined character (140). Therefore, while some immunosuppressive activity is observed *in vitro* with hCG, for example (14), the *in vivo* role of such hormones and factors is only speculation.

   In vivo and *in vitro* experiments conducted by Siiteri et al. (142) demonstrate that progesterone is capable of inhibiting inflammatory responses and prolonging the survival of skin allografts in rats. They postulated that progesterone is involved in the maintenance of pregnancy, by bringing about local immunosuppression in the vicinity of the conceptus. Progesterone is synthesized and secreted by the trophoblast in all mammalian species. High tissue concentrations of this hormone are postulated to mediate suppression of cell-mediated immune reactions against the fetus. Beer and Billingham (143) were able to extend the survival periods of skin allografts in rats, by placing silastic tubes containing progesterone over the grafts. The tissue and serum levels were reported to be equivalent to midpregnancy levels in these experiments and, therefore, these investigators suggest that progesterone is one of the factors responsible for the success of the fetal allograft by blocking the efferent limb of the immunologic reflex arc. Kitzmiller and Rocklin (144) found that estradiol, progesterone, and hCG do not suppress lymphocyte reactivity, as assessed by the production of lymphokines or the target cell response to the mediator, in the presence of these hormones. These workers, therefore, doubt a physiological role for placental steroid hormones as modulators of maternal responsiveness. Also, if higher concentrations of these hormones in the placenta were to be active, then only the effector immune response would have to be inhibited.

   Alphafetoprotein is another candidate for immunoregulation and is normally present in amniotic fluid and fetal blood. Murgita et al. (145) reported that AFP decreased lymphocyte responsiveness to mitogens, and it decreased MLR activities. Interestingly, AFP also appears to activate suppressor cells. However, it is important to obtain objective proof for these postulates by *in vivo* experimentation. Until then one cannot make unequivocal conclusions regarding the efficacy and the precise roles of these and the various other factors in pregnancy. Suffice it to say now that it is quite possible that pregnancy-specific and pregnancy-associated factors and hormones could be involved in local immunosuppression.

Local active suppression, perhaps of a nonspecific nature, mediated by immunocompetent maternal cells could be active in pregnancy; Clark and McDermott (146) have reported the presence of suppressor cells in the lymph nodes draining the uterus and these nonspecific suppressor cells could play a role in maintaining the integrity of pregnancy. This area has been dealt with in detail by Dr. David Clark in another chapter of this book.

SUMMARY

A study of this and other recent reviews reflects the state of flux the field of fetal-maternal immunology is in. Results of experiments in this area are often inconsistent and the experiments are sometimes irreproducible, with the result that it is often difficult to arrive at unequivocal conclusions regarding the factors responsible for ensuring the success of pregnancy.

This field has however advanced a great deal since Medawar's theories were put forth. The primary factors responsible for the success of pregnancy seem quite clear. The induction of cytotoxic antifetal antibodies does not appear to be appreciably strong and blocking or enhancing antibodies could conceivably inhibit or at least diminish the activity of cytotoxic antibodies. It is also clear that the generation of antifetal cellular responses is not consistent and is certainly not strong. The presence on the murine placenta of paternal H-2K and H-2D antigens, perhaps in low concentrations, combined with the absence of paternal Ia antigens, is postulated as being responsible for this anomalous immune response seen in pregnancy (12). At the same time, experimental stimulation of the maternal immune system to induce antifetal responses does not compromise pregnancy and there may be something inherent in the nature of the placenta which makes it refractory to attack and also by which the placenta may protect the fetus by serving as an anatomic or perhaps an immunologic barrier. By virtue of these properties and the ability of the placenta to serve as an immunoabsorbent for antipaternal H-2 antibodies, the placenta may actually render the fetal milieu somewhat immunologically privileged. The decidualized uterus, antigenic modulation by the trophoblast, immunosuppression in the vicinity of the conceptus, and the immunologic barrier-like characteristics of the placenta appear to be the most prominent of the mechanisms ensuring the nonrejection of the fetal allograft.

We have made considerable progress in understanding the immunology of pregnancy and we are perhaps not very far from the day when we can claim to understand this enigma completely. But the solution at this moment, to quote Loke (4), "remains tantalisingly beyond reach."

REFERENCES

1. Gorer, P. A., *J. Pathol. Bacteriol.* **47**:231, 1938.
2. Medawar, P. B., *J. Anat.* **78**:176, 1944.
3. Finn, R., and St. Hill, C. A., *Brit. Med. J.* **1**:1671, 1978.
4. Loke, Y. W., *Immunology and Immunopathology of the Human Fetal-Maternal Interactions.* New York: Elsevier/North Holland, 1978.
5. Rocklin, R. E., Kitzmiller, J. L., and Kaye, M. D., *Ann. Rev. Med.* **30**:375, 1979.
6. Gill, T. J., and Repetti, C. F., *Amer. J. Pathol.* **95**:465, 1979.
7. Edwards, R. G., and Coombs, R. R. A. In R. Gell, R. R. A. Coombs, and L. Lachman (Eds.), *Clinical Aspects of Immunology*, p. 561. Oxford: Blackwell Scientific, 1975.
8. Medawar, P. B., *Symp. Soc. Exp. Biol.* **7**:320, 1954.
9. Billingham, R. E., and Silvers, W. K., *Proc. Roy. Soc. Biol.* **61**:168, 1964.
10. Billingham, R. E., *N. Engl. J. Med.*, **270**:667, 1964.
11. Schlesinger, M., *J. Natl. Cancer Inst.* **28**:927, 1962.
12. Beer, A. E., and Billingham, R. E., *J. Reprod. Fertil.* **21**:59, 1974.
13. Edwards, R. G. In *Immunology of Reproduction*. London: International Planned Parenthood Federation, 1969.
14. Kirby, D. R. S. In F. T. Rapaport and J. Dausset (Eds.), *Human Transplantation*, p. 565. New York: Grune and Stratton, 1968.
15. Beer, A. E., and Billingham, R. E. In *Ontogeny of Acquired Immunity*, p. 149. North Holland: Excerpta Medica, 1972.
16. Kearns, M., and Lala, P. K., *J.Exp. Med.* **155**:1537, 1982.
17. Beer, A. E., and Billingham, R. E., *The Immunobiology of Mammalian Reproduction*. New Jersey: Prentice Hall, 1976.
18. Little, C. C., *J. Cancer Res.* **8**:75, 1924.
19. Heyner, S. In D. Dhindsa and G. F. B. Schumacher (Eds.), *Immunological Aspects of Fertility and Fertility Regulation*, p. 183. Amsterdam: Elsevier/North Holland, 1980.
20. Simmons, R. L., and Russell, P. S., *Ann. N.Y. Acad. Sci.* **129**:35,1966.
21. Heyner, S., and Hunziker, R. D., *Dev. Genet.* **3**:1, 1969.
22. Heyner, S., Hunziker, R. D., and Zink, G. L., *J. Reprod. Immunol.* **2**:269, 1980.
23. Heyner, S., *Transplant.* **16**:675, 1973.
24. Patthey, H. C., and Edidin, M., *Transplant.* **15**:211, 1973.
25. Webb, C. G., Gall, W. E., and Edelman, G., *J.Exp. Med.* **146**:923, 1977.
26. Hakansson, S., Heyner, S., et al., *Internatl. J. Fertil.* **3**:20, 1975.
27. Muggelton-Harris, A. L., and Johnson, M. H., *J. Embryol. Exp. Morphol.* **35**:59, 1976.
28. Heyner, S., Brinster, R. L., and Palm, J., *Nature* **22**:783, 1969.
29. Sellens, M. H., Jenkinson, E. J., and Billington, W. D., *Transplant.* **25**:173, 1978.
30. Wegmann, T. G., Singh, B., and Carlson, G. A., *J. Immunol.* **122**:270, 1979.
31. Wegmann, T. G., Mosmann, T. R., et al., *J. Immunol.* **123**:1020, 1979.
32. Wegmann, T. G., Barrington, L. J., et al., *J. Reprod. Immunol.* **2**:53, 1980.
33. Raghupathy, R., Singh, B., et al., *J. Immunol.* **127**:2074, 1981.
34. Raghupathy, R., *Expression and Relevance of Paternal MHC Antigens on the Murine Placenta*. Ph.D. Theses. University of Alberta, 1982.
35. Anderson, D. J., Sandow, B. A., Raghupathy, R., et al., *J. Reprod. Immunol.* In Press, 1983.

36. Jenkinson, E. J., and Owen, V., *J. Reprod. Immunol.* **2**:173, 1980.
37. Chatterjee-Hasrouni, S., and Lala, P. K., *J. Exp. Med.* **149**:1238, 1979.
38. Delovitch, T., Press, J. L., and McDevitt, H. O., *J. Immunol.* **120**:818, 1979.
39. Jenkinson, E. J., and Searle, R. F., *J. Reprod. Immunol.* **1**:3, 1979.
40. Chatterjee-Hasrouni, S., and Lala, P. K., *J. Exp. Med.* 1982, In Press.
41. Chatterjee-Hasrouni, S., and Lala, P. K., *J. Immunol.* **127**:2070, 1981.
42. Wegmann, T. G., *J. Reprod. Immunol.* **3**:261, 1981.
43. Goodfellow, P. N., Barnstable, C. J., Bodmer, W. F., et al., *Transplant.* **22**:595, 1976.
44. Seigler, H. G., and Metzgar, R. S., *Transplant.* **9**:478, 1970.
45. Faulk, W. P., and Temple, A., *Nature* **262**:799, 1976.
46. Faulk, W. P., Sanderson, A. R., and Temple, A., *Transplant. Proc.* **9**:1379, 1977.
47. Loke, Y. W., Joysey, V. C., and Borland, R., *Nature* **232**:403, 1971.
48. Montgomery, B., and Lala, P. K., *J. Reprod. Immunol.* (Suppl):57, 1981.
49. Wiley, L. M., and Calarco, P. G., *Dev. Biol.* **47**:407, 1975.
50. Beer, A. E., and Billingham, R. E. In *Immunobiology of Mammalian Reproduction*, p. 108. New Jersey: Prentice Hall, 1978.
51. Faulk, W. P., Lovins, R. E., et al. In B. Boettcher (Ed.) *Immunological Influence on Human Fertility*, p. 153. London: Academic Press, 1977.
52. Klopper, A., *Placenta* **1**:77, 1980.
53. Faulk, W. P., Temple, A., et al., *Proc. Natl. Acad. Sci.* **25**:1947, 1978.
54. Terry, W. D., Henkart, P. A., et al., *Transplant Rev.* **20**:100, 1975.
55. Abelev, G. I., *Transplant Rev.* **20**:1, 1975.
56. Weintraub, B. D., and Rosen, S. W., *J. Clin. Endocrinol. Metabol.* **32**:94, 1971.
57. Gooding, L. R., and Edidin, M., *J. Exp. Med.* **140**:61, 1974.
58. Calarco, P.G., and Banka, C. L., *Biol. Reprod.* **20**:699, 1979.
59. Artzt, K., Bennett, D., and Jacob, F., *Proc. Natl. Acad. Sci.* **71**:811, 1974.
60. Jacob, F., *Immunol. Rev.* **33**:3, 1977.
61. Irie, R. F., Giuiliano, A. E., and Morton, D. L., *J. Natl. Cancer Inst.* **63**:367, 1979.
62. Ray, P. K., and Seshadri, M., *Indian J. Exp. Biol.* **18**:1027, 1980.
63. Sengupta, J., and Ray, P. K., *Fed. Proc.* **38**(3):5857, 1979.
64. Salinas, F. A., Silver, H. K. B., et al., *Cancer* **42**:1654, 1978.
65. Revillard, J. P., Robert, M., et al., *Transplant. Proc.* **5**:331, 1973.
66. Jeannet, M., Werner, C., et al., *Transplant. Proc.* **9**:1417, 1977.
67. Winchester, R. J., Fu, S. M., et al., *J. Exp. Med.* **141**:924, 1975.
68. Herzenberg, L. A., and Gonzales, B., *Proc. Natl. Acad. Sci.* **48**:570, 1962.
69. Kaliss, N., and Dagg, M. K., *Transplant* **2**:416, 1964.
70. Bell, S. C., and Billington, W. D., *J. Reprod. Immunol.* **3**:3, 1981.
71. Takano, K., and Miller, J. R., *J. Med. Genet.* **9**:144, 1972.
72. Woodrow, J. C., *Ser. Haematol.* **3**:2, 1970.
73. Szulman, A. E., *Curr. Topics Develop. Biol.* **14**:127, 1980.
74. Harris, R. E., and London, R. E., *Obstet. Gynecol.* **42**:302, 1976.
75. Kruppen-Brown, K., and Wachtel, S. S., *Transplant* **27**:406, 1979.
76. Shalev, A., *Immunol.* **39**:285, 1980.
77. Hulka, J. F., and Brinton, V., *Amer. J. Obstet. Gynecol.* **86**:130, 1963.
78. Hulka, J. F., and Brinton, V., et al., *Nature* **198**:501, 1963.
79. Timmonen, T., and Saksela, E., *Clin. Exp. Immunol.* **23**:462, 1976.
80. Taylor, P. V., Gowland, G., et al., *Amer. J. Obstet. Gynecol.* **125**:528, 1976.
81. Bonnard, G. D., and Lemos, L., *Transplant. Proc.* **4**:177, 1972.
82. Finn, R., Davis, J. C., et al., *Lancet* **2**:1200, 1977.
83. Herva, E., and Tillikainen, A., *Acta Pathol. Microbiol. Scand.* **85**:33, 1977.
84. Tait, B. D., d'Apice, A. J. F., and Morris, P. J., *Tiss. Antigens* **4**:586, 1974.
85. Youtananukorn, V., and Matangkasombut, P., *Clin. Exp. Immunol.* **11**:549, 1972.

86. Hamilton, M. S., Hellström, I., and van Belle, G., *Transplant* **21**:261, 1976.
87. Smith, J. A., Burton, M. C., et al., *Transplant* **25**:216, 1978.
88. Hellström, I., and Hellström, K. E., *Internatl. J. Cancer* **15**:30, 1975.
89. Chaouat, G., Voisin, G. A., et al., *Clin. Exp. Immunol.* **35**:13, 1979.
90. Ray, P. K., and Seshadri, M., *Indian J. Exp.Biol.* **19**:405, 1981.
91. Bradbury, S., Billington, W. D., et al., *Histochem. J.* **2**:263, 1970.
92. Tighe, J. R., Garrod, P. R., and Curran, R. C., *J. Pathol. Bacteriol.* **93**:559, 1967.
93. Simmons, R. L., Lipschultz, M. L., et al., *Nature* **231**:111, 1974.
94. Taylor, P.V., Hancock, K. W., and Gowland, G., *Transplant.* **28**:256, 1979.
95. Faulk, W. P., and Galbraith, F. In W. Hemmings (Ed.), *Transport of Proteins Across Biological Membranes*, p. 55. Amsterdam: Elsevier/North Holland, 1979.
96. Hellström, I., and Hellström, K. E., *Internatl. J. Cancer* **4**:587, 1969.
97. Hellström, K. E., Hellström, I., and Brawn, J., *Nature* **224**:914, 1969.
98. Rocklin, R. E., Kitzmiller, J. L., et al., *N. Engl. J. Med.* **295**:1209, 1976.
99. Bell, S. C., and Billington, W. D., *Nature* **228**:387, 1980.
100. Pence, H., Petty, W. M., and Rocklin, R. E., *J. Immunol.* **114**:525, 1975.
101. Faulk, W. P., Jeannet, M., et al., *J.Clin, Invest.* **54**:1011, 1974.
102. Faulk, W. P., Creighton, W. D., et al., *J. Reprod. Fertil.* **21**(Suppl.):43, 1974.
103. Sjogren, H. O., Hellström, I., et al., *Proc. Natl. Acad. Sci.* **68**:1372, 1971.
104. Masson, P. L., Delire, M., and Cambiasco, C. L., *Nature* **266**:542, 1977.
105. Cambiasco, C. L., Riconi, H., and Masson, P. L., *Ann. Rheum. Dis.* 1(Suppl):40, 1977.
106. Desai, R. G., and Creger, W. P., *Blood* **21**:665, 1963.
107. Schroder, J., and de la Chapelle, A., *Blood* **39**:153, 1972.
108. Schroder, J., *Scan. J. Immunol.* **4**:279, 1975.
109. Walknowska, J., Conte, F. A., and Grumbach, M. M., *Lancet* **1**:1119, 1969.
110. Herzenberg, L. A., Bianchi, D. W., et al., *Proc. Natl. Acad. Sci.* **76**:1453, 1979.
111. Lawler, S. C., Klonda, P. T., and Bagshawe, K. D., *Amer. J. Obstet. Gynecol.* **120**:1774, 1974.
112. Minami, M., and Shreffler, D. C., *J. Immunol.* **126**:1774, 1981.
113. Billington, W. D. In P. Beaconsfield and C. Villee (Eds.), *Placenta—A Neglected Experimental Animal*, p. 267. New York: Pergamon Press, 1979.
114. Boxer, L. A., Yokoyama, M., and Lalezari, P., *J. Pediatrics* **80**:783, 1972.
115. Hitzig, H., and Gitzelman, R., *Vox. Sang.* **4**:445, 1959.
116. Lalezari, P., Nussbaum, M. et al., *Blood* **5**:236, 1960.
117. Swinburne, L. M., *Lancet* **2**:592, 1970.
118. Tongio, M. M., Mayer, S., Lebec, A., *Transplant* **20**:163.
119. Doughty, R. W., and Gelsthorpe, K., *Tissue Antigens* **8**:43, 1976.
120. Lanman, J. T., and Herod, L., *J. Exp. Med.* **122**:529, 1965.
121. Morisada, M., Yamaguchi, H., and Iizuka, R., *Amer. J. Obstet. Gynecol.* **125**:3, 1976.
122. Johnson, P. M., Natvig, J. A., et al., *Clin. Exp. Immunol.* **30**:145, 1977.
123. McIntyre, J. A., and Faulk, W. P. In P. Beaconsfield and C. Villee (Eds.), *Placenta— A Neglected Experimental Animal*, p. 294. New York: Pergamon Press, 1979.
124. McCormick, J. N., Faulk, W. P., et al., *J. Exp. Med.* **133**:1, 1971.
125. El-Alfi, O. S., and Hathout, H., *Amer. J. Obstet. Gynecol.* **103**:599, 1969.
126. Benirschke, K., and Sullivan, M. M., *The Foeto-placental Unit*, p. 37. Amsterdam: Excerpta Medica, 1969.
127. Anderson, J. M., and Ferguson-Smith, M. A., *Brit. Med. J.* **2**:166, 1971.
128. Tuffrey, M., Bishun, N. P., and Barnes, R. D., *Nature* **224**:701, 1969.
129. Billington, W. D., Kirby, D. R. S., et al., *Nature* **224**:704, 1969.
130. Beer, A. E., and Billingham, R. E., *Science* **179**:240, 1973.

131. Medawar, P. B., and Sparrow, P. M., *J. Endocrinol.* **14**:240, 1956.
132. Heslop, R. W., Krohn, P. L., and Sparrow, E., *J. Endocrinol.* **10**:325, 1954.
133. Lanman, J. T., Dinerstein, J., and Fikrig, S., *Ann. N.Y. Acad. Sci.* **99**:706, 1962.
134. Pavia, C. S., and Stites, D. P., *J. Immunol.* **123**:2194, 1979.
135. Beer, A. E., Billingham, R. E., and Scott, J. R., *Biol. Reprod.* **12**:176, 1975.
136. Pavia, C. S., Silteri, P. K., et al., *J. Reprod. Immunol.* **1**:33, 1979.
137. Gusdon, J. P. In J. R. Scott and W. James (Eds.), *Immunology of Human Reproduction*, p. 103. London: Academic Press, 1976.
138. Loke, Y. W., and Pepys, M. D., *Amer. J. Obstet. Gynecol.* **121**:37, 1975.
139. Morse, J. H., Stearn, G., et al., *Cell. Immunol.* **25**:1978, 1976.
140. Caldwell, J. L., Stites, D. P., and Fudenberg, H. H., *J. Immunol.* **115**:1249, 1975.
141. Hammarstrom, L., Fuchs, T., and Smith, C. I. E., *Acta Obstet. Gynecol. Scand.* **58**:417, 1979.
142. Siiteri, P. K., Febres, F., et al., *Ann. N.Y. Acad. Sci.* **286**:384, 1977.
143. Beer, A. E., and Billingham, R. E. In *Maternal Recognition of Pregnancy. Ciba Foundation Symposium*, Series 64, Amsterdam, Excerpta Medica, 1979.
144. Kitzmiller, J. L., Rocklin, R. E., *J. Reprod. Immunol.* **1**:297, 1980.
145. Murgita, R. A., Goidl, E. A., et al., *Nature* **267**:257, 1979.
146. Clark, D. A., and McDermott, M. R., *J. Immunol.* **127**:1267, 1981.

11
Impairment of Host Immunity and the Survival of the Fetus

David A. Clark*

In an outbred population as exemplified by man, mating produces a fetus which bears paternal antigens, some of which are transplantation antigens (1). Indeed, reproduction by sexual means almost invariably produces a fetus which bears antigens foreign to the mother. Even in syngeneic matings in inbred strains of animals where histocompatibility differences between the two parents are minimal, the fetus expresses embryonic or fetal antigens against which the maternal immune system can react (1–3). Nevertheless, the fetus, whether allogeneic of syngeneic, is not usually rejected. Thus, the fetus resembles in some respects an organ allograft which enjoys prolonged survival in an otherwise immunologically hostile host.

The normal fetus also resembles, in many respects, a malignant tumor. For example, fetal trophoblast cells invade the wall of the maternal uterus, enter blood vessels (4), and may embolize to the lungs (5). During embryogenesis, different types of embryonic cells migrate or *metastasize* to distant sites in the embryo where they develop into differentiated organs. The migration of cells from the embryonic neural crest to form the adrenal medulla is one example of this phenomenon. Malignant cell lines can also be selected to provide variants which preferentially localize at certain sites in the body (6) and can undergo differentiation into mature adult cell types (7). Malignant tumor cells express embryonic and fetal antigens on their surface (1, 8, 9), and immunization against such antigens has been shown to produce an antitumor effect in some animal model systems (10–12). Nevertheless, under normal circumstances, both the fetus and the cells of malignant tumors evade rejection. It is tempting to speculate that successful

* I thank A. Robson, A. Chaput, and D. Banwat for expert technical assistance and Dr. C. Walker and Mr. D. Tinney for performing the progesterone radioimmunoassays. I thank Drs. M. McDermott and M. Szewczuk for helpful discussions and collaboration during this work. These investigations received financial support from the World Health Organization, the Medical Research Council of Canada, the Ontario Ministry of Health, and The Banting Foundation. The author is supported by a career development award (Scholarship) from the Medical Research Council of Canada.

LIST OF ABBREVIATIONS

MHC: major histocompatibility complex (HLA or human
      leukocyte antigens in man and H-2 in the mouse)
MIF: macrophage migration inhibition factor
DLN: para-aortic and renal lymph nodes draining the uterus in the
      mouse
PLN: peripheral lymph nodes of the mouse (axillary + brachial
      + inguinal)
   T: thymus derived
EPF: early pregnancy factor
MLC: mixed lymphocyte culture
CTL: cytotoxic T lymphocyte
ADCC: antibody-dependent cell-mediated cytotoxicity
HCG: human chorionic gonadotropin
GVH: graft-versus-host reaction

malignant tumors merely exploit a preexisting behavioral phenotype that allows normal fetal development and nonrejection.

Understanding the physiologic basis for survival of the fetal allograft should provide useful insights into problems confronting tumor immunologists, and physiologic methods that might be employed to prevent rejection of other types of tissue such as kidney, skin, and heart grafts. Conversely, failure of normal physiologic protective mechanisms might explain some examples of recurrent spontaneous abortion and infertility.

In this chapter, I will review our current state of knowledge concerning mechanisms protecting the fetal allograft and describe some new findings emerging from our own studies done on inbred strains of mice. Mice provide a genetically and immunologically defined model system with a short gestation period (19 to 21 days) and have a hemochorial placental structure similar to that of man (13).

THE TROPHOBLAST BARRIER THEORY

Two contrasting models have been proposed to explain why the allogenic fetus is usually exempt from maternal rejection. The first holds that specialized cells derived from the conceptus called *trophoblast* cells lack transplantation antigens thereby enabling them to form an inert barrier or shield between the fetus and mother (14). The second model proposes that immunosuppressive mechanisms may prevent an effective immune reaction by the mother.

Antigens Expressed by Trophoblast

Prior to implantation, the murine blastocyst or egg cylinder expresses only low levels of paternal H-2 antigens which can be demonstrated by using an ultrasensitive immunoperoxidase staining method (15, 16). At the time of implantation both H-2 and non-H-2 transplantation antigens disappear from the ectoplacental cone that will give rise to the trophoblast. Whether or not strong H-2 MHC-type antigens occur on placental trophoblast cells at later times during gestation is controversial. Sellens et al. (17) using a sensitive hemadsorption technique were unable to detect H-2 alloantigens on the trophoblast giant cell outgrowths cultured from 7½ day ectoplacental cones, but both H-2 and non-H-2 antigens were detected on outgrowths from day 13 and 14 placentae. Chatterjee-Hasrouni and Lala (18, 19) using an indirect autoradiographic technique were able to show as many anti-H-2 binding sites on trophoblast cells cultured from murine placentae as on thymocytes. However, little, if any, HLA or β-2 microglobulin appears to be present on the surface of trophoblast lining human placentae (20–22). The detection of paternal H-2 antigens on murine trophoblast cells reported by Chatterjee-Hasrouni and Lala (18, 19) could have been due to the effects which enzyme treatment can have on surface antigen expression by cells. The detection of H-2 and non-H-2 antigens on trophoblast outgrowths by Sellens et al. (17) could reflect effects which cell culture can have on surface antigen expression of cells. Alternately, the findings of these investigators could be explained by the presence in the placenta of several different types of trophoblast cells (23), only some of which bear paternal transplantation antigens. Those trophoblast cells which contact maternal blood are frequently multinucleated (syncytiotrophoblast) (23) may be difficult to isolate, and do not proliferate in culture. It is thus not surprising that no one has convincingly shown paternal transplantation antigens on multinucleate syncytiotrophoblast cells *in vitro*. Wegmann et al. (24) have studied the *in vivo* localization of radioiodinated monoclonal anti-H-2 antibodies in mouse placentae. The majority of the antibody localized (25) in the lateral yolk-sac sinus area of the placenta—presumably on fetal Hoffbauer cells, but light staining could be seen on the spongiotrophoblast at the maternal-placental interface when large amounts of labeled antibody or labeled F(ab′)$_2$ against paternal H-2 antigens were injected (personal communication, submitted for publication). Lala et al. have also recently shown autoradiography binding of anti-H-2 antibody to placental trophoblast cells *in vivo* (23). Neither Lala et al. (19) nor Jenkinson and Searle (26) have found any Ia

antigens on the murine trophoblast. Taken together, these data indi̤.̤.̤.
while some types of placental trophoblast cells may express some types of
MHC and non-MHC antigens, strong paternal class I and class II MHC
antigens are not likely expressed in appreciable quantity at the fetomaternal
interface.

Some additional evidence for the lack of significant amounts of H-2 antigens
on the early embryo and trophoblast has been obtained by blastocyst transplantation studies. Murine trophoblast cells do not simulate transplantation
immunity even when pretreated with neuraminidase (27). Female mice which
have been intensively immunized by repeated skin and lymphoid grafts
from allogeneic males will reject blastocysts transplanted under the kidney
capsule (28). In this case, however, the target antigens are *weak* non-H-2
alloantigens (29). When one transplants ecotplacental cone trophoblast derived from implanted embryos 7.5 days after mating, however, the trophoblast
itself seems to be able to proliferate unharmed by preexisting immunity to
paternal antigens (30). Cells of the growing fetus express MHC antigens
on their surface however, and fetal tissue transplanted to an extrauterine
site during pregnancy appears to be rejected successfully (30). Thus, there
is good evidence that the lack of transplantation antigens on syncytiotrophoblast allows this cell type to form an inert barrier between mother and
fetus at the fetal-maternal interface. The effect would be analogous to prolongation of skin graft survival by preventing contact between the graft and
the host's lymphatics (31).

Problems with the Trophoblast Barrier Theory

Several lines of evidence now suggest that the lack of paternal transplantation
antigens on syncytiotrophoblast is not sufficient to explain survival of the
allogeneic fetus. Human trophoblast cells bear a trophoblast-specific TA1
antigen and a second TA2 antigen that is also present on lymphocytes (32,
33). Indeed, trophoblast cells appear to be susceptible to immunologic
attack *in vivo*! Passive transfer of heterologous rabbit antirodent trophoblast
serum produces abortions in rats (34). Furthermore, immunization can affect
trophoblast outgrowth from transplanted blastocysts in certain strain combinations of mice (30, 35, 36). In xenogeneic matings where female horses
are mated to donkeys, the mother develops a spontaneous immunity against
trophoblast (37). In the placenta, some of the trophoblast cells detach and
form cellular islands in the maternal decidua; these trophoblast islands in
xenogeneic matings appear to be destroyed (37) by an inflammatory cell
infiltrate. The survival of the hybrid horse × donkey fetuses is not com-
primised by this reaction. However, in goat × sheep hybrids, the embryos
are destroyed (38). In an outbred population, one can readily conceive of

situations in which there has been a sufficient genetic drift so that some matings will simulate an xenogeneic cross, in an immunocompetent mother, elicits a rejection reaction. Recently, we have observed that blastocysts obtained from *Mus caroli*, an Asian species of mouse, implant normally when transferred into *Mus musculus* females. Within 5 to 6 days the implanted site is infiltrated by maternal lymphocytes. These cells bear Thy-1.2 and kill *Mus caroli* lymphoblasts *in vitro* (39). In human systemic lupus erythematosus (SLE), an autoimmune disorder frequently seen in females, Breshihan et al. (40) found that autoantibodies to lymphocytes bind to placental trophopblast and this binding is associated with a high frequency of spontaneous abortion. Thus, lack of MHC type transplantation antigens on trophopblast does not necessarily render the trophopblast inert. It has been recently recognized that quite powerful graft rejection responses can be elicited by non-MHC antigens (41). Indeed, resistance to tumors derived from the murine placenta is determined by an antigen that is not H-2 (42). Taken together, these data suggest that trophopblast is not necessarily immunologically inert.

Some additional information strongly suggests that trophopblast may not necessarily provide an effective barrier between the mother and fetus. There is a cellular and molecular traffic between the mother and fetus. Fetal cells may be found in maternal blood (43), and maternal lymphoid cells may enter the fetus in sufficient numbers to produce the occasional chimera (44, 45), although in rodents this seems to be infrequent (46) and dependent on the strain of animal studied and on other manipulations that may increase placental porosity. There have been a few reports of a graft-versus-host (GVH) reaction occurring in the allogeneic fetus following an intrauterine blood transfusion (45) and this suggests that the fetus may be susceptible to damage by a sufficiently large graft of immunocompetent maternal lymphoid cells. Nevertheless, the magnitude with which maternal cells enter the fetus during normal pregnancy is unknown, either because affected embryos are spontaneously aborted or resorbed early in pregnancy, or because natural selection has favored the development of strain combinations where such *accidents* are infrequent.

The Immunologic Reaction of the Mother to her Fetus

Further evidence against an inert barrier separating the fetus from the mother is provided by the observation that normal allogeneic pregnancy also elicits a spontaneous cellular and humoral immunity against paternal antigens. Allogeneically mated mice produce anti-H-2 antibodies (47) and in man, anti-HLA antibodies are produced (48). Although the frequency with which serum antibodies are detected during the first pregnancy in women is not high, Chaouat and Voisin (49) and Jeannet et al. (50) have shown such antibodies can be detected by elution from the placenta. Furthermore, Baines et al. (51) have shown a rise in the number of cells forming rosettes with paternal erythrocytes in the spleens of allogeneically-mated CBA mice during the first allogeneic pregnancy. Antifetal antibodies which cross-react with trophopblast and with a spectrum of malignant tumors have also been detected in maternal blood (3). In addition to this humoral immunity that is stimulated by allogeneic pregnancy, cellular immunity to paternal antigens is signaled both in rodents (52) and humans (53, 54) by the appearance of a subset of lymphocytes which secrete the lymphokine macrophage migration inhibition factor (MIF). These sensitized T cells develop during first pregnancy in rats and during the 3rd to 4th month of human pregnancy. Ray and Seshadri have shown that sensitization to embryonal antigens by multiparity in syngeneic mice may delay mortality following inoculation of transplantable DBDN-induced fibrosarcoma (55). Unlike the protection afforded by deliberate immunization against embryonal antigens, the immunity engendered by multiparity had no effect on the time of appearance or growth rate of the fibrosarcoma (12).

Changes in Lymph Nodes Draining the Uterus in Pregnancy

Another indication of the mother's response to her allogeneic fetus that is reported has been enlargement and weight gain in the para-aortic lymph nodes draining the uterus (DLN) in rats (56–59), in mice (60–62), and in certain strains of hamsters (63). DLN enlargement has been reported to be more pronounced in allogeneic compared to syngeneic matings in mice (60), and the enlargement is abolished if the mother is rendered tolerant to paternal transplantation antigens prior to mating (59). The mechanism of DLN enlargement is unclear, but Ansell et al. (61) have suggested that one mechanism may be enhanced trapping of circulating T lymphocytes. These data suggest that the DLN enlargement in allogeneically mated mice represents an immunologic reaction to the paternal alloantigens of the fetus.

However, not all investigators have found the anticipated enlargement of the DLN in allogeneically mated mice. Chambers and Clarke (64) found as much enlargement in syngeneically pregnant CBA females as in those bearing allogeneic progeny and Humber and Hetherington (65) observed DLN enlargement in pregnant mice but could not correlate the magnitude of weight gain with the degree of histoincompatibility between mother and fetus. There are a number of possible explanations for these observations. It is clear that the size of the DLN may change during the course of pregnancy and the time chosen to make these measurements may be important (57, 60, 64). For example, in some strain combinations of mice there may be an early phase and/or a late phase of DLN enlargement (64).

There are additional influences on the cellularity of the DLN that need to be considered. The hormones of pregnancy have an involuting effect in lymphoid tissue and this involution is abrogated to some extent by immunization with paternal tissues (58, 60). These observations suggest that the tendency of DLN to enlarge results from fetal antigenic stimulation and may be counteracted to some extent by the hormonal changes of pregnancy. The assumption that H-2 or MHC alloantigens are the primary stimulus to DLN enlargement in allogeneic pregnancy and that the syngeneic fetus is nonantigeneic would seem to represent an over simplification. In addition, DLN enlargement can also occur in F_1 females when backcrossed to the male parent (65). DLN enlargement, in this situation, may represent a GVH reaction in which lymphoid cells of the fetus react against maternal antigens (56) and could occur regularly in an outbred human population where the fetus does not inherit all of the mother's HLA antigens. Alternately, DLN enlargement in F_1 females could be caused by a reaction to the idiotypic receptors on fetal lymphocytes directed against alien maternal alloantigens. These considerations illustrate the potential complexities of interpreting changes in the size of the DLN in pregnant animals.

In our own studies (66–70), we have examined the cell recovery from DLN obtained from C3H/HeJ mice mated with allogeneic DBA/2J males. Figure 11.1 shows the pooled result from five independent experiments in which the cell yield from the DLN was determined during normal pregnancy. In these studies, the mice were mated at different times and all were studied on the same day. The day of sighting the vaginal plug was denoted as day 0.5 of pregnancy. It can be seen that following mating, there was a transient increase in cellularity which declined by the time of implantation. This initial rise in DLN cellularity after mating has also been described by Forster et al. (58) and by Hetherington and Humber (65). A second peak of increased cellularity was seen on day 10.5. During the second half of pregnancy, DLN cellularity was often decreased compared to virgin control animals. Similar observations have been reported in a study of the DLN from women at the end of a normal pregnancy (71). Our findings in C3H mice, which also hold for CBA mice mated to DBA/2 males, do not appear to show the DLN enlargement in the latter half of pregnancy reported by some other investigators (60–62). It is possible that DLN weight gain that has been reported by others may reflect an increased fluid content rather than increased cellularity. However, we have noted that when few cells were recovered from the DLN of the virgin mice, the cellularity in the DLN usually increased with allogeneic pregnancy. These data suggest that an allogeneic mating stimulates an initial reaction in the DLN which subsequently subsides. If the C3H/HeJ virgin control mice have small hypocellular nodes, one may see a significant increase in cellularity in the second and third weeks of pregnancy.

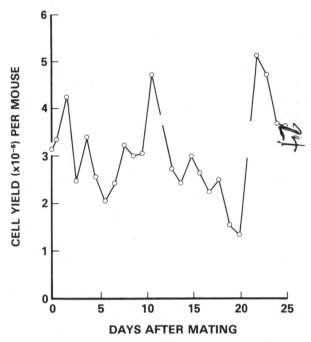

Fig. 11.1. Cell yield from lymph-node cells of C3H mice during allogeneic pregnancy.

Effect of Allogeneic and Syngeneic Pregnancy on Colony Formation by DLN Cells

Even in C3H mice where allogeneic pregnancy stimulates little change in the DLN cellularity, we have found evidence of activation of the immune system. When the PLN cells from C3H mice are plated at high concentration in methycellulose together with concanavalin A- or PHA-conditioned medium, one can readily observe the development of 5,000 to 10,000 colonies per 10^6 cells plated (72). Colony development, which is radiosensitive, does not appear to represent the growth of clones from single precursors. Rather, colony frequency is determined by the presence of non-T accessory cells that can be removed using carbonyl iron-magnet treatment (72). It was found that a small number of colonies developed when the DLN from virgin mice were tested, and colony formation was augmented to a greater extent by an allogeneic mating compared to syngeneic mating (72). Taken together with the data in Figure 11.1, these results suggest that allogeneic pregnancy in C3H mice is associated with significant immunologic changes in the DLN, both early and late in pregnancy.

Regulation of the Quality of the Immune Response in Pregnancy

The type of humoral and cellular immunity engendered by allogeneic pregnancy does not appear to be capable of producing graft rejection (73). Indeed, repeated allogeneic pregnancy appears to produce a state of tolerance to paternal antigens (74, 75). In the case of the male H-Y antigen, female C57Bl/6 mice can be immunized to H-Y and the immune cells from these mice can cause GVH disease when inoculated into neonatal male mice (76). However, multiparous C57Bl/6 females become tolerant to the paternal H-Y antigen and this tolerance can be transferred to virgin female mice by suppressor T cells (77). It has already been pointed out that the immunity to an embryonal antigen in a DBDN-induced fibrosarcoma is much weaker when induced by multiparity than that induced by deliberate immunization (12, 55). These data suggest that the immunogenicity of the fetal allograft is such that only those immunologic mechanisms that are not harmful to the fetus are activated.

Excision of the DLN appears to impair fertility (52, 78) and to prevent the generation of MIF producing cells in pregnancy (52). Although these observations suggest that the DLN may be quite important in normal pregnancy, it is unclear whether this reflects a need to activate inhibitory mechanisms which prevent the generation of transplantation immunity against fetal and trophopblast antigens or represents a positive stimulating effect on pregnancy.

We have shown elsewhere that early during allogeneic pregnancy in C3H mice, there is an inhibition of the generation of cytotoxic T lymphocytes (CTL) in the DLN following intravaginal challenge on day 7.5 of pregnancy with irradiated allogeneic paternal tumor cells (67–70). Similar inhibition was not observed when the generation of CTL in lymph nodes draining tumor-challenged footpads were studied (68). Furthermore, the generation of antibody forming cells against sheep erythrocytes inoculated into the vaginal wall on day 7.5 of pregnancy was not impaired (68). Although some investigators have found systemic antibody responses to be suppressed in mice during the latter half of pregnancy (62, 79), Fabris (80), Kennedy and Diamond (81), and Merrit and Galton (82) found normal or increased antibody responses. Murray et al. (83) also reported normal antibody responses to influenza virus vaccine in pregnant women. Taken together, these data suggest there is a localized and selective impairment of generation of CTL in the DLN early during pregnancy in allogeneically mated C3H mice.

The selective impairmant of CTL generation in lymph nodes draining the uterus of mice has some interesting implications with respect to explaining nonrejection of the allogeneic fetus. It has been observed that embryonal carcinoma cells which bear F9 antigen but lack H-2 antigens (analogous to some types of trophoblast cells) stimulate the production of anti-F-9 antibodies in normal mice (84), but this strong humoral response does not impair tumor growth. Although humoral antibody can sometimes play an important role in allograft rejection, in most model systems, acute rejection of an allograft requires infiltration with cytotoxic cells. In some situations, these cytotoxic cells are macrophages (85). In many examples, however, the dominant effector appears to be CTL (86, 87). Thus, the reduction in CTL generation in the DLN of allogeneic pregnant mice may be indicative of an important mechanism that impairs a major effector mechanism of graft rejection. CTL appear to recognize viral and non-H-2 antigens in association with H-2, and one could argue that lack of H-2 on trophoblast would render trophoblast resistant to lysis by CTL (88, 89). However, CTL which lyse targets without H-2 restriction have been generated against targets bearing either F9 or a Tla-linked antigen (90, 91, 92).

Immunostimulation of Pregnancy

There is some suggestive evidence that the type of immunity stimulated during allogeneic pregnancy may actually be helpful to the fetus. Fertility in mice usually increases after the first pregnancy (93). Some (59), but not all (94), investigators have reported that immunization against paternal antigens increases placental size and fetal weight. Palm (95) reported that the male progeny resulting from syngeneic matings in certain strains of rats suffered a high mortality. This mortality was prevented if an AgB incompatible allogeneic male was the father. These findings are supported by the high frequency of a HLA identity among couples suffering from unexplained infertility (96). Prehn and Lappe (97) have observed that deliberate immunization against H-Y may actually increase the number of male progeny if the mothers have been splenectomized. Humber et al. (98) also reported that immunization against paternal antigens increases litter size. Several possible mechanisms could underlie these effects. For example, MHC alloantigen priming may impair the generation of immunity against fetal antigens (99). In humans, immune lymphoid cells have been reported to stimulate production of chorionic gonadotropin (HCG) from trophoblast cells and may in this way enhance the production of hormones necessary for successful pregnancy (100). Beer and Billingham (56) have reported that a uterine horn that has rejected a skin allograft develops a flare when rechallenged and that this reactivity is associated with an increased frequency of implantation of allogeneic blastocysts. This latter finding suggests the beneficial effects of immunization that have been reported may represent selective enhancement of implantation of antigen-bearing blastocysts (1).

Deleterious Effects of Immunization on Pregnancy

Although certain types of immunity may benefit the fetus, one must note that immunization of the female animal in an appropriate way can impair fertility. For example, immunization against a paternal *tumor* was found by Parmiani and Della Porta (101) to reduce fertility and cause resorptions in mice. Similar results were obtained by Nista et al. (102) using neuraminidase-treated placental cells, by Hamilton et al. (103) immunizing with F9 cells in syngeneic and allogeneic mice, and by Webb (104) who immunized female mice with a teratocarcinoma. Milgrom et al. (105) immunized female rats with the skin of allogeneic males and produced intrauterine runting and postpartum GVH disease in the F1 offspring. In contrast, immunization against paternal skin alloantigens in mice was found by Humber et al. (98) to promote fertility. The most likely explanation for the variable effects of immunization on fertility (discussed in 98) would seem to be that those types of effectors capable of causing graft rejection are not always generated against the relevant antigens of the fetal allograft. Batchelor et al. (106) have shown that MHC alloantigens are not intrinsically strong antigens. Rather, the ability to generate transplantation immunity depends on regulatory signals which *amplify* the response (107). Furthermore, activation of cytotoxic effector cells within the graft itself may be a necessary step to effect rejection (108).

Where immunization is performed in an appropriate manner, maternal immunity appears to be capable, in certain cases, of overcoming the putative trophoblast barrier and destroying the fetus. We remain ignorant of the mechanism(s) causing fetal damage in these situations and have little insight into the regulatory mechanisms that control the rejection of the fetal allograft. Since antibody formation is not compromised in the DLN early in allogeneic pregnancy, it is tempting to speculate that the protective regulatory mechanisms must primarily inhibit cell-mediated immunity.

Conclusions

Three conclusions can be drawn from the above information. First, although the trophoblast interface between the fetus and the mother is deficient in strong MHC antigens, it is unlikely that the nonrejection of the fetal allograft can be attributed entirely to this feature of trophoblast. Trophoblast is neither completely inert nor an impervious barrier to maternal-fetal exchange of soluable and cellular agents. Second, the type of immunity engendered by allogeneic pregnancy is seldom harmful to the fetus and may, in some situations, exert a positive immunostimulating effect on pregnancy. In other words, the quality of the immune response is regulated so as to favor the allogeneic fetus. Third, there is good evidence from our own studies for an immunosuppressor mechanism active locally in the DLN early during first pregnancy. This suppressor mechanism selectively inhibits the generation of CTL—cells believed to play an effector role in the rejection of allografts. Three types of immunosuppressor mechanisms have been described in pregnancy by different groups of investigators. In the remainder of this chapter, I will discuss each of the three mechanisms and its relationship to the results of our studies of impaired CTL generation in allopregnant C3H/HeJ mice.

IMMUNOLOGICAL ENHANCEMENT

It has been known for many years that simultaneous grafting of an allogeneic organ or tumor and inoculation of alloantibody against the graft antigens can delay graft rejection (109). Indeed, enhancement of survival can be sufficient to allow a permanent *take*. The mechanism of enhancement is unclear. Alloantibody may prevent localization of cytotoxic effector cells (110). Alternately, alloantibody in the form of immune complexes may activate regulatory mechanisms (111) such as suppressor T cells that inhibit the immune response.

Similarities Between Enhanced Allografts and the Successful Fetal Allograft

There are several features of successful graft enhancement that resemble the situation occurring in normal allogeneic pregnancy. Enhanced grafts are resistant to rejection by transfer of immune cells and a second graft may be rejected while the first enhanced graft survives (109). Enhanced kidney grafts appear incapable of stimulating transplantation immunity in normal hosts (112). There are also certain features of normal allogeneic pregnancy that mimic immune enhancement. Immunoglobulin molecules are taken up by the blastocyst even before implantation (113). Shortly after implantation in human pregnancy, circulating immune complexes have been detected by Masson et al. (114) and Tung et al. (115), in studies of rodents, has shown that these complexes may be recovered from the kidney (109). Chaouat et al. (49) have shown that the antibody eluted from the semiallogeneic placenta can specifically enhance the growth of paternal tumor cells in normal animals. Antibody to fetal antigens can also enhance growth of syngeneic tumor cells (116). Survival of fetal bone grafts in allogeneic recipients has also been attributed to the enhancing action of anti-Ia antibodies (117). Rocklin et al. (54) have found antibody in the blood of multiparous and pregnant women which reacts with paternal leukocyte antigens. This antibody appears to be specific for HLA-D determinants, the human equivalent of murine Ia antigens, and blocks the activation of maternal MIF-producing T cells by the allogeneic cells of her husband. Rocklin et al. (54) also found that females suffering from recurrent abortion had sensitized MIF-producing T cells in their bloodstream but lacked the alloantibody blocking factor unless successful pregnancy occurred. A similar absence of blocking factor in the blood of abortion-prone women was reported by Stimson et al. (118). Taken together, these data suggest that immunological enhancement by antibody against paternal alloantigens of the fetus, particularily HLA-D and Ia antigens, and against antigens of trophoblast, could account for survival of the fetal allograft.

Evidence Against the Role Immunologic Enhancement in Fetal Allograft Survival

There are some problems which weaken the validity of the arguments for the singular importance of enhancement in allogeneic pregnancy. Trophoblast cells bear Fc receptors which bind and transport maternal IgG into the fetus (119). Wegmann et al. (25) have shown that radiolabeled anti-H-2 antibody, which reacts with paternal antigen, localizes primarily in the maternal yolk-sac sinus of the murine placenta rather than on trophoblast. The anti-H-2 antibody appears to be transported into the placenta where it too binds to paternal antigens on macrophages (Hoffbauer cells) (25). Thus, it would not be very surprising that one could elute alloantibody from the cells of the placenta. Furthermore, IgG antibody that can be detected on trophoblast in the human placenta by immunofluorescence appears to localize on the fetal side of the placental trophoblast in basement membrane (120). Jeannet et al. (50) have reported that this antibody suppresses the *in vitro* MLC response of maternal lymphoid cells without specificity for the HLA antigens of her husband. However, the observation that antibody reactive with paternal MHC antigens can also be eluted from placenta is not surprising and that this alloantibody can cause immunological enhancement of paternal tumor does not necessarily mean that such enhancement is also occurring in the pregnant animal. Lack of blocking alloantibody in women with recurrent abortion may be a *result* rather than a *cause* of the failure of successful pregnancy. Indeed, an agammaglobulinemic female who would not be expected to produce any IgG enhancing antibody have been reported to successfully undergo pregnancy (121, 153). It has recently been shown that only H-2^b type mice produce antipaternal antibody as a result of pregnancy (122). Thus, non-H-2^b strains would not be expected to produce enhancing antibody during successful pregnancy. In studies of postpartum female rats accepting paternal heart allografts, Heron (123) demonstrated that serum enhancing alloantibody was not detectable until *after* the heart had been grafted: the serum from ungrafted postpartum allopregnant females lacked enhancing activity. These data suggest that allopregnancy favors the development of immunological enhancement but that enhancement may not be elicited by the fetal allograft itself.

It is far from clear whether MIF-producing T cells in pregnant women, which are inhibited by serum blocking antibody, can cause graft rejection. In mice, MIF-producing T cells represent a T-cell subpopulation (124) distinct from cytotoxic T cells. Nomoto et al. (125) found that allosensitized lymphoid cell preparations that contained cytotoxic cells but lacked MIF-secreting cells produced tumor regression when injected into an antigenic tumor. Conversely, MIF-producing cell populations devoid of cytotoxicity did not produce regression. *In vitro* microcytotoxicity assays that have been used to detect putatively cytotoxic *aggressor lymphocytes* in pregnant and tumor-bearing mice usually involve a 48 to 72 hour coculture of lymphocytes and targets to generate a *cytotoxic* effect (126, 127) as assessed by counting the number of target cells remaining attached to the bottom of the assay well. Serum *blocking activity* has been detected by showing an inhibition of cytotoxicity when serum is present in the culture (109). The interpretation of the cytotoxic effect is often difficult (128) and may represent direct lysis, cytostasis, or nonspecific detachment of adherent targets from plastic surfaces on which they are growing. Furthermore, in studies of allopregnant mice, any cytotoxic effect demonstrable to date appears to be directed against cells of the fetus but not against trophoblast cells (126). Lysis of target cells by activated CTL occurs rapidly and is only temporarily delayed by precoating the targets with alloantibody (129). Therefore, one would not expect that alloantibody in placentae would offer much protection against the local action of CTL. It seems more likely that regulation of the generation and distribution of cytotoxic cells and of the cells which help cytotoxic cells in graft rejection (130, 131) must play a key role in protecting the fetal allograft.

SUPPRESSOR CELLS

Suppressor T cells play an important role in regulation of the immune response to antigenic tumors and allografts (132, 133). It has already been mentioned that antigen-antibody complexes can indirectly activate suppressor T cells (111) by triggering a series of T cell-T cell interactions (a suppressor T-cell circuit) and thereby producing immunologic enhancement. Suppressor T cells have also been shown to account for survival of H-2 incompatible skin grafts in mice rendered tolerant to the antigens of the graft donor (134).

In this situation, Brooks et al. (134) found a 50% reduction in the generation of CTL activity in the spleens of the grafted mice following an intraperitoneal challenge with alloantigenic donor cells. Kolsch et al. (135) have shown that very small numbers of antigenic tumor cells can activate suppressor T cells and thereby *sneak through* host defenses. A similar situation could exist in pregnant mice when the blastocyst implants. Suppressor T cells may inhibit the generation of CTL by elaboration of soluble factors. Truitt et al. (136) have described such a factor produced by H-2 specific suppressor T cells isolated from peripheral lymph nodes of mice following footpad injection of alloantigenic cells. Once produced, however, the factor non-specifically inhibits the generation of CTL to unrelated H-2 determinants. Thus, suppressor T cell regulation of CTL generation can have both a specific and nonspecific component.

A variety of non-T suppressor cells have also been described in a variety of systems. Calkins et al. (137), Nineman (138) and others (139) have described suppressor B cells. Some of these suppressor B cells may act by secreting antibody that causes immunological enhancement, whereas others (139) seem to directly stimulate the generation of suppressor T cells. Suppressor cells without surface markers, so called *null cells*, have also been described in ageing mice (140), and in murine trypanosomiasis (141).

Suppressor Cells in the Fetus

Suppressor T cells can enhance the survival and growth of antigenic malignant tumors in an otherwise immunocompetent host (49, 133), and it has been suggested that suppressor cells of various types may be present within the tumor itself (142–144). There is good evidence that the fetus (an analog of an antigenic tumor) contains suppressor cells. Skowron-Cendrzak and Ptak (145) reported that fetal liver cells could suppress a GVH reaction by maternal cells. Olding et al. (146) have similarly reported that human neonates possess suppressor cells that prevent maternal lymphoid reactivity *in vitro* against the cells of the alloantigenic fetus.

The nature of these suppressor cells is still controversial. The suppressor cell isolated from the spleens of neonatal mice appears to be a *null* cell (147) similar in some respects to natural killer cells. By the 6th postnatal day, however, Lyt-1$^+$ suppressor T cells can be demonstrated (148). The exact relationship of these suppressor T cells to the null cell population is unclear.

Fetal suppressor cells may play a very important role in pregnancy by inactivating the small number of maternal immunocompetent cells which seem to traverse the putative trophoblast barrier. This inactivation may be analogous to natural cytotoxic mechanisms that permit F1 mice to reject grafts of parental bone marrow (hybrid resistance) (149). A defense mech-anism of this type in the fetus could be overwhelmed by an increase in placental porosity that could be produced by radiation, cytotoxic drugs, or by specific antitrophoblast antibody. It has been shown (76) that male fetuses bearing the H-Y antigen usually resist aggression by inocula of maternal cells, but if one injects cells taken from a female animal primed against H-Y, then a lethal GVH reaction ensues. Therefore, there appears to be a need for mechanisms that prevent, insofar as possible, the generation of a large number of sensitized T effector cells in the mother that react with antigens of the fetoplacental unit, and a need to reduce to the lowest levels the entry of such cells into the fetus. Such mechanisms would be most likely located at the maternal side of the placenta.

Suppressor Cells in the Mother

Suppressor T cells may also arise in the mother as a result of allogeneic pregnancy, both in women (150) and in mice (49, 77, 151, 152). In these situations, however, repeated allogeneic pregnancies have been required (77, 150, 151, 152). In our own research, we have been interested in the immunological events occurring in the DLN during the *first* allogeneic preg-nancy in C3H/HeJ mice. The DLN from C3H (H-2^k) mice mated to DBA/ 2 (H-2^d) males were removed and treated with mitomycin C, an inhibitor of DNA synthesis. These cells were then shown to be able to inhibit the generation of allospecific CTL from normal lymphocytes (67, 69). When the suppressive DLN cells from pregnant mice were separated by velocity sedimentation (153), the suppressor cells were found to behave as small lymphocytes sedimenting at 3 mm/hr. (69).

We have reported elsewhere that a soluble suppressor activity can be obtained by incubating DLN in culture medium at 37° for 15 to 48 hours (68, 69). The suppression is not H-2 specific, arises in syngeneic as well as allogeneic matings, appears to act by reducing cellular proliferation (as shown in Table 11.1), and is absent from allogeneically-mated CBA strain mice undergoing spontaneous abortions (resorptions) (68–70). This activity can be obtained somewhat less frequently from peripheral lymph nodes, from thymus, and least frequently from spleen (68, 69). Velocity sedimen-tation studies have shown that the soluble suppressive activity is also elab-orated by cells sedimenting at 3 mm/hr. (69). To date, all attempts to eliminate suppressor cell activity in DLN by treatment with anti-T-cell serum and complement have failed (69, 70). These data suggest that DLN of mice undergoing their first successful allogeneic pregnancy contain a novel type of nonspecific suppressor of CTL generation that may not be a suppressor T cell. More recently we have shown that this suppressor lacks

Table 11.1. Soluble Suppressor Activity Obtained from Lymph Node Cells of Pregnant Mice

Status of Mice Used to Prepare Supernatants[a]	Cell Yield per Culture	Cytotoxic Activity per Culture[b]
—	1.3×10^6	1162 ± 82
C3H Virgin	1.4×10^6	1078 ± 73
C3H (m DBA/2)	0.73×10^6	573 ± 73^c

[a] Supernatants were prepared as described elsewhere (68) from lymph nodes of C3H mice 12.5 to 16.5 days after mating to DBA/2 males, and added at a 1/6 dilution to MLC cultures of virgin C3H PLN and mitomycin C-treated $C_3D_2F_1$ spleen cells. CTL activity was determined after 4 days of culture.

[b] CTL activity was determined by analysis of titration curves relating the lysis of 2×10^4 ^{51}Cr-labeled P-815-X2 target cells to the concentration MLC culture cells tested (67, 68). Six hundred ninety-three units of activity is equivalent to 1 Lytic Unit (the amount of activity required to lyse 50% of the target cells during the assay incubation period).

[c] Significantly suppressed compared to control value.

lyt-1 and lyt-2 markers (155). Nonspecific suppression by a variety of agents has been shown to favor the generation of suppressor T cells (in response to antigenic challenge) (156, 157). Chaouat et al. (159) have isolated an immunosuppressive molecule from murine placenta that together with antigen stimulates the development of suppressor T cells. We have reported elsewhere (70) that repeated allogeneic pregnancy in C3H/HeJ mice causes a sustained impairment of the generation of CTL against paternal alloantigens. Table 11.2 demonstrates that immunization of pregnant mice with TNP-modified C3H cells leads to a state of tolerance. These data raise the interesting possibility that the antigen-specific suppressor T cells that have been associated with repeated allogeneic pregnancies (49, 77, 150–152) may be a *result* of repeated exposure to alloantigen in the presence of a nonspecific

Table 11.2. Effect of Immunization during Pregnancy on Subsequent Generation of Anti-TNP Effector Cells

Initial Treatment	Cytotoxic Activity Generated *In Vitro* (Nat $\times 10^3 \pm$ SEM)
Untreated virgin control	50 ± 20^a
Untreated during allogeneic pregnancy[b]	40 ± 18
Virgin given TNP-C3H nucleated cells	164 ± 36
TNP-C3H cells given during allogeneic pregnancy	17 ± 15

[a] Data represents results of culturing 3×10^6 peripheral lymph-node cells with irradiated and TNP-modified syngeneic nucleated spleen cells *in vitro*. Cytotoxic cells were tested for lytic activity using 4×10^4 ^{51}Cr-labeled target cells according to the method of Sinclair and Law (158). Cytotoxicity was TNP specific and H-2 restricted (data not shown). Cytotoxic activity (lytic units) was calculated as described previously (68–70). A similar effect of immunization was observed when spleen cells were tested.

[b] Recipients were mated 7.5 days earlier to DBA/2 males and immunized with 1×10^7 TNP-modified syngeneic spleen cells intravaginally as described elsewhere (68) four weeks prior to testing.

suppressor mechanism. These suppressor T cells may play a role in regulating the maternal immune response to subsequent allogeneic pregnancies.

Further studies we have done have shown that the nonspecific suppressor appears rapidly in DLN and decidua following mating, and is maximal in DLN at the time of implantation (69, 155) —timing which is optimal to suppress an antigraft immune response. Indeed, the magnitude of suppressive activity in the DLN appears to correlate with the phases of reduced cellularity that follow the initial and midpregnancy peaks shown in Figure 11.1 (69). This correlation is in agreement with the conclusion drawn from the experiment in Table 11.1—that cell proliferation is suppressed.

Chatterjee-Hasrouni et al. (160) have described an increase in null cells in the DLN of allopregnant mice. More intriguing yet is the description by Bernard et al. (161) of a population of seven micron diameter null cells in the decidua adjacent to the mouse placenta. Seven micron diameter nucleated cells usually sediment at approximately 3 mm/hr, and this coincidence suggests the possibility that the same type of suppressor cell we have found in the DLN of allopregnant C3H mice may be present at the site of intrauterine engraftment. Indeed, in support of this idea we have recently shown that small thy-1$^-$ lyt-1$^-$ Ly-2$^-$ lymphocytes isolated from uterine venous blood and decidua of allopregnant mice are particularly potent suppressors (70, 155).

NONSPECIFIC LOCAL AND SYSTEMIC SUPPRESSOR MECHANISMS

Nonspecific Systemic Suppression

Several investigators have demonstrated a nonspecific suppressive activity in the serum of pregnant mice (162) and pregnant humans (163). The nature of the suppressive molecules in man and mouse is unknown although α_2-macroglobulins would appear to be partly responsible (164). Some suppression may also be due to *Early Pregnancy Factor* (EPF) which appears in serum shortly after fertilization (165). Systemic suppression in pregnancy may be significant in ameliorating certain autoimmune disorders such as rheumatoid arthritis (166) and experimental autoimmune encephalomyelitis (167). In addition, infection with agents such as *Herpes* virus (168), malaria (169), and other bacterial and viral agents (170) may be more severe during pregnancy. However, rejection of extrauterine paternal skin grafts is only slightly delayed by allogeneic pregnancy (56, 123, 171). It is difficult to envisage how systemic suppression without selectivity for any class of immune response, such as one may create with nonspecific immunosuppressive drugs following organ transplantation, could prevent fetal allograft rejection without lethally compromising all maternal immune defense functions. For this reason, we have found the concept of a local selective suppressive mechanism in the uterus at the maternal-fetal interface to be quite attractive.

Nonspecific Local Suppression in the Placenta

Two potential suppressor substances localized to the fetoplacental unit that have been considered are the hormone HCG, produced by human trophoblast, and alphafetoprotein, produced by the fetus itself. Alphafetoprotein suppresses the antibody response (172), unlike the pattern of suppression we observed in the DLN (68), and despite the high concentration of alphafetoprotein in its serum, the fetus is capable of rejecting skin grafts while *in utero* (173). Further analysis by Clarke et al. (174) suggests that the suppressive activity of HCG and alphafetoprotein most likely represents contamination by components of Early Pregnancy Factor.

Recent studies have focused on suppressive factors produced by trophoblast cells. Barg et al. (175) found that murine trophoblast suppressed the *in vitro* generation of CTL without affecting the antibody response,—a pattern identical to what we have found in the DLN of allopregnant mice (68). Faulk and McIntyre (176) have also described a soluble suppressor factor produced by trophoblast that inhibits allogeneic cell stimulation in the MLC reaction but does not inhibit mitogen-induced responses. Trophoblast cells in women produce large quantities of the hormone progesterone which in high local concentration can suppress graft rejection (177–179) while having only small effects on the magnitude of the antibody response (80, 177, 180). Indeed, the antibody response in pregnant (83) or hormone-treated (181) women, appears to be either normal or only slightly impaired. We, therefore, conducted some experiments to determine if progesterone could account for the soluble suppressive activity which we obtained from murine DLN. We found that addition of high concentrations of progesterone *in vitro* suppressed the generation of CTL activity. However, supernatants obtained from lymphoid cells of pregnant mice did not contain sufficient progesterone to account for their suppressive activity (69). The highest concentration of progesterone in the membranes of human syncytiotrophoblast cells as determined by radioimmunoassay has been reported to be 1 to 2 mg/g wet weight (182) whereas a concentration of 5 to 10 mg/ml was needed to substantially suppress the *in vitro* MLC response of human peripheral blood lymphocytes (183). Moreover, in rodents where rejection of skin grafts was prevented by implanting progesterone in the graft (177), serum progesterone levels were much greater than those expected during normal pregnancy (184). These data suggest that direct local suppression by progesterone in the placentae is unlikely to represent an important *in vivo* suppressive mechanism.

Intrauterine Suppression in the Absence of Trophoblast

Some additional information indicates that a significant impairment of graft rejection can occur within the uterus in the *absence* of trophoblast. Beer and Billingham (56) showed that allogeneic male skin grafted onto the decidua of pregnant and pseudopregnant rats experienced prolonged survival. Prompt rejection occurred, however, if the recipients had been immunized or were given an inoculation of immune lymphoid cells (56). The histology of this rejection has been recently studied in rabbits by Dodds et al. (185). They have reported that the cellular infiltrate at the rejection site consisted of polymorphonuclear leukocytes. This observation suggests an antibody-dependent cell mediated cytotoxicity (ADCC) rejection mechanism of the type reported to mediate the rejection of xenografts (186, 187) rather than a lymphocyte-mediated rejection. Furthermore, the work of Dodds et al. (185) suggests the possible existence of a local mechanism within the decidua that blocks the CTL-mediated rejection mechanism. Heron (188) found it particularly difficult to achieve enhanced survival of skin allografts in rats that had undergone allogeneic pregnancy in comparison to the ease with which heart allografts were protected. Skin may, therefore, provide an insensitive test graft for detecting local immunosuppression in the uterus that could readily protect less susceptible tissues from rejection. For example, pseudopregnancy dramatically enhances the growth and survival of intra-uterine tumor cell allografts (189). It has been reported that allogeneic blastocysts are rejected when implanted under the kidney capsule of immunized female mice (28). However, Kirby et al. (190) showed that allogeneic blastocysts implant successfully when placed within the uterus of immune female mice. This is perhaps one of the best pieces of evidence for the existence of a local suppressor of the graft rejection mechanism within the uterus. What is the relationship of this *in vivo* mechanism to null cells in the decidua and to our small-sized anti-T-cell serum-resistant suppressor cell in DLN and decidua? The answer to this question is being actively sought in current studies in our laboratory.

SUMMARY

The mechanisms contributing to survival of the fetal allograft that have been discussed in this chapter are summarized in Table 11.3. Although hypoantigenicity of the trophoblast may afford partial protection to the

Table 11.3. Summary

Mechanism Proposed to Protect Antigenic Fetus	Objections to the Hypothesis	References
1. Trophoblast lacks transplantation antigens and hence forms an inert barrier between fetus and mother.	Trophoblast does bear antigens.	17, 18, 19, 32, 33, 40
	Trophoblast is susceptible to antitrophoblast antibodies.	34
	Xenogeneic embryos are rejected.	38
	Mother does develop both humoral and cellular immunity to allogeneic fetus.	47, 48, 49, 51, 122, 52, 53, 54, 63
	Maternal lymphoid cells may enter fetus and fetal cells enter mother.	43, 44, 45
	Appropriately performed immunization can compromise fetal survival.	28, 29, 30, 35, 36, 101, 102, 103, 104, 105
2. Immunologic enhancement by antibody prevents rejection of fetal allograft.	Maternal antibody is not clearly localized at the maternal-fetal interface in placenta.	120
	Serum enhancing antibody detected only after completion of first allogeneic pregnancy.	123
	Agammaglobulinemic female can have normal pregnancies.	121, 154
3. Specific suppressor cells prevent the type of maternal immunity capable of, causing graft rejection.	Suppressor T cells are detected only after the first allogeneic pregnancy and multiple allogeneic pregnancies are usually required.	49, 77, 150, 151, 152
	Suppression nonspecific and a fetus is not needed for its generation.	68, 69
4. Nonspecific suppressor substances block maternal immunity:	Systemic suppression is not sufficiently potent to protect nonfetal allografts, and systemic suppression would compromise survival of mother by increasing susceptibility to infection.	56, 123, 171
Systemic serum factors		
Local progesterone	Local suppression by progesterone not likely as concentration *too* low in placenta.	69, 177, 182, 183
Alphafetoprotein	Alphafetoprotein appears later than the suppression of CTL generation in DLN and alphafetoprotein impairs antibody response.	68, 69, 70, 172
Early pregnancy factor	Fetus is not needed to generate suppression in the uterus.	56, 69, 185, 189
Trophoblast products	Suppressor cells can be isolated from the DLN during the first allogeneic pregnancy in mice.	67, 68, 69, 70

298

fetus, there is substantial evidence indicating a role for localized suppression of the maternal immune system and a degree of systemic immunosuppression may occur as exemplified by the appearance of suppressor T-cells in multiparous females. While the relevance of many of the suppressive mechanisms to successful pregnancy remains uncertain, no one has conclusively shown that immunosuppression is irrelevant to survival of the fetus.

Alterations in immune reactivity occurring in normal pregnancy have some implications in understanding problems in transplantation, tumor immunology, and in fertility regulation.

In the case of human renal allografts, there is usually some degree of histoincompatibility between the graft and the recipient. It is only after the graft has survived for some time *in vivo*, that suppressor cells are detected in peripheral blood (132, 191), a sequence not unlike that which seems to occur where *repeated* allogeneic pregnancies in a setting of nonspecific suppression antedates the generation of detectable levels of suppressor T cells.

In the case of most spontaneous neoplasms, as with trophoblast, there is little evidence for immunogenicity *in vivo* (27, 192). However, Lafferty et al. (107, 193) have shown that CTL can be generated against putatively nonantigenic syngeneic tumor cells in mice provided one adds a nonspecific T-cell growth factor. These observations suggest that antigen-bearing tumors, like the trophoblast, may survive by not stimulating certain types of immune responses. It is still unclear whether this occurs by eliciting active suppression or by the absence of the types of surface antigens on tumor cells that stimulate transplantation immunity. If certain types of immune responses, as Prehn (97) and others (59, 98, 193) suggest, can stimulate tumors and enhance fertility, it would be disadvantageous for cells of the trophoblast to be totally devoid of antigens. However, one may be able to influence the type of immune response mounted by the host to these antigens. For example, appropriately timed administration of T-cell growth factors may permit the generation of a sufficient degree of transplantation immunity against the types of antigens at the fetomaternal interface to provide an effective method for fertility control and a similar strategy could be applied in generating effective immune responses to spontaneous tumors (107, 193). On the other hand, one might achieve the same result by the local elimination of suppressor cells. Conversely, elimination of T-cell growth factors or promotion of local suppressor mechanisms within the graft should enhance graft survival and promote fertility. Indeed, experiments that determine the effect of directly altering maternal immune reactivity and suppressor-cell activity on the outcome of allogeneic pregnancy should clearly establish which immunosuppressor mechanisms are crucial for the survival of the naturally occurring fetal allograft.

REFERENCES

1. Johnson, L. V., and Calarco, P. G., *Anat. Rec.* **196**:201, 1980.
2. Hamilton, M. S., and Hellström, I., *Transplantation* **21**:261, 1976.
3. Salinas, F. A., Silver, H. K. B., Sheikh, K. M., et al., *Cancer* **42**:1653, 1978.
4. Burek, J. D., Golberg, B., Hatchins, G., et al., *Vet. Pathol.* **16**:553, 1979.
5. Douglas, G. W., Thomas, L., Carr, M., et al., *Amer. J. Obs. Gyn.* **78**:960, 1959.
6. Schirrmacher, V., *Immunobiology* **157**:89, 1980.
7. Illmensee, K., and Mintz, B., *Proc. Natl. Acad. Sci. USA* **73**:549, 1976.
8. Ting, C-C., Lavrin, D. H., Shiu, G., et al., *Proc. Natl. Acad. Sci. USA* **69**:1664, 1972.
9. Goldberg, E. H., and Tokuda, S., *Transpl. Proc.* **9**:1363, 1977.
10. Weppner, W. A., and Coggin, J. H., Jr., *Cancer Res.* **40**:1380, 1980.
11. Sikora, K., Stern, P., and Lennox, E., *Nature* **289**:813, 1971.
12. Ray, P. K., and Seshadri, M., *Ind. J. Exp. Biol.* **18**:1027, 1980.
13. Gill, T. J., and Repetti, C. F., *Amer. J. Path.* **95**:465, 1979.
14. Billingham, R. E., *Amer. J. Obs. Gyn.* **111**:469, 1971.
15. Searle, R. F., Sellens, M.H., Elson, J., et al., *J. Exp. Med.* **143**:348, 1976.
16. Webb, C. G., Gall, W. E., and Edelman, G. M., *J. Exp. Med.* **146**:923, 1977.
17. Sellens, M. H., Jenkinson, E. J., and Billington, W. D., *Transplantation* **25**:173, 1978.
18. Chatterjee-Hasrouni, S., and Lala, P. K., *J. Exp. Med.* **149**:1238, 1979.
19. Chatterjee-Hasrouni, S., and Lala, P. K., *J. Immunol.* **127**:2070, 1981.
20. Faulk, W. P., and Temple, A., *Nature* **262**:799, 1976.
21. Faulk, W. P., Sanderson, A., and Temple, A., *Transplant. Proc.* **9**:1379, 1977.
22. Goodfellow, P. N., Barnstable, C. J., Bodmer, W. F., et al., *Transplantation.* **22**:595, 1976.
23. Chatterjee-Hasrouni, S., and Lala, P. K., *J. Exp. Med.* **155**:1679, 1982.
24. Wegmann, T. G., Singh, B., and Carlson, G. A., *J. Immunol.* **122**:270, 1979.
25. Wegmann, T. G., Leigh, J. B., Carlson, G. A., et al., *J. Reprod. Immunol.* **2**:53, 1980.
26. Jenkins, E. J., and Searle, R. F., *J. Reprod. Immunol.* **1**:3, 1979.
27. Searle, R. F., Jenkins, E. J., and Johnson, M. H., *Nature* **255**:719, 1975.
28. Vandeputte, M., and Sobis, H., *Transplantation* **24**:331, 1972.
29. Searle, R. F., Johnson, M. H., Billington, W. D., et al., *Transplantation* **18**:136, 1974.
30. Simmons, R. L., and Russel, P. S., *Ann. New York Acad. Sci.* **129**:35, 1966.
31. Barker, C. F., and Billingham, R. E., *Transplantation Proc.* **5**:153, 1973.
32. Whyte, A., and Loke, Y. W., *Clin. Exp. Immunol.* **37**:359, 1979.
33. Faulk, W. P., Yeager, C., McIntyre, J. A., et al., *Proc. Roy. Soc. Lond. B.* **206**:163, 1979.
34. Beer, A. F., Billingham, R. E., and Yang, S. L., *J. Exp. Med.* **135**:1177, 1972.
35. Kaneko, Y., and Nishimura, T., *Transplantation* **25**:309, 1978.
36. James, D. A., and Yoshida, S. M., *Canadian J. Zool.* **50**:1131, 1972.
37. Allen, W. R., Maternal recognition of pregnancy and immunological implications of trophoblast-endometrium interactions in equids. In *Maternal Recognition of Pregnancy, Ciba Foundation Symposium 64*, p. 323. New York: Excerpta Medica, 1979.
38. Hancock, J. L., McGovern, P. T., and Stamp, J. T., *J. Reprod. Fert.* (Suppl.) **3**:29, 1968.
39. Croy, B. A., Rossant, J. R., and Clark, D. A., *J. Reprod. Immunol.* **4**:277, 1982.
40. Breshihan, B., Gregor, R. R., Oliver, N., et al., *Lancet* **2**:1205, 1977.
41. Halle-Pannenko, O., Pritchard, L. L., Motta, R., et al., *Biomedicine* **29**:253, 1978.
42. Log, T., Chang, K. S. S., and Hsu, Y. C., *Int. J. Cancer* **27**:365, 1981.
43. Herzenberg, L. A., Bianchi, D. W., Schroeder, J., et al., *Proc. Natl. Acad. Sci. USA*

76:1453, 1979.
44. Pollack, M. S.,Kapoor, N., Sorell, M., et al., *Transpl. Proc.* **13**:270, 1981.
45. Gill, T. G., *Transpl. Proc.* **9**:1423, 1977.
46. Trentin, J. J., Gallagher, M. T., and Priest, E. L., *Transpl. Proc.* **9**:1473, 1977.
47. Goodlin, R. C., and Herzenberg, L. A., *Transplantation* **2**:57, 1964.
48. Nymand, G., Heron, I., Jenson, K. G., et al., *Acta Pathol. Microbiol. Scand.* (B) **79**:595, 1971.
49. Chaouat, G., Voisin, G. A., Escalier, D., et al., *Clin. Exp. Immunol.* **35**:13, 1979.
50. Jeannet, M., Wernig, C., Ramirez, E., et al., *Transpl. Proc.* **9**:1417, 1971.
51. Baines, M. G., Speers, E. A., Pross, H., et al., *Immunology* **31**:363, 1976.
52. Tofoski, J. G., and Gill, T. J., *Amer. J. Path.* **88**:333, 1977.
53. Youtananukorn, V., Matankasombut, P., and Osthanondh, V., *Clin. Exp. Immunol.* **16**:593, 1974.
54. Rocklin, R. E., Kitzmiller, J. L., Carpenter, C. B., et al., *New Eng. J. Med.* **295**:1209, 1976.
55. Ray, P. K., and Seshadri, M., *Md. J. Exp. Biol.* **19**:405, 1981.
56. Beer, A. E., and Billingham, R. E., *J. Reprod. Fert.* (Suppl.) **21**:59, 1974.
57. McLean, J. M., Shaya, E. I., and Gibbs, A. C. C., *J. Reprod. Immunol.* **1**:285, 1980.
58. Forster, P. M., McLean, J. M., and Gibbs, A. C. C., *J. Anat.* **128**:837, 1979.
59. Beer, A. E., Scott, J. S., and Billingham, R. E., *J. Exp. Med.* **142**:180, 1975.
60. Maroni, E. S., and de Sousa, M. A. B., *Clin. Exp. Immunol.* **31**:107, 1973.
61. Ansell, J. D., McDougall, C. M., Speedy, G., et al., *Clin. Exp. Immunol.* **31**:397, 1978.
62. Baines, M. G., Pross, H. F., and Millar, K. G., *Obst. & Gynecol.* **50**:457, 1977.
63. Head, J. R., Hamilton, M. S., and Beer, A. E., *Fed. Proc.* **37**:2054, 1978.
64. Chambers, S. P., and Clarke, A. G., *J. Reprod. Fert.* **55**:309, 1979.
65. Hetherington, C. M., and Humber, D. P., *J. Immunogenetics* **4**:271, 1977.
66. Clark, D. A., *Clin. Exp. Immunol.* **35**:421, 1979.
67. Clark, D. A., and McDermott, M. R., *J. Immunol.* **121**:1389, 1978.
68. Clark, D. A., McDermott, M. R., and Szewczuk, M. R., *Cell. Immunol.* **52**:106, 1980.
69. Clark, D. A., and McDermott, M. R., *J. Immunol.* **127**:1267, 1981.
70. Clark, D. A., Slapsys, R., Croy, B. A., et al., Regulation of cytotoxic T-cells in pregnant mice. In T. Wegmann and T. J. Gill (Eds.), *Reproductive Immunology.* London: Oxford University Press, 1983.
71. Nelson, J. H., Lu, T., Hall, J. E., et al., *Amer. J. Obs. Gyn.* **177**:689, 1973.
72. Clark, D. A., *Cell. Immunol.* **56**:152, 1980.
73. Wegmann, T. G., Waters, C. A., Drell, D. W., et al., *Proc. Natl. Acad. Sci. USA* **76**:2410, 1979.
74. Breyere, E. J., and Barret, M. K., *J. Natl. Cancer Inst.* **27**:409, 1961.
75. Prehn, R. T., *J. Natl. Cancer Inst.* **25**:883, 1960.
76. Kuroiwa, A., Nagino, H., Miyazaki, S., et al., *Int. Arch. Allergy Appl. Immunol.* **62**:235, 1980.
77. Smith, R. N., and Powell, A. E., *J. Exp. Med.* **146**:899, 1977.
78. Beer, A. E., and Billingham, R. E., *Transplantation Proc.* **9**:1393, 1977.
79. Sasaki, K., and Ishida, N., *Tohoku J. Exp.Med.* **116**:391, 1975.
80. Fabris, N., *Experientia* **29**:610, 1973.
81. Kenney, J. F., and Diamond, M., *Infect. and Immunity* **16**:174, 1977.
82. Merritt, K., and Galton, M., *Transplantation* **7**:562, 1969.
83. Murray, D. L., Imagana, D. T., Okada, D. M., et al., *J. Clin. Microbiol.* **10**:184, 1979.
84. Damonneville, M., Morello, D., Gachelin, G., et al., *Eur. J. Immunol.* **9**::932, 1979.

85. Haskill, S. S., Key, M., Radov, L. A., et al., *J. Reticuloendothelial Soc.* **26**:417, 1979.
86. Von Willebrand, E., Soots, A., and Hayry, P., *Cellular Immunol.* **46**:327, 1979.
87. Hayry, P., Von Willebrand, E., and Soots, A., *Scand. J. Immunol.* **10**:95, 1979.
88. Bevan, M. J., *J. Exp. Med.* **142**:1349, 1975.
89. Golstein, P., Kelly, F., Avner, P., et al., *Nature* **262**:693, 1976.
90. Wagner, H., Starzinski-Powitz, A., Rollinghoft, M., et al., *J. Exp. Med.* **147**:251, 1978.
91. Lindahl, K. F., and Hausmann, B., *Eur. J. Immunol.* **10**:289,1980.
92. Wernet, D., and Klein, J., *Immunogenetics* **8**:361, 1979.
93. Bigger, J. D., Finn, C. A., and McLaren, A., *J. Reprod. Fert.* **3**:315, 1962.
94. Hetherington, C. M., Humber, D. P., and Clarke, A. G., *J. Immunogenetics* **3**:245, 1976.
95. Palm, J., *Cancer Res.* **34**:2061, 1974.
96. Gerencer, M., Kastelan, A., Drazanac, A., et al., *Tissue Antigens* **12**:223, 1978.
97. Prehn, R. T., and Lappe, M. A., *Transplant. Rev.* **7**:26, 1971.
98. Humber, D. P., Mahouy, G., Chinn, S., et al., *J. Reprod. Fert.* **41**:193, 1974.
99. Halle-Pannenko, O., Pritchard, L. L., Mota, R., et al., *Transplant. Proc.* **11**:652, 1979.
100. Dickman, W. J., and Cauchi, M. N., *Nature* **271**:377, 1978.
101. Parmiani, G., and Della Porta, G., *Nature* (New Biol.) **241**:26, 1973.
102. Nista, A., Sezzi, M. L., and Belleli, S., *Oncology* **28**:402, 1973.
103. Hamilton, M. S., Beer, A. E., May, R. D., et al., *Transpl. Proc.* **11**:1069, 1979.
104. Webb, C. G., *Biol. Reprod.* **22**:695, 1980.
105. Milgrom, F., Comini-Andrada, E., and Chaudhry, A. P., *Transpl. Proc.* **9**:1409, 1977.
106. Batchelor, J. R., Welsh, K. J., and Burgosi, H., *Nature (London)* **273**:54, 1978.
107. Warren, H. S., Woolnough, J. A., and Lafferty, K. J., *Aust. J. Exp. Biol. Med. Sci.* **56**:247, 1978.
108. Sakemi, T., Kuriowa, A., Taniguchi, K., et al., *Cell. Immunol.* **54**:321, 1980.
109. Hellström, K. E., and Hellström, I., *Ann. Rev. Microbiol.* **24**:373, 1970.
110. Chang, A. E., and Sugarbaker, P. H., *Transplantation* **29**:127, 1980.
111. Rao, V. S., Bennett, J. A., Shen, F. W., et al., *J. Immunol.* **125**:63, 1980.
112. Batchelor, J. R., Welsh, K. I., Maynard, A., et al., *J. Exp. Med.* **150**:455, 1979.
113. Bernard, O., *Immunogenetics* **5**:1, 1977.
114. Masson, P. L., Delire, M., and Cambiaso, C. L., *Nature* **286**:542, 1977.
115. Tung, K. S. K., *J. Immunol.* **112**:186, 1974.
116. Goldberg, E. H., and Tokuda, S., *Transplantation* **21**:263, 1976.
117. Segal, S., Siegal, T., Altaraz, H., et al., *Transplant.* **28**:88, 1979.
118. Stimson, W. H., Strachan, A. F., and Shepherd, A., *Brit. J. Obs. Gyn.* **86**:41, 1979.
119. Elson, J., Jenkinson, E. J., and Billington, W. D., *Nature* **255**:412, 1975.
120. Faulk, W. P., Jeannet, M., Creighton, W. D., et al., *J. Reprod. Fert.* (Suppl.) **21**:43, 1974.
121. Holland, N. H., and Holland, P., *Lancet* **2**:1152, 1966.
122. Bell, S. C., and Billington, W. D., *J. Reprod.Immunol.* **3**:3, 1981.
123. Heron, I., *Transplantation* **14**:239, 1972.
124. Kuhner, A. L., Cantor, H., and David, J. R., *J. Immunol.* **125**:117, 1980.
125. Nomoto, K., Sato, M., Yano, Y., et al., Dissociation between delayed hypersensitivity and cytotoxic activity against syngeneic or allogeneic tumor grafts. In D. Misuno, G. Chihara, F. Fukuoka, T. Yamamoto, and Y. Yamamura (Eds.), *Host Defence Against Cancer and its Potentiation*, p. 55. Baltimore: University Park Press, 1975.
126. Jenkinson, E. D., and Billington, W. D., *Transplantation* **18**:286, 1974.

127. Sjogren, H. O., Hellström, I., Bansal, S. C., et al., *Proc. Nat. Acad. Sci. USA* **68**:1372, 1971.
128. Gyongyossy, M. I. C., Liabeuf, A., and Golstein, P., *Cellular Immunol.* **45**:1, 1979.
129. Faanes, R. B., Choi, Y. S., and Good, R. A., *J. Exp. Med.* **137**:171, 1973.
130. Fernandez-Cruz, E., Woda, B. A., and Feldman, J. D., *J. Exp. Med.* **152**:823, 1980.
131. Hall, B. M., Roser, B. J., and Dorsch, S. E., *Transpl. Proc.* **11**:638, 1979.
132. Charpentier, B., Lang, B., Martin, B., et al., *Transplant. Proc.* **13**:90, 1981.
133. Broder, S., and Waldman, T. A., *New Engl. J. Med.* **299**:1335, 1978.
134. Brooks, C. G., Brent, L., Kilshaw, P. J., et al., *Transplantation* **19**:134, 1975.
135. Kolsch, E., Stumpf, R., and Weber, G., *Transplant. Rev.* **26**:56, 1975.
136. Truitt, G. A., Rich, R. R., and Rich, S. S., *J. Immunol.* **121**:1045, 1978.
137. Calkins, D. F., Orbach-Arbouys, S., Stutman, O., et al., *J. Exp. Med.* **143**:1421, 1976.
138. Nineman, J. L., *J. Immunol.* **120**:1573, 1978.
139. L'Age-Stehr, J., Teichmann, H., Gershon, R. K., et al., *Eur. J. Immunol.* **10**:21, 1980.
140. Roder, J. C., Bell, D. A., and Singhal, S. K., *Cell. Immunol.* **29**:272, 1977.
141. Roelants, G. E., Pearson, T. W., Tyrer, H. W., et al., *Eur. J. Immunol.* **9**:195, 1979.
142. Kirchner, H., *Europ. J. Cancer* **14**:453, 1978.
143. Mantovani, A., Allavena, P., Biondi, A., et al., NK activity in human ovarian carcinoma. In B. Serrou, C. Rosenfeld, and R. B. Herberman (Eds.), *Natural Killer Cells*, p. 123. Amsterdam: Elsevier Biomedical Press, 1982.
144. Caufield, M. J., and Cerney, J., *J. Immunol.* **124**:255, 1980.
145. Skowron-Cendrzak, A., and Ptak, W., *Transplantation* **24**:45, 1977.
146. Olding, L. B., Bernirschke, K., and Oldstone, M. B. A., *Clin. Immunol. Immunopathol.* **3**:79, 1974.
147. Rodriguez, G., Anderson, B., Wigzell, H., et al., *Eur. J. Immunol.* **9**:737, 1979.
148. Mosier, D. E., Mathieson, B. J., and Campbell, P. S., *J. Exp. Med.* **146**:59, 1977.
149. Cudkowicz, G., and Yung, Y. P., *J. Immunol.* **119**:483, 1977.
150. McMichael, A. J., and Sasazuki, T., *J. Exp. Med.* **146**:368, 1977.
151. Chaouat, G., and Voisin, G. A., *J. Immunol.* **122**:1283, 1979.
152. Chaouat, G., and Voisin, G. A., *Immunol.* **39**:239, 1980.
153. Miller, R. G., and Phillips, R. A., *J. Cell. Physiol.* **73**:191, 1969.
154. Kobayaski, R. H., Hyman, C. J., and Stiehm, R., *Amer. J. Dis. Children* **134**:942, 1980.
155. Slapsys, R. M., and Clark, D. A., *Amer. J. Reprod. Immunol.* **3**:65, 1983.
156. Rieger, M., Gunther, J., Kristofova, H., et al., *Folia Biol.* (Praha) **24**:145, 1978.
157. Simpson, M. A., and Gozzo, J. J., *Transplant. Proc.* **11**:452, 1979.
158. Sinclair, N. R. St. C., and Law, F. Y., *J. Immunol.* **123**:1439, 1979.
159. Chaouat, G., Chaffaux,S., Duchet-Suchaux, M., et al., *J. Reprod. Immunol.* **2**:127, 1980.
160. Chatterjee-Hasrouni, S., Santer, V., and Lala, P. K., *Cell. Immunol.* **50**:290, 1980.
161. Bernard, O., Scheid, M. P., Ripoche, M. A., et al., *J. Exp. Med.* **148**:580, 1978.
162. Harrison, M. R., *Scand. J. Immunol.* **5**:881, 1976.
163. Kaskura, S., *J. Immunol.* **107**:1296, 1971.
164. Stimson, W. H., *Clin. Exp. Immunol.* **40**:157, 1980.
165. Norman, F. P., Halliday, W. J., Morton, H., et al., *Nature* **278**:649, 1979.
166. Persellin, R. H., *Bull. Rheum. Dis.* **9** (27):922, 1977.
167. Keith, A. B., *J. Neurol. Sci.* **38**:317, 1978.
168. Young, E. J., and Gomez, C. I., *Proc. Soc. Exp. Biol. Med.* **160**:416, 1979.
169. Van Zon, A. A. J. C., and Eling, W. M., *Infect. Immunity* **28**:630, 1980.
170. Harkness, R. A., *J. Royal Soc. Med.* **73**:161, 1980.

171. Anderson, J. M., *Lancet* **2**:1077, 1971.
172. Murgita, R. A., and Tomasi, T. B., *J. Exp. Med.* **141**:269, 1975.
173. Silverstein, A. M., Ontogeny of the Immune Response: A perspective. In M. D. Cooper and D. H. Dayton (Eds.), *Development of Host Defences*, p. 1. New York: Raven Press, 1977.
174. Clarke, F. M., Morton, H., Rolfe, B. E., et al., *J. Reprod. Immunol.* **2**:151, 1979.
175. Barg, M., Burton, R. C., Smith, J. A., et al., *Clin. Exp. Immunol.* **34**:441, 1978.
176. McIntyre, J. A., and Faulk, W. P., *Proc. Natl. Acad. Sci. USA* **76**:4029, 1979.
177. Beer, A. E., and Billingham, R. E., Maternal Immunological recognition mechanisms during pregnancy. In *Maternal Recognition of Pregnancy. Ciba Foundation Symposium 64*, p. 293. New York: Excerpta Medica, 1979.
178. Siiliteri, P. K., Febres, F., Clemens, L. E., et al., *Ann. New York Acad. Sci.* **268**:384.
179. Munroe, J. S., *J. Reticuloendothelial Soc.* **9**:361, 1971.
180. Fabris, N., Piantanelli, L., and Muzzioli, M., *Clin. Exp. Immunol.* **28**:306, 1977.
181. Rojo, J. M., Portoles, M. P., and Portoles, A., *J. Reprod. Immunol.* **2**:29, 1980.
182. Smith, N. C., and Brush, M. G., *Med. Biol.* **56**:272, 1978.
183. Clemens, L. E., Siiteri, P. K., and Stites, D. P., *J. Immunol.* **122**:329, 1979.
184. Sanyal, M. K., *J. Endocrinol.* **79**:179, 1978.
185. Dodds, M., Andrew, T. A., and Coles, J. S., *J. Anat.* **130**:381, 1980.
186. Jooste, S. V., Winn, H. J., and Russel, P. S., *Transplantation Proc.* **5**:715, 1973.
187. Hamilton, D. N. H., and Gaugas, J. M., *Transplantation* **13**:620, 1972.
188. Heron, I., *Transplantation* **14**:551, 1972.
189. Moriyana, I., and Sugawa, T., *Nature* (New Biol.) **236**:150, 1972.
190. Kirby, D. R. S., Billington, W. D., and James, D. A., *Transplantation* **4**:713, 1966.
191. Thomas, J., Thomas, F., Hoffman, S., et al., *Surgery* **86**:266, 1979.
192. Hewitt, H. B., Blake, E.R., and Walder, A. S., *Brit. J. Cancer* **33**:241, 1976.
193. Warren, H. S., and Lafferty, K. J., *Scand. J. Immunol.* **10**:349, 1979.

12

Immunology of Growth and Demise of Embryo-Trophoblast Unit Indicated by Comparative Study between Abortion and Hydatidiform Mole—A Nature's Experiment System

Shoshichi Takeuchi

Immunity is the physiological state of the host enabling it to distinguish between *non-self* and *self*; it plays an important role in the protection of the individual by rejection of the non-self elements. Pregnancy has, however, been recognized to be an exception to this rule. The conceptus becomes fertilized ovum, which develops through embryo-trophoblast unit (ETU) to fetoplacental unit (FTU). It is clearly non-self to the mother, because it is endowed with paternal gene products, and the mother surely responds to some of these products as antigens, but they behave, seemingly, as an immunologically inert tissue. Furthermore, it has been reported that, in some way, this maternal reactivity against non-self alloantigens of the conceptus is normally beneficial in terms of improving its initial chance of implantation and its subsequent growth rate. Disparity in major histocompatibility complex (MHC) between mother and conceptus is apparently beneficial for the mother's reproductive performance (1).

The immunology of pregnancy thus reveals a sharply antithetic difference in behavior from transplantation immunology. Pregnancy constitutes a great exception to the general rule. However, when we consider that immunity is involved not only in the maintenance of individual survival, but also in the propagation of the species, and that both are important biological functions of the living being, reproductive immunology should, I believe, not be the

LIST OF ABBREVIATIONS

Ab: antibody
AFP: α-fetoprotein
Ag: antigen
BA: blocking antibodies
ETU: embryotrophoblast unit
FR: facilitation reaction
FTU: fetoplacental unit
GVH: graft-versus-host
HM: hydatidiform mole
Ig: immunoglobulin
IR: immune reaction
Mφ: macrophage
MHC: major histocompatibility complex
MLTC: mixed leucocyte-trophoblast culture
RR: rejection reaction
SpA: spontaneous abortion
Tc: cytotoxic T cell
Tk: killer T cell
Ts: suppressor T cell
V_H: variable segment of Ig heavy chain

exception to transplantation immunology. We clearly have to look for a general rule of the immunoregulatory mechanisms which can explain immunological facts observed in pregnancy as well as in allograft transplantation without any contradictions.

The purpose of this paper is —first, to put the emphasis on the assumption that any immunoregulatory mechanism in transplantation immunology has to explain also immunological facts observed in reproductive physiology and pathology, and vice versa, and second, to put the emphasis on the so-far neglected notion that comparative study on immunology of spontaneous abortion (SpA) and hydatidiform mole (HM) is a *Nature's Experiment Model*. This gives us an excellent clue for elucidation of the following basic problems in transplantation biology in addition to clarification of the genesis of these two diseases; (a) An immune dependency of trophoblastic growth and damage *in vivo*, (b) an immunological mechanism involved in immunologic coexistence of the antigenic conceptus in the mother, and (c) a general immunoregulatory mechanism in human beings. The final purpose is, in this context, to propose an immunoregulatory mechanism by blocking antibodies

(BA) which may play an important role in determining the destiny of trans-planted allograft, either *take* or *rejection*.

MECHANISMS TO EXPLAIN THE NONREJECTION OF ALLOGENEIC CONCEPTUS

Overview

The survival and growth of the conceptus resulting from allogeneic matings, and thus potentially alien to the mother, constitute the greatest exception to all the known laws of tissue transplantation. To explain this phenomenon, various hypotheses have been forwarded. Medawar in 1953 set forth several reasons for believing that mechanisms responsible for a successful placental graft are immunological (2). These include: (a) Conceptuses are antigenically immature (3–4), (b) the uterus is an immunologically privileged site (3–4), (c) there is a neutral barrier existing at the fetomaternal tissue interface which prevents immune interactions between the maternal and fetally derived cells (3–6), (d) histocompatibility antigens are absent from the surface of placental trophoblast cells that remain in direct contact with maternal blood (6–10), (e) there is a general nonspecific depression of the maternal immune functions possibly resulting from pregnancy-associated humoral factors and hormones (7–13), and (f) there is a specific blocking of the effector arm of the maternal immune response by antibodies (Abs) and/or suppressor T cells (Ts) to fetal antigens (Ags) (13).

The explanations that conceptuses are antigenically immature and that the uterus is an immunologically privileged site are now rendered untenable by the following evidence. Minor and subsequently major transplantation antigens appear sequentially on the plasma membranes of fertilized ovum, from at least the two-cell stage onwards (14). The uterus affords a very effective route for elicitation and expression of transplantation immunity either by solid tissue allografts or by suspensions such as dispersed leukocytes and washed epididymal spermatozoa, introduced into its lumen during the nonpregnant state (15). There is suggestive evidence that the decidual tissue may interfere with the lymphatic drainage of the early zygote (16), but this cannot account for the success of gestation in a presensitized female (15).

The explanations accepted at present will be summarized in Table 12.1. The placenta clearly plays a central role in the fetomaternal interaction. It does this by complete separation of maternal and fetal blood circulation and by acting as an immunological barrier which will be made up of immunologically privileged trophoblasts that are neutral against maternal immunological attack and are able to inactivate maternal immunologic effectors during their transmission from mother to fetus (17–18). Trophoblasts will

Table 12.1 Mechanisms to explain the nonrejection of allogeneic fetoplacental units

1. Complete separation of maternal and fetal blood circulation (17, 18)
2. Function of placenta as immunologic barrier
   2-1 trophoblast as immunologically privileged tissue through its low antigenic expression due to
      2-1-1 adaptive failure of trophoblast to synthesize antigens (19)
      2-1-2 antigenic shedding (20)
      2-1-3 antigenic modulation by maternal antibodies (21, 22)
      2-1-4 masking of surface antigens (23–25)
   2-2 inactivation of maternal immunologic effectors (28–32)
3. Suppression of maternal immune response
   3-1 nonspecific inhibitory factors (36–44)
      3-1-1 production by fetus:
          AFP, factor released from stimulated fetal lymphocytes
      3-1-2 production by placenta:
          prog. estrogens, hCG, cortisol-binding globulin
      3-1-3 production by mother:
          adrenal corticosteroids, special plasma protein (pregnancy-zone or PZ proteins), early pregnancy factors (EPF), α-2-globulins
      3-1-4 decidual tissue
   3-2 specific blocking factors
      3-2-1 synthesis of *blocking* antibodies (21, 47, 48, 58, 59, 89, 90, 92)
      3-2-2 generation of suppressor T cells (58, 59)
      3-2-3 idiotype-antiidiotype antibodies (58)

acquire an immunological privilege through their low antigenic expression of MHC by several mechanisms, such as adaptive failure in synthesis of Ags (19), antigenic shedding (20), antigenic modulation by maternal Ab (21–22), and/or surface Ags by glycocalyx which is responsible for repulsion of maternal cytotoxic T(Tc) cells (23–25). Trophoblasts do not contain the ABH blood group, Ags; the endothelium of the vessels of the placenta and umbilical cord have only the basic H structure (26). In contrast, the endothelial cells of the fetus have a large amount of these Ags. The lack of ABH Ags in trophoblast prevents attack by maternal AB isoantibodies (27). It is possible that the placental tissue may contain MHC antigens distributed in such a way that specifically sensitized lymphocytes react with placental tissue with minimal effect on placental function, but are prevented from passing into the fetal circulation (28). Passively transferred Ab to the mother is rapidly absorbed from the maternal circulation, most likely by the placenta (28). Thus the placenta may act to remove and inactivate immune reactants. When a small number of maternal lymphocytes gets across the placenta, the fetus in utero may eliminate them by an early development of immune competence. (29–30). In the human, most instances of neonatal GVH disease are associated with an immune deficiency of the fetus (29). But when maternal lymphocytes transfer massively across the placenta to the fetus, GVH can occur in them (31–32). In fact there is speculation that the high incidence of lymphomas in children may be related to production of subclinical runt

disease caused by maternal lymphocytes that infiltrate the fetus during pregnancy and are not eliminated by an immune response of the fetus (32). The
placenta surely creates a privileged refuge environment that will enable
growth and development of a histoincompatible fetus in isolation from its
mother's immune system. However, the placenta does not serve as a complete
isolating barrier and is incapable of completely preventing the escape or
the migration of maternal cells into fetal circulation or the fetal immune
factors into the mother's circulation (33–35).

The assumption that the immune system of the pregnant female is systemically suppressed and thus incapable of generating a harmful immune
response against her conceptus has been proposed. Incidence of certain
infectious diseases such as tuberculosis and small pox is increased during
pregnancy (36) and certain nonspecific inhibitory factors produced by the
fetus (37–39), the placenta (40, 44), and the mother (41–42) are also
increased during gestation. If the nonspecific suppression of the immune
system of a pregnant female plays an important role in the nonrejection of
antigenic conceptus, this may in turn result in a decrease in her ability to
resist life-threatening infection. Hence, such an assumption may be hard
to accept. In fact, there is a report that a general systemic suppression of
the immune system in pregnant females was not observed (43). Consequently
these nonspecific immunosuppressive factors may be the cause of the nonrejection of the conceptuses locally because of their high concentration near
the placenta (43–44). Furthermore, the notion that induction of specific
tolerance to paternal Ags may be responsible for the nonrejection is incompatible with the fact that a pregnant female usually rejects promptly skin
allografts of either paternal or F_1 origin (45). But, multiparity by allogeneic
male leads to a progressive weakening of the female's capacity to reject
test allografts from paternal donors or from F_1 hybrid donors (46). This
interestingly parallels the appearance of specific BAs in her serum (46).

BAs in mouse pregnancy sera were first reported by Hellström et al. in
1969 during their experiments to protect embryonal cells *in vitro* against
the action of cytotoxic lymphocytes (21). Since then, it has been suggested
that the role of serum BAs to block CMI reactions is important for immunologic coexistence even in human pregnancy. This is because such BAs
have been identified in both maternal (47–48) and neonatal plasma (47) as
well as in the eluate (49–53). They are capable of inhibiting mixed leukocyte
reaction (MLR), and are cytotoxic to paternal lymphocytes in the presence
of complement. In mice, it has been reported that a greater amount of
antibody could be bound to semiallogeneic placentas than to syngeneic
placentas, the amount of BAs on semiallogeneic placentas increased with
parity, and that IgG eluted from placentas had paternal antigen-specific
enhancing properties *in vivo* (13).

Suppressor cells have also been reported increased in the mother (55–56) and newborns (57). Janaway (1978) gave an overview of suppressor T cells (Ts) in immunoregulation (54). Two possible control mechanisms were popular as a result of work by different investigators; (a) a T cell modulates the activities of helper (Ly-1$^+$) cells and suppressor cells (Ly-2,3$^+$). Thus, Ts could be of two types—a mature cell that is committed to suppression, and an immature one that reacts to signals by an antigen. (b) In the context of the idiotypic network hypothesis of Jerne, Ts may recognize idiotypic receptors of other T or B cells and thus modulate the initial idiotypic response. But there was no description as to relations between Ts and BAs.

Peck et al. (1978) reported that AFP exerted a highly selective suppressive activity on I-region-associated immune responses, mediated predominantly by Ly-1$^+$ cells and unaffected MHC K or D region determinants, mediated predominantly by Ly-2$^+$ cells (56). The AFP suppression was suggested as being dependent, at least in part, on the ability of AFP to induce highly efficient suppressor T cells (12).

BAs may bear close relations with two other important immunoregulatory agents: Ts and antiidiotypic antibodies (Voisin 1980) (58). BAs appear to trigger Ts in some way since the inhibitory effect of anti-MHC antibodies on MLR largely disappears when Ts are eliminated from the reactive population. BAs seem to produce antiidiotypic antibodies (58).

Segal (1980) demonstrated that females are different from males in their immune capacity to react against fetal MHC determinants encoded on alloantigens. MHC expressed on a fetal tissue generated different immunogenic signals than those expressed on adult tissues, because the former produced predominantly IgG$_1$ while the latter predominantly IgG$_2$ (59). At this point, it may be worthwhile to note Voisin's view that paternal MHC-encoded antigens, which have been found to be expressed on trophoblastic tissues, can absorb specific MHC antibodies of the IgG$_1$ isotype raised during pregnancy. These antibodies were found to enhance specifically the growth of tumors of paternal origin (58). These results may indicate that the I region of fetal alloantigens controls fetal antigens in addition to Ia antigens, thus generating signals to produce BAs to fetal Ia antigens.

The BAs, Ts, and antiidiotypic antibodies, therefore, are considered the important factors for regulating the maternal immune reaction that permit fetal nonrejection. However, the issues encountered at present in reproductive immunology are the lack of evidence that maternal immunologic activity is capable of bringing about destruction of trophoblast *in vivo* (1). It is difficult to give any evidence for that because trophoblasts give sparse or absent expression of MHC, and thus any immunologic destruction of non-antigenic trophoblasts cannot be considered. Lack of evidence as to immunological destruction of trophoblasts *in vivo* may prevent us from knowing the complete story in reproductive immunology so an immunologic coexistence during pregnancy still remains enigmatic. In contrast to this, emphasis is put on the notion that *A Nature's Experiment System* regarding SpA and HM will be useful for solving the current problems in reproductive immunology.

Immunoregulatory Mechanisms in Transplantation Immunology

Transplantation immunology has received an impact from the development of reproductive immunology, which has recently made remarkable progress. Here, a brief review will be given on immunoregulatory mechanisms of transplanted allografts.

Rejection of solid tissue grafts is mainly mediated by the cellular type of allergic reaction. Humoral Ab may contribute to rejection of a tissue allograft or it may interfere with (block) the action of sensitized cells in rejection. The type of rejection of an allogeneic skin graft depends upon the degree of immune activity. An allograft to an unsensitized individual will be rejected after vascularization by a mononuclear cell infiltrate, while an autograft or synograft will *take*, that is, survive and heal into the grafted site. An allograft to a sensitized recipient will not become vascularized and will be rejected by ischemic necrosis within a few days after transplantation (60).

The paradoxical situation in which humoral antibody may also prolong graft survival was first recognized in the 1930s, when it was noted that prior immunization to tumor tissue might increase the incidence and growth of tumors in allogeneic systems (61). This phenomenon was termed *tumor enhancement*. Later it was noted that grafts of normal tissues would survive longer if the animal was preimmunized in such a way as to produce circulating humoral antibody to allograft antigens rather than delayed hypersensitivity (62) or if humoral antibody was passively transferred to the recipient (63). This effect was termed *graft facilitation* by Voisin (1971) (64). The enhancement-facilitation effect was proposed to suppress other effects of delayed hypersensitivity such as GVH reactions and to prevent rejection of fetal tissue by the mother, autoallergic diseases, and tumor growth (64–65).

The rejection reaction (RR) may be divided into three phases: Afferent, central, and efferent. Afferent phase refers to the delivery of antigens to the cells recognizing it; central phase refers to events following recognition, culminating in production of specifically sensitized cells; and efferent phase refers to the delivery of the sensitized cells to the target tissue, the reaction of these cells with target cell antigens, and the destruction of the target cell by the sensitized killer cell. The sites of action of BAs (or enhancing-facilitating antibodies) were also considered to be present in efferent sites. At present it is impossible to select one site as the most important in allograft facilitation; it is likely that more than one mechanism is operative in a given situation. In particular, BAs may mask antigenic sites so that they are not available to recognition cells (afferent effect) or to effector cells (efferent effect). Interference with effector cells by masking of target cell antigens is supported by the finding that humoral antibody to a target cell may block immune attack by killer cells *in vitro* (48). In addition to BAs, complexes of BAs, and antigen and/or free antigens may react directly with sensitized cells to block either the induction or expression of CMI.

Immune responses are regulated by two genetic regions; the MHC and the immunoglobulin V_H (variable segment of Ig heavy chain) genes. These genes and their products mediate such regulations by controlling essential cell interactions involving helper T cell (T_H) and Ts, and by determining the specificity of lymphocyte clones stimulated by antigens (66–67).

The mouse MHC located on chromosome 17 includes H-2K, H-2D genetic regions, the immune response (Ir) region, and Ss genes controlling the serum concentration of the fourth component of complement. If tissue grafts are made between strains of mice that differ at these loci, a prompt immune rejection of the graft takes place. In addition, cytotoxic T cells (Tc) or killer T cells (Tk) and antibodies to H-2 and H-2D gene products will appear in animals that have rejected such grafts or have otherwise been immunized with H-2 antigens. Thus, H-2K and H-2D regions code for cell surface antigens that serve for targets for production of antibody or generation of CMI. This recognition mechanism is used not only to identify the difference between individuals of the same species (allografts), but also to recognize the individual's own tissue cells, which become altered because of viral infection.

The human MHC located on the sixth chromosome is divided into sero-logically defined (SD) HLA-A, B, and C, and lymphocyte defined (LD) HLA-D. Recently, antisera have been prepared that permit serologic iden-tification of HLA-D determinants that are called the HLA-DR (Ia like) determinants (69). The DR antigen was found primarily on B cells and may correspond to the Ia antigens of the mouse, whereas the HLA-A,B, and C regions correspond to H-2D and H-2K. Understanding of the role of the MHC in human immune responses is as advanced as that in mouse immune responses.

The I region, where Ir genes map, controls various immune responses. The I region has been divided into at least five subregions: A, B, J, E, and C. This region also controls a series of serologically recognized antigens (Ia antigens) that are present mainly on B cells and macrophages (Mϕ). Some are, however, present on activated T cells. Blocking antibodies (BAs) are found in the antisera to Ia antigens. They have several purposes such as inhibition of MLR, blocking of Fc receptors, inhibition of antigen-induced blast formation, interference of cellular interactions (Mϕ, T, and B cell interactions), killing of B cells, and interference with T_H and Ts.

The most recent event has been the discovery of T-cell regulatory factors bearing I-region controlled determinants and of the fact that Ir genes are identical with Ia molecules. The T-cell product, referred to as the *T-cell receptor*, carries V_H determinants as shown by the binding of specific antiidiotype antibodies (Abs) and of Abs directed against V_H framework determinants (67–68). The antigen-specific T-cell products have been isolated from T-cell lysate or supernatants on affinity columns containing antigen antiidiotype or anti-V_H Ab. The general molecular properties of the isolated T-cell products bear striking resemblances, despite the diversity of systems. A large component was repeatedly found with a molecular weight between 62,000 and 68,000 daltons. The T-cell product, irrespective of its sources, may effectively display suppressor activity. A number of investigators have shown that the 62,000 to 68,000 component could be resolved into 40,000 to 45,000 and 25,000 components. The larger component bears the V_H determinants, the smaller the Ia antigenic markers. Thus, the idiotype network, postulated by Jerne to operate antibodies and B cells, has been found to be even more important for the regulation of T-cell responses in conjunction with MHC gene products. (69).

Therefore, the immune reaction (IR), as Voisin proposed, can reasonably be classified into a part for rejection (RR), which is universally found in transplantation of allografts in mammals, and a regulatory part for limiting the IR for protecting the allograft by facilitation reaction (FR): IR = RR + FR. Here, the FR may involve the production of BAs and the idiotype-antiidiotype Abs, and the generation of Ts (58).

The existence of the virtual universality of allograft rejection in mammals, which has been considered a golden rule, is apparently not always the case. In fact, several examples of prolonged survival of transplanted allografts have been reported: survival of liver grafts among certain pigs (70); prolonged survival of kidney allografts in rats, when the host had been passively immunized with antisera specifically directed against antigens on the donor kidney (71); prolonged survival of kidney grafts in certain MHC-incompatible strains of mice (72); and prolonged survival time of endocrine allografts if they could be maintained in organ culture prior to grafting (73). It was suggested that some of these exceptions are dependent on elicitation of FR.

Segal et al. showed that allograft of BM rat fetal bone, unlike allografts of adult bone, are not rejected by allogeneic recipients of the Lewis strain in spite of the existence of MHC imcompatibility between donor and host. They further showed that BM rats did reject the fetal bone of the Lewis rats because of their incapability to produce anti-Ia Abs due to a genetic defect in their capacity to respond to Ia determinants of the Lewis fetal bone. They proposed that the capacity of the Ia determinants, expressed on the cells of the embryo, to elicite anti-Ia Abs in the pregnant mother determined the capacity of the embryo to escape rejection by the histoincompatible mother (74).

In conclusion, the immunoregulatory mechanisms in transplantation immunology may be reasonably summarized at present as follows: The IR as the RR will be regulated by the I region of MHC and V_H genes and, thus, may protect the transplanted allograft from the RR when the FR elicits, depending upon the capability of the host to respond to the regulatory gene products of the graft.

From these considerations a possibility arises that pregnancy is not the exception to the rule in transplantation and there may be a general rule of immunoregulation responsible for both pregnancy and allograft transplantation.

DESTINY OF CONCEPTUSES AFTER EARLY DEMISE OF THE EMBRYO—A NATURE'S EXPERIMENT SYSTEM DURING PREGNANCY

A neglected fact which is important for pathology in the first trimester of pregnancy is that the destiny of the conceptus after early demise of the embryo will be either SpA or HM (75–76). Recognition of this fact will give us a Nature's Experiment System during human pregnancy (77). The conceptus after death of embryo clearly results in abortion, but the neoplasm concept in the nature of HM has prevented us from recognizing this important fact.

Hertig et al. (1940) (78) proposed the following hypothesis regarding the pathogenesis of HM: It is the missed abortion of a pathologic ovum, a conceptus in which an embryo is absent or dies during the third to fifth week of development, resulting in the progressive accumulation of fluid within the villi by the functioning of the trophoblast in the absence of fetal circulation. Most of the pathologic or blighted ova result in SpA, with early hydatidiform swelling showing in two-thirds of them. The sequence of events leading to SpA and HM thus considered is shown in Figure 12.1A. This hypothesis, however, has encountered quite a few objections: what is the reason responsible for a variety of hyperplasia of trophoblast in HM? What is the reason for a preponderance of female sex chromatin of chromosome found in HM? The answers to these questions were, at that time, very difficult to determine due to poor knowledge of pregnancy immunology and cytogenetics from the aspect that HM is an abortion. Park proposed a concept of primary neoplastic change of trophoblasts which easily explains

A. Hertig's Hypothesis

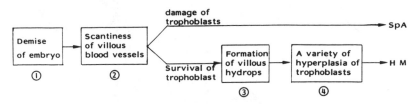

B. Park's Hypothesis

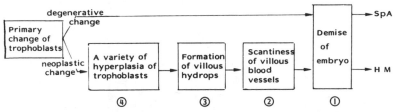

Fig. 12.1. Antithetic sequence in genesis of SpA and HM between Hertig's abortion-hypothesis and Park's neoplasm-hypothesis.

their overgrowth (79). Female preponderance would also be explained by the neoplastic concept from the analogy of the fact that females give rise to higher incidence of struma (79). The abnormality or dysplasia (neoplastic change) of the trophoblast may cause oversecretion of fluid into villi and overtaxing of the circulatory arrangement of the embryo, perhaps even causing pressure atrophy and disappearance of vessels within the villi, usually leading to the death of the embryo. This is manifested clinically either as a hydropic abortion or, if more severe, as a HM. If the abnormality of trophoblasts is a sort of degeneration, they are incapable of sustaining the life of the embryo; this is manifested clinically as a SpA (Fig. 12.1B) (79).

Therefore, the sequence of morphological events leading to a genesis of HM and SpA presents a dramatic contrast between the two hypotheses. In this context, our morphogenetic study on HM and SpA gave support to Hertig's hypotheses but not to Park's, indicating the preceding absence or presence of the pathologic embryo followed by the damage or formation of hydrops in the villi (75).

Hypotheses concerning the nature of HM so far reported are summarized in Table 12.2. In addition to *abortion* (78) or neoplasm (79) theory, *malnutrition* (80), suggested by its higher incidence in less developed countries, and *infectious etiology*, including viruses (81), and recently *malformation theory by androgenesis* have also been reported (82–84). The viral or nutritional etiology seem invalid, at least as principal causes, at present,

Table 12.2. Hypothesis Concerning Nature of HM

Nature	Author	Pathogenesis* (Formal Genesis)	Etiology (Causal Genesis)
Abortion	Hertig et al. (1940)	①→②→③→④	Early demise of the embryo due to *blighted ovum* arising from unknown causes
	Takeuchi (1971, 1980)	→③→ ①→②→④	1) Early demise of the embryo due to lethal chromosomal anomalies such as adrogenesis, triploidy, trisomy, etc. (*mainly androgenesis*). 2) *Immune survival of trophoblasts* by continuing production of BA, probably due to higher antigenicity of them
Neoplasm	Park (1971)	④→③→②→①	Unknown
Malnutrition or metabolic disturbance	Reynolds (1976)	?	Subclinical deficiency of folic acid
Infection	De Ruyck (1951)	?	Viral infection
Malformation	Kajii (1978)	?	Androgenesis of conceptuses

*① early demise of embryo, ② scantiness of blood vessels in the villi, ③ formation of villous hydrops, ④ a variety of hyperplasia of trophoblasts.
BAs: blocking antibodies.

although the possibilities are by no means excluded. Evidence of qualitative abnormality such as dysplasia in the trophoblast has never been produced in the development of HM (85). Unfortunately, however, after introduction of successful chemotherapy, neoplasm concept of HM has been accepted as a benign phase of the trophoblastic neoplasm which has been proposed by Hertz. Spectrum concept of a trophoblastic neoplasm, which is a generic term for HM, invasive mole, and choriocarcinoma, is seemingly beneficial for clinical management (86). But neoplasm concept of HM is clearly misleading now that cytogenetical study gives clear evidence of an androgenetic origin in most HM (82–84), and immunological study reveals that both damaged trophoblasts in SpA and a variety of hyperplasia of trophoblasts in HM are related to immunology (76–77). In this context, the evidence that HM is an abortion in nature is summarized in Table 12.3. It may now be very clear that HM is an abortion with trophoblastic overgrowth and not a neoplastic tumor in nature. We should now abandon the idea that HM may arise from neoplastic transformation of the trophoblastic villus. This will be mandatory for both finding a solution to the enigmatic problems encountered at present in reproductive immunology and understanding the real nature of HM.

It is, therefore, now self-evident from abortion-concept of HM that the destiny of the conceptus after the early demise of the embryo will be either SpA or HM, as already proposed by Hertig in 1940 (78). But, both the puzzling nature of HM which is an abortion with a variety of trophoblastic hyperplasia of hydropic villi and prevalence of a misleading tumor concept, which was introduced by success of chemotherapy and has been more prevailing than the abortion concept due to clinical convenience, may make it hard for us to recognize this fact clearly.

Table 12.3. Evidence That HM Is an Abortion with a Variety of Trophoblastic Hyperplasia of the Hydropic Villi

1. Evidence that early demise of the embryo precedes the formation of HM
   1-1 by pathological study on the sequence of the morphological events leading to formation of HM (78, 75)
   1-2 by clinical observation with ultrasonic echo (101,102)
2. HM shows presence of lethal chromosomal anomalies responsible for early demise of the embryo such as *androgenesis* (82, 83)
3. That the early demise of the embryo may drop out as SpA in most cases will be evidenced by the experiment that early embryectomy of the monkey resulted in SpA, but not in HM (103)
4. After the early demise of the embryo, conceptuses destined to SpA decrease their capability to produce BAs while those destined to HM continue to produce BAs, indicating immune injury of trophoblasts in SpA and immune survival of trophoblasts in HM (76, 104)
5. No evidence of neoplastic change of trophoblasts in HM evidenced by transplantation of molar tissues into nude mice (85)

The fact which is surely giving us *A Nature's Experiment System* has thus been neglected. In spite of remarkable progress in reproductive immunology, the enigmatic issues such as immunologic coexistence during pregnancy and immunologic mechanisms which regulate either survival and growth or damage of trophoblasts *in vivo* still remain to be solved. This may be responsible for lack of recognition of this excellent system.

To make a break-through in reproductive immunology, study on the Nature's Experiment System concerning SpA and HM is indispensable. Hence, we have to recognize that we are in a very complicated situation; where in order to solve the immunologic enigma during pregnancy, a clear recognition of this system is needed and in order to recognize the presence of this system, a reasonable immunological explanation for overgrowth of trophoblasts in HM, which is an abortion in nature, is requested.

Both HM and SpA are abortions as shown in Figure 12.2; SpA may arise either from primary *early death of the embryo* (Ⓐ) followed by secondary *damage of the trophoblasts* (Ⓑ) or primary Ⓑ followed by secondary Ⓐ, while HM will occur only from primary Ⓐ followed by *a variety of trophoblastic hyperplasia* (Ⓒ) with formation of villous hydrops. Hence, the destiny of the primary Ⓐ, in most cases, results in SpA with Ⓑ and the remaining cases develop into HM with Ⓒ. The mechanism selecting either SpA or HM, however, was not known. In this context, we, in 1971, proposed the hypothesis that an immune selection mechanism might play an important

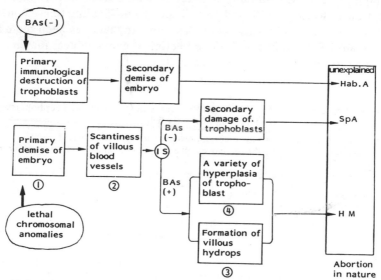

Fig. 12.2. Takeuchi's hypothesis on the formal and causal genesis of SpA and HM. IS: Immune selection by dynamic change in BAs production. BAs: blocking antibodies. Hab. A: habitual abortion. SpA: spontaneous abortion. H M: hydatidiform mole. (−): no or sparse production. (+): enough production.

role in determining the destiny of the dead embryo on the basis of comparative study on SpA and HM related to NP-1 (75). At first, embryomaternal compatibility or incompatibility after Ⓐ was considered to play an important role in immune selection of either Ⓑ or Ⓒ, because higher and no antigenic expression of the trophoblasts in SpA and HM were observed respectively. The reactivity of Abs in the patient's sera with autologous trophoblasts evidenced by immune adherence (IA) test was found more often in SpA than in NP-1, while it was observed in no cases of HM (75–76).

Further studies in our laboratory along this line gave evidence for our hypothesis, but led us to contrary views concerning the embryomaternal incompatibility: trophoblasts of HM were more antigenic than those of SpA and NP-1 in MHC, especially fetal HLA-D (Ia-like) determinants, which gave a signal for production of BAs that are necessary for successful maintenance of pregnancy. In 1980, we proposed that an immunoregulatory mechanism by a dynamic change of BAs-production might play an important role in determining the destiny of the conceptus — either SpA or HM—after Ⓐ (76).

ANTITHETIC DIFFERENCE IN IMMUNOLOGICAL FINDINGS BETWEEN SPA AND HM RELATED TO NP-1

Few immunologically comparative studies between abortion and HM have been reported. In our laboratory, as described above, a comparative study on the immunology of SpA and HM has been extensively made to determine how the immunological mechanism selects the destiny of the conceptus after the early demise of the embryo. We have found that the antigens of the ETU are immunogenic and the mother produces both humoral and cell-mediated immunity (CMI) against them in the abnormal pregnancy, such as SpA and HM, as well as in the normal pregnancy in the first trimester (NP-1).

Cell-Mediated Immunity (CMI)

The macrophage migration inhibition (MMI) assay which was performed with trophoblastic cell extracts to the maternal lymphocytes showed that percent (%) inhibition of MMI

$$\left(\left[1 - \frac{\text{migration in MLTC supernatant}}{\text{migration in control culture}} \right] \times 100 \right)$$

was 36, 16, and 30 in SpA, HM, and NP-1, respectively. This clearly indicates that CMI to the antigens of the trophoblasts or ETU by maternal lymphocytes occurs in normal and abnormal pregnancy. The response index of the mixed trophoblast-lymphocyte culture (MLTC)

$$\left(\text{MLTC response index} \ = \ \frac{\text{MLTC (cpm)}}{\text{control culture (cpm)}} \right)$$

revealed that maternal lymphocytes were toxic to autologous trophoblasts, indicating generation of Tc cells in sensitized maternal lymphocytes. But, the counts ($\times 10^4$) of H^3-thymidine uptake by one-way mixed leukocyte reaction (MLR) performed in couples (responder: maternal lymphocytes; stimulator: paternal lymphocytes treated with mitomycin) were 1.7 ± 0.7, 1.9 ± 0.6, and 2.1 ± 0.7, respectively, in SpA, HM, and NP-1, indicating no occurrence of CMI. The HLA-D(Ia like) determinants of the human MHC represent the major stimulating alloantigens in MLR. Thus the maternal lymphocytes are considered to be sensitized to produce macrophage migration inhibitory factors (MIF) and Tc cells, but not to generate T_{MLR}. It may further be worthwhile to note that the value of one-way MLC performed in couples with recurrent abortions averaged 1.0 ± 0.3, and is significantly depressed compared to 1.7 ± 0.7 in couples with SpA which was not habitual.

Humoral Immunity

The mother's humoral responses to erythrocytes and MHC of leukocytes are well known. Anti-HLA-A and B Abs were found more frequently (26%) in HM compared to NP-1 (7.1%), indicating molar trophoblasts to be more antigenic than those in NP-1. The higher antigenicity of molar trophoblast to production of anti-HLA-A and B Abs was already proposed by Lawler (88). This tendency was also observed by us in the production of anti-OFA-1 Abs. We found Abs against M-14 cells which was detected by an immune adherence (IA) test (87). M-14 cells are from a malignant melanoma cell line which has OFA-1, that are also present in fetal brain tissue (87). Anti-OFA-1 Abs were detected in 61, 73, and 46% of SpA, HM, and NP-1, respectively.

The presence of BAs in the sera from pregnant women was found by blocking beffect (BE)

$$\left(\left[1 \ - \ \frac{\text{MLC in autologous serum}}{\text{MLC in nonpregnant AB serum}} \right] \right) \ \times \ 100 \ ,$$

which will be described later in detail.

Characterization of Blocking Antibodies (BAs)

A number of investigators have recognized BAs which block the MLR in the serum of multigravid women (76, 89). BAs could be detected in unabsorbed serum, but they were markedly decreased in absorbed serum from which IgG had been removed by anti-IgG affinity chromatograpy (76, 89). Blocking effect (BE) was regained by the addition to the absorbed serum of IgG extracted from multigravid women, indicating that the main component of BAs is IgG antibody (76, 89). Thus, the higher the BE, the more BAs are present. The BAs are not removed by exhaustive absorption with pooled human platelets, and they selectively bind to human B lymphocytes but not T lymphocytes, thus showing them to be Abs to HLA-D locus, which have Ia-like determinants, but not to HLA-A, B, and C loci (77, 89).

Uncertainty, however, remains as to the individual specificity of BA. Sera from NP-1 and HM demonstrated the presence of BAs not only to the MLR in NP-1 and HM, but also to the MLR in SpA. Sera from SpA revealed absence or sparse BE even on MLC in NP-1 and HM (77).

These results indicate that the BAs are seemingly not sharp in individual-specificity and thus are likely to be pregnancy-specific Abs which are produced against organ-specific fetal antigens of the ETU. Alternatively, anti-HLA-D antibody may be inherently less individual-specific, compared with that of HLA-A, B, and C. We, however, found that individual specificity of BAs was not sharp when MLR in the couples was performed with the whole lymphocytes, but became sharp when performed with B-cell rich-lymphocyte fractions obtained by Mann's method (91–93).

Dynamic Change of Blocking Antibody Production during Normal and Abnormal Pregnancy

As described in the previous section, it has been proposed that BAs observed in the pregnant sera probably protect the ETU from the mother's CMI. This proposal was supported mainly by animal experiments and the only human evidence is that IgG eluted from pooled placentas has shown a complement-dependent cytotoxic effect on allogeneic lymphocytes and was capable of inhibiting MLR. Rocklin et al. gave support for this proposal with human evidence that BAs were absent in sera from habitual aborters as well as from nullgravid women, but present in sera from multiparous females by BE of these sera on MMI test (89). This was confirmed by Stimson using the MMI-1 blocking test (92), and by us using the MLR-blocking test (76–77). The BE(%) in sera from habitual aborters and nullgravid women was 3 ± 9 and 3 ± 8, respectively, and is significantly lower than 15 ± 7 from

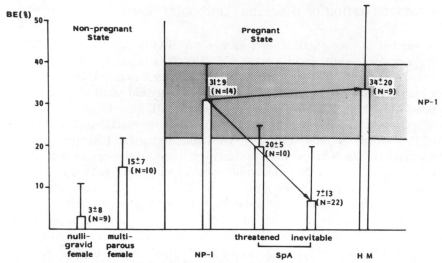

Fig. 12.3. Dynamic change in production of BAs during early pregnancy. NP-1: normal pregnancy in the first trimester. SpA: spontaneous abortion. HM: hydatidiform mole. BE: blocking effect. BAs: blocking antibodies.

multiparous females (77). These results may indicate that, in man, the nonproduction of BAs will result in SpA which is liable to occur repeatedly and that such a condition is necessary for the maintenance of a successful pregnancy. Lack of BAs production in early pregnancy may give rise to primary damage to trophoblast, which is apparently responsible for abortion. But no evidence for this has ever been given. In this context, antithetic difference of BAs production between the two states, as shown in Figure 12.3, may give strong support to the idea that BAs are indispensable for successful pregnancy by sustaining trophoblast survival, and lack of them results in abortion by destroying trophoblasts. In SpA, BAs decreased insignificantly at the threatened stage, but significantly at the inevitable stage, while, in HM, they did not decrease. The data received strong support from the difference in trophoblast-bound Abs evidenced by immunofluorescence Ab technique and the immunological properties of IgG Abs in the eluates from normal and molar trophoblasts.

Trophoblast-Bound Antibodies

Immunofluorescence Antibody Technique. To detect trophoblast-bound Abs, the indirect immunofluorescence technique was applied using antihuman

Ig-rabbit (r) antisera, antihuman IgG-r-antisera, and anithuman IgM-r-antisera in our laboratory (76).

IgG was observed in granular patterns on the cell membrane of syncytio-trophoblasts in NP-1 and HM, but not clearly in SpA. On the contrary, IgM was found in linear patterns on the syncytiotrophoblast in SpA, but not in NP-1 and HM. Aborted trophoblasts are mostly degenerated and thus are inappropriate for immunologic study of the cell membrane. But that IgM instead of IgG, associated with βIC, was observed on the cell membrane of the trophoblasts indicates the probable involvement of an immune cytotoxic reaction with damage of the aborted trophoblasts. This notion may receive support from CH50 determinations of the sera, which were significantly decreased in SpA compared with HM and NP-1.

Immunological Properties of the Ig Eluates from the Trophoblast Tissues of NP-1 and HM. Elution of the tissues was performed according to the method of Faulk et al. (51). Purified IgG was obtained by DE-32 column chromatography. The immunological properties of the eluates thus obtained were studied for their blocking effect on MLR performed in the couples and unrelated combinations in our laboratory. We found that the eluate-IgG from both normal placental tissues and molar tissues contained BAs produced against fetal HLA-DR determinants inherited from husband's MHC (93).

In man as well as mice, IgG eluted from pooled placentas has shown the immunological properties indicating the presence of BAs which are trapped on the trophoblasts by their Ab-trapping activity. These may play a protecting role for the trophoblasts in various ways, either specifically or nonspecifically. No reports, however, have been made on the molar trophoblastic tissues. Considering that molar trophoblasts show a variety of hyperplasia without the live embryo, molar trophoblast-bound BAs will become more apparent as an important factor for survival and growth of trophoblasts. Elution of IgG and IgM from the aborted placental tissues is being done in our laboratory.

PRODUCTION OF BLOCKING ANTIBODIES TO EMBRYOTROPHOBLAST UNIT AND ITS IMPLICATIONS IN PREGNANCY

Production of Blocking Antibodies

Why do the BAs not develop in women who have repeated abortions and who are undergoing SpA? Why do they continue to develop in women with HM in the absence of the embryo? Three possibilities can be considered for the production of BAs. The first possibility is a degree of histoincompatibility between ETU and mother and, therefore, the absence or presence of a sufficient stimulus, especially related to HLA-D locus. The second is the ability of the patient's genetic factors to respond to antigens of the ETU. The third is abnormality of the Ia antigens of the ETU. Fetal Ia-antigens may differ from adult Ia-determinants in their ability to induce production of BAs (59). In Segal's experiment, utilizing fetal bone graft, the BM rats did not respond to Ia antigens of Lewis fetal bone while they induced in Lewis recipients a vigorous humoral response consisting mainly of the production of IgG antibody that seemed to be directed against antigens of Ia-like specificity (74). Therefore, in his experimental system, the second possibility is correct and the third cannot be ruled out.

In our experiment described here, the first possibility is likely to be correct for the following reasons. (a) Habitual aborter's lymphocytes are less responsive to husband's lymphocytes than to fertile unrelated male's lymphocytes. (b) The fact that, after the demise of the embryo, BAs apparently begin to decrease in SpA but do not decrease and continue to be produced in HM which is more immunogenic than NP-1 and SpA. However, the third possibility may also be involved in our experiment, because embryonal or fetal Ia antigens may possibly be more capable of elicitation of BAs, by the cooperation with fetal antigens, than adult Ia antigens.

The result observed in SpA apparently indicates that presence of the live embryo may be necessary for the survival and growth of the trophoblast in an early stage of pregnancy. This may further indicate that antigenic stimulation of trophoblast without embryo is generally not enough to produce BAs in the mother. Thus most cases may result in SpA after the early demise of the embryo. But in the case of HM, only molar trophoblasts without embryo may have a capability for eliciting BAs in the patient. Contrary to this, in the case of habitual abortion, even a complete ETU may not have enough antigenic stimulation to produce BA. HM which mostly arise from pathologic ova of androgenesis and thus are complete allografts, though the usual conceptus is a semiallograft, have a strong possibility of being more antigenic than NP-1. Indeed, Aoki et al. (1981) demonstrated that cases with few MHC incompatibility were far less common in the habitual aborters (2.2%) than in the fertile couples (30.0%), but one or more compatibilities of HLA-DR antigens was significantly more common in the former (85.0%) as compared to the latter (24.4%) (94). Consequently, a sufficient antigenic stimulation of HLA-D locus is necessary for production of enough BAs for survival and growth of trophoblasts.

Komlos and Halbrecht reported that couples who shared two or three common HLA antigens were found more frequently in the fertile group than in the group of repeated aborters, proposing a hypothesis that alloimmunization of maternal cells to fetal transplantation antigens may have beneficial or adverse effects on the fetal target cells, and that it is dependent upon fetomaternal MHC interrelationship should provide a new approach for interpreting functional disturbances in certain cases of human pregnancy (95).

According to Segal et al., BAs have been defined by Davies and Stains (96), Carpenter et al. (50), and Welsh et al. (97) as equivalent to the Abs directed to Ia-like components of MHC of the rat (74). They proposed an attractive hypothesis that the trophoblast initiates the production of anti-Ia alloantibodies in the mother and subsequently absorbs these as BAs (74). Wegmann (1977) supports the idea that the trophoblastic epithelium of the placenta can serve as a paternal antigen-bearing immunoabsorbent (98). Barg et al. (1978) suggests that the trophoblast may promote the synthesis of local T-cell-dependent BAs and an effective Ab-trapping mechanism on an immunologically specific basis by the trophoblasts (100). These results strongly suggest that BAs can be produced only by trophoblasts after the early demise of the embryo.

Further, our study indicated that fetal MHC-encoded alloantigens, especially HLA-D determinants might have an immunogenicity to the mother to produce BAs more efficiently compared to adult ones. In this context, a potentially important immunoregulatory role of fetal antigens such as alphafetoprotein (AFP) may be taken into consideration, because Peck et al. suggested that AFP appears to regulate T-cell-dependent IR *in vivo* in a highly selective manner (56).

Implications of Blocking Antibody Production in Normal and Abnormal Pregnancy

As described above, it is apparent that antigenic stimulation of HLA-D (Ia-like determinants) expressed on the ETU to elicit and continue to produce BA is necessary for successful pregnancy. When the conceptus does not give enough antigenic stimulation to produce BA, SpA may occur. The woman in this situation is prone to be a habitual aborter, because the conceptus is less antigenic. Alternatively, patients may have some genetic defect in their response to the HLA-D determinants of the conceptus. When the mother does not develop BAs to the conceptus, she is prone to be a habitual aborter. When the conceptus develops BAs, it continues to grow into an ETU. However, when early demise of the embryo occurs due to lethal chromosomal aberrations, BAs begin to decrease because the antigenic capacity of the remaining trophoblast is not enough to elicit them and in turn SpA results. In a few cases, BAs do not decrease, but continue to be produced because the stronger antigenic capacity of the remaining trophoblast is enough to elicit them and thus the trophoblast develops into HM. Needless to say that, when the embryo survives and continues to produce BA, the ETU successfully develops through FTU to delivery of the infant.

Therefore, we can now reasonably conclude that the active immune recognition and generation of BAs against fetal MHC, especially HLA-D determinants, is one of the physiological immunoregulatory mechanisms ensuring survival and development of the conceptus through the ETU to the FTU.

The Mode of the Facilitating Activity of Blocking Antibodies

The mode of the facilitating action of BAs in the immunoregulatory aspect of pregnancy is not fully understood at present, but two factors are assumed; one is protection of the trophoblastic cells and the other is specific suppression of RR from the immunological center. As is strongly suggested by our study, immune-injury of the trophoblast in SpA by failure of production of BA, and immune-survival of the trophoblast in NP-1 and HM by production of BA, concerns the first mode of action of BAs. But, in pregnancy, we have not yet studied the second mode of action of BAs, which clearly needs to be studied. It has been reported that BAs can inhibit the generation of Tc or Tk cells and suppress the stimulating capacity of human lymphocytes with primed allogeneic cells (99). The generation of Tk has also been reported to be dependent upon cooperation between lymphocytes recognizing SD and those recognizing LD determinants (100). Hence, masking of LD determinants by BAs may inhibit generation of Tk cells.

AN IMMUNOREGULATORY MECHANISM DEDUCED FROM STUDY ON THE NATURE'S EXPERIMENT SYSTEM IN HUMAN PREGNANCY

Our immunological study on the Nature's Experiment System regarding SpA and HM led us to the conclusion that BAs produced against HLA-D determinants of conceptuses are necessary for survival and growth of trophoblasts. These play an immunological barrier function between ETU or FTU and the mother, and they, therefore, are indispensable for successful continuation of pregnancy. Antigenic expression of trophoblasts has been generally considered to be low, but this property should be considered as changeable depending upon maternal immunological environment. Our study strongly suggested that where production of BAs did not occur, trophoblasts became antigenic in terms of MHC and OFA and thus they underwent immunological destruction by maternal CMI and/or humoral immune cytotoxicity. Furthermore, our study suggested that fetal MHC, especially Ia determinants, were more prone to produce BAs than the adult MHC, suggesting that fetal antigens such as AFP may play some role in production of BAs by cooperation with Ia antigens.

BAs may play the most important role as FR by regulation of Ts generation and antiidiotypic Abs production or by cooperation with them. Thus the destiny of transplanted allograft, either *take* or *rejection*, may be determined by the capability of the graft's antigenicity to elicite BAs in the recipient and the ability of the host to produce BAs to the graft's antigens.

There were, however, the following puzzling results in our study. (a) HM was more antigenic in terms of Ab production than NP. But antigenic expression of molar trophoblasts was far less than that of normal trophoblasts, evidenced by IA test performed with autologous sera. (b) CMI of the mother to ETU was clearly demonstrated by MMI test and MLTC, but not demonstrated by MLR. (c) Individual specificity of BAs was not sharp when MLRs in the couples were performed with the whole lymphocytes but became sharp when performed with T-cell rich-or B-cell rich-lymphocyte fractions as stimulation. Wegmann et al. showed that trophoblasts, even without the embryo, were a highly effective immunoabsorbent and had an Ab-trapping activity (98). In fact, we demonstrated that BAs bound on the trophoblasts in HM as well as NP. Therefore, the BAs could play important roles in masking and/or modulation of Ags of the trophoblasts. Thus the possibility may be proposed that the more the trophoblasts are antigenic, the more BAs are produced, which lessens the antigenic expression of the trophoblast. This may be reasonable explanation for the first result. But, at present, no reasonable explanations can be given for the second and third results. We may find a reasonable explanation in the future when immunoregulatory effects of BAs are clarified in more detail. We are tempted to speculate that BAs may give a unified explanation for the immunological results obtained in our laboratory, and thus BAs may play the most important role in the immunoregulatory mechanisms during pregnancy.

SUMMARY

The enigmatic issues such as coexistence of the antigenic embryo in the immunologically competent mother still remain unsolved in spite of the recent developments in reproductive immunology. This is mainly due to the lack of evidence for immune damage and immune survival of trophoblasts *in vivo*, which may prevent us from finding a complete story of the immunology of pregnancy. Conversely, transplantation immunology, which treated pregnancy as an exception, has been developed to the point where a general rule of immunoregulation is responsible for both allograft transplantation and pregnancy.

In this context, this paper puts an emphasis on the recognition that comparative study on immunology of SpA and HM as a Nature's Experiment System gives us a clue for solving the enigmatic issues encountered by present reproductive immunology. Further intensive study on this system may lead us, we believe, to a complete understanding of the immunobiology of transplantation, cancer, and pregnancy.

The neoplasm concept of HM has misled us in the development of pregnancy immunology and the understanding of the real nature of HM. HM is now clearly an abortion in nature. The conceptuses are destined to abortion including HM after the early demise of the embryos. The destiny is selected immunologically into either *SpA* or *HM*. Our study on this Nature's Experiment System indicates that both immune survival and immune damage of trophoblasts are regulated by the dynamic change of BAs production against HLA-D (Ia like) determinants of ETU. Embryonal HLA-D antigens were suggested to be different from adult HLA-D in their capability of elicitation of BAs. The more the embryonal allograft is different in MHC from the mother, the more BAs are produced by the mother. Thus, disparity in MHC between mother and conceptus is beneficial by producing BAs for the mother's reproductive performance.

The immunoregulatory mechanisms related to immunology of pregnancy have been clarified; immune reaction is regulated by facilitation reaction involving not only production of BAs but also generation of Ts and antiidiotypic Abs. Further studies on this Nature's Experiment System are required regarding the relationship of BAs with Ts and antiidiotypic Abs in the immunoregulatory mechanisms and, in addition, for clarification of the mechanism of immune survival and immune injury of trophoblasts by BAs.

REFERENCES

1. Beer, A. E., and Billingham, R. E., *Folia Biologica* 26:225, 1980.
2. Medawar, P. B., *Symp. Soc. Exp. Biol.* 7:320, 1953.
3. Billingham, R. E., *N. Eng. J. Med.* 270:667, 1964.
4. Kirby, D. R. S., *Transplantation* (Baltimore) 6:1005, 1968.
5. Bardawil, W. A., and Toy, B. L., *Transplantation* (Baltimore) 5:444, 1957.
6. Kirby, D. R. S., Billingham, R. E., Bradbury, S., and Goldstein, D. J., *Nature* (London) 204:548, 1964.
7. Currie, G. A., and Bagshaw, K. D., *Lancet* 1:708, 1967.
8. Simmons, R. L., and Russell, P. S., *Ann. N.Y. Acad. Sci.* 99:717, 1962.
9. Faulk, W. P., and Temple, A., *Nature* (London) 262:399, 1976.
10. Faulk, W. P., Sanderson, A. R., and Temple, A., *Transplant. Proc.* 9:1379, 1977.
11. Kanazawa, K., Takahashi, T., Kajiwara, S., Arai, M., Ohno., M., and Takeuchi, S., *Acta Obstet. Gynaecol. Jpn*, Engl. ed. 213:143, 1974.
12. Murgita, R. A., Goidl, E. A., Kontiainen, S., and Wigzell, H., *Nature* (London), 267:257, 1977.

13. Voisin, G. A., and Chaout, G., *J. Reprod. Fertil.* (Suppl.) **21**:89, 1974.
14. Webb, C. G., Gall, W. E., and Edelman, G. M., *J. Exp. Med.* **146**:923, 1977.
15. Beer, A. E., and Billingham, R. E., *J. Reprod. Fert.* (Suppl.) **21**:59, 1974.
16. Padykula, H. A., *Anat. Rec.* **184**:49, 1976.
17. Billington, W. D., and Jeukinson, E. J., Antigen expression during early mouse development. In M. Balls, and A. E. Wild (Eds.), *Early Development of Mammals*, p. 219. London: British Society University Press, 1979.
18. Swineburne, L. M., *Lancet* **2**:592, 1970.
19. Billington, W. D., *Ups. J. Med. Sci.* (Suppl.) **22**:51, 1978.
20. Alexander, P., *Cancer Res.* **34**:2077, 1974.
21. Hellström, K. E., Hellström, I., and Brawn, J., *Nature* (London) **224**:914, 1969.
22. Wegman, T. G., Carlson, G. A., and Singh, B., The placenta as a paternal antigen-bearing immunoabsorbent barrier between mother and fetus. In *21st Annual Meeting of Canadian Federation of Biological Societies*, p. 87. London and Canada: University of Western Ontario, 1978.
23. Bradbury, S., Billingham, W. D., Kirby, D. R. S., and Williams, E. A., *Histochem. J.* **2**:263, 1970.
24. Borland, R., Loke, Y. W., and Wilson, D., Immunological privilege resulting from endocrine activity of trophoblast activity *in vivo*. In R. G. Edwards et al. (Eds.), *Immunobiology of Trophoblast*, p. 157. Cambridge, Engl.: Cambridge University Press, 1975.
25. Braunotein, G. D., Grodin, J. M., Vaitukaitis, T., and Ross, G. T., *Amer. J. Obstet. Gynec.* **115**:447, 1973.
26. Szulman, A. E., *N. Engl. J. Med.* **286**:1028, 1972.
27. Edidin, M., Histocompatibility genes, transplantation antigens and pregnancy. In M. Edidin (Ed.), *Transplantation Antigens*, p. 75. New York: Academic Press, 1972.
28. Wegmann, T. D., and Carlson, G. A., *J. Immunol.* **119**:1659, 1977.
29. Kadowaki, J., Thompson, R. J., and Zueler, W. W., *Lancet* **2**:1152, 1965.
30. Turner, J. H., Wald, N., and Quinlivan, W. L. G., *Am. J. Obstet. Gynec.* **95**:831, 1966.
31. Beer, A. E., *Symposium on Perinatal Medicine*. San Diego, California, 1964.
32. Fialkow, P. J., Thomas, E. D., Bryant, J. I., and Neiman, P. E., *Lancet* **1**:251, 1971.
33. Benirschke, K., and Driscoll, S. G. (Eds.), *Pathology of the Human Placenta*. New York: Springer-Verlag, 1967.
34. Woodrow, J. C., Clarke, C. A., Donohoe, W. T. A., Finn, R., McConnell, R. B., Sheppard, P. M., Lehene, D., Russel, S. H., Kulke, W., and Durkin, C. M., *Brit. Med. J.* **1**:279, 1965.
35. Walknoswska, J., Contre, F. A., and Grumbach, M. M., *Lancet* **1**:1119, 1969.
36. Beer, A. E., and Billingham, R. E., *Transpl. Proc.* **9**:1357, 1977.
37. Tomasi, T. B., *Cell. Immunol.* **37**:459, 1978.
38. Bankhurst, A. D., Witemeyer, S., and Williams, R. C., *Immunol. Commum.* **7**:187, 1978.
39. Skowron-Cendrzak, A., and Ptak, W., *Transplan.* **24**:45, 1977.
40. Adcock, E. N., Teasdale, F., August, C. S., Cox, C., Meschia, G., Battaglia, F. C., and Naughton, M. A., *Science* **181**:845, 1973.
41. Grill, T. J., and Repetti, C. F., *Am. J. Path.* **20**:605, 1979.
42. Noonan, F. P., Halliday, W. J., Morton, H., and Clunie, G. T. A., *Nature* (London) **278**:649, 1979.
43. Clemens, L. E., Siteri, P. K., and Stites, D. P., *J. Immunol.* **122**:1978, 1979.
44. Siteri, P. K., Febres, F., Clements, L. E., Chang, J. R., Gondos, B., and Stites, D., *Ann. N.Y. Acad. Sci.* **286**:384, 1977.
45. Beer, A. E., and Billingham, R. E., *Transpl. Proc.* **9**:1393, 1977.

330   Immunobiology of Transplantation, Cancer and Pregnancy

46. Breyere, E. J. and Barrett, M. E., *J. Natl. Cancer Inst.* **24**:699, 1975.
47. Bernard, O., *Immunogenetics* **5**:1, 1977.
48. Feldman, J. D., *Adv. Immunol.* **15**:167, 1972.
49. McCormick, J. N., Faulk, W. P., Fox, H., and Fudenberg, H. H., *J. Exp. Med.* **133**:1, 1971.
50. Carpenter, C. B., Soulillou, J. P., D'Apice, A. F., Strom, T. B., and Grarovoy, M. R., *Transpl. Proceed.* **8**:199, 1976.
51. Faulk, W. P., Jeannet, M., Creighton, W. D., and Carbonara, A., *J. Clin. Invest.* **54**:1011, 1974.
52. Riggio, R. R., Saal, S. D., Stenzel, K. H., and Rubin, A. J., *Transpl. Proc.* **8**:281, 1976.
53. Revillard, J. P., Brocier, J. Robert, M., Bonneau, M., and Traeger, J., *Transpl. Proc.* **8**:275, 1976.
54. Janaway, C. A., *Transpl. Proc.* **10**:355, 1978.
55. Stahn, R., Fabricius, H., and Hartleithner, W., *Nature* **276**:831, 1978.
56. Peck, A. B., Murgita, R. A., and Wigzell, H., *J. Exp. Med.* **147**:667, 1978.
57. Oldstone, M. B. A., and Tishon, A., *Nature* (London) **269**:333, 1977.
58. Voison, G. A., *Immunol. Rev.* **49**:3, 1980.
59. Segal, S., Tartakovsky, B., Katzav, S., and DeBaetselier, P., *Transpl. Proc.* **12**:582, 1980.
60. Sell, S., *Immunology, Immunopathology and Immunity*, 3rd ed., p. 316. New York: Harper & Row, 1980.
61. Sasey, A. E., *Proc. Soc. Exp. Biol. Med.* **29**:816, 1932.
62. Billingham, R. E., and Sparrow, E. M., *J. Embryol. Exp. Morphol.* **3**:265, 1955.
63. Waksman, B. H., and Namba, Y., *Cell. Immunol.* **2**:161, 1976.
64. Voisin, G. A., *Prog. Allergy* **5**:328, 1971.
65. Hellström, K. E., and Hellström, I., The role of serum factors ('blocking antibodies') as mediators of immunological nonreactivity to cellular antigens. In *Ontogeny of Acquired Immunity*, p. 133. Elsevier, NY: Ciba Foundation Symposium, 1972.
66. Reinherz, E. L., and Shlossman, S. F., *Immunology Today* **2**(4):69, 1981.
67. Benaceraff, B., Genetic control of the specificity of T lymphocytes and their regulatory products. In M. Fougerean, and J. Dausset (Eds.), *Fourth International Congress of Immunology, Progress in Immunology III*, p. 419. New York: Academic Press, 1980.
68. Sachs, D. H., Genetic control of idiotypic expression. In M. Fougerean, and J. Dausset (Eds.), *Fourth International Congress of Immunology, Progress in Immunology III*, p. 478. New York: Academic Press, 1980.
69. Sela, M., Genetic regulation of immune responsiveness. Summary of theme 7. In M. Fougerean and J. Dausset (Eds.), *Fourth International Congress of Immunology, Progress in Immunology III*, p. 496. New York: Academic Press, 1980.
70. Calney, R. Y., Sells, R. A., Pene, J. R., Davis, D. R., Millard, R. P., Herberston, B. M., et al., *Nature* (London) **223**:472, 1969.
71. Batchelor, J. R., and Welsh, K. L., *Brit. Med. Bull.* **32**:113, 1976.
72. Russell, P. S., Chase, C. M., Colvin, P. B., and Plate, J. M. D., *J. Exp. Med.* **147**:1449, 1978.
73. Lafferty, K. J., and Woolnongh, J., *Immunol. Rev.* **35**:231, 1979.
74. Segal, S., Siegal, T., Altaraz, H., et al., *Transplan.* **28**:88, 1979.
75. Takeuchi, S., Hando, T., Honda, T., Ohno, M., and Kanazawa, K., *J. Asian Fed. Obstet. Gynecol.* **2**:218, 1971.
76. Takeuchi, S., *Am. J. Reprod. Immunol.* **1**:23, 1980.
77. Takeuchi, S., *An immunoregulatory mechanism implicated by the blocking factors in serum from pregnancy.* In T. Aoki, I. Urushizaki, and E. Tsubura, (Eds.), *Manipulation*

of Host Defense Mechanisms, pg. 147. *Excerpta Medica*, International Congress Series 576, 1981.

78. Hertig, A. T., and Edmond, H. W., *Arch. Pathol.* **30**:260, 1940.
79. Rark, W. W., (Ed.), *Choriocarcinoma; A Study of its Pathology*. Philadelphia: F. A. Davis, 1971.
80. Reynolds, R. W., *Obs. Gyn.* **47**:244, 1976.
81. De Ruyck, R., *Bull Assoc. franc. étade cancer* **38**:252, 1951.
82. Kajii, T., and Ohama, K., *Nature* **268**:633, 1977.
83. Wake, N., Takagi, N., and Sasaki, M., *J. Natl. Cancer Inst.* **60**:51, 1978.
84. Yamashita, K., Wake, N., Araki, T., et al., *Am. J. Obstet. Gynecol.* **135**:597, 1979.
85. Kato, M., Tanaka, K., and Takeuchi, S., *Am. J. Obstet. Gynecol.* **142**:497, 1982.
86. Hertz, R., *Choriocarcinoma and Related Gestational Trophoblastic Tumors in Woman*. New York: Raven Press, 1971.
87. Takeuchi, S., Higuchi, M., Takeuchi, Y., and Naveshima, Y., Immunochemical characterization of antibody-like substance in the sera from the patients with gynecologic malignancies and from pregnant or pregnancy related patients reacted with oncofetal antigen on UCLASO M14 cell membrane. In E. G. Lehman (Ed.), *Carcino-Embryonic Protein*, Vol. 2, p. 873. New York: Elsevier/North Holland, 1979.
88. Lawler, S. D., *Brit. Med. Bull.* **34**:305, 1978.
89. Rocklin, R. E., Kitzmiller, J. L., Carpenter, C. B., Garovoy, M. R., and David, J. R., *New Engl. J. Med.* **285**:1209, 1976.
90. Taylor, A. V., *Am. J. Obstet. Gynec.* **138**:293, 1980.
91. Kajino, T., Kanazawa, K., and Takeuchi, S., *Am. J. Reprod. Immunol.*, in press, 1983.
92. Stimson, W. H., Strachan, A. F., and Shephered, A., *N. Engl. J. Med.* **295**:1209, 1976.
93. Hanaoka, J., *Am. J. Reprod. Immunol.* **3**, 1983.
94. Aoki, K., Katahira, T., Nakane, S., et al., Search for HLA, especially DR antigen-antibody system in the couples of the unexplained habitual abortions (in Japanese). In *Proceedings of 33rd General Meeting of Japan Society of Obstetrics and Gynecology*, p. 113, 1981.
95. Komlos, L., and Halbrecht, I., *Medical Hypothesis* **5**:901, 1979.
96. Davis, D. A. L., and Stains, N. A., *Transplant. Rev.* **30**:18, 1976.
97. Welsh, K. I., Burgos, H., and Batchelor, J. R., *Europ. J. Immunol.* **7**:267, 1977.
98. Wegmann, T. G., Singh, B., and Carlson, G. A., *J. Immunol.* **122**:270, 1979.
99. Moe. T., David, C. S., Rijinbeek, A. M., et al., *Tran. Proc.* 7 (Suppl.):127, 1975.
100. Barg, M., Burton, R. C., Smith, J. A., Luckenbach, G. A., Decker, J., and Metchell, G. F., *Clin. Exp. Immunol.* **34**:441, 1978.
101. Smith, C., Gregori, C. A., and Breen, J., *Obstet. Gynec.* **51**:173, 1978.
102. Yoshizawa, H., and Takeuchi, S., To be published.
103. Lewis, J., and Hertz, R., *Proc. Soc. Exp. Biol. Med.* **123**:805, 1966.
104. Takeuchi, S. In *Host Resistance to Cancer and Its Manipulation*, 1983.

PART V
IMMUNOBIOLOGY OF TRANSPLANTATION, CANCER, AND PREGNANCY—SIMILARITIES AND CONFUSIONS

13
Possible Roles of Natural Killer Cells in Transplantation and Cancer

Ronald B. Herberman

Natural killer (NK) cells are attracting an increasing amount of attention by tumor immunologists, basic immunologists, oncologists, and microbiologists. What are these cells and why has there been so much recent interest in them? Such questions are particularly relevant since their existence has only been known for about 7 years. Studies on natural cell-mediated cytotoxicity began as a rather restricted effort to understand a puzzling series of observations made during investigations of cell-mediated cytotoxicity in individuals that were tumor-bearing or immunized against tumors. The expected finding was specific cytotoxic activity against autologous tumor cells or against tumors of the same histologic or etiologic type. It was assumed in the initial studies that lymphoid cells from normal individuals would be unreactive and thus would serve as good baseline controls for comparison. Indeed, mice or rats immunized against various tumors, especially those induced by type C oncornaviruses, were found to have increased cytotoxic reactivity against the immunizing tumor or against tumor cells sharing the relevant tumor-associated antigens (1–4). Similarly, a considerable proportion of patients with various types of cancer appeared to react selectively against cell lines derived from tumors of the same organ or of the same histologic type (4, 5).

Although this concept of almost ubiquitous, specific tumor-associated, cell-mediated cytotoxicity against tumors became generally accepted, some exceptions to the expected specificity in clinical testing began to be noted by a few investigators. Normal individuals, including those unrelated or unexposed to cancer patients, were found to react against leukemic cells (6) or against cell lines derived from tumors (7–9). During this period, most investigators in the field attributed this anomalous control reactivity to a variety of *in vitro* artifacts (e.g., see discussion in 10). However, it was not possible to eliminate the cytotoxic reactivity of normal individuals by technical modifications in the assays, and gradually more and more investigators, including some of those initially describing good cancer-patient-restricted specificity, reported on cytotoxic reactivity by normal individuals and a lack of complete histologic type-specific reactivity by cancer patients (11–16).

Concurrent with the initial recognition of cytotoxic reactivity by normal human donors were similar observations in rodent systems. When spleen cells from young, 6- to 8-week-old normal rats were tested as controls for studies of immunity to a Gross virus-induced leukemia, they were found to frequently give substantial levels of lysis above the medium control, often as high as those from tumor-immune rats (17). Shortly thereafter, similar observations were made with normal mice (18).

Shortly after the phenomenon of natural cell-mediated cytoxicity was recognized in studies with human and rodent tumor cells, intensive efforts were begun to identify the nature of the responsible lymphoid cells. It was soon found that much of the reactivity was attributable to a particular sub-population of nonadherent cells, which have been termed NK cells. Within a short period of time, studies on NK cells have expanded into a broad and multifaceted research area, ranging from a series of problems in rather fundamental immunobiology to practical issues related to host resistance against tumors and infectious diseases, prognostic indicators, immune surveillance, and immunotherapy. I will here attempt to focus on the available information on the characteristics of NK cells and on their possible *in vivo* roles. For a more detailed and comprehensive summary of the current state of the field, the reader may refer to a recent book on NK cells and other natural cell-mediated effector mechanisms (19).

CHARACTERISTICS OF NK CELLS

Since NK cells have been detected by their cytotoxic reactivity, the definition of these cells has been mainly a functional one. However, extensive efforts have been made to determine the cell surface markers and other morphologic and functional properties of NK cells. Of particular interest has been the quest for unique features of these effector cells that would allow them to be readily and definitively distinguished from other cytotoxic effector cells. In addition to the importance in understanding the nature of various cell-mediated cytotoxic reactions, NK-specific markers would allow identification and enumeration of this subpopulation by direct means separate from these functional activities. The other main objective in the characterization studies has been to determine the possible relationship of NK cells to better known and characterized subpopulations of lymphoid cells. Satisfactory resolution of these issues has been quite elusive. Although considerable progress has been achieved, findings with these effector cells have repeatedly raised major challenges to the accepted classification of lymphoid cells. Attempts to solve these problems have helped to delineate the limitations of cell separation techniques and of cell surface markers as reliable indicators of the lineage of a given cell type.

The General Phenotype of NK Cells

In initial characterization studies, NK cells were found to lack almost all of the markers and properties that were tested for. They were shown to be nonadherent and nonphagocytic (20–26) and they appeared to lack surface immunoglobulins (20, 21, 23, 27, 28), receptors for the Fc portion of IgG (FcγR) (20, 21), Thy 1 antigen (20, 21) (with mouse NK cells), or receptors for sheep erythrocytes (29, 30) (with human NK cells). However, by using more sensitive techniques, evidence has accumulated for the consistent expression of several markers on NK cells.

The FcγR has been found to be a general feature of NK cells. Although mouse and rat NK cells initially appeared to lack these receptors, more sensitive procedures for depletion of FcγR-bearing cells resulted in removal of more than half of the lytic activity of NK cells (31, 32). FcγR have been more readily detectable on human NK cells and depletion of FcγR+ cells has been associated with virtual elimination of NK activity (25, 29, 30). The finding of FcγR on NK cells of each of these species raised questions about the relationship between NK cells and K cells mediating antibody-dependent cell-mediated cytotoxicity (ADCC). One possible explanation for NK activity is that it is produced by K cells, which are *armed* with *in vivo*-bound natural antibodies (33), or which react against target cells that become coated with antibodies secreted during the *in vitro* assay (34). However, extensive studies in my laboratory (35–37) and in some others (38) have failed to confirm that IgG plays a major role in natural cell-mediated cytotoxicity. Despite this, NK and K cells appear to share many characteristics and both activities appear to be associated with the same subpopulation of lymphocytes (35, 39–42). On the basis of experiments in which some target cells sensitive to NK activity were able to inhibit ADCC, it appears that much of the NK and ADCC activities may be mediated by the same cells (43, 44). The ability to deplete a considerable portion of the human K cells by selective adsorption of NK cells on target cell monolayers (38, 45) has supported this possibility. The overall pattern of results that has been obtained, with the lack of a major role for antibodies in NK activity despite the overlap between NK and K cells, suggests that the same cell may produce cytotoxic effects either by interaction with antibody-coated target cells via its FcγR or with some target cells via separate *NK receptors*. Such a dissociation between the two mechanisms of cytotoxicity has been supported by several situations in which NK and ADCC activities have not correlated (e.g., 37, 41). Kim et al. (46) have shown that the development of ADCC activity in germ-free piglets occurs several weeks earlier than the development of NK activity. There have also been some indications that at least some of the NK and ADCC activities may reside in discrete subsets of cells. Neville (47) has shown some physical separation of the activities in human peripheral blood mononuclear cells, based on differences in the affinities of the FcγR on NK and K cells. Also, the leukemic cells of a patient with chronic lymphocytic leukemia were found to mediate ADCC, but had no detectable NK activity (48).

Expression of Markers Restricted to NK Cells

For detailed studies of NK cells, in regard to the size and differentiation of this population of cells and the regulation of its activity, it would be very helpful to identify markers that are restricted to, or are at least highly associated with, NK cells. If such markers would provide a basis for purifying NK cells and separating them from other lymphoid cells, it would then be possible to definitively study their physical, biochemical, and functional characteristics and to compare these properties to those of other cell types. Recent findings with human and rat NK cells have indicated that these objectives can now be approached, if not completely fulfilled.

Timonen et al. (49) found that the majority of human lymphocytes binding to NK-sensitive target cells and thereby forming conjugates were large lymphocytes with an indented nucleus and prominent azurophilic granules in the cytoplasm (large granular lymphocytes, LGL). It has been possible to enrich for LGL on discontinuous Percoll density gradients (50, 51) and this has allowed detailed examination of the degree of association between LGL and NK cells (52). Most of the NK activity against K562 [a highly NK-sensitive target cell derived from a patient with chronic myelogenous leukemia in blast crisis (53)] has been found in the Percoll fractions with 75 to 85% LGL, whereas these fractions contained only 10 to 20% of the input peripheral blood lymphocytes. In contrast, the fractions containing most of the small-medium lymphocytes have been virtually devoid of NK activity. Thus, this procedure consistently results in at least fivefold enrichment of NK activity. The possibility that the LGL are solely responsible for NK activity has been supported by observations that, in the LGL-enriched fractions, only the LGL were able to form conjugates with K562 and that most of these conjugate-forming LGL had the capacity to kill the attached target cells (52, 54). It was of note in these studies that a considerable portion (up to 20 to 25%) of non-LGL cells in some of the other Percoll fractions could form conjugates with K562, but this was not accompanied by any detectable lysis of the target cells. Thus, since LGL comprise only about 5% of the peripheral blood mononuclear cells (PBL), the majority of conjugate-forming cells in the total population are non-LGL and do not accurately reflect the NK activity.

In parallel studies with Percoll-fractionated human PBL, LGL were also shown to be responsible for all of the ADCC activity against antibody-coated tumor target cells (52). This was compatible with a previous report by Ault and Weiner (55), indicating an association between K cells and cells with this morphology. It was then of interest to determine whether LGL were also the effector cells for natural cytotoxicity against human monolayer target cells derived from carcinomas, as well as against K562 and other leukemia cell lines that grow in suspension. This was of particular concern because of reports that the natural effector cells in mice that react against monolayer target cells differ from NK cells in regard to cell surface markers and organ distribution and to their expression in mice of various ages and strains (56–58). However, only LGL-enriched Percoll fractions of human PBL were reactive against all of the monolayer target cells tested, as well as against the leukemia target cells (59). Thus, in man, LGL appear to account for K-cell activity and for natural cell-mediated cytotoxicity against both suspension and monolayer targets. Any heterogeneity among the effector cells for the different types of targets would thus have to reside within this population of cells with similar morphology.

Having established that all human NK- and K-cell activities are due to LGL, it has been of importance to obtain more highly enriched populations of such cells. Two different methods have been found to be quite useful. Since almost all LGL were found to have $Fc\gamma R$, exposure of LGL-enriched Percoll fractions to monolayers of immune complexes has resulted in fractions containing 90% LGL and most of the NK activity of the PBL (52). LGL could also be discriminated from other lymphocytes by rosetting with sheep erythrocytes (E). About one-half of the LGL had low-affinity E receptors, forming rosettes at 4°C, not at 29°C, and the remainder lacked detectable receptors. In contrast, most other nylon-nonadherent lymphocytes had high-affinity E receptors, rosetting at 29°C as well as at 4°C. This has provided the basis for an alternative procedure for further purification of NK cells (52). Removal of high-affinity, E-rosette-forming cells from the LGL-containing Percoll fractions has resulted in a subpopulation containing ⩾95% LGL.

To further establish the degree of association between LGL and NK and K cells, it has been important to determine the proportion of LGL that have cytotoxic activity. It was possible that only a small subpopulation of LGL expressed such functions, which would make the enumeration of LGL less useful as a correlate of NK or ADCC activities. However, it was found that about 50% of LGL could form conjugates with K562 or antibody-coated target cells (52) and that a lower percentage formed conjugates with monolayer target cells (59). Thus, recognition and cytotoxicity of target cells seems to be a major function of LGL. It remains to be determined whether all LGL have this potential, or whether a subpopulation of LGL is unrelated to NK cells.

LGL have also been detected in rats and, as in man, these cells appear to play a central role in mediating NK activity (60). The highest percentages of LGL were found in peripheral blood (7%) and in suspensions of cells from the lungs (7%), followed by the spleen (4%), peritoneal exudates (3%), and lymph nodes (1%). Few if any LGL were detected in the thymus or bone marrow. This pattern was the same as the distribution of NK activity, except for the cells from the lungs that had no detectable activity. Discontinuous density gradients of Percoll, similar to those used for human studies, were found to be useful to highly enrich or deplete LGL from either spleen or peripheral blood. Only the LGL-enriched fractions had NK activity and within the fractions only the LGL formed conjugates with NK-susceptible target cells. Essentially the same results were obtained in studies with a variety of target cells, including monolayers of sarcomas or carcinomas (Reeds, Reynolds, and Herberman, 1983, in press). Among the LGL in the blood or spleen of young rats with high NK activity, up to 22% of LGL could form lytic conjugates with NK-sensitive lymphoma target cells. Thus, in rats, LGL also appear to account for virtually all NK activity and a considerable portion of such cells have the potential to express this function. However, as indicated above for LGL in the lungs, NK activity has not been invariably associated with LGL. This is probably, at least in part, a reflection of factors regulating the cytotoxic activity of NK cells. NK activity in rats has been shown to be age dependent, with rats older than 12 weeks of age usually having low levels of reactivity in the spleen (22, 61). In contrast, spleen cells from older rats were found to have the same frequency of LGL as from young rats with high NK activity. Since NK activity of older rats can be substantially augmented by interferon (62) and such treatment can increase the proportion of lytically active LGL (63), it appears that the age-related differences in NK activity are related to the degree of activation of the pool of NK cells rather than to differences in the size of the population of potential effector cells.

Once the association between LGL and human and rat NK cells was noted, it was of interest to determine whether LGL were also present in other species. A preliminary study has indicated that most mammalian species and chickens have 1 to 10% LGL in their peripheral blood (64). This correlated in most cases with the parallel detection of NK and/or ADCC activity. Of all the species examined, it has been most difficult to detect LGL in the

blood or spleen of mice. This was quite surprising, since mice have considerable levels of NK activity and have been one of the main experimental
animal systems for studies of NK cells. It now appears, however, that this
was related to some technical problems in identification and separation of
mouse LGL, rather than to a deficit of such cells in the mouse. By maintaining
blood or spleen cells at 4°C and by centrifuging on discontinuous Percoll
gradients of high density, Luini et al. (65) have been able to isolate cell
fractions enriched in LGL-like cells and in NK activity. The cells had cytoplasmic granules with the same appearance as in LGL, but they were
smaller and had a lower cytoplasmic to nuclear ratio. Since their size was
closer to that of typical lymphocytes, they have been considerably more
difficult to identify in unfractionated cell suspensions.

With mouse NK cells, considerably more effort has been directed toward
the identification of NK cell-associated surface antigens. Several markers
have been found to be expressed, with some selectivity, on most or all
mouse NK cells. Glimcher et al. (66) found that some alloantisera contained
antibodies which, in the presence of complement, abrogated much of the
NK activity but had no detectable effect on cytotoxic T cells or some other
cell types or functions. The detected alloantigen has been termed NK 1.1
and has been considered a specific marker for mouse NK cells (66–68).
However, it still needs to be documented that only NK cells, and interferon-
inducible pre-NK cells, have this marker. Some data on this important point
have been reported by Tam et al. (67), indicating that 17% of NK 1.1+
cells formed conjugates with YAC-1, a highly NK-sensitive lymphoma target
cell. However, it is not clear what proportion of the conjugate-forming
cells could lyse the bound target cells. Although the NK 1.1+ cells were
enriched in NK activity, it would be necessary to perform single cell cytotoxicity assays, such as that developed by Grimm and Bonavida (69), to
enumerate the effector cells. In addition, it remains to be determined whether
the remaining 85% of NK 1.1+ cells could, under some circumstances,
also react with or lyse NK-susceptible targets. Resolution of these issues
is needed for adequate evaluation of the available data on the incidence of
NK 1.1+ cells in various situations. For example, Tam et al. (67) found
that older mice with low NK activity have the same numbers of NK 1.1+
cells as do young, high NK-reactors. These data appear analogous to the
findings with LGL in rats, but are at variance with the report of Roder and
Kiessling (70), showing a decrease in conjugate-forming cells in older mice.
Such discrepancies can only be settled by better determination of the specificity of each of the procedures.

Burton (58) has developed other mouse alloantisera that appear to be
selective for mouse NK cells. As with anti-NK 1.1, these reagents, in the
presence of complement, could eliminate most NK activity against the YAC-
1 lymphoma target cell. However, these reagents appeared to mark a smaller

subpopulation of spleen cells, with only 1 to 4% being positive by immunofluorescence (58), in contrast to 20 to 30% of nylon wool-passed spleen
cells being reactive with anti-NK 1.1 (71). From this, one might expect
that a higher proportion of cells positive with the other anti-NK alloantisera
would actually function as NK cells. However, analyses of conjugate formation and single cell cytoxicity will be needed to directly answer this
question.

It is important to note that, in contrast to the findings with LGL, the
alloantigenic markers have only been associated with the effector cells for
natural cell-mediated cytotoxicity against lymphoma targets. The effector
cells that mediate lysis of various monolayer targets of sarcoma cell lines
have been unreactive with these antisera (57).

Several other cell markers (Qa-4, Qa-5, asialo GM1, Ly-5) have been
associated with mouse NK cells and, in the presence of complement, each
has been useful for depletion of NK activity without affecting the majority
of lymphoid cells, including cytotoxic T cells (68, 72–75). However, it is
clear that most of these markers are not completely selective for NK cells.
For example, Ly-5 has been detected on some cells of most types with
hematopoietic origin (76) and asialo GM1 has been found in macrophages
(Habu and Okumura, personal communication). As with the alloantisera
discussed above, it will be necessary to more clearly define the extent of
the association of each marker with NK cells.

Cell Lineage of NK Cells

Since the initial placement of NK cells into the ill-defined and heterogeneous
population of null cells, there have been many efforts to find cell surface
markers and/or other characteristics that would indicate the relationship of
NK cells to the three main classes of lymphoid cells, i.e., T cells, B cells,
and macrophages. Most of the evidence and consequent debate have focused
on whether NK cells belong to the T-cell or macrophage lineage. Initial
studies in rodents indicated that NK cells were distinct from typical macrophages or T cells, since they were nonadherent and nonphagocytic and
they were detected with high activity in athymic (nude) mice (77, 78) and
in neonatally thymectomized mice and rats (23, 79). However, since then
NK cells in mice and humans have been found to have several characteristics
in common with T cells and macrophages.

Possible Relationship to T Cells. Over the last few years, an increasing
amount of evidence as accumulated for a relationship of NK cells to the T-
cell lineage (Table 13.1). By use of optimal conditions for formation of E
rosettes, 50 to 80% of human NK cells were found to have low-affinity

Table 13.1. Evidence for Relationship of NK Cells to T-Cell Lineage

Sharing of cell surface markers
  Human: E receptors, HTLA, reactivity with T-cell-associated monoclonal antibodies (LyT3, OKT10, 3A1), gp 120
  Mouse: Thy-1, Ly-1, Qa-4, Qa-5, Ly-11
  Rat: OX-8
Growth in response to T-cell growth factor (TCGF or interleukin 2).
Proliferative response to T-cell mitogens, Con A, and PHA.
Production of TCGF.
Depression of NK activity by left cerebral decortication.
Increase in NK in nude rats due to increase in LGL.
Alteration in NK activity by humoral thymic factors.

receptors for E (25). Such receptors have been universally utilized as a reliable marker for human T cells and have yet to be clearly demonstrated on lymphoid cells of other lineages. As a further indication that human NK cells are related to T cells, treatment with specific heterologous anti-T-cell sera (anti-HTLA) plus complement has been shown to abrogate cytotoxic activity (80). Based on the findings of T-cell-associated markers on human NK cells, mouse NK cells were carefully examined for their expression of Thy 1 antigen. Although Thy 1 has been found in brain and on a myelo-monocytic leukemia cell line (71), with normal lymphoid cells, it has appeared to be a quite reliable and useful marker for cells in the T lineage. Treatment with high concentrations of anti-Thy 1 plus complement, or repeated treatments, eliminated an appreciable amount of mouse NK activity (81, 82). In addition, it has been possible to positively select for a portion of NK cells from nude or euthymic mice, using a monoclonal anti-Thy 1 antibody and the fluorescence-activated cell sorter (82). Similarly, Koo and Hatzfeld (68) have reported that monoclonal antibodies to Lyt1 can react with about one-fourth of mouse NK cells and that Qa 4 and Qa 5, which are mainly restricted to T cells, are expressed on most or all mouse NK cells. Also, Ly 11.2, which appears to be restricted to the T-cell lineage (83), has been detected on most or all NK cells of the appropriate mouse strains (84).

The strong association between LGL and human and rat NK cells has provided the opportunity to more extensively and directly examine the phenotype of these effector cells and to compare it with small T lymphocytes. Human LGL have been tested with a series of monoclonal antibodies (85), using the fluorescence-activated cell sorter. A considerable proportion of LGL reacted with anti-LyT3 (86) and 3A1 (87), which have appeared to detect only T-cell-associated antigens. Further, it was of considerable interest that most LGL reacted with OKT10, a monoclonal antibody that has been shown to react mainly with thymocytes (88), whereas this antibody was virtually unreactive with all other PBL. About one-fourth of the LGL also reacted with OKT8, which has been associated with T-cell suppressor activity (89). LGL have also been found to express gp 120, a protein which appears to be specific for mature T cells (50). In contrast, OKT3 (90) and some other monoclonal antibodies that react with a high proportion of T cells were almost completely negative with LGL. Thus, the phenotype of human LGL is clearly distinct from most typical T cells, yet there is considerable sharing of several T-cell-associated markers.

The presence of both E receptors and FcγR on about half of human LGL indicates that an appreciable portion of these cells can be categorized as T-gamma (T_G) cells. In fact, Ferrarini et al. (91) have isolated T_G cells by rosetting with antibody-coated erythrocytes and found that most of the cells had the morphology of LGL. However, by analysis of LGL and T cells separated on Percoll gradients, T_G cells could be identified in both fractions (52). This was accompanied by a functional division, with only the T_G cells with LGL morphology having NK and ADCC activities. Studies are now in progress to determine the distribution between the two cell types of other immune functions that have been associated with T_G cells, particularly suppressor activity.

Rat LGL also have been tested with a series of monoclonal antibodies to determine whether they expressed T-cell-associated antigens (92). LGL lacked the W3/25 antigen, which has been found on about two-thirds of peripheral T cells (93). In contrast, a large proportion of LGL from both athymic and euthymic rats were positive for OX-8 (94), which is expressed on about one-third of T cells and is undetectable on monocytes or granulocytes. It is of particular interest, in view of the close association of human LGL and T_G cells and the presence of OKT8 on a subset of LGL, that the OX-8 antigen has been associated with the subpopulation of T cells that have suppressor activity but neither helper nor immune cytotoxic functions (94, 95).

The association in the rat of LGL with NK activity has also allowed a detailed study of the factors responsible for increased cytotoxic reactivity in athymic individuals (63). In nude rats as well as in euthymic animals, LGL appeared to account for virtually all of the NK activity. The NK activity of nude rats was incrased severalfold over that in euthymic littermates and this was associated with a parallel increase in the frequency of LGL in the spleen and peripheral blood. Thus, the higher NK activity in rats lacking a thymus appeared attributable to an expansion in the effector-cell population, rather than to a diminution in thymic-dependent suppression of their activity. These observations are most consistent with the hypothesis that NK cells are in the T-cell lineage, but they are prethymic T cells or develop along a thymic-independent pathway. In further support of this hypothesis, it has recently been shown that a soluble thymic factor, facteur thymique serique, can modulate NK activity in mice, with either this factor or a thymus graft causing a decrease in NK activity of thymectomized mice to normal levels (96).

Another line of evidence for a relationship between NK cells and T cells has come from studies with T-cell growth factor (TCGF or interleukin 2). TCGF has been shown to be produced by T cells (97) and to stimulate the *in vitro* proliferation of T cells (98). It has recently been found that human LGL can produce TCGF, upon stimulation with concanavalin A (Con A) plus phorbol myristate acetate (99). Furthermore, highly enriched populations of human LGL have been shown to proliferate for a few weeks in the presence of a purified preparation of TCGF as well as supernatants containing TCGF (100, 101). The proliferating cells have retained the morphology of LGL and their characteristic NK and ADCC activities. However, the surface phenotype of the cells changed within 7 days of culture (102), becoming reactive with the OKT3 monoclonal antibody and unreactive with OKT10 and OKM1, which reacts with an antigen on myelomonocytic cells (see below). Thus, LGL in culture become more similar to typical cells, while retaining their cytotoxic functions.

There are also recent indications that LGL can proliferate well in response to Con A or PHA (101), which are generally accepted as T-cell mitogens.

In analogy to the ability of human LGL to grow in culture, mouse NK cells also can apparently grow in the presence of TCGF. It has even been possible to obtain clones of these cells, which retain most of the characteristic features of NK cells (103, 104). Some of these clones of NK-like cells have been shown to also express the Lyt2 antigen (104).

A further, interesting study that supports the association of NK cells with the T-cell lineage has been recently reported by Bardos et al. (105). Ablation of the left cerebral cortex of mice caused a severe depression in T-cell-mediated responses. This treatment also caused a substantial decrease in NK activity but had no detectable effect on the function of macrophages or other immune cells.

Based on the above information, one can speculate on the possible placement of NK cells within the T-cell lineage. With the initial indications that the development of NK cells was thymic-independent, it seemed likely that these cells might be prethymic T cells (79). However, several of the various features that have been found to be shared with cells in the T-cell lineage have been more typical of peripheral T cells. This suggests that NK cells may not be early T cells or precursors of typical T cells but rather more differentiated cells that have developed along a thymic-independent pathway. In individuals with a thymus, only a small proportion of T lineage cells may follow this route. In contrast, in nude or neonatally thymectomized animals, more cells would be likely to differentiate in this direction.

In the context of the suggested relationship of NK cells to T cells, it is of interest to consider the possible relationship between NK cells and cytotoxic T cells (CTL). It has been postulated that they may share certain features, including similar types of recognition structures (106, 107). Although some relationship is possible, there is considerable evidence that the receptors on NK cells differ substantially from those on CTL. With CTL, recognition of the major histocompatibility complex (MHC) appears to be a major attribute of their receptors (108), whereas with NK cells there is no apparent MHC restriction. For example, mouse NK cells can have appreciable cytotoxicity against xenogeneic as well as allogeneic targets (109, 110). Furthermore, there does not even appear to be a need for NK-susceptible target cells to express MHC products, with some cell lines, e.g., K562, lacking such determinants (111) being highly susceptible to lysis. Such apparent differences between NK cells and CTL do not, however, rule out the possibility that NK cells might, under some circumstances, develop into CTL, or vice versa. The current studies with proliferating clones of NK cells and CTL may lead to some evidence for such transitions.

Possible Relationship to Macrophages or Monocytes. Initially, when NK cells of mice, rats, and humans were shown to be nonphagocytic and non-adherent (20–26), they were considered to be quite distinct from macrophages. However, it has become clear that macrophages or monocytes, including those from normal individuals (112–114), can have cytotoxic activity against tumor cells, and some features have been found to be shared by macrophages and NK cells. The activity of both NK cells and macrophages can be augmented by interferon (115) and can be inhibited by prostaglandins and phorbol esters (116–121). Furthermore, a possible role for proteases in the mechanism of cytotoxicity by both effectors has been suggested (122, 123). Thus, recently, questions have been raised as to whether NK cells may be in the macrophage lineage.

Table 13.2 summarizes the main lines of evidence that point to a possible relationship of NK cells to the macrophage lineage. The monoclonal antibody OKM1 was found to react with a high proportion of human monocytes, granulocytes, and NK cells, but was unreactive with most typical T cells (124–126). OKM1 was also found to react with a considerable portion of T_G cells, but this in conjunction with the lack of reactivity of these cells with OKT3 was taken as an argument for the monocytic nature of T_G cells (127). In confirmation of the reactivity of OKM1 with human NK cells, a

Table 13.2. Evidence for Relationship of NK Cells to Macrophage Lineage

Sharing of cell surface markers.
  Human: asialo GM1, reactivity with OKM1, Mac 1, and anti-Ia monoclonal antibodies
  Mouse: Mph 1
  Rat: asialo GM1
Some morphologic resemblance between LGL and macrophages.
Development of NK activity from mouse bone-marrow cells cultured with supernatants containing
  colony stimulating factor.
Depression of NK activity by *in vivo* treatment with silica or carrageenan.

high proportion of LGL were found to be reactive with this antibody (85). Both human NK cells and monocytes have also been found to express Mac 1 (128) and asialo GM1 (85). Similarly, rat LGL, monocytes, and granulocytes were found to express asialo GM1 (92). Also, Lohmann-Matthes and Domzig (129) reported that an anti-Mph 1, an antimacrophage mouse alloantiserum, plus complement appreciably inhibited mouse NK activity. This last piece of evidence is in dispute, since Gidlund et al. (130) failed to observe an effect of anti-Mph 1 on mouse NK activity.

For adequate interpretation of these results, the central question is whether any of the above markers are in fact reliable markers for cells of the macrophage lineage. Although the antiasialo GM1 used in the above study (72) did not react with human peripheral blood T cells, it did react well with a considerable proportion of rat T cells (92). Thus, asialo GM1 and possibly the other antigens may in some situations be expressed on cells of various lineages. The loss of reactivity to OKM1 by cultured human LGL suggests that expression of this antigen may reflect the stage of differentiation of the cells rather than their derivation. An interesting possibility to be carefully examined is whether the OKM1 antibody is directed against some portion of the FcγR, which is known to be expressed on monocytes, granulocytes, NK cells, and T_G cells, but is difficult to detect on cultured LGL (101).

Another series of studies to be carefully considered is that of Lohmann-Matthes and Domzig (129) on the relationship of mouse NK cells to cells early in the macrophage lineage. They observed that after a few days of culture of mouse bone-marrow cells in the presence of culture medium containing colony stimulating factor, nonadherent, nonphagocytic cells appeared which had NK-like activity. Since typical macrophages developed a short time later, the effector cells were considered to be promonocytes. However, it was not clearly demonstrated that the effector cells were precursors of macrophages or that the appearance of cells with NK activity was a consistent phase in the *in vitro* development of macrophages (19). Against the relationship of the cultured effector cells to NK cells was the considerable reactivity of cultured cells from A strain and beige mice (129, 131, 132), which have low NK activity.

An additional line of suggestive evidence for an association of NK cells with macrophages has been the observation that treatment of mice or rats with the selective macrophage toxic agents, silica or carrageenan, caused substantial inhibition of NK activity (133–135). However, *in vitro* treatment of mouse spleen cells with these agents, under conditions that remove or inactivate macrophages, had no effect on NK activity (136). Administration of poly I:C to animals previously treated with silica or carrageenan failed to induce interferon to augment NK activity, whereas interferon itself was effective in boosting NK activity in such animals. These results suggested that macrophages were needed to produce interferon in response to certain stimuli but were not directly related to the effector cells. An additional possible mechanism for the depressed NK activity after *in vivo* treatment with silica or carrageenan is that such agents can induce suppressor cells for NK activity (137).

One must also consider some major differences between cytotoxicity by NK cells and by macrophages that have been observed. The selectivity of cytolytic activity by mouse NK cells and by activated bone-marrow macrophages was found to be substantially different, with some target cells highly sensitive to one type of effector cell but not to the other (131). Similarly, peritoneal macrophages and NK cells were shown to have different specificity patterns (138). In addition, the strain distribution of high or low NK reactivity is substantially different from that of macrophage-mediated cytolytic activity (114, 131). C3H/HeJ mice, which have low macrophage reactivity, have high levels of NK reactivity, similar to those of C3H/HeN mice which lack the deficit in macrophage function. Conversely, SJL/J and A strain mice, which have quite low NK activity, have high levels of macrophage reactivity (131, 139). Beige mice also appeared to have a quite selective deficit in NK activity, with normal function of macrophages and CTL (132). However, this distinction has become less clear, with evidence on the one hand that macrophages from beige mice have reduced cytotoxic activity at early time points (140) and on the other hand that NK cells from beige mice are not completely unreactive (141) and function almost as well as those from normal mice when the assay period is prolonged (142). Studies on cells from patients with the Chediak-Higashi syndrome, who have the human analogue of the beige mutation, have indicated a selective and severe deficit in NK activity, with normal levels of monocyte-mediated cytotoxicity (143). However, this distinction may also not be clear-cut. It has already been found that in prolonged NK assays the NK reactivity of the patients became substantial, although still lower than that of normal donors (144).

Interpretation of Available Evidence Regarding Lineage of NK Cells. The available evidence, as summarized above, does not provide a definitive answer to the question of the cell lineage of NK cells. In fact, it points out the inadequacy of the available and widely used markers for definitively characterizing lymphoid cells. Several of the markers that have been generally considered to indicate a particular cell type may in fact be differentiation antigens that may be expressed on cells of various lineages. Despite these problems, my own tentative conclusions are that NK cells are in some way related to the T-cell lineage and that the apparent monocyte-associated or other paradoxical markers are differentiation markers. However, it should be noted that others have been more impressed with the data supporting an association of NK cells with the macrophage or myelomonocytic lineage (125, 126, 129). Another group of investigators has taken a more middle-of-the-road hypothesis, that NK cells and LGL are are derived from a separate cell lineage (91) which shares some properties with both T cells and macrophages. Resolution of this issue may come from current studies in my laboratory on the *in vitro* growth of LGL or on the *in vivo* transfer of LGL to lethally irradiated recipients. One of the main objectives in these studies is to determine whether LGL can be induced to develop into cells with typical and characteristic functions of T cells and/or macrophages.

POSSIBLE *IN VIVO* ROLES OF NK CELLS

The most important practical issue to be settled is the role of NK cells *in vivo*. Most of the attention has been directed toward the *in vivo* resistance to growth of NK-susceptible tumor cell lines. However, other and potentially more important roles have come up for consideration: (a) role in resistance against growth of primary tumors; (b) role in immune surveillance against development of spontaneous or carcinogen-induced tumors; (c) role in natural resistance against microbial infections; (d) role in natural resistance against bone-marrow transplants; (e) role in graft-versus-host disease; (f) role in regulation of differentiation of normal hemotopoietic or other cells; and (g) role as secretory and immunoregulatory cells.

Role in Resistance Against Tumor Cell Lines

There is substantial evidence for an important role of NK cells in *in vivo* resistance against established cell lines of tumors, particularly those that show susceptibility to *in vitro* cytolysis by NK cells (summarized in Table 13.3).

A major approach has been to look for correlations between *in vivo* resistance to the growth of the tumor cell lines and the levels of NK activity in the recipients. In several different situations, a good correlation was observed. Some NK-sensitive tumor lines have produced a lower incidence of tumors, and have grown more slowly, in nude or thymectomized mice than in euthymic mice with the same genetic background (79, 145, 146). Fewer transplantable tumors have also been induced in 5- to 10-week-old mice, at the peak of NK activity, than in older mice with low NK activity (79, 147). Some recent studies have examined the effects of age on growth of several transplantable tumors in nude mice. A much higher incidence of metastases, after either intravenous or subcutaneous transplantation, was seen in 3-week-old nude mice, which had low NK activity, than in 6-week-old nude mice, which had high NK activity. A high rate of pulmonary metastases in young nude recipients was seen with xenogeneic as well as

Table 13.3. Evidence for *In Vivo* Role of NK Cells Against Tumor Cell Lines

1. Variations in growth of NK-sensitive cell lines in recipients with different levels of NK activity.
   a. Less growth in nudes than in euthymic mice of same strain.
   b. Less growth in 5 to 10-week-old than in older mice.
   c. Less growth in F_1 hybrids with high NK activity than in those with low activity.
   d. Less growth in radiation chimeras reconstituted with bone marrow from high NK strains.
   e. Increased growth in beige mice.
2. Local and systemic adoptive transfer of resistance to tumor growth, by NK-cell-enriched populations.
3. Increased tumor growth in mice treated with anti-asialo GM1.
4. Correlation between *in vivo* elimination of ^{125}IUdR labeled NK-susceptible tumor cells and levels of NK activity in recipients.
   a. More rapid clearance of radioisotope in high NK strains.
   b. More rapid clearance in 4 to 8-week-old mice than in older mice.
   c. Augmentation of clearance in mice with NK activity boosted by interferon, poly I:C, *C. parvum*, pyran, or tumor cells.
   d. Depression of clearance in mice with NK activity inhibited by cyclophosphamide, lethal irradiation, corticosteroids, silica, carrageenan, pyran.
   e. Ability to reconstitute both NK activity and *in vivo* clearance in cyclophosphamide-treated mice by intravenous transfer of cells with characteristics of NK cells.

allogeneic tumor cell lines (148, 149). Augmentation of NK activity in the 3-week-old nude mice by treatment with poly I:C or *C. parvum* inhibited the development of metastases. The apparent major role for NK cells in resistance in nude mice against growth of transplantable tumors, and the ability to circumvent this by using nude mice with low NK activity, has practical implications for the strong interest in utilizing nude mice for growth of human tumors. Many investigators have noted the difficulty of growing some tumors in nude mice and the rarity of metastases, even when metastatic deposits of human tumors were transplanted (150–155). The findings that some human tumor cells are susceptible to mouse NK activity (109, 110) are consistent with a role for NK cells in this resistance.

Kiessling and his associates (156, 157) performed an extensive series of experiments which demonstrated a correlation between the levels of NK activity in different strains of mice and the resistance of F_1 hybrids between each strain and A mice to the A strain lymphoma, YAC, the cultured line of which is highly sensitive to NK activity. Mice which were thymectomized, irradiated, and reconstituted with fetal liver also showed this resistance (145). Haller et al. (158) extended this approach by transferring bone-marrow cells from high or low NK strains to lethally-irradiated low NK recipients. Recipients of cells from high NK donors developed high NK activity and had increased resistance to growth of YAC.

The various types of correlations described above have only been observed with tumor lines with some susceptibility to lysis by NK cells. The growth of completely NK-resistant cell lines has not been affected by the levels of NK activity in the recipients (e.g., 146). It is of interest in this regard that in a study of two sublines of a mouse lung tumor, the metastatic subline was resistant to NK activity, whereas the nonmetastatic subline showed some susceptibility (159).

Beige mice, with low NK activity associated with their recessive point mutation (160), have also provided a convenient model for examining the role of NK cells in resistance to growth of transplantable tumor lines. Talmadge et al. (161) found that an NK-susceptible syngeneic melanoma cell line grew more rapidly and produced more metastases in beige compared to normal mice. This difference was not seen with an NK-resistant subline of the same tumor. Using a similar approach, Karre et al. (162) found that two NK-susceptible syngeneic lymphomas produced a higher incidence of tumors and grew more rapidly in beige than in normal heterozygous littermates.

Another approach to the *in vivo* role of NK cells in the growth of transplantable tumors has been the attempt to transfer increased resistance by NK cell-enriched populations. Kasai et al. (163) enriched for Ly 5+ spleen cells and depleted Thy 1+ and B cells and showed that this small subpopulation of cells had high NK activity. Mixture of these Ly 5+ cells with an NK-sensitive lymphoma cell line resulted in reduced tumor incidence after transplantation. Similarly, local adoptive transfer of NK-1+ cells suppressed growth of the YAC lymphoma (67). Systemic adoptive transfer of cells, with the characteristics of NK cells, from normal or nude mice was also found, in an immunochemotherapy model system, to increase protection against a transplantable leukemia (164).

In an alternative approach that utilized information about selective markers on mouse NK cells, Habu et al. (165) administered antiasialo GM1 to nude mice. The treated mice had almost no detectable NK activity and showed increased susceptibility to transplantation of syngeneic, allogeneic, and human tumors.

Although the above studies point to a significant role of NK cells in resistance against tumor growth, they do not conclusively show that NK cells are the actual *in vivo* effector cells. Since these studies relied on measurement of tumor incidence or growth rate, at a considerable time after tumor challenge, one cannot rule out the possibility that NK cells helped to induce or recruit other effector mechanisms, such as T cells or activated macrophages. To obtain more direct information about the role of NK cells in the direct and rapid *in vivo* elimination of tumor cells, ^{125}I-iododeoxyuridine ([125]IUdR)-labeled tumor cells were inoculated intravenously and clearance from the lungs and other organs was measured (166–168). In young mice of strains with high NK activity, there was a greater clearance of radioactivity when measured at 2 to 4 hours after inoculation than was seen in strains with low reactivity. In parallel with the decline of NK activity in mice 10 to 12 weeks of age, *in vivo* clearance of intravenously inoculated tumor cells was also found to decrease. Furthermore, treatment of mice with a variety of agents that produced augmented or decreased *in vitro* reactivity also resulted in similar shifts in *in vivo* reactivity (Table 13.3). Such correlations were observed with several NK-susceptible tumor lines and not with some completely NK-resistant lines (167).

As further confirmation of the role of NK cells in resistance to growth of NK-susceptible transplantable tumors, transfer of NK cell-containing populations into mice with cyclophosphamide-induced depression of NK activity was shown to significantly restore both *in vivo* clearance and NK reactivity (169, 170). The effectiveness of the transfer correlated with the levels of NK activity of donor cells in a variety of situations. (a) NK-reactive spleen cells were able to transfer reactivity whereas NK-unreactive thymus cells were ineffective; (b) spleen cells from young mice of high NK strains were considerably more effective than cells from older mice or from strains with low NK activity; (c) the cells responsible for transfer had the characteristics of NK cells, being nonadherent, nonphagocytic, expressing asialo GM1, and lacking easily detectable Thy 1 antigen; and (d) cells from donors with drug-induced depression of NK activity were unable to transfer reactivity. These results extend the recent findings of Hanna and Fidler (171), who showed that the transfer of NK-reactive spleen cells to cyclophosphamide-treated mice could decrease the number of metastases developing in the lungs after challenge with NK-susceptible solid tumor cells.

A similar pattern of results was obtained when radiolabeled cells were inoculated subcutaneously into the footpads of mice (172). Clearance correlated in several ways with the levels of NK activity in the recipients and cells with the characteristics of NK cells were effective in local adoptive transfer. However, in contrast to NK activity and the results with intravenously inoculated tumor cells, no decrease in clearance was observed in older or beige mice. Those results suggest that other effector cells may also be involved in reactivity in subcutaneous tissues [e.g., the natural cytotoxic cells described by Stutman et al. (56, 57)] or that in some situations local factors may augment the NK cell activity.

Although the results in some studies, particularly those with intravenously-inoculated radiolabeled tumor cells, suggested that NK cells may be particularly involved in resistance against hematogenous metastatic spread of tumors (171), the results with the footpad assay (172) and the various demonstrations of NK-related differences in outgrowth of subcutaneous tumors indicate that natural effector cells can also enter and be active at sites of local tumor growth. This is supported by the direct demonstration of NK cells in cell suspensions prepared from small tumors growing at subcutaneous or intramuscular locations (173). Thus, NK cells have the potential to be involved in the primary line of defense against both the local outgrowth as well as the metastatic spread of transplanted tumors. However, it appears that the effectiveness of this natural resistance mechanism is rather limited. Even with tumor cells that are highly susceptible to NK activity, development of progressively growing tumors can occur in animals with high NK activity. The mechanisms for such escape from complete elimination by NK cells are not clear, but the possible explanations include: (a) development of resistance of the tumor cells to lysis by NK cells. NK-susceptible cultured tumor lines have been shown to become relatively NK-resistant after growth *in vivo* (174, 175). The nature of this resistance is not well defined, but there have been some indications that it is reversible (174). Treatment of some NK-resistant cell lines with inhibitors of RNA or protein synthesis has been found to make them sensitive to lysis by NK cells (176, 177). Interferon has been found to be one of the mediators of induction of NK-resistance of target cells, since pretreatment of some NK-sensitive target cells with interferon can render them resistant (178, 179). (b) Inhibition of NK activity in tumor-bearing individuals. Tumor-bearing mice (77, 180) and cancer patients with advanced disease (181–185) have been found to have low NK activity. This may be due, at least in part, to the development of suppressor cells. Cell suspensions prepared from large tumors in mice (186) and from some human tumors (173, 187–189) have been shown to contain macrophages or other lymphoid cells which could inhibit NK activity. Prostaglandin production by such suppressor cells or by the tumor cells might be responsible for some of the depressed NK activity, since treatment of mice bearing murine sarcoma virus-induced tumors with inhibitors of prostaglandin synthesis (indomethacin or aspirin) partially or completely restored NK activity to normal levels (119).

Role in Resistance Against Growth of Primary Tumors

From the available evidence that was summarized above, it seems likely that NK cells play an important role in resistance to growth and metastatic spread of some tumor cell lines. Although such results are encouraging, they do not indicate whether NK cells also can have a similar role in defense against growth and metastasis of primary tumors. To obtain evidence in support of such a function, it would be desirable to document the following predictions: (a) Primary tumor cells should have some demonstrable susceptibility to recognition by NK cells. (b) The NK cells of tumor-bearing individuals should be able, under some circumstances, to interact with the autologous tumor. (c) Selective alterations in NK activity in tumor-bearing individuals should affect the growth or degree of metastatic spread of the tumors.

Unfortunately, information relevant to any of these points is quite scanty and, to my knowledge, no clear data exist for the last prediction. Before

Table 13.4. Evidence for Reactivity of NK Cells Against Primary Tumors

1. Low levels of susceptibility of some primary tumors to lysis by NK cells
   Mouse: AKR lymphomas, C3H mammary tumors
   Human: Some leukemias, carcinomas, and other tumors
2. Cold target inhibition of NK activity by some primary mouse and human tumors.
3. *In situ* localization of mouse NK cells in small spontaneous mammary tumors and in primary murine sarcoma virus-induced tumors.
4. Low levels of NK reactivity of syngeneic, and even autologous tumor-bearing individuals, against some primary tumor cells.

reviewing the available evidence regarding NK reactivity against primary tumor cells, I would like to point out the difficulties that would be anticipated were NK cells playing a significant role in growth of primary tumors. For such studies, one would have to obtain tumors of sufficient size to prepare adequate numbers of tumor cells. By definition, such tumors had to have been at least relatively successful in evading host defense mechanisms. Therefore, if NK cells play an important role in resistance, one would predict that tumor outgrowth would only occur in the face of relative resistance to lysis by NK cells and/or depression of NK activity. Thus, the data most consistent with these qualifications of the earlier stated predictions would be detectable but low levels of interaction between NK cells and tumor cells.

As summarized in Table 13.4, some evidence has been accumulated in this direction. The majority of spontaneous mammary tumors of C3H mice (190) and of spontaneous lymphomas in AKR mice (191) have been found to have detectable, albeit low, susceptibility to lysis by NK cells. Similarly, some human leukemias (6, 192, 193), a myeloma (192), and some carcinomas, sarcomas, and melanomas (194, 195) have been significantly lysed by NK cells. Such lysis has been appreciably augmented, and thereby evident with a higher proportion of tumors, when the effector cells were pretreated with interferon (192–195). As further support for the ability of NK cells to recognize primary tumor cells, Ortaldo et al. (196) showed that a variety of human tumor cells could cold target inhibit the lysis of radiolabeled K562 cells. Most of these positive results were obtained with NK cells from normal allogeneic donors. In fact, Vanky et al. (194) detected NK reactivity only against allogeneic human tumor cells and concluded that the NK cells of the tumor-bearing individual lacked the ability to recognize the autologous tumor cells. They postulated that recognition of foreign histocompatibility antigens was involved in lysis by NK cells, particularly those stimulated by interferon. If correct, their hypothesis would virtually preclude a role for NK cells in resistance against primary tumor growth. However, such restriction of NK reactivity to allogeneic tumors does not fit the many examples of tumor cell lines being susceptible to syngeneic NK cells (e.g., 77, 78). Similarly, normal C3H mice have been found to be reactive against some syngeneic mammary tumors (190), and some cancer patients also have had detectable, interferon-augmentable, NK activity against their autologous tumor cells (195). The reasons for the discrepancies among the human studies are not clear. The positive results were obtained with ovarian carcinoma cells, mainly in 20-hour cytotoxicity assays (195), whereas the allorestricted results involved other types of tumors, tested only in 4-hour assays. The greater sensitivity of the prolonged assay would seem sufficient to account for the differences. In addition, it is possible that the subpopulation of NK cells that are required to interact with certain types of tumors may be selectively inhibited in the autologous tumor-bearing host.

Another line of evidence in support of the possibility for NK cells to interact *in vivo* with autologous primary tumor cells is the demonstration that NK cells can enter and accumulate at the site of tumor growth. NK cells have been detected in small spontaneous mouse mammary carcinomas (173) and in small primary mouse tumors induced by murine sarcoma virus (173, 197). In contrast, NK activity has usually been undetectable in large tumors in mice (173) or in clinical tumor specimens. This may be due, at least in part, to the presence of suppressor cells, which have been demonstrated in some cell suspensions from some tumors (173, 186–189).

To further support the possible role of NK cells in resistance against the growth of primary tumors, it would be very helpful to examine the effects of selective alterations of NK activity in tumor bearers. However, very few experiments specifically designed to examine this issue have been reported. Suggestive evidence has come from the administration of indomethacin to mice bearing primary murine sarcoma virus-induced tumors (119). With a treatment schedule that augmented the depressed NK reactivity, tumor incidence and size were reduced and a higher proportion of tumors completely regressed. Similarly, one could invoke the therapeutic efficacy of interferon for some primary tumors, a treatment known to augment NK reactivity. The limitations of such data are that such agents have pleiotropic effects and it is not possible to determine whether the alterations in other functions had the more important influence on tumor growth. Studies with more selective alterations in NK activity will be needed to settle this issue. Such experiments probably should be performed in individuals with only a small amount of tumor present, to allow the detection of effects on tumor growth that might be more likely during a phase when the host is not already overwhelmed by extensive tumor burden.

Role in Immune Surveillance Against Tumors

Of paramount interest is whether NK cells may be involved in immune surveillance against the initial development of spontaneous or carcinogen-induced tumors. Such a consideration is particularly pertinent at this time, since the whole concept of immune surveillance is being questioned (198, 199). The original formulations of the immune surveillance hypothesis emphasized the central importance of the immune system in prevention of spontaneous tumors (200, 201). Later, the theory was modified to stress the key role of thymus-dependent immunity in immune surveillance (202). The frequent, recent criticisms of the hypothesis have focused on two main issues: (a) The inability of the modified theory to account for a number of observations in T-cell-deficient mice. For example, much attention has been given to the decreased incidence of mouse mammary tumors in neonatally thymectomized mice and to the failure to observe more rapid tumor growth or even higher incidences of spontaneous or chemical carcinogen-induced tumors in nude mice (203, 204). (b) The failure to find evidence for tumor-associated transplantation antigens on many spontaneous tumors (205). The latter problem has led to the suggestion that immune surveillance may only be operative against tumors induced by oncogeneic viruses, which usually have strong transplantation antigens (206). The major exceptions to the central role of immune T cells in resistance to tumor development has led many investigators to more generally question the theory of immune surveillance. Even a counter theory of immunostimulation has been formulated (207), suggesting that the immune system may have mainly enhancing effects on tumor induction and growth.

Postulation of an important role of NK cells in immune surveillance offers possible solutions for both of the major difficulties with the theory. The observations that nude or neonatally thymectomized mice or rats have high levels of NK activity would then be compatible with their relatively low incidence of tumors. Furthermore, susceptibility of tumor cells to attack by NK cells seems to be independent of the expression of tumor-associated transplantation antigens, thus leaving open the possibility for surveillance against tumors lacking such classically defined and immune T-cell-dependent antigens.

Given such attractive theoretical arguments for the possible participation of NK cells in immune surveillance, what then is the available supportive evidence? Thus far, very few well designed experiments have been performed to directly address this issue. However, before turning to those, it is of interest to summarize several pieces of circumstantial evidence that are consistent with, or suggestive of, a role for NK cells (Table 13.5): (a) NK activity has been shown to be substantially augmented by retinoic acid (121), which has been reported to retard the development of some primary tumors (208). In support of this possibility, cells with the characteristics of NK cells have been found to inhibit the *in vitro* proliferation of autologous EBV-infected B cells (209). (b) Patients with the genetically determined Chediak-Higashi syndrome have a high risk of development of lymphopro-

Table 13.5. Circumstantial Evidence for a Role of NK Cells in Immune Surveillance

1. High NK activity in nude or neonatally thymectomized consistent with their low incidence of spontaneous mammary tumors or chemical carcinogen-induced tumors.
2. Augmentation of NK activity by retinoic acid, a tumor preventive agent, and inhibition of NK activity by tumor promoters.
3. High incidence of lymphoproliferative diseases in patients with Chediak-Higashi syndrome, who have a selective deficit in NK activity.
4. High incidence of lymphomas in a colony of beige mice, which also have a selective deficit in NK activity.
5. Low NK activity in patients with X-linked lymphoproliferative disease.
6. Low NK activity in kidney allograft recipients, who have a high risk of development of lymphoproliferative and other tumors.

liferative diseases (210). In recent detailed studies on several patients with this disease (143, 144), all were found to have profound deficits in NK- and K-cell activities, whereas a variety of other immune functions, including cytotoxicity against tumor cells by T cells, monocytes, and granulocytes, was essentially normal. (c) Similarly, beige mice, which have an analogous genetic defect, also have a substantial (132, 160), but incomplete (141, 142), selective deficiency in NK activity. A small colony of aged beige mice have recently been reported to have a high incidence of lymphomas (211). (d) Another human genetic abnormality, X-linked lymphoproliferative disease (212), has been associated with a defect in the ability to control proliferation of B cells infected with Epstein-Barr virus (EBV). Recently, low NK activity has been found in such individuals and this deficit has been suggested to be involved in the pathogenesis of the disease (213). (e) Patients on immunosuppressive therapy after kidney allotransplants have a high risk of developing tumors, both reticuloendothelial tumors and also a variety of carcinomas (214). Patients on such treatment regimens have recently been found to have very low NK activity and this has been suggested as a contributing factor to the subsequent development of tumors (215). Each of these lines of evidence fits one of the major predictions of the immune surveillance theory, that tumor development would be associated with, and in fact preceded by, depressed immunity.

A related prediction of the immune surveillance theory is that carcinogenic agents would cause depressed immune function, thereby impairing the ability of the host to reject the transformed cells. This postulate has been examined by many investigators in regard to the possible role of mature T cells and humoral immunity, and conflicting results have been obtained (203). In contrast, the initial and still fragmentary data on this point in relation to NK cells are promising. (a) Urethane, which produces lung tumors in only some strains of mice, caused transient and marked depression of NK activity in a susceptible strain (216) but not in resistant strains (217). Administration of normal bone-marrow cells, which, as discussed earlier, can reconstitute

NK activity, to urethane-treated mice reduced the subsequent development of lung tumors (218; Gorelik and Herberman, unpublished observations). Also, infection during the latent period with various viruses, each known to induce interferon and thereby augment NK activity, also reduced the incidence of lung tumors induced by urethane. (b) Carcinogenic doses of dimethylbenzanthracene also were found to produce depression of NK activity during the latent period (219). (c) Sublethal irradiation of mice has been found to cause considerable depression of NK activity (220). Of particular interest, the schedule of multiple, low doses of irradiation of C57BL mice, which has been highly effective in inducing leukemia in this strain, was found to produce a substantial deficit in NK activity (221; Gorelik and Herberman, unpublished observations). The depressed NK activity could be restored by transfer of normal bone-marrow cells (Gorelik and Herberman, unpublished observations), a procedure which has been reported to interfere with radiation-induced leukogenesis (222). (d) NK activity also has been strongly inhibited by two different classes of potent tumor promoters, phorbol esters (120, 121) and teleocidin (Goldfarb, Sugimura, and Herberman, unpublished observations). All of these observations support the possibility that one of the requisites for tumor induction by carcinogenic agents may be interference with host defenses, including those mediated by NK cells.

Further studies are needed to more directly demonstrate a role for NK cells in immune surveillance. Ideally, one would like to show increased tumorigenesis when NK activity is selectively depressed and reduced tumor formation when such deficiencies are selectively reconstituted or normal levels of reactivity are selectively augmented. However, there are several practical problems which limit vigorous pursuit of such experimental protocols. In addition to the long periods of time needed for such studies and difficulties in identifying the most relevant experimental carcinogenesis models, completely selective and sustained alterations of NK activity are not easily found or produced. For example, as discussed above, much attention is currently being given to the beige mouse model as a test system for oncogenesis in NK-deficient animals. However, beige mice have some residual NK activity, which can be augmented by interferon (141) and which can approach normal levels upon prolonged incubations with target cells (142). Furthermore, they appear to have normal levels of natural cytotoxic activity *in vitro* against some monolayer tumor target cells (58) and *in vivo* against subcutaneous inoculations of both lymphoma and carcinoma cell lines (172). In addition, the rate of cytotoxicity by macrophages is also somewhat retarded (140), so that an increased tumor incidence in beige mice could not be definitively attributed to the deficit in NK activity. Conversely, induction of interferon or other procedures to augment NK activity generally also alter other immune functions. Yet another, and perhaps the most central, limitation to the use of beige mice or other NK-deficient mice to evaluate the role of NK cells in prevention of carcinogenesis is that, as discussed above, many of the carcinogens themselves can strongly inhibit NK activity. Thus, after treatment with a carcinogen, the normal recipients may have as low NK activity as the beige mice and, therefore, differences in tumor development might not be seen. The most convincing protocol might be to reconstitute animals with depressed NK activity, by adoptive transfer of purified NK cells, and determine the effects on carcinogenesis.

Role in Natural Resistance Against Microbial Infections

There have been increasing numbers of suggestions that NK cells may play some role in resistance against microbial infections. Most of the studies have related to viruses, with several investigators showing that cells infected by a variety of viruses become considerably more sensitive to lysis by NK cells (223, 224). In parallel, Bloom et al. (223) have found that persistently virus-infected tumor cells grow poorly in nude mice, apparently as a result of interferon induction and reactivity by NK cells. Furthermore, as summarized in Table 13.6, in vivo resistance to infection by several types of viruses has been found to correlate with NK activity. Lopez (225) has accumulated considerable evidence for a role of NK cells in genetic resistance of mice to severe infection by herpes simplex virus type 1: (a) The strain distribution of resistant and susceptible mice was similar, with nude mice of a resistant strain also being resistant; (b) resistance could be transferred to susceptible recipients by bone marrow; (c) resistance developed rapidly at 3 weeks of age; (d) resistance was impaired by treatment of mice with macrophage-toxic agents or with [89]strontium. It also seems likely that NK cells play an important role in natural resistance to infection by mouse cytomegalovirus (226). In all but one of eleven inbred strains tested, NK reactivity correlated with resistance to this virus. This included the observations that beige mice were considerably more susceptible to infection

Table 13.6. Evidence for Possible Role of NK Cells in Natural Resistance Against Microbial Infections

Direct Correlations between NK Activity and Resistance	Some Consistent Data for a Role but No Direct Correlations	Evidence against a Role for NK Cells
Herpes simplex virus type 1	Malaria	Lymphocytic chorio-meningitis virus
		Influenza and
Mouse cytomegalovirus	Candida	related viruses
Vaccinia virus	Listeria	
Marek's disease virus	Brucella	
Babesia		
Cryptococcus		

than normal C57BL/6 mice. Also, as pointed out by Bloom et al. (223), the findings of Schellekens et al. (227) of protection against vaccinia infection *in vivo* but not *in vitro* by interferon were quite compatible with mediation by NK cells. There have also been some indications that natural genetic resistance to another herpes virus, Marek's disease virus in chickens, may be mediated by NK cells. Cells with the characteristics of NK cells were found to transfer resistance to susceptible, newborn chicks (228). In contrast to these suggestions for an important role of NK cells in protection against infection by several viruses, it should be noted that there is evidence against a role for NK cells in resistance against some other viruses. Welsh and Kiessling (229) found no increased NK activity against target cells infected by lymphocytic choriomeningitis virus, and beige mice and normal C57BL/ 6 mice had similar resistance to *in vivo* infection. Similarly, Haller et al. (230) performed detailed studies on the nature of natural genetic resistance of mice to lethal infection by influenza and other orthomyxoviruses and obtained some evidence against an important role of NK cells. Although nude mice were resistant and interferon was involved in protection, resistance was not depressed by cyclophosphamide or ^{89}Sr and it could not be transferred with bone-marrow cells.

NK cells may also be involved in resistance against some other types of microbial infections. Ruebush et al. (231) have recently found a correlation between NK activity and resistance of mice to the malarial parasite, *Babesia microti*. Beige mice were highly susceptible to infection whereas heterozygous, normal mice were resistant. There has also been suggestive evidence for a role of NK cells in malaria infection (H. Wigzell, personal communication). NK cells may also play a role in natural resistance of mice to infection by the fungus, *Cryptococcus neoformans*. During the first 2 weeks after infection, nude mice were found to be more resistant to growth of the organism than euthymic mice (232). This observation raised the question of possible involvement of NK cells, and to examine the mechanism of resistance parallel *in vitro* studies were performed on the characteristics of NK cells and on the lymphoid cells mediating inhibition of colony formation by the fungus (233). In several respects, a good correlation has been noted. Relative resistance of nude mice to infection may be a useful clue to investigate the possible role of NK cells in resistance against other microbial agents. It is of interest that nude mice have been found to be relatively resistant to another fungus, *Candida albicans* (234), and to the bacteria, *Listeria monocytogenes* (235, 236) and *Brucella abortus* (235). In addition, initial resistance to infection of mice by *Listeria* has been shown to be impaired in ^{89}Sr-treated mice (237), a treatment which has been shown to cause a rather selective deficit in NK activity (238). Although other mechanisms of resistance have been suggested, and as with the orthomyxoviruses may indeed be responsible for resistance, it seems worthwhile to at least carefully consider a possible role of NK cells with these agents.

Role in Natural Resistance Against Bone-Marrow Transplants

For many years, it has been recognized that mice have natural resistance to transplantation of normal bone marrow and that the characteristics of this phenomenon did not conform to the well-established rules governing transplantation of other tissues. A major exception was that parental hematopoietic or lymphoid grafts failed to survive in lethally irradiated F_1 hybrids of certain inbred strains of mice, even though the F_1 hybrid has been found to be a universal recipient of transplants of other parental tissues. With the development of information about the characteristics of NK cells, it soon became clear that NK cells might account for such hybrid resistance. In direct comparisons between the characteristics of natural resistance to bone-marrow transplants and of NK cells, an excellent correlation has been found and it is now generally agreed by investigators in this area that NK cells are the main effector cells for this *in vivo* phenomenon (133, 142, 239, 240). Such findings have potential implications for clinical bone-marrow transplants.

The *in vivo* resistance to bone-marrow transplants has been measured primarily by inhibition of proliferation and of colony formation of donor cells in the spleens of the recipients. The evidence for a role of NK cells implied that NK cells could interact with at least a subpopulation of normal bone-marrow cells. This is supported by *in vitro* findings of NK reactivity against a portion of normal bone-marrow cells (191). Furthermore, Hansson and Kiessling (241) have recently shown that colony-forming stem cells may be among the subpopulation of human bone-marrow cells that are susceptible to lysis by NK cells.

To obtain some direct evidence for the *in vivo* ability of NK cells to eliminate a portion of bone-marrow cells, Riccardi et al. (242) measured the rapid *in vivo* clearance of ^{125}IUdR-labeled bone-marrow cells after intravenous inoculation. There had been previous indications that rapid elimination of radiolabeled normal or leukemia cells was greater in allogeneic or semisyngeneic recipients (243–246) and a role for NK cells was suggested. As with tumor target cells, Riccardi et al. (170, 242) found that young mice of high NK strains eliminated a higher proportion of bone-marrow cells than did older mice or those of a low NK strain. Furthermore, both *in vivo* and *in vitro* reactivities against the normal cells were modulated in parallel by NK-augmenting or inhibitory treatments. Also, the extent of elimination of radiolabeled parental bone-marrow cells by F_1 radiation chimeras was dependent on the genotype of the bone-marrow cells used to produce the chimera, with parental F_1 chimeras less effective than syngeneic F_1 chimeras. The one exception in the correlation between bone-marrow transplantation data and the evidence for *in vitro* and *in vivo* NK activity against bone-marrow cells is that some cytotoxic reactivity has been seen against syngeneic cells, in addition to the stronger reactivity against allogeneic or parental cells. This indicates at least some autoreactivity of NK cells and it will be of interest to determine whether NK cells can discriminate between homozygous and heterozygous cells or whether separate subpopulations with different specificity and function mediate the recognition of syngeneic or parental cells.

Role in Graft-Versus-Host Disease

Another association between NK cells and bone-marrow transplants has been related to the occurrence of graft-versus-host (GVH) disease. Lopez et al. (247) first noted, and it has been confirmed in a larger series of patients (248), that GVH disease after bone-marrow transplantation is more likely to occur in recipients who had high pretransplant levels of NK activity against virus-infected target cells. Dokhelar et al. (249) have also recently reported that the occurrence of acute GVH disease was associated with an early reappearance of NK activity, within 4 weeks after grafting. In contrast, in patients not developing acute GVH disease, NK activity returned a few weeks later. Although other explanations for these observations are possible, they raise the possibility that reactivity of either donor or host NK cells against normal tissues of the recipients may contribute to the manifestations of GVH disease.

Role in Regulation of Differentiation of Normal Hematopoietic or Other Cells

Several of the above observations, including the finding that NK cells can react *in vivo* and *in vitro* against normal syngeneic bone-marrow cells, have raised the possibility that NK cells may act as regulators of differentiation of normal hematopoietic cells (142, 168, 192). This hypothesis has been further supported and extended by evidence that NK cells can react against subpopulations of thymocytes (191, 250) and adherent peritoneal cells (191, 251). Although cytotoxicity has been greatest against allogeneic normal target cells, syngeneic cells have also been susceptible (168, 191, 242). Differentiation antigens may be the target structures recognized by NK cells, since fetal cells and less differentiated cells appear to be particularly susceptible to attack (168, 192). This reactivity against fetal cells and thymocytes, as well as against bone-marrow cells, has been shown to occur *in vivo* as well as *in vitro* (168). Thus, it seems possible that NK cells may in some way regulate the growth and differentiation of thymocytes, bone-marrow cells, and possibly other normal cells. It is of interest that the subpopulation of NK-sensitive cells in the thymus have been shown to be immature, cortisone-sensitive cortical thymocytes (250). This may provide an explanation for the finding that most normal thymocytes die rapidly and never leave the thymus (252). In addition, one may speculate that *in vivo* NK cells may have cytostatic or other regulatory effects on normal cells, rather than or in addition to the cytolytic effects observed *in vitro*.

Role as Secretory and Immunoregulatory Cells

In addition to their cytotoxic effects against tumor cells, virus-infected cells, and some normal cells, there are increasing indications that NK cells may have secretory and immunoregulatory functions. Best documented is the ability of NK cells to produce interferon (IFN). This was initially suggested to occur when it was observed that *in vitro* or *in vivo* exposure to NK-susceptible target cells led to the production of IFN (253, 254). Recent studies with human and rat LGL, highly enriched for NK activity by Percoll density gradient centrifugation, have confirmed that these cells can produce high levels of IFN upon overnight incubation with various tumor cell lines (254–256). LGL also produced IFN in response to viruses, mitogens and adjuvants, BCG, *C. parvum*, and poly I:C. Of particular note was that during these short-term incubations, only the LGL, and not T cells or monocytes, produced IFN in response to most of these stimuli. The main exception was poly I:C, which appeared to be capable of inducing IFN with each of the cell populations. These observations are of considerable significance from at least three standpoints. First, they indicate that NK cells can serve as important immunoregulatory cells, providing accessory function for a variety of immune responses that are augmented by IFN (e.g., activation of macrophages) and likewise inhibiting some immune functions that are depressed by IFN (e.g., lymphoproliferative responses and antibody production) (257–259). Second, it appears that NK cells are able to defend against foreign materials in a multifaceted way, by producing soluble factors that can induce antiviral resistance and cytostasis of tumor cells, as well as by direct cytotoxic effects. Further, the ability of NK cells to rapidly produce IFN upon contact with target cells provides a mechanism for positive self regulation. The IFN induced by initial contact can then lead to augmented cytotoxic activity against the target cells. However, one note of caution about this proposed sequence needs to be mentioned. Although cells with the same morphology have been shown to have cytotoxic activity and the ability to produce IFN, it is not clearly established that the same cells have both functions. Only about 50% of human LGL have been found to form conjugates with a susceptible target cell and a similar proportion reacted with anti-IFN (255), suggesting that the two functions do overlap.

NK cells also appear to be able to produce other lymphokines. Human LGL, upon stimulation with a mitogen and PMA, produced high levels of TCGF (99). This implies that NK cells can also facilitate the growth of T cells and thereby augment the magnitude of immune reactions to various stimuli. Furthermore, since LGL with NK activity seem to be able to proliferate in response to TCGF (100, 101), this appears to be another form of positive self regulation.

CLINICAL CORRELATIONS

One major issue of practical importance has been whether measurement of NK activity in cancer patients would provide information that could help in the management of the disease. Depressed NK activity has been observed in mice (77, 180) and patients (181–185) bearing various types of tumors, and this has been particularly associated with large tumor burdens. This raises the possibility that determination of NK activity in cancer patients might have prognostic value and studies to directly address this question seem warranted. Depressed NK activity has also been associated with other diseases, e.g., active multiple sclerosis (260) and systemic lupus erythematosus (261), and thus this parameter may have more general clinical applicability.

Another aspect of potential clinical importance is the possible effects of therapy on NK activity. This is of interest from two different standpoints. On the one hand, various forms of conventional therapy might inhibit NK activity and thereby have potentially deleterious effects on resistance against tumor growth. On the other hand, some treatments could actually cause an augmentation of NK activity and such an effect might contribute to the therapeutic efficacy of the agent. NK activity in mice and rats has been found to be relatively but not completely resistant to high doses of radiation (133–135). Even when investigators have found little or no effect on NK activity shortly after radiation, a later and relatively prolonged depression in reactivity was seen (220). In regard to chemotherapeutic agents, mouse or rat NK cells have been shown to be quite sensitive to cyclophosphamide, hydrocortisone, and some other agents (134, 135). However, these agents did not interfere with boosting of NK activity by poly I:C, suggesting the existence of treatment-resistant pre-NK cells. On a clinical level, there is a surprising paucity of information on the effects of radiotherapy or chemotherapy on NK activity. The few reports that have dealt with this issue have suggested some, but not impressive, treatment-related decreases in activity (9, 184, 185, 262). There is almost no information on the ability of interferon or other agents to boost the depressed reactivity of treated patients, and as a possible analogy to the rodent data, this would seem to be quite worthwhile to examine. In fact, one report has indicated that cyclosporin A strongly inhibited human NK activity but had no effect on boosting by interferon (263). It should be noted that some chemotherapeutic agents have not depressed NK activity (135, 264) and others, depending on the route and dosage, could induce either increased or decreased reactivity. Adriamycin has been shown to fall into this last category. Initial studies indicated that this drug had little or no inhibitory effect on NK activity (135, 264). However, a later, more detailed study indicated that adriamycin could depress splenic NK activity, apparently due to the activation of suppressor macrophages, whereas it led to a substantial augmentation of NK activity in the peritoneal cavity, bone marrow, and lymph nodes (265).

REFERENCES

1. Oren, M. E., Herberman, R. B., and Canty, T. G., *J. Natl. Cancer Inst.* **46**:621, 1971.
2. Leclerc, J. C., Gomard, E., and Levy, J. P., *Int. J. Cancer* **10**:589, 1972.
3. Lavrin, D. H., Herberman, R. B., Nunn, M., and Soares, N., *J. Natl. Cancer Inst.* **51**:1497, 1973.
4. Herberman, R. B., Cell-mediated immunity to tumor cells. In G. Klein and S. Weinhouse (Eds.), *Advances in Cancer Research*, Vol. 19, p. 207. New York: Academic Press, 1974.
5. Hellström, K. E., and Hellström, I., *Adv. Immunol.* **18**:209, 1974.
6. Rosenberg, E. B., Herberman, R. B., Levine, P. H., Halterman, R. H., McCoy, J. L., and Wunderlich, J. R., *Int. J. Cancer* **9**:648, 1972.
7. Oldham, R. K., and Herberman, R. B., *J. Immunol.* **111**:1862, 1973.
8. McCoy, J. L., Herberman, R. B., Rosenberg, E. B., Donnelly, F. C., Levine, P. H., and Alford, C., *Natl. Cancer Inst. Monogr.* **37**:59, 1973.
9. Rosenberg, E. B., McCoy, J. L., Green, S. S., Donnelly, F. C., Siwarski, D. F., Levine, P. H., and Herberman, R. B., *J. Natl. Cancer Inst.* **52**:345, 1974.
10. Herberman, R. B. and Gaylord, C. E. (Eds.), *Natl. Cancer Inst. Monogr.* **37**:1, 1973.
11. Takasugi, M., Mickey, M. R., and Terasaki, P. I., *Cancer Res.* **32**:2898, 1973.
12. Skurzak, H. M., Steiner, L., Klein, E., and Lamon, E. W., *Natl. Cancer Inst. Monogr.* **37**:93, 1973.
13. Heppner, G., Henry, E., Stolbach, L., Cummings, F., McDonough,, E., and Calabresi, P., *Cancer Res.* **35**:1931, 1975.
14. Peter, H. H., Kalden, J. R., Seeland, P., Diehl, V., and Eckert, G., *Clin. Exp. Immunol.* **20**:193, 1975.
15. Kay, H. D., Thota, H., and Sinkovics, J. G., *Clin. Immunol. Immunopathol.* **5**:218, 1976.
16. Canevari, S., Fossati, G., and DellaPorta, G., *J. Natl. Cancer Inst.* **56**:705, 1976.

17. Nunn, M., Djeu, J., Lavrin, D., and Herberman, R. B., *Proc. Amer. Assoc. Cancer Res.* **14**:87, 1973.
18. Herberman, R. B., Ting, C. C., Kirchner, H., Holden, H., Glaser, M., Bonnard, G. D., and Lavrin, D. H., Effector mechanisms in tumour immunity. In L. Brent and J. Holborow (Eds.), *Progress in Immunology, II*, p. 285. Amsterdam: North Holland, 1974.
19. Herberman, R. B. (Ed.), *Natural Cell-mediated Immunity Against Tumors*. New York: Academic Press, 1980.
20. Herberman, R. B., Nunn, M. E., Holden, H. T., and Lavrin, D. H., *Int. J. Cancer* **16**:230, 1975.
21. Kiessling, R., Klein, E., Pross, H., and Wigzell, H., *Eur. J. Immunol.* **5**:117, 1975.
22. Nunn, M. E., Djeu, J. Y., Glaser, M., Lavrin, D. H., and Herberman, R. B., *J. Natl. Cancer Inst.* **56**:393, 1976.
23. Shellam, G. R., *Int. J. Cancer* **19**:225, 1977.
24. Levin, A., Massey, R., Deinhardt, F., Schauf, V., and Wolter, J., Use of a ^{51}Cr release microcytotoxicity assay for the study of lymphocytotoxicity and inhibition of lymphocytotoxicity in human breast cancer. In R. G. Crispen (Ed.), *Neoplasm Immunity: Theory and Application*, p. 107. Chicago: ITR, 1975.
25. West, W. H., Cannon, G. B., Kay, H. D., Bonnard, G. D., and Herberman, R. B., *J. Immunol.* **118**:355, 1977.
26. Hersey, P., Edwards, A., Edwards, J., Adams, E., Milton, G. W., and Nelson, D. S., *Int. J. Cancer* **16**:173, 1975.
27. Pape, G. E., Troye, M., and Perlmann, P., *J. Immunol.* **118**:1925, 1977.
28. Bakacs, T., Gergely, P., Cornain, S., and Klein, S., *Int. J. Cancer* **19**:441, 1977.
29. Pross, H. F., and Jondal, M., *Clin. Exp. Immunol.* **21**:226, 1975.
30. Peter, H. H., Pavie-Fischer, J., Fridman, W. H., Aubert, C., Cesarini, J. P., Roubin, R., and Kourilsky, F. M., *J. Immunol* **115**:539, 1975.
31. Herberman, R. B., Bartram, S., Haskill, J. S., Nunn, M., Holden, H. T., and West, W. H., *J. Immunol.* **119**:322, 1977.
32. Oehler, J. R., Lindsay, L. R., Nunn, M. E., and Herberman, R. B., *Int. J. Cancer* **21**:204, 1978.
33. Koide, Y., and Takasugi, M., *J. Natl. Cancer Inst.* **59**:1099, 1977.
34. Troye, M., Perlmann, P., Pape, G. R., Spiegelberg, H. L., Naslund, J., and Gidlöf, A., *J. Immunol.* **119**:1061, 1977.
35. Kay, H. D., Bonnard, G. D., and Herberman, R. B., *J. Immunol.* **122**:675, 1979.
36. Kay, H. D., Fagnani, R., and Bonnard, G. D., *Int. J. Cancer* **42**:141, 1979.
37. Kay, H. D., Differential effects of immune complexes on human natural and antibody-dependent cell-mediated cytotoxicity. In R. B. Herberman (Ed.), *Natural Cell-mediated Immunity Against Tumors*, p. 329. New York: Academic Press, 1980.
38. Koren, H. S., and Jensen, P. J., Natural killing and antibody-dependent cellular cytotoxicity: Independent mechanisms mediated by overlapping cell populations. In R. B. Herberman (Ed.), *Natural Cell-mediated Immunity Against Tumors*, p. 347. New York: Academic Press, 1980.
39. West, W. H., Boozer, R. B., and Herberman, R. B., *J. Immunol.* **120**:90, 1978.
40. Santoni, A., Herberman, R. B., and Holden, H. T., *J. Natl. Cancer Inst.* **62**:109, 1979.
41. Santoni, A., Herberman, R. B., and Holden, H. T., *J. Natl. Cancer Inst.* **63**:995, 1979.
42. Herberman, R. B. Holden, H. T., West, W. H., Bonnard, G. D., Santoni, A., Nunn, M. E., Kay, H. D., and Ortaldo, J. R., Cytotoxicity against tumors by NK and K cells. In F. Spreafico and R. Arnon (Eds.), *Tumor-associated Antigens and Their Specific Immune Response*, p. 129. London: Academic Press, 1979.
43. Ojo, E., and Wigzell, H., *Scand. J. Immunol.* **7**:297, 1978.

44. Bonnard, G. D., Kay, H. D., Herberman, R. B., Ortaldo, J. R., Djeu, J., Pfiffner, K. J., and Oehler, J. R., Models for the mechanisms of natural cell-mediated cytotoxicity. I. Relationship to antibody-dependent cell-mediated cytotoxicity. In G. Riethmuller, F. Wernet, and G. Gudkowicz (Eds.), *Natural and Induced Cell-mediated Cytotoxicity. Effector and Regulatory Mechanisms*, p. 63. New York: Academic Press, 1979.

45. Landazuri, M. O., Silva, A., Alvarez, J., and Herberman, R. B., *J. Immunol.* **123**:252, 1979.

46. Kim, Y. B., Huh, N. D., Koren, H. S., and Amos, D. B., *J. Immunol.* **125**:755, 1980.

47. Neville, M. E., *J. Immunol.* **126**:2604, 1980.

48. Pandolfi, F., Strong, D. M., Slease, R. B., Smith, M. L., Ortaldo, J. R., and Herberman, R. B., *Blood* **56**:653, 1980.

49. Timonen, T., Saksela, E., Ranki, A., and Hayry, P., *Cell. Immunol.* **48**:133, 1979.

50. Saksela, E., and Timonen, T., Morphology and surface properties of human NK cells. In R. B. Herberman (Ed.), *Natural Cell-mediated Immunity Against Tumors*, p. 173. New York: Academic Press, 1980.

51. Timonen, T., and Saksela, E., *J. Immunol. Methods* **36**:285, 1980.

52. Timonen, T., Ortaldo, J. R., and Herberman, R. B., *J. Exp. Med.* **153**:569, 1981.

53. Lozzio, C. B., and Lozzio, B. B., *Blood* **45**:321, 1975.

54. Timonen, T., Ortaldo, J. R., and Herberman, R. B., *J. Immunol.* **128**:2514, 1982.

55. Ault, K. A., and Weiner, H. L., *Clin. Immunol. Immunopathol.* **11**:60, 1978.

56. Paige, C. J., Figarella, E. D., Cuttito, M. J., Cahan, A., and Stutman, O., *J. Immunol.* **121**:1827, 1978.

57. Stutman, O., Figarella, E. F., Paige, C. J., and Lattime, E. C., Natural cytotoxic (NC) cells against solid tumors in mice: General characteristics and comparison to natural killer (NK) cells. In R. B. Herberman (Ed.), *Natural Cell-mediated Immunity Against Tumors*, p. 187. New York: Academic Press, 1980.

58. Burton, R. C., Alloantisera selectively reactive with NK cells: Characterization and use in defining NK cell classes. In R. B. Herberman (Ed.), *Natural Cell-mediated Immunity Against Tumors*, p. 19. New York: Academic Press, 1980.

59. Landazuri, M. O., Lopez-Botet, M., Timonen, T., Ortaldo, J. R., and Herberman, R. B., *J. Immunol.* **127**:1380, 1981.

60. Reynolds, C. W., Timonen, T., and Herberman, R. B., *J. Immunol.* **127**:282, 1981.

61. Shellam, G. R., and Hogg, N., *Int. J. Cancer* **19**:212, 1977.

62. Reynolds, C. W., and Herberman, R. B., *J. Immunol.* **126**:1581, 1981.

63. Reynolds, C. W., Timonen, T., Holden, H. T., Hansen, C. T., and Herberman, R. B., *Eur. J. Immunol.* **12**:577, 1982.

64. Herberman, R. B., Brunda, M. J., Domzig, W., Fagnani, R., Goldfarb, R. H., Holden, H. T., Ortaldo, J. R., Reynolds, C. W., Riccardi, C., Santoni, A., Stadler, B. M., Taramelli, D., Timonen, T., and Varesio, L., Immunoregulation involving macrophages and natural killer cells. In M. E. Gershwin and L. N. Ruben (Eds.), *The Biological Significance of Immune Regulation*, p. 139. New York: Marcel Dekker, 1982.

65. Luini, W., Boraschi, D., Alberti, S., Aleotti, A., and Tagliabue, A., *Immunol.* **43**:663, 1981.

66. Glimcher, L., Shen, F. W., and Cantor, H., *J. Exp. Med.* **145**:1, 1977.

67. Tam, M. R., Emmons, S. L., and Pollack, S. B., FACS analysis and enrichment of NK effector cells. In R. B. Herberman (Ed.), *Natural Cell-mediated Immunity Against Tumors*, p. 265. New York: Academic Press, 1980.

68. Koo, G. C., and Hatzfeld, A., Antigenic phenotype of mouse natural killer cells. In R. B. Herberman (Ed.), *Natural Cell-mediated Immunity against Tumors*, p. 105. New York: Academic Press, 1980.

69. Grimm, E., and Bonavida, B., *J. Immunol.* **123**:2861, 1979.

70. Roder, J. C., and Kiessling, R., *Scand. J. Immunol.* **8**:135, 1978.
71. Tai, A., and Warner, N. L., Biophysical and serological characterization of murine NK cells. In R. B. Herberman (Ed.), *Natural Cell-mediated Immunity Against Tumors*, p. 241. New York: Academic Press, 1980.
72. Kasai, M., Iwamori, M., Nagai, Y., Okumura, K., and Tada, T., *Eur. J. Immunol.* **10**:175, 1980.
73. Young, W. W., Jr., Hakomori, S.-I., Durdik, J. M., and Henney, C. S., *J. Immunol.* **124**:199, 1980.
74. Cantor, H., Kasai, M., Shen, H. W., Leclerc, J. C., and Glimcher, L., *Immunol. Rev.* **44**:1, 1979.
75. Pollack, S. B., Tam, M. R., Nowinski, R. C., and Emmons, S. L., *J. Immunol.* **123**:1818, 1979.
76. Scheid, M. P., and Triglia, D., *Immunogenetics* **9**:423, 1979.
77. Herberman, R. B., Nunn, M. E., and Lavrin, D. H., *Int. J. Cancer* **10**:216, 1975.
78. Kiessling, R., Klein, E., and Wigzell, H., *Eur. J. Immunol.* **5**:112, 1975.
79. Herberman, R. B., and Holden, H. T., *Adv. Cancer Res.* **27**:305, 1978.
80. Kaplan, J., and Callewaert, D. M., *J. Natl. Cancer Inst.* **60**:961, 1978.
81. Herberman, R. B., Nunn, M. E., and Holden, H. T., *J. Immunol.* **121**:304, 1978.
82. Mattes, M. J., Sharrow, S. O., Herberman, R. B., and Holden, H. T., *J. Immunol.* **123**:2851, 1979.
83. Meruelo, D. M., Paolino, A., Flieger, N., and Offer, M., *J. Immunol.* **125**:2713, 1980.
84. Meruelo, D. M., Paolino, A., Flieger, N., Offer, M., Dworkin, J., Hirayama, N., and Ovary, Z., *J. Immunol.* **125**:2719, 1980.
85. Ortaldo, J. R., Sharrow, S. O., Timonen, T., and Herberman, R. B., *J. Immunol.* **127**:2401, 1981.
86. Kamoun, M., Martin, P. J., Hansen, J. A., Brown, M. A., Siadek, A. N., and Nowinski, R. C., *J. Exp. Med.* **153**:207, 1981.
87. Eisenbarth, G. S., Haynes, B. F., Schroer, J. A., and Fauci, A. S., *J. Immunol.* **124**:1237, 1980.
88. Reinherz, E. L., Kung, P. C., Goldstein, G., Levey, R. N., and Schlossman, S. F., Discrete stages of human intrathymic differentiation: Analysis of normal thymocytes and leukemic lymphoblasts of T-cell lineage. *Proc. Natl. Acad. Sci. USA* **77**:1588, 1980.
89. Reinherz, E. L., Kung, P. C., Goldstein, G., and Schlossman, S. F., *J. Immunol.* **124**:1301, 1980.
90. Hoffman, R. A., Kung, P. C., Hansen, W. P., and Goldstein, G., *Proc. Natl. Acad. Sci. USA* **77**:4914, 1980.
91. Ferrarini, M., Cadoni, A., Franzi, T., Ghigliotti, C., Leprini, A., Zicca, A., and Grossi, C. E., Ultrastructural and cytochemical markers of human lymphocytes. In F. A. Aiuti (Ed.), *Thymus, Thymic Hormones, and T Lymphocytes*, p. 39. New York: Academic Press, 1980.
92. Reynolds, C. W., Sharrow, S. O., Ortaldo, J. R., and Herberman, R. B., *J. Immunol.* **127**:2204, 1981.
93. Williams, A. F., Galfre, G., and Milstein, C., *Cell* **12**:663, 1977.
94. Mason, D. W., Brideau, R. J., McMaster, W. R., Webb, M., White, R. A. H., and Williams, A. F., Monoclonal antibodies that define T-lymphocyte subsets in the rat. In R. H. Kennett and T. J. McKearn (Eds.), *Monoclonal Antibodies. Hybridomas: A New Dimension in Biological Analysis*, p. 251. New York: Plenum Press, 1980.
95. Brideau, R. J., Carter, P. B., Mason, D. W., McMaster, W. R., and Williams, A. F., *Eur. J. Immunol.* **10**:690, 1980.
96. Bardos, P., Tursz, T. and Bach, J. F.: Thymic influence on NK activity. In B. Serrou

and R. B. Herberman (Eds.), *NK Cells: Fundamental Aspects and Role in Cancer. Human Cancer Immunology*, Vol. 4, p. 139. Amsterdam: Elsevier/North Holland, 1982.

97. Bonnard, G. D., and Alvarez, J. M., *Behring Inst. Mitt.* **67**:230, 1980.
98. Smith, K. A., T cell growth factor. *Immunol. Rev.* **51**:337, 1980.
99. Domzig, W., Timonen, T. T., and Stadler, B. M., *Proc. Amer. Assoc. Cancer Res.* **22**:309, 1981.
100. Ortaldo, J. R., Timonen, T., and Bonnard, G. D., *Behring Inst. Mitt.* **65**:258, 1980.
101. Timonen, T., Ortaldo, J. R., Bonnard, G. D., and Heberman, R. B., Culture of human natural killer cells in the presence of T cell growth factor (TCGF) containing medium (CM). In *Proc. 14th International Leukocyte Culture Conference*, p. 289, 1982.
102. Ortaldo, J. R., and Timonen, T. T., Modification of antigen expression and surface receptors on human NK cells grown *in vitro*. In *Proc. 14th International Leukocyte Culture Conference*, p. 286, 1982.
103. Dennert, G., *Nature* **287**:47, 1980.
104. Kedar, E., Herberman, R. B., Gorelik, E., Sredni, B., Bonnard, G. D., and Navarro, N., Antitumor reactivity *in vitro* and *in vivo* of mouse and human lymphoid cells cultured with T cell growth factor. In A. Fefer and A. Goldstein (Eds.), *The Potential Role of T Cells in Cancer Therapy*, p. 173. New York: Raven Press, 1981.
105. Bardos, P., Biziere, K., Degenne, D., and Renoux, G., Regulation of NK activity by the cerebral neocortex. In B. Serrou and R. B. Herberman (Eds.), *NK Cells: Fundamental Aspects and Role in Cancer. Human Cancer Immunology*, Vol. 4, p. 1. Amsterdam: Elsevier/North Holland, 1982.
106. Kaplan, J., and Callewaert, D. M., Are natural killer cells germ line V-gene encoded prothymocytes specific for self and nonself histocompatibility antigens? In R. B. Herberman (Ed.), *Natural Cell-mediated Immunity Against Tumors*, p. 893. New York: Academic Press, 1980.
107. Klein, E., Masucci, M. G., Masucci, G., and Vank, F., Natural and activated lymphocyte killers which affect tumor cells. In R. B. Herberman (Ed.), *Natural Cell-mediated Immunity against Tumors*, p. 909. New York: Academic Press, 1980.
108. Doherty, P. C., Blanden, R. V., and Zinkernagel, R. M., *Transpl. Rev.* **29**:89, 1976.
109. Haller, O., Kiessling, R., Örn, A., Kärre, K. Nilsson, K., and Wigzell, H., *Int. J. Cancer* **20**:93, 1977.
110. Nunn, M. E., and Herberman, R. B., *J. Natl. Cancer Inst.* **62**:765, 1979.
111. Klein, G., Zeuthen, J., Eriksson, I., Terasaki, P., Bernocco, M., Rosen, A., Masucci, G., Povey, S., and Ber, R., *J. Natl. Cancer Inst.* **64**:725, 1980.
112. Keller, R., *Brit. J. Cancer* **37**:732, 1978.
113. Mantovani, A., Jerrells, T. R., Dean, J. H., and Herberman , R. B., *Int. J. Cancer* **23**:18, 1979.
114. Tagliabue, A., Mantovani, A., Kilgallen, M., Herberman, R. B., and McCoy, J. L., *J. Immunol.* **122**:2363, 1979.
115. Herberman, R. B., Ortaldo, J. R., Djeu, J. Y., Holden, H. T., Jett, J., Lang, N. P., and Pestka, S., *Ann. N.Y. Acad. Sci.* **350**:63, 1980.
116. Schultz, R. M., Stoychkov, J. N., Pavlidis, N., Chirigos, M. A., and Olkowski, Z. L, *J. Reticuloendothel. Soc.* **26**:93, 1979.
117. Russel, S. W., Taffet, S. M., and Pace, J. L., The roles of lymphokine and prostaglandin in the regulation of mouse macrophage activation for tumor cell killing. In M. A. Chirigos, M. Mitchell, M. J. Mastrangelo and M. Krim (Eds.), *Mediation of Cellular Immunity in Cancer by Immune Modifiers*, p. 49. New York: Raven Press, 1981.
118. Droller, M. J., Schneider, M. V., and Perlman, P., *Cell Immunol.* **39**:165, 1978.
119. Brunda, M. J., Herberman, R. B., and Holden, H. T., *J. Immunol.* **124**:2682, 1980.

120. Keller, R., *Nature* **282**:729, 1979.
121. Goldfarb, R. H., and Herberman, R. B., *J. Immunol.* **126**:2129, 1981.
122. Goldfarb, R. H., and Herberman, R. B., Characteristics of natural killer cells and possible mechanisms for their cytotoxic activity. In G. Weissman (Ed.), *Advances in Inflammation Research*, p. 45. New York: Raven Press, 1981.
123. Hudig, D., Haverty, T., Fulcher, C., Redelman, D., and Mendelsohn, J., *J. Immunol.* **126**:1569, 1981.
124. Zarling, J. M., and Kung, P. C., *Nature* **288**:394, 1980.
125. Kay, H. D., and Horwitz, D. A., *J. Clin. Invest.* **66**:847, 1980.
126. Breard, J., Reinherz, E. L., O'Brien, C., and Schlossman, S. F., *Clin. Immunol. Immunopathol.* **18**:145, 1981.
127. Reinherz, E. L., Moretta, L., Roper, M., Breard, J. M., Mingari, M. C., Cooper, M. D., and Schlossman, S. F., *J. Exp. Med.* **151**:969, 1980.
128. Ault, K. A., and Springer, T. A., *J. Immunol.* **1267**:359, 1981.
129. Lohmann-Matthes, M.-L., and Domzig, W., Natural cytotoxicity of macrophage precursor cells and of mature macrophages. In R. B. Herberman (Ed.), *Natural Cell-mediated Immunity against Tumors*, p. 117. New York: Academic Press, 1980.
130. Gidlund, M. Haller, O., Orn, A., Ojo, E., Stern, P., and Wigzell, H., Characteristics of murine NK cells in relation to T lymphocytes and K cells. In R. B. Herberman (Ed.), *Natural Cell-mediated Immunity Against Tumors*, p. 79. New York: Academic Press, 1980.
131. Roder, J. C., Lohmann-Matthes, M.-L., Domzig, W., Kiessling, R., and Haller, O., *Eur. J. Immunol.* **9**:283, 1979.
132. Roder, J. C., Lohmann-Matthes, M.-L., Domzig, W., and Wigzell, H., *J. Immunol.* **24**:2174, 1979.
133. Kiessling, R., Hochman, P. S., Haller, O., Shearer, G. M., Wigzell, H., and Cudkowicz, G., *Eur. J. Immunol.* **7**:655, 1977.
134. Oehler, J. R., and Herberman, R. B., *Int. J. Cancer* **21**:221, 1978.
135. Djeu, J. Y., Heinbaugh, J. Vieira, W. D., Holden, H. T., and Herberman, R. B., *Immunopharmacology* **1**:231, 1979.
136. Djeu, J. Y., Heinbaugh, J. A., Holden, H. T., and Herberman, R. B., *J. Immunol.* **122**:182, 1979.
137. Cudkowicz, G., and Hochman, P. S., *Immunol. Rev.* **44**:13, 1979.
138. Wiltrout, R. H., Brunda, M. J., and Holden, H. T., *Int. J. Cancer*, in press.
139. Gallily, R., and Haran-Ghera, N., *Develop. Compar. Immunol.* **3**:523, 1979.
140. Mahoney, K. H., Morse, S. S., and Morahan, P. S., *Cancer Res.* **40**:3934, 1980.
141. Brunda, M. J., Holden, H. T., and Herberman, R. B., Augmentation of natural killer cell activity of beige mice by interferon and interferon inducers. In R. B. Heberman (Ed.), *Natural Cell-mediated Immunity Against Tumors*, p. 411. New York: Academic Press, 1980.
142. Cudkowicz, G., in preparation.
143. Roder, J. C., Haliotis, T., Klein, M., Korec, S., Jett, J. R., Ortaldo, J., Herberman, R. B., Katz, P., and Fauci, A. S., *Nature* **284**:553, 1980.
144. Roder, J. C., Laing, L., Haliotis, T., and Kozbor, D., Genetic control of human NK function. In B. Serrou, C. Rosenfeld and R. B. Herberman (Eds.), *NK Cells: Fundamental Aspects and Role in Cancer. Human Cancer Immunol.*, Vol. 4, p. 169. Amsterdam: North Holland, 1982.
145. Kiessling, R., Petranyi, G., Klein, G., and Wigzell, H., *Int. J. Cancer* **17**:275, 1976.
146. Riesenfeld, I., Örn, A., Gidlund, M., Azberg, I., Alm, G. V., and Wigzell, H., *Int. J. Cancer* **25**:399, 1980.
147. Sendo, F., Aoki, T., Boyse, E. A., and Buofo, C. K., *J. Natl. Cancer Inst.* **55**:603, 1975.

148. Hanna, N., *Int. J. Cancer* **26**:675, 1980.
149. Hanna, N., and Fidler, I. J., *Cancer Res.* **41**:438, 1981.
150. Rygaard, J., and Poulsen, C. O., *Acta Pathol. Microbiol. Scand.* **77**:758, 1969.
151. Castro, J. E., *Nature New Biol.* **239**:83, 1972.
152. Ozzello, L., Sordat, B., Merenda, C., Carrel, S., Hurlimann, J., and Mach, J. P., *J. Natl. Cancer Inst.* **52**:1669, 1974.
153. Schmidt, M., and Good, R. A., *Lancet* **1**:39, 1976.
154. Maguire, H., Jr., Outzen, H. C., Custer, R. P., and Prehn, R. T., *J. Natl. Cancer Inst.* **57**:439, 1976.
155. Sharkey, F. E., and.Fogh, J., *Int. J. Cancer* **24**:733, 1979.
156. Kiessling, R., Petrányi, G., Klein, G., and Wigzell, H., *Int. J. Cancer* **15**:933, 1975.
157. Petrányi, G., Kiessling, R., Povey, S., Klein, G., Herzenberg, E., and Wigzell, H., *Immunogenetics* **3**:15, 1976.
158. Haller, O., Kiessling, R., Örn, A., and Wigzell, H., *J. Exp. Med.* **145**:1411, 1977.
159. Gorelik, E., Fogel, M., Feldman, M., and Segal, S., *J. Natl. Cancer Inst.* **63**:1397, 1979.
160. Roder, J. and Duwe, A., *Nature* **278**:451, 1979.
161. Talmadge, J. E., Meyers, K. M., Prieur, D. J., and Starkey, J. R., *Nature* **284**:622, 1980.
162. Kärre, K., Klein, G. O., Kiessling, R., Klein, G., and Roder, J. C., *Nature* **284**:624, 1980.
163. Kasai, M., Leclerc, J. C., McVay-Boudreau, L., Shen, F. W., and Cantor, H., *J. Exp. Med.* **149**:1260, 1979.
164. Cheever, M. A., Greenberg, P. D., and Fefer, A., *J. Immunol.* **124**:2137, 1980.
165. Habu, S., Fukui, H., Shimamura, K., Kasai, M., Nagai, Y., Okumura, K., and Tamaoki, N., *J. Immunol.* **127**:34, 1981.
166. Riccardi, C., Puccetii, P., Santoni, A., and Herberman, R. B., *J. Natl. Cancer Inst.* **63**:1041, 1979.
167. Riccardi, C., Santoni, A., Barlozzari, T., Puccetti, P., and Herberman, R. B., *Int. J. Cancer* **25**:475, 1980.
168. Riccardi, C., Santoni, A., Barlozzari, T., and Herberman, R. B., Role of NK cells in rapid *in vivo* clearance of radiolabeled tumor cells. In R. B. Herberman (Ed.), *Natural Cell-mediated Immunity Against Tumors*, p. 1121. New York: Academic Press, 1980.
169. Riccardi, C. Barlozzari, T., Santoni, A., Herberman, R. B., and Cesarini, C., *J. Immunol.* **126**:1284, 1981.
170. Riccardi, C., Santoni, A., Barlozzari, T., Cesarini, C., and Herberman, R. B., *In vivo* role of NK cells against neoplastic or non-neoplastic cells. In B. Serrou and C. Rosenfeld (Eds.), Human Cancer Immunology, Vol. 4, p. 57. *NK Cells: Fundamental Aspects and Role in Cancer.* Amsterdam: North Holland, 1982.
171. Hanna, N., and Fidler, I. J., *J. Natl. Cancer Inst.* **65**:801, 1980.
172. Gorelik, E., and Herberman, R. B., *Int. J. Cancer* **27**:709, 1981.
173. Gerson, J. M., Systemic and in situ natural killer activity in tumor-bearing mice and patients with cancer. In R. B. Herberman (Ed.), *Natural Cell-mediated Immunity Against Tumors*, p. 1047. New York: Academic Press, 1980.
174. Becker, S., Kiessling, R., Lee, M., and Klein, G., *J. Natl. Cancer Inst.* **61**:1495, 1978.
175. Durdik, J. M., Beck, B. N., and Henney, C. S., The use of lymphoma cell variants differing in their susceptibility to NK cell mediated lysis to analyze NK cell-target interactions. In R. B. Herberman (Ed.), *Natural Cell-mediated Immunity Against Tumors*, p. 805. New York: Academic Press, 1980.
176. Collins, J. L., Patek, P. Q., and Cohn, M., *J. Exp. Med.* **153**:89, 1981.

177. Kunkel, L. A., and Welsh, R. M., *Int. J. Cancer* **27**:73, 1981.
178. Trinchieri, G., and Santoli, D., *J. Exp. Med.* **147**:1314, 1978.
179. Welsh, R. M., Jr., and Kiessling, R. W., Modification of target susceptibility to activated mouse NK cells by interferon and virus infections. In R. B. Herberman (Ed.), *Natural Cell-mediated Immunity Against Tumors*, p. 963. New York: Academic Press, 1980..
180. Becker, S., and Klein, E., *Eur. J. Immunol.* **6**:892, 1977.
181. McCoy, J., Herberman, R., Perlin, E., Levine, P., and Alford, C., *Proc. Amer. Assoc. Cancer Res.* **14**:107, 1973.
182. Takasugi, M. Ramseyer, A., and Takasugi, J., *Cancer Res.* **37**:413, 1977.
183. Hersey, P., Edwards, A., and McCarthy, W. H., *Int. J. Cancer* **25**:187, 1980.
184. Forbes, J. T., Greco, F. A., and Oldham, R. K., Natural cell-mediated cytotoxicity in human tumor patients. In R. B. Herberman (Ed.), *Natural Cell-mediated Immunity Against Tumors*, p. 1031. New York: Academic Press, 1980.
185. Pross, H. F., and Baines, M. G., Natural killer cells in tumor-bearing patients. In R. B. Herberman (Ed.), *Natural Cell-mediated Immunity Against Tumors*, p. 1063. New York: Academic Press, 1980.
186. Gerson, J. M., Varesio, L., and Herberman, R. B., *Int. J. Cancer* **27**:243, 1981.
187. Vose, B. M., Natural killers in human cancer: Activity of tumor-infiltrating and draining node lymphocytes. In R. B. Herberman (Ed.), *Natural Cell-mediated Immunity Against Tumors*, p. 1081. New York: Academic Press, 1980.
188. Eremin, O., NK cell activity in the blood, tumour-draining lymph nodes and primary tumours of women with mammary carcinoma. In R. B. Herberman (Ed.), *Natural Cell-mediated Immunity Against Tumors*, p. 1011. New York: Academic Press, 1980.
189. Allavena, P., Introna, M., Mangioni, C., and Mantovani, A., *J. Natl. Cancer Inst.* **67**:319, 1981.
190. Serrate, S., and Herberman, R. B., *Fed. Proc.* **40**:1007, 1981.
191. Nunn, M. E., Herberman, R. B., and Holden, H. T., *Int. J. Cancer* **20**:381, 1977.
192. Axberg, I., Gidlund, M., Örn, A., Pattengale, P., Riesenfeld, I., Stern, P., and Wigzell, H., In F. Aiuti (Ed.), *Thymus, Thymic Hormones and T Lymphocytes*, p. 154. New York: Academic Press, 1980.
193. Zarling, J. M., Eskra, L., Borden, E. C., Horoszewica, J., and Carter, W. A., *J. Immunol.* **123**:63, 1979.
194. Vanky, F. T., Argov, S. A., Einhorn, S. A., and Klein, E., *J. Exp. Med.* **151**:1151, 1980.
195. Mantovani, A., Allavena, P., Biondi, A., Sessa, C., and Introna, M., Natural killer activity in human ovarian carcinoma. In B. Serrou and R. B. Herberman (Eds.), *NK Cells: Fundamental Aspects and Role in Cancer. Human Cancer Immunology*, Vol. 4, p. 123. Amsterdam: North Holland, 1980.
196. Ortaldo, J. R., Oldham, R. K., Cannon, G. C., and Herberman, R. B., *J. Natl. Cancer Inst.* **59**:77, 1977.
197. Becker, S., Intratumor NK reactivity. In R. B. Herberman (Ed.), *Natural Cell-mediated Immunity Against Tumors*, p. 985. New York: Academic Press, 1980.
198. Prehn, R. T., *Prog. Exp. Tumor Res.* **14**:1, 1971.
199. Schwartz, R. S., *N. Eng. J. Med.* **293**:181, 1975.
200. Burnet, F. M., *Brit. Med. J.* **1**:779, 1957.
201. Thomas, L., Discussion. In H. S. Lawrence (Ed.), *Cellular and Humoral Aspects of the Hypersensitive State*, p. 529. New York: Harper, 1959.
202. Burnet, F. M., *Prog. Exp. Tumor Res.* **13**:1, 1970.
203. Stutman, O., Immunodepression and malignancy. In G. Klein, S. Weinhouse and A. Haddow (Eds.), *Advances in Cancer Research* Vol. 22, p. 261. New York: Academic Press, 1975.

204. Stutman, O., *J. Natl. Cancer Inst.* **62**:353, 1979.
205. Hewitt, H. B., Blake, E. R., and Walker, A. S., *Brit. J. Cancer* **33**:241, 1976.
206. Klein, G., and Klein, E., *Transpl. Proc.* **9**:1095, 1977.
207. Prehn, R. T., and Lappe, M. A., *Transpl. Rev.* **7**:26, 1971.
208. Lotan, R., *Biochim. Biophys. Acta* **605**:33, 1980.
209. Shope, T. C., and Kaplan, J., *J. Immunol.* **123**:2150, 1979.
210. Dent, P. B., Fish, L. A., White, J. F., and Good, R. A., *Lab. Invest.* **15**:1634, 1966.
211. Loutit, J. R., Townsend, K. M. S., and Knowles, J. F., *Nature* **285**:66, 1980.
212. Purtilo, D. T., De Florio, D., Hutt, L. M., Bhawan, J., Yang, J. P. S., Otto, R., and Edwards, W., *N. Eng. J. Med.* **297**:1077, 1977.
213. Sullivan, J. L., Byron, K. S., Brewster, F. E., and Purtilo, D. T., *Science* **210**:543, 1980.
214. Penn, I., and Starzl, T. E., *Transpl. Proc.* **4**:719, 1972.
215. Lipinski, M., Tursz, T., Kreis, H., Finale, Y., and Amiel, J. L., *Transplantation* **29**:214, 1980.
216. Gorelik, E., and Herberman, R. B., *J. Natl. Cancer Inst.* **66**:543, 1981.
217. Gorelik, E., and Herberman, R. B., *Fed. Proc.* **40**:1093, 1981.
218. Kraskovsky, G., Gorelik, L., and Kagan, L., *Proc. Acad. Sci. BSSR* **11**:1052, 1973.
219. Ehrlich, R., Efrati, M., and Witz, I. P., Cytotoxicity and cytostasis mediated by splenocytes of mice subjected to chemical carcinogens and of mice bearing primary tumors. In R. B. Herberman (Ed.), *Natural Cell-mediated Immunity Against Tumors*, p. 997. New York: Academic Press, 1980.
220. Hochman, P. S., Cudkowicz, G., and Dausset, J., *J. Natl. Cancer Inst.* **61**:265, 1978.
221. Parkinson, D. R., Brightman, R. P., and Waksal, S. D., *J. Immunol.* **126**:1460, 1981.
222. Kaplan, H. S., Brown, M. B., and Faull, J., *J. Natl. Cancer Inst.* **14**:303, 1953.
223. Bloom, B. R., Minato, N., Neighbour, A., Reid, L., and Marcus, D., Interferon and NK cells in resistance to virus persistently infected cells and tumors. In R. B. Herberman (Ed.), *Natural Cell-mediated Immunity Against Tumors*, p. 505. New York: Academic Press, 1980.
224. Santoli, D., Perussia, B., and Trinchieri, G., Natural killer cell activity against virus-infected cells. In R. B. Herberman (Ed.), *Natural Cell-mediated Immunity Against Tumors*, p. 1171. New York: Academic Press, 1980.
225. Lopez, C., Genetic resistance to herpes virus infections: Role of natural killer cells. In E. Skamene, P. A. L. Kongshawn and M. Landy (Eds.), *Genetic Control of Natural Resistance to Infection and Malignancy*, p. 253. New York: Academic Press, 1980.
226. Bancroft, G. J., Shellam, G. R., and Chalmer, J. E., *J. Immunol.* **126**:988, 1981.
227. Schellekens, H., Weimar, W., Cantell, K., and Stitz, L, *Nature* **278**:742,, 1979.
228. Lam, K. M., and Linna, T. J., *J. Immunol.* **125**:715, 1980.
229. Welsh, R. M., Jr., and Kiessling, R. W., *Scand. J. Immunol.* **11**:363, 1980.
230. Haller, O., Arnheiter, H., and Lindenmann, J., Natural resistance of mice toward orthomyxoviruses. In R. B. Herberman (Ed.), *Natural Cell-mediated Immunity Against Tumors*, p. 1145. New York: Academic Press, 1980.
231. Ruebush, M. J., and Burgess, D. E. Induction of natural killer cells and interferon production during infection of mice with Babesia microti of human origin. In R. B. Herberman (Ed.), *NK Cells and other Natural Effector Cells*, p. 1483. New York: Academic Press, 1982.
232. Cauley, L. K., and Murphy, J. W., *Infect. Immun.* **23**:644, 1979.
233. Murray, J. W., Natural cell mediated resistance in cryptococcosis. In R. B. Herberman (Ed.), *NK Cells and other Natural Effector Cells*, p. 1503. New York: Academic Press, 1982.
234. Cutler, J. E., *J. Reticuloendothel. Soc.* **19**:121, 1976.
235. Cheers, C., and Waller, R., *J. Immunol.* **115**:844, 1975.

236. Newborg, M. F., and North, R. J., *J. Immunol.* **124**:571, 1980.
237. Bennett, M., and Baker, E. E., *Cell Immunol.* **33**:203, 1977.
238. Haller, O., and Wigzell, H., *J. Immunol.* **118**:1503, 1977.
239. Datta, S. K., Gallagher, M. T., Trentin, J. J., Kiessling, R., and Wigzell, H., *Biomedicine* **31**:62, 1979.
240. Clark, E. A., and Harmon, R. C., *Adv. Cancer Res.* **31**:227, 1980.
241. Hansson, M., and Kiessling, R., NK surveillance of primitive normal cells in the thymus and bone marrow. In B, Serrou, C. Rosenfeld, and R. B. Herberman (Eds.), NK Cells: *Fundamental Aspects and Role in Cancer. Human Cancer Immunology*, Vol. 4. Amsterdam: North Holland, 1982.
242. Riccardi, C., Santoni, A., Barlozzari, T., and Herberman, R. B., *Cell Immunol.* **60**:136, 1981.
243. Carlson, G. A., and Wegman, T. G., *J. Immunol.* **118**:2130, 1977.
244. Carlson, G. A., Melnychok, D., and Meeker, M. J., *Int. J. Cancer* **25**:111, 1980.
245. McNeilage, L. J., and Heslop, B. F., *Cell. Immunol.* **50**:58, 1980.
246. Pincott, C. E., and Bainbridge, D. R., *Eur. J. Immunol.* **10**:250, 1980.
247. Lopez, C., Kirkpatrick, D., Sorell, M., O'Reilly, R. V., and Ching, C., *Lancet* **2**:1103, 1979.
248. Lopez, C., Kirkpatrick, D., Livnat, S., and Storb, R., *Lancet* **2**:1025, 1980.
249. Dokhelar, M.-C., Lipinski, M., Gluckman, E., and Tursz, T., Early recovery of NK cell activity in bone-marrow recipients with acute graft-versus-host disease. In B. Serrou, C. Rosenfeld, and R. B. Herberman (Eds.), *NK Cells: Fundamental Aspects and Role in Cancer. Human Cancer Immunology*, Vol. 4, p. 53. Amsterdam: North Holland, 1982.
250. Hansson, M., Kärre, K. Kiessling, R. Roder, J., Andersson, B., and Häyry, P., *J. Immunol.* **123**:765, 1979.
251. Welsh, R. M., Zinkernagel, R. M., and Hallenbeck, L., *J. Immunol.* **122**:475, 1979.
252. Scollay, R. G., Butcher, E. C., and Weissman, I. L., *Eur. J. Immunol.* **10**:210, 1980.
253. Trinchieri, G., Santoli, D., Dee, R. R., and Knowles, B. B., *J. Exp. Med.* **147**:1299, 1978.
254. Djeu, J. Y., Timonen, T., and Herberman, R. B., Augmentation of natural killer cell activity and induction of interferon by tumor cells and other biological response modifiers. In M. A. Chirigos, M. Mitchell, M. J. Mastrangelo, and M. Krim (Eds.), *Progress in Cancer Research and Therapy. Mediation of Cellular Immunity in Cancer by Immune Modifiers*, Vol. 19, p. 161. New York: Raven Press, 1981.
255. Saksela, E., Timonen, T., Virtanen, I., and Cantell, K., Regulation of human natural killer activity by interferon. In R. B. Herberman (Ed.), *Natural Cell-mediated Immunity Against Tumors*, p. 645. New York: Academic Press, 1980.
256. Djeu, J. Y., Reynolds, C. W., and Herberman, R. B., in preparation.
257. Schultz, R. M., Papamatheakis, J. D., and Chirigos, M. A., *Science* **197**:674, 1977.
258. Jett, J. R., Mantovani, A., and Herberman, R. B., *Cell. Immunol.* **54**:425, 1980.
259. Johnson, H. M., and Baron, S., *Pharmac. Ther. Part A* **1**:349, 1977.
260. Benczur, M., Petrányi, G. G., Pálffy, G., Varga, M., Tálas, M., Kotsky, B., Földes, I., and Hollán, S. R., *Clin. Exp. Immunol.* **39**:657, 1980.
261. Hoffman, T., *Arthritis and Rheumatism* **23**:30, 1980.
262. Herberman, R. B., Rosenberg, E. B., Halterman, R. H., McCoy, J. L., and Leventhal, B. G., *Natl. Cancer Inst. Monogr* **35**:259, 1972.
263. Introna, M., Allavena, P., Spreafico, F., and Mantovani, A., *Transplantation* **31**:113, 1981.
264. Mantovani, A., Luini, W., Peri, G., Vecchi, A., and Spreafico, F., *J. Natl. Cancer Inst.* **61**:1255, 1978.
265. Santoni, A., Riccardi, C., Sorci, V., and Herberman, R. B., *J. Immunol.* **124**:2329, 1980.

14

The Clinical Relevance of Circulating Immune Complexes in Cancer, Kidney Transplantation, and Pregnancy

Nicole A. Carpentier and Peter A. Miescher*

The formation of antigen-antibody complexes *in vivo* and their subsequent removal by the reticuloendothelial system is an important component of the normal defense against pathogens and other foreign substances. This physiological process is designed to eliminate or neutralize antigens and thus protect the host. Under some circumstances, however, immune complexes persist in large amounts in biological fluids and have pathogenic consequences when they localize in tissues. Recent advances in immunological research have identified many of the factors involved in the formation, removal, and tissue localization of immune complexes, and have clarified the mechanisms of immune complex-induced inflammatory lesions. The most important model for understanding the pathogenesis of these lesions has been experimentally-induced serum sickness in rabbits (1). Using this model, Dixon et al. have shown that antigen-antibody complexes are present in the circulation at the time animals develop glomerulonephritis, vasculitis, synovitis and heart injury. Furthermore, the development of these lesions was associated with the deposition of antigen and antibody in the glomeruli and in other vascular sites, where they were detected by immunofluorescence microscopy. On the basis of these observations, a number of human diseases (2–4) have been linked to immune complex formation and deposition. This is particularly

* This work has been supported by grants no. 3.908.080 and 3838-0.81 of the Swiss National Science Foundation and by the Dinu Lipatti-Dubois-Ferrière Fund. We are very grateful for the advice of Prof. P. H. Lambert and for the collaboration of Dr. M. Jeannet and Mr.G. Benzonana. The secretarial assistance of Mrs. J. Ringrose is appreciated.

the case for immunological and infectious disorders in which the pathological manifestations obviously implicate immune complexes.

The formation of immune complexes also has been demonstrated in other disease states, notably malignancies (5,6) and renal failure even of non-immunological origin (7–10), as well as during pregnancy (11). In these situations, the potential pathogenic role of immune complexes has yet to be defined. In cancer patients, several studies have provided evidence of an association of circulating immune complexes (CIC) with an unfavorable course of the disease. Conversely, in patients with renal failure undergoing transplantation, CIC have been found to represent a favorable prognostic factor for the graft survival. These observations, as well as experimental data in animals, have suggested that CIC may aid tumor growth in cancer patients and protect allograft in kidney recipients by modulating the afferent phase and impairing some effector mechanisms of the host immune response to foreign antigens. CIC may indeed participate in the regulation of the immune response either at the stage of lymphocyte activation or during the effector phase. Such biological functions of CIC could also be involved in the mechanisms which protect the fetus from maternal rejection.

CIRCULATING IMMUNE COMPLEXES IN CANCER PATIENTS

Tumor immunology over the past 15 years has become one of the most studied fields in clinical and experimental medicine. A great deal of knowledge has been accumulated regarding tumor antigens and host tumor-cell destruction mechanisms including the immune response. Several studies have suggested that immune complexes in cancer may favor tumor progression, since an association between the detection of CIC and poor prognosis has been found in malignancies.

The occurrence of CIC in cancer patients was first indicated by the finding of deposits of Ig and complement in the renal glomeruli of some patients with malignancy (12–22). Further evidence of their presence was the demonstration in individuals with growing neoplasms of humoral factors capable of inhibiting *in vitro* host lymphocyte reactivity to tumor cells (23–27). Some of these factors could have been immune complexes, although tumor antigens were also implied.

More recently, with the availability of many sensitive methods for detection of soluble immune complexes (38), material with biological and physico-chemical properties analogous to those of antigen-antibody complexes has been demonstrated in the blood of cancer patients. To date, a great many studies have been concerned with the incidence of CIC in patients with various malignancies. Some of the reports documented the prevalence of CIC at certain stages of cancer and gave information on the physicochemical properties of CIC found in cancer patients.

One of the early studies was conducted by Samayoa and co-workers (29). These investigators looked for CIC in a group of 146 patients with different malignant diseases using monoclonal rheumatoid factor assay and a precipitin test. They recorded positive results in 29 percent of patients, and in women with breast cancer reactive material was mostly found in patients with metastatic disease.

Teshima et al. (30) and Rossen et al. (31), using more sensitive methodology, i.e., the C1q deviation and the C1q binding assays, detected CIC in 50 to 83% of patients with various types of cancer. The C1q reactive material was found to be greater than 19S, or of intermediate, between 7S and 19S, size. In the study of Teshima and colleagues, the presence of IC in 67 to 77% of sera was associated with a lowered total hemolytic complement activity or reduced levels of C3 and C1q.

Theofilopoulos and colleagues (32), using the Raji cell assay that they have devised, demonstrated CIC in 16 to 52% of patients according to the type of malignant solid tumor. In this study, the overall incidence of CIC reached 41%. Furthermore, of 251 patients with available clinical data, 109 had CIC and all but 5 had clinically evident disease, i.e., localized tumor or metastatic cancer. In melanoma patients, higher levels of CIC were detected in association with larger tumors. Moreover, in some cases, the level of CIC fluctuated with the tumor mass. Similar fluctuations in CIC levels recently observed in tumor-bearing animals were shown to have a directly proportional relationship with the tumor burden (33).

Jerry et al. (34), who also studied patients with melanoma for the presence of CIC by measuring the binding to polyclonal rheumatoid factor and the C1q deviation, found complexes in early as well as in advanced stages of cancer. It was shown that serum C1q deviating material sedimented as an intermediate 7S-19S or greater than 19S material on sucrose density gradient. In this study, the fluctuations in the CIC levels which were observed could be related to the therapy given. After chemotherapy, the levels of CIC dropped to within the normal range but increased again in the following weeks. Immunotherapy with BCG was associated with continuous variations in CIC levels but not complete disappearance of complexes.

In a recent study on patients with bronchial carcinoma (35), no significant changes in CIC levels could be observed in patients after radio-, chemo-, or immunotherapy. However, at the time of diagnosis, patients with metastatic cancer exhibited CIC more frequently than those with localized tumors.

In women with ovarian cancer, Poulton et al. (36) found CIC only in cases where the tumor had recurred. Similarly, CIC in postoperative cancer

Table 14.1. Incidence of Circulating Immune Complexes in Patients with Leukemia

Type of Leukemia	Clq-binding Activity	Patients with CIC*	
(No. of sera)	Mean ± 1 SD (%)	No	%
Acute myeloid (395)	8.3 ± 15.3	98/224	43.8
Acute lymphatic (100)	6.1 ± 16.1	17/60	28.3
Blastic crisis (110)	6.3 ± 10.0	26/64	40.6
Chronic myeloid (191)	2.1 ± 5.5	17/74	23.0
Chronic lymphatic (104)	7.5 ± 17.8	14/70	20.0

* Patients with serum C1q BA > 3 SD above the mean normal value.

patients were more frequent in individuals with residual tumor than those assumed to be cured (31, 32, 37–39).

In children with neuroblastoma (40), a close correlation was observed between the amount of serum immune complexes and the tumor mass. Levels of complexes increased with the extent of the disease and were significantly higher in stage 4 then in all other stages combined. In cancer patients at stage 4, the amount of CIC decreased as treatment progressed.

Brandeis and collaborators also (41) reported recently the correlation between the levels of CIC, assayed by the Raji cell method, total hemolytic complement activity, C1q and C3 levels with the clinical stage, the histological type, age, sex, and treatment, in 86 children with Hodgkin's disease studied over a 4-year period. The most significant findings were the changes in these levels during disease activity and following treatment. Prior to therapy, 81% of children had elevated CIC levels. During treatment, 33% were still positive; during the year after cessation of treatment, 37% remained above the normal level. At relapse, 63% again had CIC which reached higher levels than at other periods. Changes in total hemolytic complement activity related mostly to treatment periods. This activity, elevated in untreated patients, dropped to normal during and after therapy. In sera from children at first, second, or third relapse, total hemolytic complement levels were significantly different to those in controls and to levels during treatment periods.

Over the past 6 years, we have investigated (42–49) a large number of patients with leukemia, malignant lymphoma, or solid tumor for the presence

Table 14.2. High Incidence of Circulating Immune Complexes during Florid Stage of Acute Leukemia

	Clq Binding Activity	Patients with CIC*	
Stage of Leukemia	Mean ± 1 SD (%)	No.	%
Diagnosis	15.1 ± 12.3	116/187	62.0
Complete remission	7.2 ± 11.2	34/112	30.4
Relapse	14.2 ± 12.2	42/64	65.6

*Patients with serum Clq BA > 3 SD above the mean normal value.

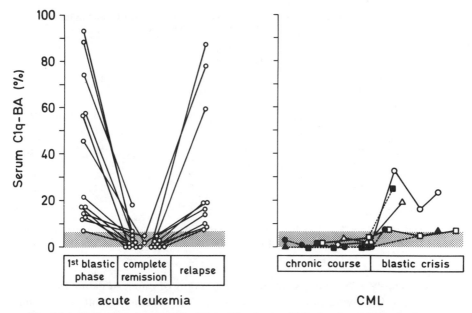

Fig. 14.1. Evolution of serum C1q-BA in 27 patients with leukemia according to the stage of the disease; in the left part of the figure, serum C1q-BA of 21 patients with AML, ALL, or BC; in the right part of the figure, serum C1q-BA in 6 patients with CML who developed blastic crisis.

of CIC, using primarily the C1q binding assay (5). In leukemia, we found serum C1q-binding material in 41% of patients with acute leukemia and in 22% of those with chronic leukemia (Table 14.1). In acute myeloid leukemia (AML) and acute lymphatic leukemia (ALL) as well as in blastic crisis (BC) of chronic myeloid leukemia (CML), CIC were mostly detected in patients at the blastic stage (Table 14.2). This association of CIC with the acute phase of the disease was particularly evident when CIC were measured serially (Fig. 14.1). In 13 cases in which immune complexes were present during the acute phase, C1q-BA was no longer detectable after induction of complete remission. Conversely, in 10 patients in complete remission and in 6 cases with CML, circulating immune complexes appeared but at the time of relapse or of blastic transformation, respectively. However, CIC could also be demonstrated in some patients during the period of complete remission.

We also found serum C1q binding material in 28% of patients with Hodgkin's disease, 38% of patients with non-Hodgkin malignant lymphoma, and in 37% of patients with various solid tumors. The patients were all studied at the time of diagnosis prior to any active therapy. Comparative analysis of the results with regard to the extent of the tumor indicated that CIC were

Table 14.3. Circulating Immune Complexes in Patients with Malignant Lymphoma: Relation to the Stage of the Disease

Type and Stage of Tumor[a] (No. Patients)		Serum Clq-Binding Activity Mean ± 1 S.D.(%)	Patients with CIC	
			No.	%
Hodgkin's disease	(65)	4.7 ± 6.9	18	27.7
Localized	(33)	2.9 ± 4.0	5	15.2
Disseminated	(32)	6.5 ± 8.8	13	40.6
A	(30)	3.6 ± 5.6	5	16.7
B	(35)	5.7 ± 7.9	13	37.1
Non-Hodgkin				
Lymphoma	(94)	6.5 ± 12.9	36	38.3
Localized	(33)	1.2 ± 3.2	4	12.1
Disseminated	(61)	9.2 ± 15.2	32	52.5
A	(54)	2.5 ± 5.6	11	20.4
B	(40	11.8 ± 17.5	25	62.5
Blood donors	(76)	0.0 ± 1.5	0	0.0

* Localized: stages 1 and 2; disseminated: stages 3 and 4; subgroup A: patients without general symptoms; B: patients with general symptoms.

predominantly associated with advanced stages of cancer (Table 14.3 and Fig. 14.2). CIC were more frequent in patients with malignant lymphoma at stage 3 or 4 and in patients with widespread malignant solid tumors. In this small series of solid tumors, the highest incidence of CIC was recorded in patients with bronchial carcinoma, which could be explained by the large number of cases with disseminated tumor in this group.

In another group of patients with lung cancer (49), we found CIC in 36% of cases. As previously observed, CIC were mostly present in patients with metastatic or unresectable cancer; 46% of 48 patients with high tumor burden had CIC at the time of diagnosis as compared to 21% of 38 with low tumor load. The relationship between CIC and the tumor mass became particularly evident when comparing individual pre- and postoperative levels of CIC in patients who had undergone curative surgery. Of 17 patients with high amounts of CIC before surgery, 71% had levels that decreased or returned to normal after tumor resection.

In a recent series of 136 women with breast carcinoma (47), comparative analysis of the CIC levels in relation to the clinical cancer stage at the time of sampling also showed the prevalence of CIC in the disseminated tumor group (Table 14.4). Also, among metastatic breast cancers, higher incidence and levels of CIC were recorded in cases with evolutive disease than in those considered to be in complete (100% regression) or partial (more than 50% regression) remission. In localized breast tumors, the CIC level at diagnosis did not correlate with tumor size. However, CIC were more frequent in patients with bilateral rather than unilateral tumors.

In our studies, for comparative purposes, a number of serum samples were assayed for immune complexes by the Raji cell assay (32) and the conglutinin

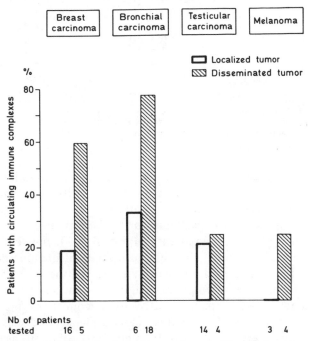

Fig. 14.2. Incidence of circulating immune complexes in 70 patients with malignant solid tumor according to the extent of cancer. The number of patients tested in each group is indicated in the lower part of the figure.

binding test (51) in parallel to the C1q binding method. The high degree of correlation obtained between the results of the three assays indicated that the serum material reacting with C1q also involved Ig and C3. Furthermore, the physicochemical properties of this material were analogous with those of immune complexes. In density gradients, the material sedimented as 10-28S macromolecules (Fig. 14.3a,b) which dissociated into 7S molecules containing IgG after treatment at acid pH (Fig. 14.4). Removal of IgG by immunoabsorption or by ultracentrifugation at acid pH resulted in the abrogation of the ability of the material to bind C1q. While the possibility that unknown polyanionic substances accounted for the C1q-BA of some cancer sera cannot be ruled out, interference of DNA could be excluded as could that of endotoxins or C-reactive protein complexes (50).

Taken together, the results of the studies to date provide good evidence for the presence of CIC in cancer patients. However, in most studies, there is little information concerning the specificity of the complex antibody

Table 14.4. Incidence of Circulating Immune Complexes in Breast Carcinoma:
High Incidence in Widespread Tumor

Stage of Cancer	Clq Binding Activity Mean ± 1 SD (%)	Patients with CIC* No	%
Localized	2.9 ± 3.6	14/84	17
T1 or T2, N + or −	2.6 ± 3.1	7/49	14
T3 or T4, N + or −	2.4 ± 2.8	3/26	12
Bilateral	4.3 ± 5.9	4/9	44
Metastatic	5.8 ± 6.1	22/52	42
Evolutive	9.3 ± 7.2	14/23	61
Nonevolutive**	3.1 ± 4.0	8/29	28

*Patients with serum Clq BA > 3 SD above the mean normal value.
**Patients in complete or partial remission, i.e., with 100% or > 50% tumor regression.

moiety and, hence, the nature of the antigens involved. Complexed antigens have only rarely been identified. CIC involving antilymphocyte antibodies were found in a case of chronic lymphatic leukemia (52). More recently, leukemia-specific antigens, probably in the form of immune complexes, were demonstrated in certain patients with AML (53). In two patients with African Burkitt's lymphoma, IgG eluted from renal immune deposits had a specificity for viral capsid and early antigens of the Epstein Barr virus (EBV) (54). In this type of lymphoma and in nasopharyngeal cancer, Heimer and Klein showed that antigens in CIC were glycoproteins, possibly EBV-associated antigens (55). In infectious mononucleosis, a disease which resembles in many ways a malignant lymphoproliferative disease, we found that some of the complexed antibodies were directed against viral capsid antigen (56).

In patients with Hodgkin's disease, it was claimed that CIC and antibodies from these complexes could react specifically with cultured cells derived from lymphoma (57). According to Theofilopoulos et al. (38) and others (58, 59), immune complexes in some patients with colon cancer contained carcinoembryonic antigen (CEA). The occurrence of CIC involving CEA in patients with gastrointestinal malignant tumors was confirmed in recent reports (39, 60–61). Some months ago, Pascal and Slovin (62) identified CEA and corresponding antibodies in renal glomeruli of a patient who had died of gastric carcinoma but with no evidence of nephrotic syndrome. IgG antibodies eluted from the kidney were also found to be reactive with the patient's tumor as well as another patient's colonic carcinoma. These findings led investigators to conclude that CIC containing CEA produced by the gastric carcinoma had resulted in the formation of glomerular subendothelial immune deposits without significant renal damage. Recently, tumor-specific antigen and antibodies were also found in kidney eluates of a patient with disseminated malignant melanoma, who had developed membranoproliferative glomerulonephritis with renal failure (63). It has also been reported

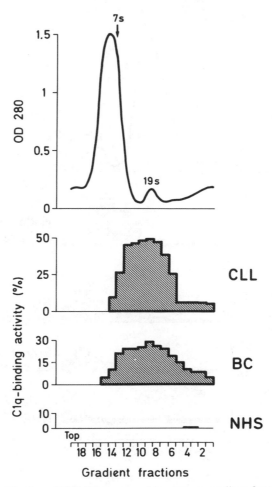

Fig. 14.3a. Distribution of C1q-BA measured in sucrose gradient fractions obtained by density ultracentrifugation of serum samples from a patient with CLL, a patient with BC, and a healthy blood donor (NHS). C1q-BA is represented by the shaded columns in the lower part of the figure. The optical density (OD) pattern and the position of 7 S and 19 S markers are indicated in the upper part.

that tumor-associated antigens could be detected by xenogeneic antisera on the surface of Raji cells incubated in sera from some patients with sarcoma, melanoma, or colon carcinoma (39).

Characterization of CIC has also been done in patients with retinoblastoma (64). Affinity chromatography and analytical polyacrylamide gel electrophoresis demonstrated that IgG was the predominant immunoglobulin in these immune complexes. In addition, affinity of the complexes for Sepharose-concanavalin A indicated the glycoprotein nature of the antigenic constituents.

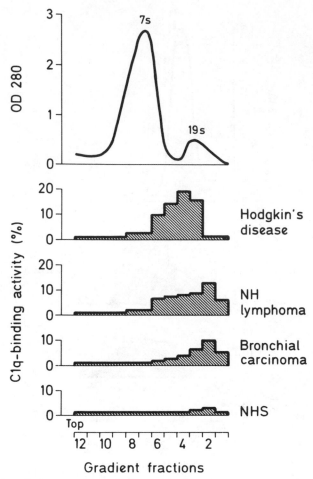

Fig. 14.3b. Distribution of C1q-BA measured in sucrose gradient fractions obtained by density ultracentrifugation of C1q-binding material partially purified from serum samples of patients with Hodgkin's disease, non-Hodgkin (NH) lymphoma or bronchial carcinoma and of a healthy blood donor (NHS). C1q-BA is represented by the shaded columns in the lower part of the figure. The optical density (OD) pattern obtained with a 4% PEG precipitate of NHS and the position of 7 S and 19 S markers are indicated in the upper part of the figure.

One of the most interesting observations to emerge from the clinical studies on CIC in human cancer is the frequent association of these complexes with an unfavorable course of the disease. We (42, 48), and recently others (65), have found that leukemic patients positive for CIC at the time of diagnosis or during remission had a worse prognosis than those without complexes.

First, when assessing the incidence of complete remission among 187 patients studied at diagnosis of AML, ALL, or BC, we recorded a response

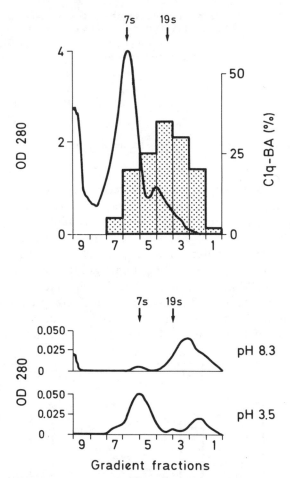

Fig. 14.4. Dissociation of the C1q-binding material at acid pH. The upper part of the figure represents the optical density (OD) pattern and the distribution of C1q-BA (shaded columns) in gradient fractions obtained by density ultracentrifugation of partially purified C1q-binding material from a leukemic patient. The fractions with C1q-BA were pooled, divided in 2 aliquots and analysed by density ultracentrifugation at either pH 8.3 or 3.5. The OD patterns observed are shown in the lower part of the figure.

rate much higher in patients without than in those with initial CIC (Table 14.5). Complete remission took place in 75% of the former patients but in only 26% of the latter group. Moreover, in 16% of patients with CIC at diagnosis who responded to therapy, the duration of complete remission was shorter than 6 months. The poorer response rate to treatment of the patients with initial CIC was unrelated to unfavorable prognostic features such as age, sex, hematological parameters, or sepsis. For instance, analysis of response rate in patients separated into age groups showed that the incidence

Table 14.5. Response to Therapy in Patients with Acute Leukemia According to the Presence of Circulating Immune Complexes at Diagnosis

Type of leukemia	No	Patients with CIC* Complete Remission		No	Patients without CIC complete Remission	
		>6 mo.	<6 mo.		>6 mo.	<6 mo.
Acute myeloid	88	10%	17%	53	70%	8%
Acute lymphatic	11	27%	27%	10	100%	—
Blastic crisis	17	—	6%	8	25%	—
Total	116	10%	16%	71	69%	6%

*Patients with serum Clq-BA > 3 SD above the mean normal value.

of complete remission decreased with increasing age regardless of whether or not the patients had CIC (Fig. 14.5). Thus, age and CIC appeared as two independent prognostic factors which could be combined to evaluate prognosis. The low incidence of complete remission in patients with CIC at diagnosis of leukemia was also unrelated to the cytological type of leukemia. Analysis of the response rate in the patients grouped according to the cytological variety of AML, as defined by the French-American-British (FAB) classification (66), showed that the incidence of complete remission was much lower in all the groups of patients with CIC than in those without CIC, regardless of the cytological type of the leukemic cells (48). The

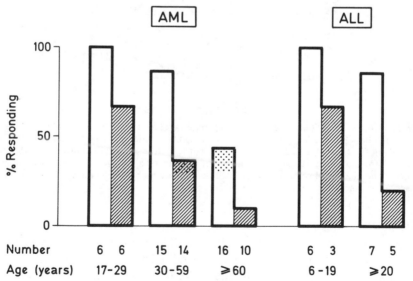

Fig. 14.5. Incidence of remission in relation to the presence of immune complexes in various age groups of patients with AML (left-hand side) and ALL (right-hand side). Patients with detectable circulating immune complexes at onset of leukemia are represented by the shaded columns and those without such complexes by the plain columns. In each column, the dotted areas indicate the proportion of patients who responded to treatment by partial remission.

difference in response of patients according to the presence or absence of CIC at diagnosis of acute leukemia was reflected in the survival times. The median survival times within the five year study period in patients without CIC at diagnosis were: 16 months in AML, 20 months in ALL, and 7 months in BC. The corresponding survival times in patients with CIC at this time were much lower: 72, 140, and 100 days, respectively.

Second, the clinical course of 45 patients tested during the first 2 months of complete remission of acute leukemia was also examined in relation to the presence of IC within this period. Eighteen (40%) of these patients had CIC during this period. With one exception, all these positive patients experienced a complete remission shorter than 6 months. Conversely, in the 27 patients without CIC at this time, only 4 relapsed within the first year of complete remission. The median duration of complete remission in the CIC-positive patients was 4 months, while it was 15.5 months in the patients without CIC.

Third, the detection of CIC appeared also to be of prognostic significance in patients maintained in complete remission more than 1 year and whose serum was negative during the first several months of remission. CIC occurred from 3 weeks to 5.5 months prior to relapse in 9 of 14 patients studied sequentially before relapse.

Correlation of CIC with poor prognosis has also been observed in patients with malignant lymphoma or solid tumor. In malignant lymphomas, several studies (67, 68) including our own (43, 45) have indicated that the presence of CIC correlates not only with the tumor extent but also with other features, such as general symptoms, known to adversely affect prognosis. For example, about 51% (38 out of 75) of our patients with general symptoms had positive results as compared to 19% (16 out of 84) of patients with no symptoms (Table 14.3). However, when examining the levels of CIC in relation to both the extent of the disease and the presence of general symptoms, it appeared that the detection of CIC was much more often related to the dissemination of the disease than to the systemic symptoms. In patients with Hodgkin's disease, Amlot and coworkers (68) further found a relationship between the presence of CIC and the histological types of tumor carrying poor prognosis.

Rossen et al. (31) reported that in patients with bronchial carcinoma followed up 7 months after serum testing for immune complexes, those who had high levels of CIC at the first test were more likely to have tumors that grew rapidly or recurred. Dent and collaborators (69), who studied 50 patients with lung cancer for the prognostic value of increased serum levels of immune complexes and CEA, recorded a two- to threefold longer median survival time in patients with normal postoperative levels than in those with elevated values. In a recent study (70) on CIC in 53 patients with a variety of cancers, CIC levels in lung-cancer patients showed a marked correlation with the survival time, and appeared to be a better prognostic indicator than performance status (Karnofsky scale) at the time of diagnosis. Serial serum analysis performed in this study showed that CIC levels decreased concomitantly with good response to therapy and increased with, and sometimes prior to, clinical evidence of cancer progression. In the patients with bronchial cancer studied by us, no evidence of disease was noted during the period of observation after surgery in 73% of patients without CIC at diagnosis, whereas 65% of patients with initial CIC had progressing disease or died from cancer during this period.

The predictive value of the CIC level with regard to the clinical evolution was also obvious in patients with breast cancer. Among the women with localized breast tumor, we recorded long-term (3 years or more) complete remission in 80% of those without initial CIC, but in only 43% of those positive for CIC at diagnosis. The other patients had tumors which recurred and progressed early after the initial treatment. Analysis of the response in patients grouped according to both the CIC level and the tumor extent at diagnosis revealed a poorer incidence of long-term complete remission in patients positive for CIC regardless of the initial tumor extent (Table 14.6). Tumor burden and CIC level at diagnosis appeared as two independent prognostic features. The survival times in patients with localized breast cancer correlated inversely with initial CIC levels. The median survival time was more than 5.5 years in patients without CIC and 3 years and 4 months in those with CIC; all patients positive for CIC at diagnosis died within 4 years. In the patients with metastatic breast cancer, the course of the disease differed also in relation to the patient's CIC level at the time of the first serum sampling. Cancer progression occurred in 91% of patients with CIC at this time as compared to 43% in those without such complexes. Furthermore, serial serum analysis showed that in most of the patients whose cancer progressed during the period of observation, CIC appeared, or their levels increased, during the 6-month period preceding clinical evidence of tumor progression. (Fig. 14.6). These findings confirmed data

Table 14.6. Prognosis in Patients with or without Circulating Immune Complexes at Diagnosis of Localized Breast Cancer

	Incidence of Long-Term Complete Remission*			
	Patients with CIC**		Patients without CIC	
	No	%	No	%
T1, T2, N + or −	4/7	57	36/42	86
T3, T4, bilateral, N + or −	2/7	29	20/28	71
Total	6/14	43	56/70	80

*Complete remission maintained 3 years or more.
**Patients with serum Clq BA > 3 SD above the mean normal value.

IC and BREAST CANCER PROGRESSION

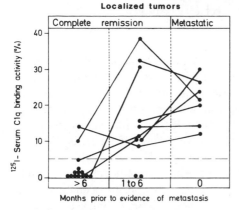
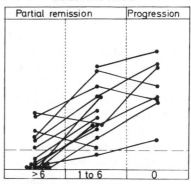

Fig. 14.6. Serum C1q-binding activity at various times before relapse among patients with breast cancer studied during remission and whose cancer progressed. Left part: patients with localized breast tumors, right part: patients with metastatic breast cancer.

reported in a previous retrospective study (37) which showed that in women with breast cancer, serum levels of immune complexes correlated with the clinicopathological prognosis of the tumor and indicated that sequential measurement of complexes could be useful for the identification of patients with residual tumor and for estimating the prognosis. Indeed, in patients without lymph node involvement at mastectomy, i.e., with good prognosis, the levels of complexes returned to normal within a year after removal of the primary tumor. In contrast, the levels remained abnormal 12 months or more after surgery in women with poor prognosis (lymph node metastases at mastectomy) and, regardless of clinicopathological staging, in those with recurrent tumor or fatal outcome within 22 months after surgery.

Similarly, CIC in women with ovarian cancer were found only in patients who relapsed after surgery (36). Serial analysis of serum in three of these patients showed that the levels of immune complexes which had decreased to undetectable amounts during a period of remission rose before tumor recurrence was clinically detectable.

In patients with gastrointestinal carcinoma (61), preoperative circulating CEA immune complexes proved to be a marker with regard to tumor extent and prognosis. In addition, their occurrence during the postoperative period of surveillance appeared as an indicator of relapse. It was also observed that the survival time of children with neuroblastoma (40) and of patients with retinoblastoma (64) or brain tumors (71) was significantly shorter when high levels of CIC were present.

CIRCULATING IMMUNE COMPLEXES IN KIDNEY TRANSPLANT RECIPIENTS

Clinical and experimental evidence indicates that glomerular deposition of immune material plays a basic role in the pathogenesis of the majority of glomerulonephritides (2, 7). Glomerular deposits of immunoglobulins of different classes and of complement components could be visualized by immunofluorescence procedures and immunoelectron microscopy in a large number of patients with membranoproliferative glomerulonephritis. Seventy to 80% of glomerulonephritides of immunological nature result from the deposition of antibodies complexed to circulating antigens in kidney vessels and filtering structures. Immune complex glomerulonephritis is characterized by a broken, granular pattern of immune deposits which contrasts with the linear deposition of anti-GBM antibodies seen in Goodpasture's syndrome. Exogenous antigens such as infectious agents (54, 72–80) or drugs, as well as endogenous antigens such as DNA (81–84) and tubular (85, 86) or tumor antigens (58, 59, 62, 63) may be implicated in the formation of nephrotoxic immune complexes.

One particularity of immune complex-induced nephropathy is the relatively rare detection of CIC so far noted in this disease. Most patients with immune complex glomerulonephritis complicating systemic disease, in particular SLE, have CIC which are detectable by different assays (87, 88). Conversely, in patients with primary glomerulonephritis, especially the chronic forms, such complexes are infrequent (89–91). This low incidence of serum immune complexes in certain types of immune glomerulonephritis suggests that most of the nephrotoxic complexes formed in these patients are undetectable by the current assays used or are trapped rapidly in renal glomeruli after brief passages into the circulation.

Besides their pathological role in inducing primary kidney lesions, immune complexes are increasingly recognized as factors possibly influencing the outcome of renal allograft in transplant recipients. Most of these patients undergo one or more clinical episodes of acute graft rejection and there is evidence that both cell-mediated and humoral immune mechanisms are involved in the rejection phenomena. The participation of immune complexes was demonstrated by immunofluorescence studies showing granular deposits of immunoglobulins and complement in the glomeruli of the grafted kidney (92–97). In many cases, the structural features of the nephropathy at the site of transplant resembled those observed in recipients' kidneys before grafting. In other cases, the immunopathological lesions of the grafted kidney could not be related to the underlying original renal disease (98–100).

Evidence of CIC also exists in patients with kidney transplant (98–108). In certain cases, such complexes appear to reflect the acute rejection process. Ooi et al. (98), using the C1q binding assay, investigated the presence of CIC in 24 allografted patients undergoing acute rejection characterized by deposition of fibrin in the kidney vasculature. The other patients with the cellular pattern of acute renal rejection and those with graft in a quiescent phase had no detectable CIC. In 8 of the positive patients, serial serum analysis further showed a close correlation between the occurrence of serum immune complexes and the episodes of rejection. The levels of the serum complexes decreased to within the normal range when the rejection process was reversed by therapy. In this study, the serum C1q binding material found in 6 patients was characterized. On sucrose density gradient, it sedimented as a 15-18S material and, after acid dissociation, was found to contain IgG. In 5 patients with CIC whose transplant biopsy was studied by immunofluorescence, granular deposits of immunoglobulins and, sometimes, complement were found in the glomeruli and tubular basement membranes. In 10 of the positive patients, the basic renal pathology was of a *nonimmunological* nature, thus excluding in these cases the involvement in the graft rejection of immune complexes related to the recipient's original disease. Moreover, in 6 patients studied sequentially, the presence of CIC could not be demonstrated prior to the period of graft rejection. Smith and colleagues (103), using the Raji cell assay for detection of CIC, found them in 7 out of 12 patients with renal transplant. Contrary to findings in the preceding study, CIC were already present in 5 patients prior to the clinical diagnosis of acute rejection. An association of complexes with the type of acute rejection involving glomerular fibrin deposition was also noted as well as a rapid disappearance of complexes after treatment of the rejection phase. Similarly, in a recent study (104), CIC could be demonstrated in 5 patients with normal graft function. Elevation of the CIC levels occurred during some rejection crises and correlated to some extent with lowered serum C3, C4, and properdin factor B levels.

Association of CIC with the rejection of renal grafts was questioned in other studies. Matl et al. (105), using a polyethylene glycol precipitation procedure, found CIC in only two of eleven patients studied during acute transplant rejection. The results of this study corroborated the findings of Dandavino et al., who used the same method to detect serum immune complexes in patients with renal graft (106).

Junor et al. (99), who measured the levels of CIC by the C1q binding assay in 147 renal transplant recipients, also observed an inconsistent relationship between the presence of these complexes and the rejection phenomena. Like Ooi and collaborators, they did not find evidence of a relationship between the formation of CIC in the patients after transplantation and the basic renal disease.

Two recent studies also failed to document a cause-effect relationship between CIC and acute kidney graft rejection. Jordan et al. (100), who measured CIC with the C1q solid phase and the Raji cell assays in 27 pediatric allograft recipients, found CIC at some stages of posttransplantation period in only 8 recipients. They observed an increase in CIC concomitant with allograft rejection in only 2 patients who also had CIC levels which dropped following antirejection therapy. Allograft immunohistological examination in 3 recipients demonstrated characteristic features of acute rejection but no significant deposits of immunoglobulins or complement components. Further experiments supported the supposed immune-complex nature of the reactive material found in patients' sera, but provided no evidence that antilymphocyte globulins are the immunogen in patients with CIC. In the other study conducted by Johny et al. (107), serial serum samples from 26 patients before renal transplantation and from 28 kidney graft recipients were assayed by four methods for the presence of soluble immune complexes. CIC were found in 54% of patients tested prior to grafting, glomerulonephritis being the primary disease in only half of the group. After transplantation, 68% of patients had CIC. In 14 recipients, complexes could be demonstrated during the entire observation period, while in 5 instances their detection was spasmodic. CIC were present during 39% (9 out of 23) of rejection episodes, but their occurrence in association with rejection process was only observed in 5 cases.

Recently, we determined (108) the incidence of CIC among 48 patients with renal failure before and after kidney grafting, and, in particular, examined the evolution of renal graft in relation to CIC levels. Before transplantation, 54% of the patients studied had CIC demonstrable by both the C1q binding assay and the conglutinin binding test. During the 3-month period following grafting, 69% of these patients still had CIC, while patients without complexes prior to transplantation remained negative (Fig. 14.7). As in previously mentioned studies, we did not find a correlation between the presence of CIC in the grafted patients and the rejection of the transplant; only 3 out of 16 patients who were studied during the period of irreversible graft rejection had serum immune complexes at this time.

The presence of CIC in the patients before transplantation appeared unrelated to the type of nephropathy; 48 and 52% of patients, with glomerulonephritis or renal failure of other origin respectively, had CIC. Furthermore, in the majority of patients, the detection of CIC could not be related to a viral infection. Abnormal levels of antibodies to cytomegalovirus, chickenpox, or Epstein Barr viruses were found in 20% (3 out of 15) of sera containing immune complexes and in 13% (3 out of 23) of sera without complexes. Of 11 patients whose serum contained hepatitis B antigens, 5 were positive and 6 negative for CIC. In addition, there was no correlation between the detection of CIC and blood transfusions given to patients prior

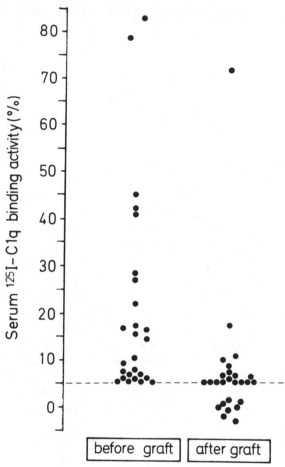

Fig. 14.7. Highest values of serum ^{125}I-C1q binding activity before and after grafting in patients with circulating immune complexes prior to transplantation. The upper limit of normal serum C1q binding activity is indicated by the horizontal line.

to transplantation. CIC were found in 52% of 27 patients who received blood transfusions, but also in 4 out of 6 patients never transfused. Furthermore, we did not note variations in the level of CIC after blood transfusions in 8 patients studied sequentially during a transfusion program before grafting. Sera tested for CIC were also investigated for the presence of lymphocytotoxic antibodies. Such antibodies were detected in 115 samples: 49 out of 132 (37%) positive and 66 out of 252 (26%) negative for CIC. There was also no correlation between individual CIC levels and serum amounts of IgG or IgM.

Table 14.7. Survival Rate of Renal Grafts with Respect to Circulating Immune Complexes before Transplantation

Patients	(n)	% (n) Grafts Surviving at 3 Months		% (n) Grafts Surviving at 12 months	
		%	(n)	%	(n)
with CIC	(26)	92	(24)	92	(22)
without CIC	(24)	41.5	(10)	41.5	(9)
TOTAL	(50)	68	(34)	68	(31)
SWISSTRANSPLANT	(315)	80	(229)	68	(188)

When examining the final outcome of renal grafts with respect to CIC levels, the presence of CIC prior to grafting was associated with a better graft survival (108). Of the 26 grafts performed in 24 positive patients, only 2 (8%) were rejected during the first year after transplantation; 2 grafts of 10 and 11 months' duration functioned normally at the time of evaluation; 22 survived for between 1 and 7 years after grafting. Among the 24 patients negative before transplantation, 14 (58%) grafts were rejected within the first 3 months, 1 graft was still functioning after 11 months, and 9 survived for more than 1 year. There was a significant difference in the number of grafts rejected at 3 and 12 months post-transplantation between the patients CIC-positive before transplantation and those who were CIC-negative at that time. The median survival time of the renal grafts was more than 18 months in patients with CIC as compared with only 2.5 months in those without CIC. The survival rates (68%) of the grafts at 3 and 12 months in the patients we studied were comparable to those observed (80% and 68%) in 315 patients included in the Swiss transplant program, who were transplanted during the same period. (Table 14.7).

CIRCULATING IMMUNE COMPLEXES IN PREGNANCY

Inheriting half of its histocompatibility phenotype from the father, the fetus represents an allograft capable of eliciting immune recognition in the mother. Preservation of the fetus from the potential immune rejection by the mother constitutes one of the most intriguing phenomena in immunology. Many hypotheses have been advanced to explain this phenomenon, but little to date has been conclusively proved. Studies have shown that the mother is sensitized to the paternal histocompatibility antigens (109, 110); thus, blocking of the recognition or effector stages of the maternal immune response do occur.

    A number of data ascribe the protection of the fetus to the presence in the maternal blood of factors capable of masking placental and fetal antigens and of impairing cell-mediated immune reactions (111–119). The ability of maternal humoral factors to suppress immune response was first shown with mixed leukocyte cultures. The reactivity of the latter could be abolished by maternal plasma (111, 112). IgG eluted from human placenta were found to have the same capacity (113). In another study (116), plasma from multiparous women inhibited the production of MIF by autologous lymphocytes stimulated with paternal cells as antigens. Gel filtration analysis indicated that the serum 7S IgG fraction was responsible for the inhibiting activity, which in addition could be absorbed on paternal cells. It was further found that this blocking effect was absent in serum of women with recurrent abortion (117). Addition of maternal serum to the system also provoked a complete inhibition of the lysis *in vitro* of human trophoblastic cells by the mother's lymphocytes (118). In this study, it was shown that the removal of IgG from serum caused a significant decrease of the preventive activity and preincubation experiments indicated that the blocking effect on the lysis involved interaction of maternal IgG with the target trophoblastic cells rather than with the effector lymphoid cells.

Contrary to these findings which implicate maternal blocking antibodies rather than immune complexes in the fetal preservation phenomenon, other data support the participation of serum antigen-antibody complexes in the maternal tolerance to fetus. In pregnant mice (119), the characterization of serum factors responsible for inhibiting K-cell activity to syngeneic tumors indicated that these factors consisted mostly of fetal antigens complexed with corresponding mouse antibodies. In the renal glomeruli of normal pregnant mice and guinea pigs (120), granular deposits of Ig and C3 could be observed. In humans, Masson and co-workers (121) found high levels of a material which inhibited agglutination of IgG-coated latex by rabbit rheumatoid factor in the serum of 55 women at various stages of normal pregnancy. They observed that the inhibition titres of the pregnant sera dropped to the levels recorded in nonpregnant women at 3 to 4 weeks prior to delivery. Fractionation of maternal sera by gel filtration indicated that the inhibitory material involved 7S IgG or *heavy* IgG in association with C3 factor of complement. Whether the complexed antigens originated from placental or fetal tissues was not determined in the study, but the molecular size of antigenic constituents was estimated to be about 400,000 daltons. In contrast, using different techniques for the detection of CIC, other investigators were unable to demonstrate CIC in women with normal pregnancy (122, 123). In these studies, CIC were detected, by the Raji cell assay or the polyethylene glycol precipitation assay, in only some women whose pregnancy was complicated by pre-eclamptic toxemia or diabetes, or in cases with habitual abortion. In these pregnant women, CIC disappeared after delivery.

Recently, using the C1q binding assay, we looked for the presence of CIC in 16 pregnant women at 39 to 41 weeks of normal gestation and 9 women at 3 to 7 days postpartum. None of these women had serum C1q binding level above the normal range (mean serum C1q binding: $5.5 \pm 2.1\%$ in pregnant women; $5.8 \pm 2.4\%$ in age-matched nonpregnant women). Plasma levels of C3, C3d, and C4 complement components were also measured in this group using the immunodiffusion technique. These levels were also found to be normal.

DISCUSSION

Protection against foreign and altered autologous antigens results from humoral and cell-mediated mechanisms. Following antibody release, immune complexes are formed which aid rapid elimination or neutralization of the antigens. For the most part, immune complexes are cleared via the phagocytic system without damaging the host. In unusual situations, however, the formation of immune complexes becomes deleterious. When complexes deposit in vascular and filtering structures, they activate inflammatory mediators such as the complement pathways with the subsequent emergence of so-called immune-complex diseases. In other pathological circumstances, evidence substantiates the harmful effects of immune complexes in exerting regulatory influences on both humoral and cellular immune responses. Which factors determine the pathogenicity of immune complexes in these situations is still unclear. The events do depend on the nature, ratio, and production rate of antigen and antibody, the physicochemical properties of the complexes formed, and on the state of the reticuloendothelial system.

Because of the involvement of soluble IC in the pathogenesis of many human diseases and their immunoregulatory role, methods for their detection have evolved rapidly. These methods, which have been described extensively in recent reports (3, 28), include either physical procedures based on increased molecular size, changes of solubility and electric charge of antigens and/or antibodies as a result of complex formation, or assays based on the interaction of immune complexes with humoral or cellular components. Thus, the assays most commonly used are based on the interaction of immune complexes with complement components (e.g., C1q binding test), rheumatoid factors, receptors on cells for complement components (e.g., Raji cell radioimmunoassay) or for the Fc portion of immunoglobulin molecules, and with conglutinin (e.g., conglutinin-binding test). It is clear that the sensitivity of each method varies according to the nature, affinity, and concentration of both constituents of immune complexes. Furthermore, it is likely that the structure of immune complexes as well as the kinetics of their formation may differ in individual cases or change during the course of the disease. Hence, it is not too surprising to record an incidence of CIC in patients with specific diseases differing from one study to another according to the method used for detection and the stage of the disease studied. Furthermore, it should be emphasized that the techniques used for detecting CIC also give positive results with nonspecifically aggregated immunoglobulins or are susceptible to interference by substances other than immune complexes. Therefore, the identification of circulating antigen-antibody complexes requires the use of methods which preclude nonspecific aggregation of Ig. Additional tests are needed to distinguish between immune complexes and possible interfering substances. Therefore, the search should continue for a specific, sensitive, and easily reproducible assay which can detect CIC of all sizes, regardless of immunoglobulin class and whether or not they fix complement.

Despite imperfect methodology, a great many studies indicate a high incidence of immune complex-like material in the serum of cancer patients. While characterization of the Ig moiety of CIC can be achieved in many instances, the specificity of the antibody and identification of the complexed antigen remains an extremely difficult task. The techniques used for the isolation of complexed antibodies have several limitations. First, the antibodies may be modified or denatured by the dissociation procedure in such a way that they become unable to react with the corresponding antigens. Second, antibodies are often obtained in such small amounts that investigation of their specificity is difficult or impossible. Third, they may have been selected for their low affinity or avidity for the antigen. In addition, since immune complexes found in cancer patients may involve a variety of antigens, it is necessary to test the reactivity of the complexed antibodies against a variety of antigens, using methods such as double immunodiffusion, radioimmunoassay, and adsorption to insoluble substrates or cells carrying antigens. Preparation of purified antigens, including tumor cell-associated antigens, are a prerequisite for such investigations. Recently, however, techniques for the isolation of large amounts of soluble immune complexes have been developed. Complement fixing complexes can be purified from human serum by binding to substrates such as C1q, conglutinin-coated beads, rheumatoid factor, Staph. A, or cells with Fc and complement receptors such as Raji cells (124–127). Subsequently, constituents of the complexes may be obtained by dissociation and then characterized, for example, by sucrose density gradient fractionation and SDS polyacrylamide gel electrophoresis. Using these procedures, work is in progress to identify the composition of the complexes found in patients.

Although it is not possible to precisely identify the complexed antigens in patients with leukemia, clinical data may be relevant to this question. In acute leukemia, CIC are most commonly found during overt, untreated leukemia and decrease with therapy and achievement of complete remission. However, even during the remission period, certain patients have detectable levels of CIC. From follow-up data in these patients, it is conceivable that the presence of CIC at this stage of leukemia also reflects active disease. Almost all patients who relapse soon after entering complete remission have increased levels of CIC from the beginning of this period. This suggests that CIC during remission may be associated with residual active disease. In patients who relapse after long-term complete remission, one may view the occurrence of CIC some time prior to overt relapse as indicating reemergence of proliferating leukemic cells. This concept is supported by data from three recent studies (128–130) which report the appearance of features reflecting the reemergence of leukemic cells in the bone marrow at a time before overt relapse similar to that recorded for the appearance of CIC. These data, which indicate a temporal relationship between CIC and the malignant cell proliferation, suggest that leukemia-associated antigens or antigens related to the proliferative stage of cells, are involved in CIC in patients with acute leukemia (52, 53). Several groups have demonstrated the existence in leukemic patients of leukemia-specific antigens and nuclear antigens expressed in proliferating cells and capable of inducing specific antibodies (131—138). Recently, it was also found that significant amounts of circulating DNA in leukemia patients correlate with the malignant cell turnover (139). It is likely that, in part, DNA forms immune complexes with anti-DNA antibodies that these patients often develop (140). However, similar to previous observations in melanoma patients (34), one observes no rise but a fall in CIC levels in leukemic patients after destruction of malignant cells by chemotherapy (42). This could mean that at the initiation of chemotherapy, all available antibodies to leukemia-related antigens are already saturated. Another possibility is that antibodies complexed to antigens of cells killed by therapy are quickly processed by the phagocytic system and thus never actually appear as CIC. It is also possible that immunosuppressive effects of drugs abolish the production of antibodies. IgG-anti-IgG complexes, including idiotype-antiidiotypes, have also been demonstrated in patients with different types of cancer (141–144). Since leukemic patients are particularly susceptible to infections (145, 146), exogenous antigens, such as bacterial or viral antigens, may possibly account for the formation of CIC in these cases. Indeed, in children with acute lymphatic leukemia, a correlation could be shown between the occurrence of CIC and a history of recent infection (147). However, bacterial or viral infection may be held responsible for the presence of CIC in only some cases of adult leukemia (42, 65).

In patients with malignant lymphoma or solid tumor, several studies, including our own, also indicate an association of CIC with the activity and extent of the malignant cell proliferation. Moreover, tumor-associated antigens could be identified in CIC of some of these patients. Nevertheless, as in leukemia, further biochemical characterization of the complexed material is necessary to positively conclude that tumor-associated antigens participate in the formation of most CIC in patients with lymphoma or solid tumors, since autoantibodies and bacterial or viral antigens may also be involved.

A similar question may be posed as to the nature of complexed antigens in patients with renal insufficiency and in kidney graft recipients. As already mentioned, the demonstration of immunoglobulin and complement deposition in kidney structures directly implicates immune complexes in the etiology of a large number of renal diseases (2, 7–10). However, recognition of antigens responsible for the formation of complexes has proved difficult. The immune complex nature of the renal lesions is often tacitly assumed from the pattern of immune deposits in kidney. Although CIC are mostly detected in patients with glomerulonephritis, acute rather than chronic, a significant number of individuals with nonimmune nephropathy show detectable levels of CIC (107, 108). For example, in patients studied by us prior to transplantation (108), incidence of CIC was similar among the glomerulonephritis group and the group with renal failure of other origin. From these observations, one may assume that CIC occurring in patients could be different in their properties and composition, notably their antigenic constituent, to nephrotoxic complexes. In addition, an immune nature of the underlying original disease is not necessarily precluded when CIC occur during graft rejection episodes in certain kidney graft recipients (98–100, 107, 108). In these cases, it remains unclear whether the appearance of CIC is subsequent to graft damage by the rejection events, or to the therapy. However, there has been no evidence to date of induction of immune complexes by immunosuppressive treatment. Similarly, it is unlikely that anti-lymphocyte globulins (ALG) administered to some renal transplant recipients are involved in the detected complexes (98, 100). CIC occur in these patients independent of ALG administration. It would be logical to assume an involvement of histocompatibility antigens in CIC of repeatedly transfused uremic patients or of graft recipients. This has yet to be demonstrated, and blood transfusions were not shown to influence the CIC levels, nor did the latter correlate with patients' lymphocytotoxic antibody levels (108). On the other hand, the absence of clinical and laboratory features of infection in most patients with CIC minimizes the likelihood of a bacterial or viral origin of most CIC. Chronic renal failure may be responsible for an increased release of nuclear antigens in the patient's blood. Nuclear material, presumably from damaged cells, has been found on used dialysis membranes (148) and in the circulation of uremic patients (149) in whom a high incidence of antinuclear antibodies has also been recorded (150). Of interest are the falls in antibody titers of these patients observed after hemodialysis or in the immediate post-transplantation period. These sudden changes in the number of antibodies suggest an antibody trapping or immune-complex formation during dialysis or after grafting.

Although little to date has been conclusively proved, the absence of infections in pregnant women with CIC and the disappearance of CIC after delivery suggest that an antibody response to fetal antigens provokes CIC (121–123).

The clinical relevance of the demonstration of CIC in cancer patients is still difficult to assess. The biological basis for the unfavorable disease course of cancer patients with CIC is unclear. Several studies in experimental animal systems have shown that immune mechanisms can play an important role in *chemotherapeutic cure* of cancer (151, 152). If similar mechanisms are operative in humans, they may be impaired by immune complexes (25, 153, 154). Regardless of the nature of the complexed antigens, immune complexes may favor tumor progression by modulating the immune responses of the host against the malignant cells, either at the stage of lymphocyte activation or during the effector phase. It has been reported that immune complexes may either enhance or suppress B- or T-lymphocyte activation (155–161). These differences may be explained by the composition and configuration of the complexes, which in turn determine whether the interaction of complexes with lymphocytes occurs in a specific way through the antigenic determinants, or in a nonspecific way through the Fc portion of the antibodies. For instance, synthesis of antibody by B lymphocytes is sharply reduced after exposure to the corresponding antigen-antibody complexes (156). Antigen-antibody complexes can also affect the effector phase of the immune response. In certain experimental systems (162–165) selective inactivation of helper T cells and inhibition of antibody-dependent or natural cell-mediated cytotoxicity appear to be due to cell-bound antigen-antibody complexes. In animals and some humans bearing growing tumors, at least some of the so-called serum blocking factors, which inhibit host lymphocyte cytotoxicity to tumor, consist of immune complexes (23, 25–27, 154). CIC may also antigen specifically suppress delayed hypersensitivity reaction in mice (166). In addition, immune complexes are particularly efficient in activating suppressor T cells (161) and inducing the production of rheumatoid factors or antiidiotypic antibodies (167–169). The latter, which can function as antireceptor antibodies for lymphocyte receptors with similar determinants, may exert a suppressive effect on immune responses (167, 170, 171). Their presence has been demonstrated in patients with malignancy (141–144, 172–174).

The following observations are particularly in agreement with the effectiveness *in vivo* of these regulatory mechanisms which can facilitate tumor growth. First, in patients with acute leukemia, complete remission is not achieved in most cases positive for CIC at the time of diagnosis. Second, there is a high rate of early recurrence among cancer patients who enter remission but have CIC either before or at the beginning of remission. An alternative hypothesis is that CIC do not affect the course of the disease but rather represent a phenomenon associated with the more refractory cases. For instance, the presence of CIC in some cancer patients may reflect a particular immune status of the host (175, 176). A defective immune competence of the patient can indeed favor both the progression of cancer and the formation and persistence of CIC (177). However, at present, no evidence exists linking the detection of CIC with immunological abnormalities in patients or particularly aggressive forms of cancer.

It is still uncertain whether the presence of immune complexes during pregnancy represents a physiologic state or a pathological one when occurring under special conditions such as toxemia. However, blocking factors have been found in maternal sera during normal pregnancy (111, 112, 114–119). Antithetically, regarding their enhancing effect on tumors, serum blocking factors in pregnancy appear capable of protecting the fetoplacental allograft from maternal immune rejection. As in neoplasia, some of these factors probably consist of immune complexes. Suppressor T-cell activity could also be important in stopping potential immunologic rejection of the fetus by the maternal host. This possibility is suggested by a recent work which indicates that human cord blood contains increased suppressor T-cell reactivity which is capable of preserving fetal integrity (178). In experiments supporting this theory, using nonblocked mixed leukocyte cultures with cord-blood lymphocytes from male babies and maternal lymphocytes, only the male babies' lymphocytes proliferated. These were identified using male chromosome markers. Later it was shown that cord blood contained an increased proportion and physiological activity of $T\gamma$ or T suppressor cells (179). A report by Murgita et al. (180) indicates that fetal blood-cord suppressor cells may be activated through mechanisms involving α-fetoprotein. As mentioned, CIC may be good inducers of suppressor T cells.

The presence of CIC in patients undergoing renal transplantation has been found to be associated with a considerably better graft survival. As in pregnancy and in contrast to the situation in cancer, CIC in kidney recipients may protect the allograft from the host immune response. Thus, by similar mechanisms, CIC may work in opposite ways in pregnancy and transplantation as compared to malignancy. However, as in cancer patients, the formation of CIC in individuals with renal failure and prognosis of the kidney graft could also be two unrelated phenomena, reflecting a deficiency in the host immune status.

Despite the uncertainties concerning the pathophysiology of CIC in cancer patients and renal transplant recipients, the data indicate that measurement

402 Immunobiology of Transplantation, Cancer and Pregnancy

of CIC may be of prognostic value in certain conditions. The association of CIC in cancer patients with the disease activity may, in particular, have clinical implications. The rate of cure in malignancies depends to a large extent on the difficulty in detecting residual or minimal disease. Identification of features closely associated with the disease activity, such as CIC, may lead to modification of treatment schedules with subsequent improved therapeutic results. In patients with CIC during apparent complete remission, intensified chemotherapy combined with a treatment designed to reduce the level of CIC might prove to be beneficial. For instance, immunoadsorption has proved to be of benefit in some tumor-bearing individuals (181–187). In addition, since prognosis in certain cancers correlates closely with the detection of CIC at the time of diagnosis (188), it would appear desirable to stratify patients in new therapeutic trials according to the presence or absence of CIC before treatment.

Assays to detect CIC do not require invasive procedures and are relatively simple to perform. Therefore, measurement of CIC appears suitable for routine use in monitoring, particularly cancer patients. It may prove useful as a prognostic tool both during initial evaluation of patients and in their follow-up after treatment.

REFERENCES

1. Dixon, F. J., Vazquez, J. J., Weigle, W. O., et al., *Arch. Pathol.* **65**:18, 1958.
2. Cochrane, C. G., and Koffler, D., *Adv. Immunol.* **16**:185, 1973.
3. WHO Report of a Scientific Group, *The Role of Immune Complexes in Disease.* WHO Technical Report Series, No. 606, Geneva, Switzerland, 1977.
4. Casali, P., Perrin, L. H., and Lambert, P. H., Immune complexes in tissue injury. In G. Dick (Ed.), *Immunological Aspects of Infectious Diseases.* Chap. 9, p. 1. London: MTP, 1978.
5. Theofilopoulos, A. N., and Dixon, F. J., Immune complexes associated with neoplasia. In R. Herberman (Ed.), *Immunodiagnosis of Cancer*, p. 1. New York: Marcel Dekker, 1979.
6. Carpentier, N. A., Louis, J. A., Lambert, P. H., and Cerottini, J. C., Immune complexes in leukemia and adult malignancies. In B. Serrou and C. Rosenfeld (Eds.), *Immune Complexes and Plasma Exchanges in Cancer Patients*, p. 111. Amsterdam, Holland: Elsevier/North Holland, 1981.
7. Wilson, C. B., and Dixon, F. J., The renal response to immunological injury. In B. M. Brenner and F. C. Rector (Eds.), *The Kidney*, p. 838. Philadelphia: W. B. Saunders, 1976.
8. Ooi, Y. M., Vallota, E. H., and West, C. D., *Kidney Int.* **11**:275, 1977.
9. Levinsky, R. J., Malleson, P. N., Barratt, T. M., et al., *N. Engl. J. Med.* **298**:126, 1978.
10. Pussel, B. A., Lockwood, A. M., Scott, D. M., et al., *Lancet* **2**:359, 1978.
11. Gleicher, N., and Theofilopoulos, A. N., *Diagn. Gynecol. Obstet.* **2**:7, 1980.
12. Lee, J. C., Yamauchi, H., and Hopper, J., *Ann. Int. Med.* **64**:41, 1966.
13. Kiely, J. M., Wagoner, R. D., and Holley, K. E., *Ann. Intern. Med.* **71**:1159, 1969.

14. Lewis, M. G., Loughridge, L. W., and Phillips, T. M., *Lancet* 2:134, 1971.
15. Plager, J., and Stutzman, L., *Amer. J. Med.* **50**:56, 1971.
16. Sherman, R. L., Susin, J., Weksler, M. E., et al., *Am. J. Med.* **52**:699, 1972.
17. Hyman, L. R., Burkholder, P. J., Too, P. A., and Segar, W. T., *J. Pediatr.* **82**:207, 1973.
18. Lokich, J. J., Galvanek, E. G., and Moloney, W. C., *Arch. Intern. Med.* **132**:597, 1973.
19. Sutherland, J. C., Markham, R. V., Jr., Ramsey, H. E., and Mardiney, M. R., Jr., *Cancer Res.* **34**:1179, 1974.
20. da Costa, C. R., Dupont, E., and Hamers, R., *Clin. Nephrol.* **2**:245, 1974.
21. Pascal, R. R., Iannacone, P. M., Rollwagen, F. M., Harding, T. A., and Bennett, S. J., *Cancer Res.* **36**:43, 1976.
22. Helin, H., Pasternack, A., Hakala, T., Penttinen, K., and Wager, O., *Clin. Nephrol.* **14**:23, 1980.
23. Sjogren, H. O., Hellström, I., Bansal, S. C., and Hellström, K. E., *Proc. Natl. Acad. Sci. USA* **68**:1372, 1971.
24. Currie, G. A., and Basham, C., *Br. J. Cancer* **26**:427, 1972.
25. Baldwin, R. W., Embleton, M. J., Price, M. R., and Robins, R. A., *Cancer* **34**:1452, 1974.
26. Jose, D. G., and Seshadri, R., *Int. J. Cancer* **13**:824, 1974.
27. Mantovani, A., and Spreafico, F., *Europ. J. Cancer* **11**:451, 1975.
28. Theofilopoulos, A. N., and Dixon, F. J., *Adv. Immunol.* **28**:89, 1979.
29. Samayoa, E. A., McDuffie, F. C., Nelson, A. M., Go, V. L. W., Luthra, H. S., and Brumfield, H. W., *Int. J. Cancer* **19**:12, 1977.
30. Teshima, H., Wanebo, H., Pinsky, C., and Day, N. K., *J. Clin. Invest.* **59**:1134, 1977.
31. Rossen, R. D., Reisberg, M., Hersh, E. M., and Gutterman, J. V., *J. Nat. Cancer Inst.* **58**:1205, 1977.
32. Theofilopoulos, A. N., Wilson, C. B., and Dixon, F. J., *J. Clin. Invest.* **57**:169, 1976.
33. Jennette, J. C., *Am. J. Pathol.* **100**:403, 1980.
34. Jerry, L. M., Rowden, G., Cano, P. O., et al., *Scand. J. Immunol.* **5**:845, 1976.
35. Gropp, C., Havemann, K., Schärfe, T., Schultz, H., and Schaumlöffel, E., *Klin. Wochenschr.* **57**:401, 1979.
36. Poulton, T. A., Crowther, M. E., Hay, F. C., and Nineham, L. J., *Lancet* 2:72, 1978.
37. Hoffken, K., Meredith, I. D., Robins, R. A., Baldwin, R. W., Davies, C. J., and Blamey, R. W., *Brit. Med. J.* 2:218, 1977.
38. Theofilopoulos, A. N., Andrews, B. S., Vrist, M. M., Morton, D. L., and Dixon, F. J., *J. Immunol.* **119**:657, 1977.
39. Staab, H. J., Anderer, F. A., Stumpf, E., and Fischer, R., *Klin. Wochenschr.* **58**:125, 1980.
40. Brandeis, W. E., Helson, L., Wang, Y., Good, R. A., and Day, N. K., *J. Clin. Invest.* **62**:1201, 1978.
41. Brandeis, W. E., Tan, C., Wang, Y., Good, R. A., and Day, N. K., *Clin. Exp. Immunol.* **39**:551, 1980.
42. Carpentier, N. A., Lange, G. T., Fière, D. M., Fournié, G. J., Lambert, P. H., and Miescher, P. A., *J. Clin. Invest.* **60**:874, 1977.
43. Heier, H. E., Carpentier, N. A., Lange, G., Lambert, P. H., and Godal, T., *Int. J. Cancer* **20**:887, 1977.
44. Heier, H. E., Carpentier, N. A., Lambert, P. H., and Godal, T., *Int. J. Cancer* **21**:695, 1978.
45. Carpentier, N. A., Lambert, P. H., and Miescher, P. A., Circulating immune complexes in patients with malignancies. In S. Ferrone, S. Gorini, R. B. Herberman, and R. A.

Reisfeld (Eds.), *Current Trends in Tumor Immunology*, pp. 165–174. New York and London: Garland STPM Press, 1979.

46. Mod, A., Carpentier, N., Fust, G., et al., *J. Clin. Lab. Immunol.* **4**:15, 1980.
47. Chollet, P., Carpentier, N., Chassagne, J., Betail, G., Bidet, J. M., Lambert, P. H., and Plagne, R., Clinical relevance of circulating immune complexes in breast cancer. In B. Serrou and C. Rosenfeld (Eds.), *New Trends in Human Immunology and Cancer Immunotherapy*, pp. 496–503. Paris: Doin, 1980.
48. Carpentier, N. A., Fière, D. M., Schuh, D., Boye, J., Lambert, P. H., and Miescher, P. A., Circulating immune complexes in human acute leukemia: relation to prognosis over a 5 year period. In B. Serrou and C. Rosenfeld (Eds.), *New Trends in Human Immunology and Cancer Immunotherapy*, pp. 465–477. Paris: Doin, 1980.
49. Carpentier, N. A., Egeli, R., Chollet, P., Maurice, P., and Lambert, P. H., Circulating immune complexes as markers for human neoplasia. In M. Colnaghi, G. Buraggi and M. Ghione (Eds.), *Markers for Diagnosis and Monitoring of Human Cancer*, pp. 9–20. Academic Press, London, 1982.
50. Zubler, R. H., Lange, G., Lambert, P. H., and Miescher, P. A., *J. Immunol.* **116**:232, 1976.
51. Casali, P., Bossus, A., Carpentier, N. A., and Lambert, P. H., *Clin. Exp. Immunol.* **29**:342, 1977.
52. Day, N. K., Winfield, J. B., Gee, T., Teshima, H., and Kunkel, H. G., *Clin. Exp. Immunol.* **26**:189, 1976.
53. Faldt, R., and Ankerst, J., *Int. J. Cancer* **26**:309, 1980.
54. Oldstone, M. B. A., Theofilopoulos, A. N., Klein, G., and Guven, P., *Intervirology* **4**:292, 1975.
55. Heimer, R., and Klein, G., *Int. J. Cancer* **18**:310, 1976.
56. Carpentier, N. A., Docquier, C. E., Pugin, P., Lambert, P. H., and Miescher, P. A., *Schweiz. Med. Wschr.* **108**:1601, 1978.
57. Long, J. C., Hall, C. L., Brown, C. A., Stamatos, C., Weitzman, S. A., and Carey, K., *New Engl. J. Med.* **297**:295, 1977.
58. Constanza, M. E., Pinn, V., Schwartz, R. S., and Nathanson, L., *N. Engl. J. Med.* **289**:520, 1973.
59. Couser, W. G., Wagonfeld, J. B., Spargo, B. H., and Lewis, E. J., *Ann. J. Med.* **57**:962, 1974.
60. Kapsopoulou-Sominos, K., and Anderer, F. A., *Clin. Exp. Immunol.* **37**:25, 1979.
61. Staab, H. J., Anderer, F. A., Stumpf, E., and Fischer, R., *Brit. J. Cancer* **42**:26, 1980.
62. Pascal, R. R, and Slovin, S. F., *Hum. Pathol.* **11**:679, 1980.
63. Olson, J. L., Philips, T. M., Lewis, M. G., and Solez, K., *Clin. Nephrol.* **12**:74, 1979.
64. Stein, P. C., Christensen, M., and Char, D. H., *Invest. Ophthalmol. Vis. Sci.* **19**:302, 1980.
65. Hubbard, R. A., Aggio, M. C., Lozzio, B. B., and Wust, C. J., *Clin. Exp. Immunol.* **43**:46, 1981.
66. Bennett, J. M., Catovsky, D., Daniel, M. T., et al., *Br. J. Haemat.* **33**:451, 1976.
67. Amlot, P. L., Slaney, J. M., and Williams, B. D., *Lancet* **1**:449, 1976.
68. Amlot, P. L., Pussell, B., Slaney, J. M., and Williams, B. D., *Clin. Exp. Immunol.* **31**:166, 1978.
69. Dent, P. B., Louis, J. A., McCulloch, P. B., Dunnett, C. W., and Cerottini, J. C., *Cancer* **45**:130, 1980.
70. Poskitt, P. K., and Poskitt, T. R., *Int. J. Cancer* **24**:560, 1979.
71. Martin-Achard, A., de Tribolet, N., Louis, J. A., and Zander, E., *Surg. Neurol.* **13**:161, 1980.
72. Treser, G., Semar, M., McVicar, M., et al., *Science* **163**:676, 1969.

73. Lange, K., Ahmed, U., Kleinberger, H., et al., *Clin. Nephrol.* **5**:207, 1976.
74. Dobrin, R. S., Day, N. K., Quie, P. G., et al., *Am. J. Med.* **59**:660, 1975.
75. Knieser, M. R., Jenis, E. H., Lowenthal, D. T., et al., *Arch. Pathol.* **97**:193, 1974.
76. Dayan, A. D., and Stokes, M. I., *Br. Med. J.* **2**:374, 1972.
77. Sutherland, J. C., and Mardiney, M. R., Jr., *J. Nat. Cancer Inst.* **50**:633, 1973.
78. Pascal, R. R., Finney, R. P., Rifkin, S. I., and Kahana, L., *Hum. Pathol.* **11**:391, 1980.
79. Andres, G. A., Kano, K., Elwood, C., et al., *Int. Arch. Allergy Appl. Immunol.* **52**:136, 1976.
80. Lambert, P. H., and Houba, V., Immune complexes in parasitic diseases. In L. Brent and J. Holborow (Eds.), *Progress in Immunology II*, Vol. 5, p. 57. Amsterdam, Holland: North Holland, 1974.
81. Krishnan, C., and Kaplan, M. H., *J. Clin. Invest.* **46**:569, 1967.
82. Koffler, D., Agnello, V., Thoburn, R., et al., *J. Exp. Med.* **134**:169, 1971.
83. Izui, S., Lambert, P. H., Fournié, G. J., et al., *J. Exp. Med.* **145**:1115, 1977.
84. Izui, S., Lambert, P. H., and Miescher, P. A., *J. Exp. Med.* **144**:428, 1976.
85. Naruse, T., Kitamura, K., Miyakawa, Y., et al., *J. Immunol.* **110**:1163, 1973.
86. Strauss, J., Pardo, V., Koss, M. N., et al., *Am. J. Med.* **58**:382, 1975.
87. Rossen, R. D., Reisberg, M. A., Singer, D. B., et al., *Kidney Int.* **10**:256, 1976.
88. Tung, K. S. K., Woodroffe, A. J., Ahlin, T. D., et al., *J. Clin. Invest.* **62**:61, 1978.
89. Ooi, Y. M., Ooi, B. S., Pollak, V., *J. Lab. Clin. Med.* **90**:891, 1977.
90. Woodroffe, A. J., Border, W. A., Theofilopoulos, A. N., et al., *Kidney Int.* **12**:268, 1977.
91. Woodroffe, A. J., and Wilson, C. B., *J. Immunol.* **118**:1788, 1977.
92. Porter, K. A., Andres, G. A., Calder, M. W., et al., *Lab. Invest.* **18**:159, 1968.
93. Porter, K. A., Dossetor, J. B., Marchioro, T. L., et al., *Lab. Invest.* **16**:153, 1967.
94. Dixon, F. J., McPhaul, J. J., and Lerner, R. L., *Arch. Intern. Med.* **123**:554, 1969.
95. Seibel, H. R., Weymouth, R. J., Craig, S. S., et al., *Virchows Arch.* **371**:5, 1976.
96. McLean, R. H., Geiger, H., Burke, B., et al., *Am. J. Med.* **60**:60, 1976.
97. Berger, J., Yaneva, H., Nabarra, B., et al., *Kidney Int.* **7**:232, 1975.
98. Ooi, Y. M., Ooi, B. S., Vallota, E. H., First, M. R., and Pollak, V. E., *J. Clin. Invest.* **60**:611, 1977.
99. Junor, B. J., d'Apice, A. J., Kincaid-Smith, P., *Transplantation* **30**:111, 1980.
100. Jordan, S. C., Sakai, R., Malekzadeh, M. H., et al., *Transplantation* **31**:190, 1981.
101. Palubuo, T., Kano, K., Anthone, S., Gerbasi, J. R., and Milgrom, F., *Transplantation* **21**:312, 1976.
102. Vincent, C., Fortier, M., Revillard, J. P., and Traeger, J., *Transplant Proc.* **11**:1274, 1979.
103. Smith, M. D., Verroust, P. J., Griffin, P. J., and Salaman, J. R., *Clin. Exp. Immunol.* **39**:141, 1980.
104. Schena, F. P., Pertosa, G., Manno, C., Losuriello, V., and Pastore, A., *Minerva Chir.* **35**:709, 1980.
105. Matl, I., Haskova, V., and Kaslik, J., *Transplantation* **27**:358, 1979.
106. Dandavino, R., Trunet, P., Descamps, B., and Kreis, H., *Transplant Proc.* **10**:655, 1978.
107. Johny, K. V., Dasgupta, M. K., Kovithavongs, T., and Dossetor, J. B., *Kidney Int.* **19**:332, 1981.
108. Carpentier, N., Benzonana, G., Jeannet, M., Leski, M., and Lambert, P. H., *Transpl.* **33**:181, 1982.
109. Youtananukorn, V., and Matangkasombut, P., *Clin. Exp. Immunol.* **11**:549, 1972.
110. Rocklin, R. E., Zuckerman, J. E., Alpert, E., and David, J. R., *Nature* **241**:130, 1973.

111. Leventhal, B. G., Buell, D. N., Yankee, R., Rogentine, G. N., and Terabaki, P., The mixed leucocyte response: effect of maternal plasma. In J. E. Harris (Ed.), *Proc. of the 5th Leucocyte Culture Conference*, p. 473. New York: Academic Press, 1970.
112. Kasakura, S., *J. Immunol.* **107**:1206, 1971.
113. Faulk, W. P., *Excerpta Medica* **281**:18, 1973.
114. Youtananukorn, V., and Mantangkasombut, P., *Nature* **242**:110, 1973.
115. Hill, C. A., Sr., Finn, R., and Denye, V., *Brit. Med. J.* **3**:513, 1973.
116. Pence, H., Petty, W. M., and Rocklin, R. E., *J. Immunol.* **114**:525, 1975.
117. Rocklin, R. E., Kitzmiller, J. L., Carpenter, C. B., et al., *N. Engl. J. Med.* **295**:1209, 1976.
118. Taylor, P. V., and Hancock, K. W., *Immunology* **28**:973, 1975.
119. Tamerius, J., Hellström, I., and Hellström, K. E., *Int. J. Cancer* **16**:456, 1975.
120. Tung, K. S. K., *J. Immunol.* **112**:186, 1974.
121. Masson, P. L., Delire, M., and Cambiaso, C. L., *Nature* **266**:542, 1977.
122. Gleicher, N., Theophilopoulos, A. N., and Beers, P., *Lancet* **2**:1108, 1978.
123. D'Amelio, R., Bilotta, P., Pachi, A., and Aiuti, F., *Clin. Exp. Immunol.* **37**:33, 1979.
124. Chenais, F., Virella, G., Patrick, C. C., and Fudenberg, H. H., *J. Immunol. Methods* **18**:183, 1977.
125. Svehag, S. E., and Burger, D., *Acta Pathol. Microbiol. Scand. (C)* **85**:45, 1976.
126. Theofilopoulos, A. N., Eisenberg, R.A., and Dixon, F. J., *J. Clin. Invest.* **61**:1570, 1978.
127. Casali, P., and Lambert, P. H., *Clin. Exp. Imm.* **37**:295, 1979.
128. Baker, M. A., Falk, J. A., Carter, W. H., and Taub, R. N., *N. Engl. J. Med.* **301**:1353, 1979.
129. Hittelman, W. N., Broussard, L. C., Dosik, G., and McCredie, K. B., *New Eng. J. Med.* **303**:479, 1980.
130. Stryckmans, P., Debusscher, L., Ronge-Collard, E., Socquet, M., and Zittoun, R., *Leukemia Res.* **4**:79, 1980.
131. Harris, P., *Nature* **241**:95, 1973.
132. Mann, D. L., Halterman, R., and Leventhal, B., *Cancer* **34**:1446, 1974.
133. Fefer, A., Mickelson, E., and Thomas, E. D., *Clin. Exp. Immunol.* **18**:237, 1974.
134. Baker, M. A., Ramachandar, K., and Taub, R. N., *J. Clin. Invest.* **54**:1273, 1974.
135. Mohanakumar, T., Metzgar, R. S., and Miller, D. S., *J. Nat. Cancer Inst.* **52**:1435, 1974.
136. Brown, G., Capellaro, D., and Greaves, M., *J. Nat. Cancer Inst.* **5**:1281, 1975.
137. Steiner, M., Klein, E., and Klein, G., *Clin. Immunol. and Immunopathol.* **4**:374, 1975.
138. Russel, A. R., and Pope, J. H., *Clin. Exp. Immunol.* **23**:83, 1976.
139. Carpentier, N. A., Izui, S., Rose, L. M., Lambert, P .H., and Miescher, P. A., *Human Lymphocyte Differentiation* **1**:93, 1981.
140. Izui, S., Lambert, P. H., Carpentier, N., and Miescher, P. A., *Clin. Exp. Immunol.* **24**:379, 1976.
141. Hartmann, D., and Lewis, M. G., *Lancet* **2**:1318, 1974.
142. Levine, G. B., Mills, P. E., and Epstein, W. V., *J. Lab. Clin. Med.* **69**:749, 1967.
143. Lewis, M. B., Phillips, T. M., Cook, K. B., and Blake, J., *Nature* **232**:52, 1971.
144. Gilboa, N., Durante, D., Guggenheim, S., et al., *Nephron.* **24**:223, 1979.
145. Bodey, G., Rodriguez, V., Chang, H.-Y., and Narboni, G., *Cancer* **42**:1610, 1978.
146. Nedelkova, M., Bagalova, S., and Gerogieva, B., *Eur. J. Cancer* **17**:617, 1981.
147. Clague, R. B., Kumar, S., Hann, I. M., Morris Jones, P. H., and Lennox Holt, P. J., *Int. J. Cancer* **22**:227, 1978.
148. Nolph, K. D., Husted, F. C., Sharp, G. C., and Siemsen, A. W., *Am. J. Med.* **60**:673, 1976.

149. Steinman, C. R., and Ackad, A., *Am. J. Med.* **62**:693, 1977.
150. Nolph, K. D., Ghods, A. J., Sharp, G. C., and Siemsen, A. W., *J. Lab. Clin. Med.* **91**:559, 1978.
151. Burnet, F. M., *Prog. Exp. Tumor Res.* **13**:1, 1970.
152. Mathé, G., and Pouillart, P., Active immunotherapy of L 1210 leukemia applied after the graft of tumor cells. In G. Mathé (Ed.), *Advances in the Treatment of Acute (Blastic) Leukemias. Recent Results in Cancer Research*, pp. 64–75. Berlin, Heidelberg, and New York: Springer-Verlag, 1970.
153. Baldwin, R. W., and Robins, R. A., *Brit. Med. Bull.* **32**:118, 1976.
154. Hellström, K. E., Hellström, I., and Nepom, J. T., *Biochem. Biophys. Acta* **473**:121, 1977.
155. Revoltella, R., Pediconi, M., Bertolini, L., and Bosman, C., *Cell. Immunol.* **20**:117, 1975.
156. Morgan, E. L., and Templis, C. H., *J. Immunol.* **120**:1669, 1978.
157. Bloch-Shtacher, N., Hirschhorn, K., and Uhr, J. W., *Clin. Exp. Immunol.* **3**:889, 1968.
158. Oppenheim, J. J., *Cell. Immunol.* **3**:341, 1972.
159. Playfair, J. H. L., *Clin. Exp. Immunol.* **17**:1, 1974.
160. Kilburn, D. G., Fairhurst, M., Levy, J. G., and Whitney, R. B., *J. Immunol.* **117**:1612, 1976.
161. Moretta, L., Webb, S. R., Grossi, C. E., Lydyard, P. M., and Cooper, M. D., *J. Exp. Med.* **146**:184, 1977.
162. MacLennan, I. C. M., *Clin. Exp. Immunol.* **10**:275, 1972.
163. Stockinger, B., and Lemmel, E. M., *Cellular Immunol.* **40**:395, 1978.
164. Waksman, B. H., *Clin. Exp. Immunol.* **28**:363, 1977.
165. Kontiainen, S., and Mitchison, N. A., *Immunol.* **28**:523, 1975.
166. Mackaness, G. B., Lagrange, P. H., Miller, T. E., and Ishibashi, T., The formation of activated T cells. In W. H. Wagner, E. Hahn, and R. Evans (Eds.), *Activation of Macrophages*, pp. 193–209. Amsterdam: Excerpta Medica, 1974.
167. McKearn, T. J., *Science* **183**:94, 1974.
168. Klaus, G. G. B., *Nature* **272**:265, 1978.
169. Johnson, P. M., and Page Faulk, W., *Clin. Immunol. Immunopathol.* **6**:414, 1976.
170. Binz, H., Lindenmann, J., and Wigzell, H., *Nature* **246**:146, 1973.
171. Nisonoff, A., and Bangasser, S. A., *Transplant. Rev.* **27**:100, 1975.
172. Lewis, M. G., Hartmann, D. P., and Jerry, L. M., *Ann. N.Y. Acad. Sci.* **276**:316, 1976.
173. Hartmann, D., Lewis, M. G., Proctor, J. W., et al., *Lancet* **2**:1481, 1974.
174. Pyrhonen, S., Timonen, T., Heikkinen, A., et al., *Eur. J. Cancer* **12**:87, 1976.
175. Hersh, E. M., Mavligit, G. M., and Gutterman, J. V., *Med. Clin. North Am.* **60**:623, 1976.
176. Serrou, B., Gauci, L., Caraux, J., et al., *Recent Results Cancer Research* **75**:41, 1980.
177. Soothill, J. F., and Steward, M. W., *Clin. Exp. Immunol.* **9**:193, 1971.
178. Olding, L. B., and Oldstone, M. B. A., *J. Immunol.* **116**:682, 1976.
179. Oldstone, M. B. A., Tishon, A., and Moretta, L., *Nature* **269**:333, 1977.
180. Murgita, R. A., Goidl, E. A., Kontiainen, S., et al., *Nature* **267**:257, 1977.
181. Bansal, S. C., Bansal, B. R., Thomas, H. L., et al., *Cancer* **42**:1, 1978.
182. Ray, P. K., Idiculla, A., Rhoads, J. E., Jr., et al., Specific immunoadsorption of plasma immunoglobulin G or its complexes—A new modality of treatment for abnormal IgG or immune complex related disorders. In *Proc. First Annual Apheresis Symposium*, pp.203–215. Chicago, IL, October 1979.
183. Ray, P. K., McLaughlin, D., et al., Ex vivo immunoadsorption of IgG or its complexes—

A new modality of cancer treatment. In B. Serrou and C. Rosenfeld (Eds.), *Immune Complexes and Plasma Exchanges in Cancer Patients*, Vol. 1, p. 197. Amsterdam, Holland: Elsevier/North Holland, 1981.

184. Terman, D. S., Young, J. B., Shearer, W. T., et al., *N. Engl. J. Med.* **305**:1195, 1981.
185. Ray, P. K., Idiculla, A., Mark, R., Rhoads, J. E., Jr., Thomas, H., Bassett, J. G., and Cooper, D. R., *Cancer* **49**(9):1800, 1982.
186. Jones, F. R., Yoshida, L. H., Ladiges, W. C. and Kinny, M. A., *Cancer* **46**:675, 1980.
187. Ray, P. K., Raychadhuri, S., and Allen, P., *Cancer Res.* **42**: 4970, 1982.
188. Chapuis, B., Louis, J., Barrelet, L., et al., *Schweiz Med. Wochenschr.* **110**(21):796, 1980.

15

Immune Rejection and Acceptance Phenomena in Transplant Recipients, Tumor Hosts, and Pregnancy

Prasanta K. Ray

The evolution of the immune system probably began with certain cells developing the ability to recognize *non-self* material, that is *foreign* to the body. These cells could attack the non-self material, either directly or through their products. Eventually, the immune system developed to meet the ever-changing problems of protection of the *self*. This immune system is designed to reject all foreign material entering the body. There are times when the body rejects material from a foreign source, as with a tissue allograft. In other instances the body partially or totally accepts tissues having foreign biological markers, as with a fetus or tumor.

An allograft is recognized by active immune phenomena: immune components of the host are sensitized against the allograft antigens, the graft is attacked, and rejected. This is the normal, expected course of events. However, we find a unique situation in the survival of the fetus (an allograft) in the foreign environment of the mother. In this case, there is limited acceptance of the allograft (fetus), at least for a 9-month period. Although there is ample evidence in the literature that spontaneous abortion of the fetus may have some relationship with the immune recognition and rejection process, there is also the question as to whether or not normal delivery is due, at least in part, to immunological rejection with attendant physiological and other biochemical phenomena. This premise leads to two questions: (a) How does the fetus avoid immunologic recognition during pregnancy? and (b) How and why, if at all, is it recognized at the end of pregnancy? It may be that there is immunological stimulation of the mother through the afferent arc of the immune system, but that the efferent arc remains non-functional.

However, with transplanted tissues, both arcs of the immune system are operative, leading to the rejection process. Even so, depending on the nature of graft, the length of time for rejection may vary. Perhaps some of the grafts which take a long time to be rejected induce immune mechanisms similar to those seen during fetal development. If the intricate immune mechanisms related to fetal development are well elucidated, and then utilized for grafts or organ transplantation, the transplants may be accepted. Compartmentalization, trophoblastic and placental barriers may contribute to the maintenance of the fetus in the mother. Creation of a similar environment might help an allograft survive. Modern scientific techniques, with the development of new nontoxic and nonantigenic materials would, at least theoretically, allow the fabrication of inert devices for use inside the body, avoiding immune recognition and rejection.

In tumor growth we see a very interesting phenomenon. Tumor cells, in spite of having *neoantigens*, are not rejected. They grow, and eventually kill the host. Occasionally, however, tumors like hypernephroma, choriocarcinoma, malignant melanoma, and neuroblastoma undergo spontaneous regression. This might result from immunological recognition of the tumor as foreign, with its subsequent rejection. In animal tumor models a number of studies have shown that tumors can be made to regress by a variety of manipulations. Experimental cancer immunotherapy in man has not yet achieved this result. This may be attributed directly to the fact that we do not know what immune mechanisms make a tumor regress.

It is known that during the progressive growth of a tumor immune reactions are initiated in two opposing directions: antitumor immunity and protumor immunity. The latter mechanism works through both humoral and cellular arc of the immune system. The former mechanism is also related to these two arcs. Since the balance is toward the latter mechanism, the tumor survives, and the antitumor immune components become nonfunctional. Thus, we must learn how to shift the balance of the immune system towards antitumor reactions. This might help control and even destroy tumors.

If delivery of a child is established to be an immunological rejection phenomenon (rejection of the non-self after a limited period of acceptance), then, with the other biochemical, hormonal, and physiological support seen during pregnancy, the same mechanism might be induced to cause tumor regression. These concepts are hypothetical at this point, although some supporting data are available in the literature.

Nature's Experimental System—Extremes and Compromise

In the arena of nature's experimental system, we see the following extremes and compromise:

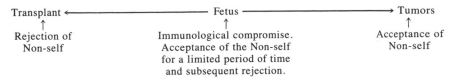

Fig. 15.1. Acceptance and/or rejection of *self* and *non-self* tissues.

In the above figure we find two extremes in immune reaction to transplants and tumors. In the former case, we see the immunological rejection of non-self, in the latter case the immunological acceptance of the non-self. In fetal development we see a compromise between these two extremes: a period of limited acceptance of non-self, then its rejection.

If all the mechanisms and sequence of events related to rejection and destruction of non-self tissue are elucidated, then we may be able to induce them to destroy tumors, and block them to allow transplants to survive.

Immunological phenomena related to transplant rejection, tumor growth, and fetal development are dealt with in detail in several chapters of this volume. In addition to immunological mechanisms, each of these events also involves biochemical, hormonal, and physiological phenomena, which are outside the scope of this volume. I will try to outline briefly some aspects of immunological rejection of transplant and of immune phenomena as they relate to tumor growth and fetal development.

ALLOGRAFT REJECTION—A PHENOMENON OF REJECTION OF NON-SELF

The immunological basis of allograft rejection was established by the studies of Gorer in 1937 and 1938 (1, 2) in the mouse, and later by the studies of Sir Peter Medawar, in 1944 and 1945, in the rabbit (3, 4). Gibson and Medawar demonstrated in 1943 that in man the second set of skin allograft is rejected faster than the first set (5). These observations have since been confirmed in a large number of laboratories.

The immune reactions related to the rejection of an allograft are primarily, though not exclusively, cellular. Humoral immunity is also involved in the process. Some early studies indicated that allograft immunity could be transferred with lymphoid cells from a sensitized individual to a nonsensitized individual; the same can be done only with difficulty with serum from sensitized individuals (6, 7).

In 1971 Elves (8) divided the process of allograft reactions into three parts: (a) Afferent arc—the antigen comes in contact with the lymphocytes and sensitizes them. (b) Central phase—stimulated lymphocytes undergo blast transformation, release various lymphokines, and recruit noncommitted cells to mediate the desired functions. These reactions usually take place in the regional lymph nodes with skin allografts. With organ transplants these reactions can take place in the spleen or even in the graft itself. (c) Efferent arc—effector cells come in contact with the graft and induce the rejection reactions.

Of these three parts of rejection reactions the central phase is the most critical. If the activity of this phase can be controlled, there will be no *armed* or *committed* effector lymphocytes produced to effect destruction of the transplanted tissue. Immunosuppressive antimetabolites react on proliferative cells to cause their destruction or halt their proliferation. In this approach a generalized immunosuppression is usually induced, making the individual immunologically compromised and susceptible to infection. Antilymphocyte serum has been used to eliminate a particular type of lymphocyte, thus blocking the afferent arc of the immune response. There is much specific and well-substantiated work in these areas. A good account may be obtained in Dr. Santiago's chapter in this volume.

Specific Inhibition of Allograft Rejection

It is very interesting that not much attention has been given to tolerance induction for a transplanted tissue. If a graft is to be maintained in a functional stage, at least two aspects must be given adequate considerations: (a) prevention of the sensitization of the host against the histocompatibility antigens of the graft; and (b) induction of a state of tolerance to the graft in a specific manner, without causing generalized immunosuppression.

Grafts can be categorized into three types according to the immune reactions they induce: (a) free grafts which do (skin grafts) or do not (cartilage, cornea) become vascularized; (b) grafts whose blood vessels can connect directly to the circulation of the host (liver, kidney); and (c) grafts of a particulate type (white blood cells, red blood cells).

In case of grafts, or transfusion of cell suspension, an immediate and good antibody response is seen. However, with solid tissue grafts antibody response is delayed. It may be that in the latter case the sensitization occurs peripherally in the graft (9), or it occurs in lymph nodes through histocompatibility antigens of the graft (10).

Neonatal thymectomy (11), thoracic duct drainage (12), and antilymphocyte serum (ALS) treatment (13) have profound effects on the host's reaction to an allograft. Depletion of recirculating lymphocytes will have two advantages: (a) it will remove the opportunity to sensitize the lymphocytes peripherally and (b) it will eliminate the opportunity for contact between lymphocytes and the histocompatibility antigens or tissue-specific antigens of the graft.

The central issue is how and where do lymphocytes come in contact with the graft antigens. It is not fully known if histocompatibility antigens or tissue-specific antigens from the graft can migrate to sensitize lymphocytes. Even though this question is not fully resolved, the apparent mechanics of facilitating an allograft would involve blocking most or all the reactions induced by the tissue-specific antigens, and creating an environment of tolerance to the graft. To reach this goal we must understand the mechanism of graft rejection. The total immune reaction against any foreign substance can be divided into two components: Total Immune Reaction (TIR) = Effector Reaction (ER) + Regulatory or Suppressor Reaction (RSR). Using this formula we might be able to explain rejection-acceptance phenomena related to transplantation, cancer, and pregnancy.

In the normal situation of allograft rejection TIR and ER maintain a unique balance, causing the destruction of the allograft. This balance is maintained because RSR, which has the ability to either counteract or limit the ER, is usually not induced in the case of allografts. If the strength and degree of RSR could be potentiated so that it could overpower ER, the allograft could be made to survive for a long time. Two inducible control mechanisms can potentiate RSR: (a) induction of enhancing factors and (b) induction of immunological tolerance.

Immunological enhancement can be mediated by antibody against the tissue-specific antigens. This can inhibit immunization (14) (afferent inhibition) or protect target tissue from attack by sensitized lymphocytes (15) (efferent inhibition). Tolerance can be induced by antigen in appropriate form and quantity. Both passive immunization and tolerance induction have been shown to prolong experimental kidney and allograft survival (16, 17). This phenomenon of antigen-induced immune tolerance can be further potentiated by reducing the population of antigen-reacting cells using drugs or ALS (18).

Immunosuppressive drugs have been used to facilitate the induction of tolerance in adult animals (19, 20). Treatment of kidney allograft recipients with drugs such as Imuran and Prednisolone has given good results (21).

Mitchison's experiments (22–24), showing that unresponsiveness to bovine serum albumin (BSA) can be induced by either one high dose or repeatedly given extremely low doses, brought a new dimension to these areas of transplantation immunology. A number of attempts were made to induce tolerance against an allograft using extracted transplantation antigen as the immunizing tolerogen. These attempts met with mixed successes. Owen and colleagues (25–27) prolonged survival of kidney allografts by injecting crude liver extract for a period of 5 weeks prior to transplantation. The data were even more impressive when injections were continued after the grafting, and when Imuran was given to the recipient animals. However, Graft and Kandutch (28) and Wheeler et al. (29) could not demonstrate significant prolongation of skin graft survival after immunization of the recipients with low doses of extracted antigen.

Several attempts have been made with ALS to induce immune unresponsiveness to allografts (30–35). ALS did prolong the survival of skin and other allografts, but did not induce immunological unresponsiveness. This was achieved only when ALS was combined with other procedures, such as thymectomy, or inoculation of large or small doses of lymphoid cells or antigen extract.

Mechanism of Tolerance

A number of hypotheses have been put forth to explain the cellular mechanisms which may lead to an unresponsive immune status in an individual. An exhaustive treatment of this subject can be found in the monograph edited by Landy and Brawn (36).

The main question unanswered in this field is whether (a) the lymphocytes of a tolerant animal are truly unresponsive or completely absent or (b) they are present and have their normal reactivity, but these reactivities are not expressed because of the presence of serum blocking factors. There are reports in the literature supporting both possibilities.

The phenomenon of tolerance is believed to be due to a central failure of the immunological response. The failure is thought to be one of immunocytes failing to recognize or to respond to the foreign antigens. This could be caused either by the elimination of the cells ordinarily responsible for antigen processing, or by the functional inactivation of these cells. Evidence supporting the latter suggestion comes from several sources.

Lymphoid cells from tolerant animals have been described as nonreactive in graft-versus-host studies (37, 38). It has also been reported that immunosuppressive drugs, having the ability to inhibit antibody production, do not interfere with tolerance induction (39, 40). Tolerance could be abrogated by inoculation of sensitized syngeneic cells (37, 41, 43). Moreover, tolerance can be induced very easily in immunologically immature animals. Diener and Feldman (44–46) have reported that a very small amount of specific antibody can induce unresponsiveness to polymerized flagellin in vitro. Immunological responses have been found to be inhibited by antibody (47). Passively transferred hyperimmune serum has been shown to extend the survival times of rat kidney allografts and F_1 hybrid kidneys (48–50).

The Hellströms and their colleagues (51) showed that lymphocytes from both tumor-bearing animals and humans can show specific antitumor immune reactions when cultured in vitro in the absence of host serum. This lymphocyte activity was inhibited by host serum (48).

Evidence of tolerance induction has also been found in fetal studies. It has been reported that serum from pregnant Balb/c mice that have been mated with C3H males contains blocking factors that nullify the *in vitro* reactivity of maternal lymphocytes to C3H embryonic cells (50). Thus, it seems to be possible that blocking serum factors provide protection for the fetus. Anderson (52) reported that skin grafts transplanted from offspring to mother survive longer than expected in some species, suggesting a possible role of serum enhancing factors.

Voisin and colleagues (53) described the presence of hemagglutinating antibodies against donor strain cells in tolerant mice. Hellström and colleagues (54) described that lymphocytes from mice made tolerant at birth by intraperitoneal injection of hybrid spleen cells showed *in vitro* cytotoxicity against fibroblasts from the donor strain. Sera from the tolerant animals had a blocking effect. These authors have also reported (55) that blood lymphocytes from dogs receiving allogeneic bone marrow following X-irradiation (about 15,000 rads) inhibited fibroblast colony formation in culture. Serum could inhibit this effect.

New data have been presented indicating that blocking factors may not play a detectable *in vivo* role in tolerant animals (56–58). Beverley and colleagues (59) reported that the appearance of blocking factors was a function of partial, rather than complete tolerance. This may explain why both cytotoxic cells and blocking factors have been demonstrated in unresponsive hosts (56, 60, 61).

Mechanism of Immune Enhancement

A number of reviews are available on this topic. Feldman's article is one of the most comprehensive (62).

In 1941 Casey (63) described that animals immunized with nonviable tumor tissues could show enhanced tumor growth when challenged with the same type of tumor cells. The involvement of antibody in the enhancement phenomena was described by Kaliss and Molomut (64). Thus, enhancement can be brought about by active immunization or by passive transfer of immune serum. The antibodies which take part in the enhancing activity are believed to be IgG_2 type.

Controversy exists regarding the mode of action of these enhancing antibodies. Literature information suggests that they can work at the afferent, efferent, or central levels (62, 65, 66). Both the afferent and efferent hypotheses are supported by observations that enhancing antibody can coat the target cell surface *in vivo* and *in vitro*. T lymphocytes cannot recognize the alloantigens on the target cells if they are coated with enhancing antibody. On the other hand, the presence of autologous immunoglobulins on the surfaces of target cells may interfere with the cell contact required for target cell damage. While these mechanisms may play a role during the early phases of transplant reactions, the enhancement at the central level has also been given much emphasis (62, 65).

A large body of data suggests that the life of both normal and malignant tissues could be prolonged by enhancing procedures. Unfortunately, the prolongation of survival, at least in the case of normal tissues, has not been successful. However, the success of infusion of hyperimmune sera in prolonging the life of rat kidney allografts offers promise that this procedure may be helpful in maintaining survival of other allografts (63, 67). In general, long-term allograft survival still remains an elusive goal. Promising progress is being made in the area of transplantation immunology by the partial success obtained with the procedures that induce tolerance and prolong allograft survival.

Induction of tolerance has so far involved only humoral tolerance-inducing factors; the role of cellular suppressor factors has not been adequately considered. We have learned from tumor immunology and immunology of pregnancy that suppressor cells play a predominant role in the overall host immunosuppression process. An understanding of these phenomena, and application of this knowledge may result in further achievements in allograft transplantation.

TUMOR GROWTH–A PHENOMENON OF ACCEPTANCE OF NON-SELF

During tumor growth, the antigens on the tumor may induce an immune reaction which favors RSR rather than ER, so that antitumor reactions are reduced. To understand this phenomenon, we must first know the nature of tumor antigens, and the immune reactions which facilitate or inhibit the growth of tumors.

Tumor Antigens

Tumor cells differ from their normal counterparts in a variety of ways: morphology, mitotic index, biochemistry, and antigenic expression. More and more information accumulating in the literature suggests that tumor cells contain neoantigens which are normally not expressed on their normal cell counterparts (68, 69). These tumor-associated antigens (TAA) have been found on a wide variety of animal and human neoplastic cells. While most of the naturally occurring neoplasms have low antigenicity, they differ in terms of the total immune reactions they induce in the host. Besides the antigenicity of the tumors, the immune ability of the host also plays an important role in tumor growth. Whatever the tumor antigenicity, antitumor immunity does exist in the host against autochthonous tumor, but is usually not strong enough to counter the progression of the tumor. If ER is strong enough, spontaneous regression can occur. Spontaneous regression of a wide variety of tumors has been reported in the literature (70, 71). This includes both primary and metastatic tumors. Spontaneous regressions of chemically and virally induced neoplasms have been reported in animals (72, 73). Complete spontaneous regression of lung carcinoma after incomplete surgical removal of the primary tumor (74), and regression of pulmonary metastases after surgical resection of carcinoma of the kidney (75) have been reported in man. Thus, these spontaneous and/or induced tumor regressions suggest that if an appropriate environment is created, tumors can be made to regress.

In many patients, metastatic tumors develop 10 to 20 years after the successful treatment of the primary tumor (70, 75, 76). The small metastatic tumor remained dormant for a long period then, at an opportune time, started growing. This raises the question, what held it in check for so long? Although various biochemical factors may contribute to this phenomenon, immune functions of the body may also play a major role.

Griffiths and colleagues (77) have reported that even though they could identify tumor cells in the lymphatics, pleural cavity, and peripheral blood of cancer patients, many of the patients never developed metastases. This observation suggests that these tumor cells may have been destroyed internally, or that their proliferation may have been restricted. Host immune reactivity obviously could be suspected of playing a role. Some types of cancer, such as carcinoma of the thyroid and prostate, and neuroblastoma, detected at postmortem, did not appear to cause any problems or complications in their hosts that could be related to the malignancy (78).

Thus, in normal individuals, tumors may be developing and regressing quite often. While tumor destruction may be mediated by an active immunological process, tumor establishment or growth may be due to an aberration or defect of the normal immune process.

Antitumor Immune Reactions in the Host

It is widely known that tumors, perhaps with the help of released antigens, can induce cellular and humoral immune reactions both *in vivo* and *in vitro*. Both cytotoxic lymphocytes and macrophages have been detected in immune animals, as well as cytotoxic antitumor antibody activity. Antitumor immune reactions can also be mediated by soluble mediators, such as macrophage migration inhibition factor (MIF) and macrophage chemotactic factor (MCF), which are produced by sensitized lymphocytes in the presence of specific antigen. Many other factors, like miogenic factors, macrophage activating factor (MAF), and specific macrophage arming factor also take part in various immune processes. Natural immunity to tumors may be effected, perhaps at the very early phase of tumor cell proliferation, by a cell type known as natural killer (NK) cells. This topic is discussed in greater detail by R. B. Herberman in another chapter in this volume.

Humoral antibodies of IgG, IgM, and IgA classes can take part in antibody-dependent cell-mediated cytotoxicity (ADCC) against tumor cells. Complement-fixing IgG and IgM antibody molecules can also directly destroy tumor cells.

However, in spite of immune surveillance and antitumor immune reactions, the tumor can grow and kill the host. This apparent paradox has not been well understood until recently.

Enhancement of Tumor Growth

Immune response can stimulate, as well as inhibit, tumor growth (79). As discussed with transplants, tumor growth can also be facilitated in the presence of specific antibody (80). Antibodies raised against extracted tumor antigen and tumor tissue can function in such manner. Antibodies raised in an allogeneic or in a xenogeneic species can also serve this purpose. The exact mechanism of action of antibody-mediated enhancement is not known. Several possibilities have been described earlier. In afferent enhancement the antibody may bind with tumor antigens, and prevent the recognition of the tumor antigen by the immunocytes, thus blocking the immunological processing step. In the central enhancement step an antibody can bind directly with the immunocompetent cells and inhibit the activity. In efferent enhancement an antibody may coat the antigenic sites on the tumor cells, preventing contact between the tumor target and effector lymphocytes.

A variety of plasma blocking factors from plasma of cancer patients has been described which is capable of abrogating the body's defense mechanisms (82–84). Blocking factors may include antibodies (85–87), free tumor antigen (88–90), and/or antigen-antibody complex (91, 92).

Soluble tumor antigens can block the surface receptors on T lymphocytes, which then lose their ability to bind antigens on the surface of the tumor cells. Serum samples from cancer patients have been found to have inhibitory properties against mitogen-induced blastogenic response of lymphocytes from normal donors (81). Antigen-antibody complexes can block lymphocyte activity by binding the antigen-binding receptor on the lymphocyte; binding may occur through the antibody part of the complex, as well as through the antigen part.

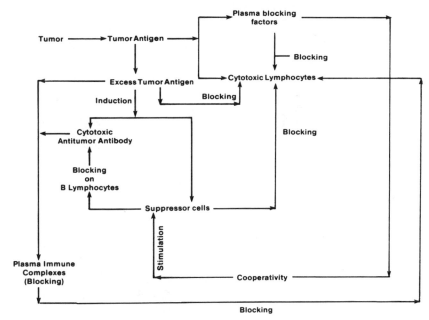

Fig. 15.2. Possible mechanism of induction of blocking and effector immune mechanisms by tumor antigen.

Immune complexes are also known to activate suppressor T cells (86, 93). Suppressor cell-mediated blocking of the immune reactivities of the tumor host has been widely reported (86, 89, 90, 93–95). Thus it appears that there may be a high degree of cooperation between the humoral and cellular RSR mechanisms, leading to the enhancement of tumor growth (Fig. 15.2). It appears to be highly logical, therefore, that any intervention in these tumor-induced RSR's should be detrimental to the tumor and beneficial to the host. Removal of serum blocking factors from the plasma of a tumor-bearing host should *unblock* and activate both cellular and humoral immunity against the tumor. Several methods for counteracting or removing serum blocking factors have been proposed (95–100). Some have been tested experimentally in animals (101–106) and also in humans (98–100, 102–104, 106–109). This approach is discussed in greater detail in the chapter by Ray and Raychaudhuri.

Ray and colleagues have reported therapeutic effect in rat, dog, and human tumor models (98–109) employing the technique of immunoadsorption of plasma IgG and/or its complexes with heat-killed and formalin-stabilized Protein A-containing *Staphylococcus aureus* Cowan I. They have also reported (103) that combined therapy using cyclophosphamide and immunoadsorption gave better therapeutic benefit than cyclophosphamide alone in rats bearing

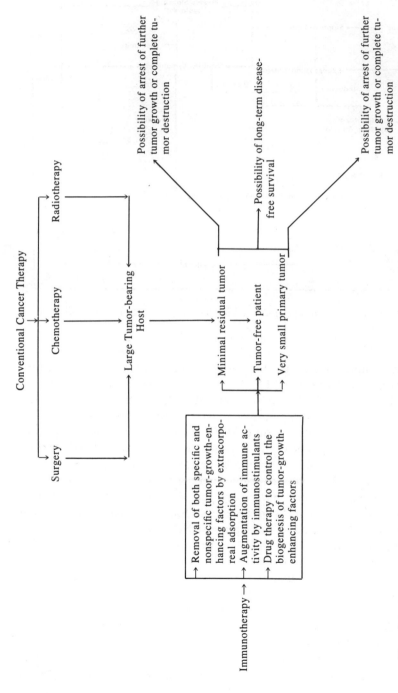

Fig. 15.3. A suggested scheme of treatment strategy for cancer with the possibility of arrest and/or complete destruction of tumor mass.

420

primary mammary adenocarcinomas. Subsequent to these reports, other laboratories (111–113) confirmed that immunoadsorption of plasma from tumor-bearing hosts with *S. aureus* could induce a tumoricidal response.

These studies (98–113) indicate that control of tumor-induced RSR can offer therapeutic benefit to the tumor-bearing host. Ray et al. also reported (103, 105, 107, 110) that immunoadsorption of plasma of cancer patients with *S. aureus* can augment the immune reactivity. In the rat tumor model immunoadsorption can augment cytotoxic antibody activity, and result in increased antibody-dependent cell-mediated cytotoxicity (114, 115).

It has been observed that using a dosage of cyclophosphamide low enough to be immunostimulatory can inhibit the growth of a transplantable methylcholanthrene-induced fibrosarcoma (116). This same dose of cyclophosphamide has eliminated suppressor-cell precursors (117). Thus, the greater therapeutic effect observed with immunoadsorption and cyclophosphamide (103) in primary mammary tumor-bearing rats, as compared to immunoadsorption alone, might have been due to the removal of both humoral and cellular blocking factors.

These studies offer a promise that, under suitable circumstances, control of both arcs of the suppressor mechanisms (humoral and cellular) may be therapeutically useful.

Besides the specific humoral and cellular tumor growth-facilitating factors (reviewed by Yamagashi and colleagues in a separate chapter of this volume), a large number of other humoral and cellular suppressor components were observed in tumor-bearing hosts. In this case, control of a few suppressor factors may not remove all the suppressive effects and augment the host's immune reactivities enough to destroy the tumor. In order to achieve total tumor destruction the following scheme may be useful (Fig. 15.3). Unfortunately, the current practice of tumor therapy does not involve protocols which take appropriate care of all the aspects of treatment strategy. Unless all these factors are properly controlled, complete eradication of the disease by immunological means may not be possible.

However, if delivery of a child has anything to do with the loss of tolerance and with the induction of immune rejection phenomena, then our knowledge of these mechanisms may be helpful in establishing strategies for successful cancer therapy.

FETAL DEVELOPMENT—A PHENOMENON OF LIMITED ACCEPTANCE OF NON-SELF

The fetus, with its foreign antigens, is an allograft on the mother and, according to the laws of transplantation immunology, should be rejected. In reality, the fetus survives and thrives, at least for a limited period of time, in the normally hostile immune environment of the mother. This apparent revocation of transplantation immunologic principles puzzled scientists for a long time.

Sir Peter Medawar's concept (118) of fetal growth considers several possibilities as to how a fetus can survive: (a) the fetus grows in an immunologically privileged site (the uterus), where antifetal antibodies and sensitized lymphocytes from the mother cannot gain access; (b) the fetus may be nonimmunogenic, so that it cannot trigger an immune response; (c) the mother may be somehow less immunologically competent to induce antifetal immune reaction; and (d) the fetus may be shielded by the placental barrier. These concepts provided for a long time, although questioned later, some very ingenious explanations about how the fetus can survive in the mother's body.

It is not clear that the uterus can truly be considered a privileged site for fetal growth, since (a) allogeneic tumor transplants are rejected when transplanted in the uterine horn of pregnant rats (119) and (b) intrauterine transfer of allogeneic tissues or cells can sensitize the host against these antigens (120). However, it has been reported that allogeneic embryos are not rejected when transplanted into the uterus, but they are rejected when transplanted into ectopic sites (121). It is suspected that some physiological, biochemical, endocrinological, and immunological alterations take place in the uterus during pregnancy, since the host cannot be sensitized by intrauterine injection of antigenic material during pregnancy. However, the same antigen can sensitize the host when inoculated by the same route in a nonpregnant animal (122). The present knowledge in the field suggests that the uterus may not be a conventional immunologically privileged site, but the privileged uninterrupted growth the fetus enjoys may be due to protection rendered by the placenta.

Antigenic Nature of the Embryo and Embryonic Tissues

A large number of studies indicate that the embryo or embryonic tissues contain a variety of antigens which are foreign to the mother. Foreign histocompatibility antigens have been detected on embryos (123–126), placental cells (127–129), and trophoblasts (130, 131). Several other antigens, broadly categorized as oncofetal antigens, such as carcinoembryonic antigen (132), alpha fetoprotein, human chorionic gonadotropin, and human chorionic somatomammotropin, also should give antigenic stimulus to the mother. Thus, the early suggestions that the fetus is antigenically inert may not be true.

These oncofetal antigens have also been detected on tumor tissues, indicating considerable similarity between fetuses and tumors. Neither is rejected by the host, in spite of being antigenic to the system. Like tumor, fetuses also can induce RSR, which protects them from their host's immunological attack.

Maternal Immune Response Against the Conceptus

Antibodies against paternal histocompatibility antigens have been detected in the mother (132–135). These antibodies can prevent mixed leukocyte culture reactions, and perhaps also function *in vivo* as blocking agents for maternal lymphocytes (133). Cytotoxic antibodies have been detected against histocompatibility antigens in pregnant hosts (135–137). Antibodies against human blood group antigens (A, B, and H) have also been detected in women (138). Spontaneous abortions may be due to anti-RBC antigens (139). Congenital abnormalities may be related to anti-HLA antibodies (140).

Like immune humoral components, immune cells capable of reacting against fetal tissues have been detected in pregnant females (141–146). Thus, both humoral and cellular immune reactions against fetal tissues can occur. In spite of this, the fetus can grow without interruption. Obviously, these reactions do not occur at all or are inhibited. Part of this protection may come from the trophoblast, which is somewhat antigenically inert. This may be due to a mucoprotein coating on the trophoblast (147). The placental microvilli are also covered with a mucopolysaccharide (148), which may be involved in the shielding.

As in tumor-bearing hosts, blocking antibodies have been described in pregnant women (149), multiparous mice (150), and pregnant mice (151); blocking immune complexes have also been demonstrated in pregnant hosts (152, 153). It is postulated that the fetus and a tumor may use similar mechanisms for protection against the host's immunological attack.

Placenta can act as an antibody filter, allowing beneficial natural antibody to pass through, while adsorbing antibodies against paternal antigens (154). These antibodies can be eluted off placenta and are detectable in the mother's blood, but not in fetal blood, nor in neonatal blood (155). Thus, it appears that the placenta may protect the fetus.

There are conflicting reports as to whether or not maternal lymphocytes can reach the fetus (156–159). It has been reported that transplacental passage of natural lymphocytes can cause a graft-versus-host reaction (159). However, several reports have indicated that sensitization of the mother by paternal histocompatibility antigens does not cause any harm to the fetus (160).

Impairment of Immune Functions in Pregnant Hosts

There are reports indicating that allogeneic pregnancy does not produce humoral and cellular immunity capable of rejecting the graft (161). Repeated allogeneic pregnancy produces tolerance, instead of immunity, to paternal antigens (162). This state of tolerance has been adoptively transferred from multiparous female animals to virgin females (163) by cell transfer. There are also reports that human neonates possess suppressor cells that prevent maternal lymphoid activity (164) *in vitro*. Soluble suppressor activity has also been noted in allopregnant mice (165).

Nonspecific immunosuppressive activity has been found in sera of pregnant mice (166) and pregnant humans (167). The immunosuppression may be due to some early pregnancy factors (168). A soluble suppressor factor, produced by the trophoblast, has also been described (169); this factor may be the hormone progesterone.

Thus, a number of immunosuppressive components have been found in pregnant mothers, as well as in fetal tissues. It is not certain in what sequence the biological events progress that allow the survival of the fetus. Whatever the sequence, it appears that blocking serum factors (specific and nonspecific), suppressor cells, and antiidiotypic antibodies (170) may have a pronounced regulatory role on the maternal immune response, permitting fetal growth.

Immunologic Aspects of Abortion

Blocking factors, humoral and cellular, discussed above, may have a protective role for the fetus against maternal immune reactions. Interestingly, habitual aborters and nulligravidae do not appear to have these blocking factors (171–173). Thus, lack of induction of blocking phenomena in early pregnancy may result in immune attack, damaging the fetus, and causing abortion. IgM type antibodies have been found on aborted trophoblasts, suggesting immunological damage. However, conclusive evidence linking immune reactions to spontaneous abortion has not yet been forthcoming.

SUMMARY

Fetal growth has points in common with both tumor growth and allograft. Like a tumor, the fetus is able to grow in an antigenically foreign environment. This ability may be due to immunosuppressive phenomena induced by both fetus and tumor. However, unlike a tumor, fetal growth is interrupted by rejection, sometimes prematurely. This rejection may be mediated, at least in part, by immune mechanisms like the ones that cause allograft rejection.

Thus, elucidation of the phenomena which allow a fetus and tumor to survive may help in the development of methods to maintain allograft. Conversely, determination of the reactions which result in rejection of fetus and allograft may lead to methods of tumor rejection by the host.

REFERENCES

1. Gorer, P. A., *Brit. J. Exp. Path.* **18**:31, 1937.
2. Gorer, P. A., *J. Path. Bact.* **47**:231, 1938.
3. Medawar, P. B., *J. Anat.* (London) **78**:176, 1944.
4. Medawar, P. B., *J. Anat.* (London) **79**:175, 1945.
5. Gibson, T., and Medawar, P. B., *J. Anat.* (London) **77**:299, 1943.
6. Herbertson, B. M., The allograft reaction. In R. Y. Calne (Ed.), *Clinical Organ Transplantation*, p. 3. Oxford: Blackwell Scientific, 1971.
7. Brent, L., Pathogenic role of delayed hypersensitivity and antibody in allograft reactions. In 2nd Int. Convoc. Immunol. Buffalo, New York: *Cellular Interactions in the Immune Response*, p. 250. Basel: S. Karger, 1971.
8. Elves, M. W., The afferent arc. The route of sensitization in the homograft reaction. In N. W. Nisbet and M. W. Elves (Eds.), *Immunological Tolerance to Tissue Antigens*, pp. 1–18. Oswestry, England: Orthopedic Hospital, 1971.
9. Medawar, P. B., *Brit. Med. Bull.* **21**:97, 1965.
10. Burwell, R. G., *Ann. N.Y. Acad. Sci.* **99**:821, 1962.
11. Miller, J. F. A. P., and Osoba, D., *Physiol. Rev.* **47**:437, 1967.
12. McGregor, D. D., and Gowans, J. L., *Lancet* **1**:629, 1964.
13. Mannick, J. A., Davies, R. C., Cooperland, S. R., et al., *New Engl. J. Med.* **284**:1109, 1971.
14. Kaliss, N., *Cancer Res.* **18**:992, 1958.
15. Billingham, R. E., Brent, L., and Medawar, P. B., *Phil. Trans. B.* **237**:357, 1956.
16. French, M. E., and Bachelor, J. R., *Lancet* **2**:1103, 1969.
17. Brent, L., and French, M. E., *Transpl. Proc.* **5**:1001, 1973.
18. Lance, E. M., and Medawar, P. B., *Proc. Roy. Soc.* B **173**:447, 1969.
19. Schwartz, R. S., and Damashik, W., *Nature* (London) **183**:1682, 1959.
20. Schwartz, R. S. In F. T. Rapaport and J. Dausset (Eds.), *Human Transplantation*, p. 440. New York and London: Grune and Stratton, 1968.
21. Murray, J. E., Barnes, B. A., and Atkinson, J. C., *Transplantation* **11**:328, 1971.
22. Dresser, D. W., and Mitchison, N. A., *Adv. Immunol.* **8**:129, 1968.
23. Mitchison, N. A., *Transplant. Proc.* **3**:953, 1971.
24. Mitchison, N. A. In B. Cinader (Ed.), *Regulation of the Antibody Response*, p. 54. Springfield, IL: Charles C. Thomas, 1968.
25. Owen, E. R., *Nature* **219**:970, 1968.
26. Owen, E. R., Slome, D., and Watuston, D. J., Prolongation of rabbit kidney allograft survival by 'desensitization'. In *Advance in Transplantation*, p. 385. Proceedings of the 1st Int'l Congress of the Tranplant. Soc., Paris, June 27–30, 1967. Copenhagen: Munksgaard, 1968.
27. Owen, E. R., *Ann. Roy. Coll. Surg. Engl.* **45**:63, 1969.
28. Graff, R. J., and Kundutch, A. A., *Transplantation* **8**:162, 1969.

426   Immunobiology of Transplantation, Cancer and Pregnancy

29. Wheeler, H. B., de Fronzo, A., and Corson, J. M., *Transplantation* **9**:78, 1970.
30. Woodruff, M. F. A., and Anderson, N. A., *Nature* **200**:702, 1963.
31. Wolstenholme, G. E. W., and O'Connor, M. (Eds.), *Antilymphocyte Serum*, pp. 1–165. London: J. & A. Churchill, 1967.
32. Amos, B. D., Brillingham, R. E., Lawrence, H. S., et al. (Eds.), Conference on Antilymphocytic serum. *Fed. Proc.* **29**:97–229, 1970.
33. Monaco, A. P., Geozzo, J. T., Wood, H. L., and Liegeors, A., *Transpl. Proc.* **3**:680, 1971.
34. Brent, L., Hansen, J. A., and Kilshaw, P. J., *Nature* **227**:898, 1970.
35. Brent, L., Hansen, J. A., and Kilshaw, P. J., *Transplantation Proc.* **3**:684, 1971.
36. Landy, M. and Brawn, W. (Eds.), *Immunological Tolerance*, pp. 1–352, New York and London: Academic Press, 1969.
37. Michie, D., Woodruff, M. F. A., and Zeiss, I., *Immunology* **4**:413, 1961.
38. Gowans, J. L., McGregor, D. D., and Cowen, D. M. In G. E. W. Wolstenholme and J. Knight (Eds.), *The Immunologically Competent Cell*, p. 20. London: J. & A. Churchill, 1963.
39. Schwartz, R. S. In F. T. Rapaport and J. Dausset (Eds.), *Human Transplantation*, p. 440. New York and London: Grune & Stratton, 1968.
40. Medawar, P. B., *Proc. Roy. Soc. B* **176**:155, 1969.
41. Billingham, R. E., Brent, L., and Medawar, P. B., *Phila. Trans. Roy. Soc. (B).* **239**:357, 1956.
42. Billingham, R. E., Silvers, W. K., and Wilson, D. B., *J. Exp. Med.* **118**:397, 1963.
43. Gowans, J. E., McGregor, D. D., Cowan, D. M., and Ford, C. E., *Nature* **196**:651, 1962.
44. Feldman, M., and Diener, E., *J. Exp. Med.* **131**:247, 1970.
45. Diener, E., and Feldman, M., *J. Exp. Med.* **132**:31, 1970.
46. Diener, E., and Feldman, M., *Transplantation Proc.* **3**:663, 1971.
47. Uhr, J. W., and Moller, G., *Adv. Immunol.* **8**:81, 1968.
48. Hellström, I., Hellström, K. E., Evans, C. A., Heppner, G. H., Pierce, G. E., and Young, J. P. S., *Proc. Natl. Acad. Sci. USA* **62**:362, 1969.
49. Allison, A. C., On the absence of tolerance in virus oncogenesis. In L. Saveri (Ed.), *Immunity and Tolerance in Oncogenesis*, pp. 563–574. Proc. 4th Perugia Quadrennial Internat'l Conf. on Cancer, June 26-July 1, 1969. Perugia, Italy: Perugia University, 1970.
50. Hellström, K. E., Hellström, I., and Brawn, J., *Nature* (London) **226**:914, 1969.
51. Hellström, K. E., and Hellström, I., *Ann. Rev. Microbiol.* **24**:373, 1970.
52. Anderson, J. M., *Proc. Roy. Soc. B.* **176**:115, 1970.
53. Voisin, G. A., *Prog. Allergy* **15**:328, 1971.
54. Hellström, I., Hellström, K. E., and Allison, A. C., *Nature* (London) **230**:49, 1971.
55. Hellström, I., Hellström, K. E., Stromb, R., and Thomas, E. D., *Proc. Natl. Acad. Sci.* **66**:65, 1970.
56. Rouse, B. T., and Warner, N. L., *Eur. J. Immunol.* **2**:102, 1972.
57. Brent, L., Hansen, J. A., Kilshaw, P. J., and Thomas, A. V., *Transplantation* **15**:160, 1973.
58. Atkins, R. C., and Ford, W. L., *Transplantation* **13**:442, 1972.
59. Beverley, P. C. L., Brent, L., Brooks, C., Medawar, P. B., and Simpson, E., *Transplant. Proc.* **5**:679, 1973.
60. Hellström, I., Hellström, K. E., and Trentin, J. J., *Cell. Immunol.* **8**:365, 1973.
61. Wood, M. L., Heppner, G., Gozzo, J. J., and Monaco, A. P., *Transpl. Proc.* **5**:691, 1973.
62. Feldman, J. D., *Adv. Immunol.* **15**:167, 1972.

63. Casey, A. E., *Cancer Res.* **1**:134, 1941.
64. Kaliss, N., and Molomut, N., *Cancer Res.* **12**:110, 1952.
65. French, M. E., and Batchelor, J. R., *Transpl. Rev.* **13**:115, 1972.
66. Brent, L., and French, M. E., *Transpl. Proc.* **5**:1001, 1973.
67. French, M. E., and Batchelor, J. R., *Lancet* **2**:1103, 1969.
68. Prehn, R. T., *Cancer Conf.* **5**:387, 1963.
69. Sengupta, J., and Ray, P. K., *Fed. Am. Soc. Exp. Biol.* **38**(3): 5857, 1979.
70. Everson, T. C., and Cole, W. H., *Spontaneous Regression of Cancer*. Philadelphia: W. B. Saunders, 1966.
71. Boyd, W., *The Spontaneous Regression of Cancer*. Springfield, IL: Charles C. Thomas, 1966.
72. Young, S., and Cown, D. M., *Brit. J. Cancer* **17**:85, 1963.
73. Russell, S. W., and McIntosh, A. T., *Nature* **268**:69, 1977.
74. Abbey Smith, R., *Brit. Med. J.* **2**:563, 1971.
75. Woodruff, M. F., *The Interaction of Cancer Host: its Therapeutic Significance*. New York: Grune and Stratton, 1980.
76. Cochrane, A. J., *Man, Cancer and Immunity*. New York: Academic Press, 1978.
77. White, H., and Griffiths, J. D., *Proc. Roy. Soc. Med.* **69**:467, 1976.
78. Currie, G., *Cancer and the Immune Response*. 2nd ed. An Edward Arnold Publication. Chicago: Year Book Medical Publishers, 1980.
79. Prehn, R. T., *J. Natl. Cancer Inst.* **59**:1043, 1977.
80. Morton, D. L., Sparks, F. C., and Haskill, C. J., Oncology. In S. I. Swarts, G. T.Shires, F. C. Spencer and E. H. Stoper (Eds.), *Principles of Surgery*. 3rd ed. New York: McGraw Hill, 1979.
81. Rangel, D. M., Golub, S. H., and Morton, D. L., *Surgery* **82**:224, 1977.
82. Ray, P. K., *Plasma, Therapy* **3**:101, 1982.
83. Hellström, K. E., and Hellström, I., *Adv. Immunol.* **81**:209, 1974.
84. Herberman, R. B., *Adv. Cancer Res.* **19**:207, 1974.
85. Ankerest, J., *Cancer Res.* **31**:997, 1971.
86. Raychaudhuri, S., Ray, P. K., Bassett, J. G., and Cooper, D. R., *Fed. Proc.* **39**:696, 1980.
87. Witz, I. P., *Curr. Top. Microbiol. Immunol.* **61**:151, 1973.
88. Alexander, P., *Cancer Res.* **34**:2077, 1974.
89. Ray, P. K., and Raychaudhuri, S., *Fed. Am. Soc. Exp. Biol.* **39**(3): 696, 1980.
90. Saha, S., and Ray, P. K., *Fed. Am. Soc. Exp. Biol.* **41**(3): 411, 1982.
91. Baldwin, R. W., and Pimm, M. V., *Natl. Cancer Inst. Monogr.* **31**:11, 1973.
92. Sjogren, H. O., Hellström, I., Bansal, S. C., *Proc. Natl. Acad. Sci.* **63**:1372, 1971.
93. Gershon, R. K., *J. Allergy Clin. Immunol.* **66**:18, 1980.
94. David, N., *Adv. Cancer Res.* **29**:45, 1979.
95. Bansal, S. C., Bansal, B. R., and Thomas, H. L., *Cancer* **43**:1, 1978.
96. Israel, L., Edelstein, R., and Mannoni, P., *Cancer* **40**:3146, 1977.
97. Isbister, W. H., Noonan, F. P., and Halliday, W. J., *Cancer* **35**:1465, 1975.
98. Ray, P. K., Idiculla, A., Rhoads, J. E., Jr., et al., Extracorporeal immunoadsorption of pathologic plasma immunoglobulin G or its complexes. A novel approach for their selective removal from the plasma. In *Proceedings of the First Annual Apheresis Symposium. Current Concepts and Future Trends*, pp. 203–215. Chicago: American Red Cross Blood Services, University of Illinois Blood Bank, 1979.
99. Ray, P. K., Idiculla, A., Rhoads, J. E., Jr., et al., *Clin. Exp. Immunol.* **42**:308, 1980.
100. Ray, P. K., Besa, E., Idiculla, A., et al., *Cancer* **45**:2633, 1980.
101. Ray, P. K., Cooper, D. R., Bassett, J. G., and Mark, R., *Fed. Proc.* **38**:4558,1979.
102. Ray, P. K., McLaughlin, D., Mohammed, J., et al., *Ex vivo* immunoadsorption of IgG

or its complexes —A new modality of cancer treatment. In B. Serrou and C. Rosenfeld (Eds.), *Immune Complexes and Plasma Exchanges in Cancer Patients*, p. 197. Amsterdam, Holland: Elsevier/North Holland, 1981.

103. Ray, P. K., Raychaudhuri, S., Mark, R., et al., *Amer. Assoc. Cancer Res.* **72**:1124, 1981.
104. Ray, P. K., Idiculla, A., Rhoads, J. E., Jr., et al., Abstract #10.5.57. Fourth Intl. Immunol. Congr., Paris, July 1980.
105. Ray, P. K., Mohammed, J., Raychaudhuri, S., et al., Abstract #10.7.25. Fourth Intl. Immunol. Congr., Paris, July, 1980.
106. Ray, P. K., Idiculla, A., Rhoads, J. E., Jr., et al., Extracorporeal immunoadsorption using protein A containing *Staphylococcus aureus* column. A method for quick removal of abnormal IgG or its complexes from the plasma. In H. Borberg and P. Reuther (Eds.), *Plasma Exchange Therapy. International Symposium*, Wiesbaden, 1980, pp. 150–154. New York and Stuttgart, West Germany: Georg-Thieme Verlag, 1981.
107. Ray, P. K., Clarke, L., McLaughlin, D., et al., Immunotherapy of cancer. Extracorporeal adsorption of plasma blocking factors using nonviable *Staphylococcus aureus* Cowan I. In J. H. Beyer, H. Borberg, Ch. Fuchs, and G. A. Nagel (Eds.), *Plasmapheresis in Immunology and Oncology*, pp. 102–113. Munich: S. Karger, 1982.
108. Ray, P. K., Raychaudhuri, S., McLaughlin, D., et al., *Cancer Res.* **41**:5010, 1981.
109. Ray, P. K., Idiculla, A., Mark, R., et al., *Cancer* **49**:1800, 1982.
110. Ray, P. K., Idiculla, A., Clarke, L., et al., Immunoadsorption of IgG and/or its complexes from colon carcinoma patients —An adjunct therapy for cancer. In *Proc. Intl. Conf. on Adjuvant. Therapy of Cancer*, p. 29. Tucson, Arizona, March 18–21, 1981.
111. Terman, D. S., Yamanoto, T., Mattioli, M., et al., *J. Immunol.* **126**:795, 1980.
112. Terman, D. S., Yamanoto, T., Tillquist, R. L., et al., *Science* **209**:1257, 1980.
113. Jones, F. R., Yoshida, L. H., Ladiges, W. C., and Kenny, M. A., *Cancer* **46**:675, 1980.
114. Ray, P. K., Raychaudhuri, S., McLaughlin, D., et al., *Cancer Res.* **41**:5010, 1981.
115. Ray, P. K., and Raychaudhuri, S., *Fed. Am. Soc. Exp. Biol.* **39**(3):696, 1980.
116. Saha, S., and Ray, P. K., *Fed. Am. Soc. Exp. Biol.* **41**(3): 411, 1982.
117. Ray, P. K., Raychaudhuri, S., Bassett, J. G., and Cooper, D. R., Abstract #17.4.13, *Proc. Fourth Intl. Congress of Immunol.*, Paris, July 21–26, 1980. New York: Academic Press, 1980.
118. Medawar, P. B., *Symp. Soc. Exp. Biol.* **7**:320, 1954.
119. Schlesinger, M., *J. Natl. Cancer Inst.* **28**:927, 1962.
120. Bur, A. E., and Billingham, R. E., *J. Reprod. Fertil.* **21**:59, 1974.
121. Kirby, D. R. S., Transplantation and pregnancy. In F. T. Rapaport and J. Dausset (Eds.), *Human Transplantation*, p. 565. New York: Grune and Stratton, 1968.
122. Bur, A. E. and Billingham, R. E., Concerning the uterus and a graft site and the fetus as a natural parabiotic organismic homograft. In A. E. Bur and R. E. Billingham (Eds.), *Ontogeny of Acquired Immunity*, p. 149. Amsterdam, Holland: Excerpta Medica, North Holland, 1972.
123. Simmons, R. L., and Russell, P. S., *Ann. N.Y. Acad. Sci.* **129**:35, 1966.
124. Heyner, S., *Transpl.* **16**:675, 1973.
125. Patley, H. C., and Edidin, M., *Transpl.* **15**:211, 1973.
126. Rocklin, R. E., Kitzmiller, J. L., and Kaye, M. D., *Ann. Rev. Med.* **30**:375, 1979.
127. Sellers, M. H., Jenkinson, E. J., and Billington, W. D., *Transpl.* **25**:173, 1978.
128. Wegmann, T. G., Mosmann, T. R., Carlson, G. A., et al., *J. Immunol.* **123**:1020, 1979.
129. Wagman, T. G., Barrington, L. J., Carlson, G. A., et al., *J. Reprod. Immunol.* **2**:53, 1980.

130. Loke, Y. W., Joysey, V. C., and Borland, R., *Nature* **232**:403, 1971.
131. Montgomery, B., and Lala, P. K., *J. Reprod. Immunol.* (Suppl.) **57**:329, 1981.
132. Sengupta, J., and Ray, P. K., *Fed. Am. Soc. Exp. Biol.* **38**:5857, 1979.
133. Salinas, I. A., Silver, H. K. B., Sheith, K. M., and Chander, S. B., *Cancer* **42**:1654, 1978.
134. Revillard, J. P., Robert, M., DuPont, E., et al., *Transplant. Proc.* **5**:331, 1973.
135. Jennet, M., Werner, C., Ramirez, E., et al., *Transplant. Proc.* **9**:1417, 1977.
136. Herzenberg, L. A., and Gonzal, S. B., *Proc. Natl. Acad. Sci.* **48**:570, 1962.
137. Kaliss, N., and Dogg, M. K., *Transpl.* **2**:416, 1964.
138. Takano, K., and Miller, J. R., *J. Med. Genet.* **9**:144, 1972.
139. Szulman, A. E., *Curr. Topics, Develp. Biol.* **14**:127, 1980.
140. Harris, R. E., and Lordon, R. E., *Obstet. Gynecol.* **43**:302, 1976.
141. Chaouat, A., Voisin, G. A., Escalier, D., and Ropert, P., *Clin. Exp. Immunol.* **34**:13, 1979.
142. Hellström, I., and Hellström, K. E., *Int. J. Cancer* **15**:30, 1975.
143. Hamilton, M. S., Hellström, I., and Van Belle, G., *Transpl.* **21**:261, 1976.
144. Maroni, E. S., and Parrot, D. M. V., *Clin. Exp. Immunol.* **13**:253, 1973.
145. Smith, J. A., Burton, R. C., Barg, M., and Mitchell, G. F., *Transpl.* **25**:216, 1978.
146. Timmonen, T., and Saksela, E., *Clin. Exp. Immunol.* **23**:462, 1976.
147. Bradbury, S., Billington, W. D., Kirby, D. R. S., and William, E. A., *Histochem. J.* **2**:263, 1970.
148. Tigne, J. R., Garrod, P. R., and Curran, R. C., *J. Pathol. Bacteriol.* **93**:559, 1967.
149. Rocklin, R. E., Kitzmiller, J. L., Carpenter, C. B., et al., *N. Engl. J. Med.* **295**:1209, 1976.
150. Hellström, K. E., Hellström, I., and Brawn, J., *Nature* (London) **224**:914, 1969.
151. Bill, S. C., and Billington, W. D., *Nature* (London) **288**:387, 1980.
152. Masson, P. L., Deline, M., and Cambiasco, C. L., *Nature* **266**:542, 1977.
153. Cambiasco, C. L., Riconi, H., and Masson, P. L., *Ann. Rheum. Disease* (Suppl.) **1**:40, 1977.
154. Swinburne, L. M., *Lancet* **2**:592, 1970.
155. Morisada, M., Yamaguchi, H., and Iizuka, R., *Amer. J. Obstet. Gynec.* **125**:3, 1976.
156. Desai, R. G., and Creger, W. P., *Blood* **21**:665, 1963.
157. Tuffrey, M., Bishun, N. P., and Barnes, R. D., *Nature* (London) **224**:701, 1969.
158. Billington, W. D., Kirby, D. R. S., Owen, J. J., et al., *Nature* (London) **224**:704, 1969.
159. Bur, A. E., and Billingham, R. E., *Science* **179**:240, 1973.
160. Lanman, J. T., Dinerstein, J., and Fikrig, S., *Ann. N.Y. Acad. Sci.* **99**:706, 1962.
161. Wegmann, T. G., Waters, C. A., Drill, D. W., and Carlson, G. A., *Proc. Natl. Acad. Sci. USA* **76**:2410, 1979.
162. Prehn, R. T., *J. Natl. Cancer Inst.* **25**:883, 1960.
163. Smith, R. N., and Powell, A. E., *J. Exp. Med.* **146**:899, 1977.
164. Olding, L. B., Birnirschke, K., and Oldstone, M. B. A., *Clin. Immunol. Immunopathol.* **3**:79, 1974.
165. Clark, D. A., McDermott, M. R., and Szewczuk, M. R., *Cell. Immunol.* **52**:106, 1980.
166. Harrison, M. R., *Scand. J. Immunol.* **5**:881, 1976.
167. Kaskura, S., *J. Immunol.* **107**:1296, 1971.
168. Noonan, F. P., Halliday, W. J., Morton, H., and Clunie, G. J. A., *Nature* **278**:649, 1979.
169. McIntyre, J. A., and Faulk, W. P., *Proc. Natl. Acad. Sci. USA* **76**:4029, 1979.
170. Voisin, G. A., *Immunol. Revs.* **49**:3, 1980.

171. Rocklin, R. E., Kitzmiller, J. L., Carpenter, C. B., et al., *New Engl. J. Med.* **295**:1209, 1976.
172. Stimson, W. H., Strachon, A. F., and Shepherd, A., *New Engl. J. Med.* **295**:1209, 1976.
173. Takeuchi, S., *An immunoregulatory mechanism implicated by the blocking factors in serum from pregnancy.* In T. Aoki, I. Urushizaki, and E. Tsubura, (Eds.), *Manipulation of Host Defense Mechanisms*, p. 147. *Excerpta Medica*, International Congress Series 576, 1981.

Index

The Contributors

C. JOHN ABEYOUNIS — Department of Microbiology, School of Medicine, State University of New York at Buffalo, Buffalo, New York

CHARLES B. CARPENTER — Department of Medicine, Harvard Medical School, Boston, Massachusetts

NICOLE A. CARPENTIER — Division of Hematology, Centre de Transfusion, Hôpital Cantonal, 1211 Genève 4, Switzerland

DAVID A. CLARK — Department of Medicine and Host Resistance Program, McMaster University Medical Center, Hamilton, Ontario, Canada L8N 3Z5

RISHAB K. GUPTA — Division of Oncology, Department of Surgery, UCLA Medical School, Los Angeles, California, and Surgical Service Veterans Administration Medical Center, Supulveda, California

RONALD B. HERBERMAN — Laboratory of Immunodiagnosis, National Cancer Institute, Bethesda, Maryland

BARRY D. KAHAN — The University of Texas Medical School at Houston, Division of Organ Transplantation, Department of Surgery, Houston, Texas

G. MATHÉ — Institut de Cancérologie et d'Immunogénétique, Hôpital Paul Brousse, 94800 Villejuif, France

PETER A. MIESCHER — Division of Hematology, Centre de Transfusion, Hôpital Cantonal, 1211 Genéve 4, Switzerland

FELIX MILGROM — Department of Microbiology, School of Medicine, State University of New York at Buffalo, Buffalo, New York

DONALD L. MORTON — Divison of Oncology, Department of Surgery, UCLA Medical School, Los Angeles, California

DONNA M. MURASKO — Department of Microbiology, The Medical College of Pennsylvania and Hospital, Philadelphia, Pennsylvania

L. OLSSON — Institut de Cancérologie et d'Immunogénétique, Hôpital Paul Brousse, 94800 Villejuif, France

444

NEAL R. PELLIS — The University of Texas Medical School at Houston, Division of Organ Transplantation, Department of Surgery, Houston, Texas

RICHMOND T. PREHN — Institute for Medical Research, San Jose, California

RAJGOPAL RAGHUPATHY — Department of Biochemistry and Molecular Biology, Harvard University, Cambridge, Massachusetts

PRASANTA K. RAY — Department of Surgery, Microbiology and Immunology, The Medical College of Pennsylvania and Hospital, Philadelphia, Pennsylvania

SYAMAL RAYCHAUDHURI — Department of Surgery, The Medical College of Pennsylvania and Hospital, Philadelphia, Pennsylvania

P. REIZENSTEIN — Karolinska Hospital, Stockholm, Sweden

EDUARDO A. SANTIAGO-DELPIN — University of Puerto Rico Medical School, Veterans Administration Hospital, San Juan, Puerto Rico

SHOSHICHI TAKEUCHI — Department of Obstetrics and Gynecology, Niigata University, School of Medicine, 1-757 Asahimachi Niigata, Japan

G. P. TALWAR — Department of Biochemistry, All India Institute of Medical Sciences, New Delhi, India

HISAKAZU YAMIGISHI — Kyoto Prefectural University Medical School, Department of Surgery, Kyoto, Japan

EDMUND J. YUNIS — Division of Immunogenetics, Sidney Farber Cancer Institute, Harvard Medical School, Boston, Massachusetts